# Harrison's
# PRINCIPLES OF
# INTERNAL MEDICINE

## PreTest® Self-Assessment and Review

# NOTICE

Medicine is an ever-changing science. As new research and clinical experience broaden our knowledge, changes in treatment and drug therapy are required. The editor and the publisher of this work have checked with sources believed to be reliable in their efforts to provide information that is complete and generally in accord with the standards accepted at the time of publication. However, in view of the possibility of human error or changes in medical sciences, neither the editor nor the publisher nor any other party who has been involved in the preparation or publication of this work warrants that the information contained herein is in every respect accurate or complete, and they are not responsible for any errors or omissions or for the results obtained from use of such information. Readers are encouraged to confirm the information contained herein with other sources. For example and in particular, readers are advised to check the product information sheet included in the package of each drug they plan to administer to be certain that the information contained in this book is accurate and that changes have not been made in the recommended dose or in the contraindications for administration. This recommendation is of particular importance in connection with new or infrequently used drugs.

# Harrison's
# PRINCIPLES OF INTERNAL MEDICINE

## *PreTest® Self Assessment and Review*

## FOURTEENTH EDITION

For use with the 14th edition of
HARRISON'S PRINCIPLES OF INTERNAL MEDICINE

*Edited by*

## RICHARD M. STONE, MD

*Dana-Farber Cancer Institute*
*Brigham and Women's Hospital*

*Associate Professor of Medicine, Harvard Medical School*
*Boston, Massachusetts*

## McGRAW-HILL
*Health Professions Division*

PreTest Series

New York  St. Louis  San Francisco  Auckland  Bogotá  Caracas  Lisbon  London
Madrid  Mexico City  Milan  Montreal  New Delhi  San Juan  Singapore  Sydney  Tokyo  Toronto

**McGraw-Hill**

*A Division of The **McGraw·Hill** Companies*

**Harrison's Principles of Internal Medicine**
PreTest ® Self- Assessment and Review
International Editions 1998

1 2 3 4 5 6 7 8 9 0 BJE UPE 9 8 7

This book was set in Times Roman by V & M Graphics.
The editors were Martin J. Wonsiewicz and Mariapaz Ramos Englis.
The production supervisor was Helene G. Landers.
Malloy was printer and binder.

The Appendix, Plate B, and figures accompanying questions 11-8 and 1X-2 are from Isselbacher et al: Harrison's Principles of Internal Medicine. 13/e New York, McGraw-Hill, 1994, with permission.

Color plates I, J, L, N, O, P, R, S, T, and X are from Fitzpatrick et al: *Color Atlas and Synopsis of Clinical Dermatology*, 3/e, New York, McGraw-Hill, 1997 with permission.

**Library of Congress Cataloging-in-Publication Data**

Harrison's principles of internal medicine : PreTest self-assessment
    and review / edited by Richard Stone --14 ed.
        p.    cm.
    " For use with the 14th edition of Harrison's principles of internal
    medicine."
        Includes bibliographical reference and index.
        ISBN 0-07-052537-4 (alk. paper)
        1. Internal medicine -- Examinations, questions, etc.    I . Harrison.
        Tinsley Randolph. 1900 --  II.  Stone, Richard M.        III. Harrison's
    principles of internal medicine.
            (DNLM: I. Internal Medicine --- examination questions.      WB 115 H322
    1997 Suppl.)
    RC46.H333    1998 Suppl.
    616'.0076--dc21
        DNLM/DLC
        for Library of Congress                                      97-35730

**When ordering this title, use ISBN 0-07-115846-4**

Printed in Singapore

# CONTENTS

*Contributors  vii*
*Introduction  ix*

I. Infectious Diseases
   *Questions  1*
   *Answers, Explanations, and References  19*

II. Disorders of the Heart and Vascular System
   *Questions  49*
   *Answers, Explanations, and References  69*

III. Disorders of the Kidney and Urinary Tract
   *Questions  91*
   *Answers, Explanations, and References  103*

IV. Disorders of the Nervous System and Muscles
   *Questions  115*
   *Answers, Explanations, and References  132*

V. Disorders of the Respiratory System
   *Questions  157*
   *Answers, Explanations, and References  165*

VI. Endocrine, Metabolic, and Genetic Disorders
   *Questions  179*
   *Answers, Explanations, and References  197*

VII. Immunologic, Allergic, and Rheumatic Disorders
   *Questions  227*
   *Answers, Explanations, and References  238*

VIII.  Disorders of the Alimentary Tract and Hepatobiliary System
*Questions   257*
*Answers, Explanations, and References   272*

IX.  Hematopoietic Disorders and Neoplasia
*Questions   293*
*Answers, Explanations, and References   311*

X.  Dermatologic Disorders
*Questions   339*
*Answers, Explanations, and References   343*

Appendix
*Laboratory Values of Clinical Importance   349*

Bibliography   *357*

Color Plates

# CONTRIBUTORS

**Richard M. Stone, MD**
*Associate Professor of Medicine*
*Harvard Medical School*
*Medical Director, Dana-Farber/Partners Cancer Care*
  *Inpatient Unit*
*Brigham and Women's Hospital*
*Department of Adult Oncology*
*Dana-Farber Cancer Institute*
*Boston, Massachusetts*

**Jorge Plutsky, MD**
*Instructor in Medicine*
*Harvard Medical School*
*Director, The Vascular Disease Prevention Program*
*Brigham and Women's Hospital*
*Boston, Massachusetts*

**Karen Miller, MD**
*Research Fellow in Medicine*
*Harvard Medical School*
*Research and Clinical Fellow*
*Endocrine Unit, Massachusetts General Hospital*
*Boston, Massachusetts*

**Dara Nachmanoff, MD**
*Clinical Fellow in Neuropathology*
*Departments of Pathology and Neurology*
*Children's Hospital*
*Harvard Medical School*
*Boston, Massachusetts*

**Craig Bunnell, MD**
*Instructor in Medicine*
*Harvard Medical School*
*Dana-Farber Cancer Institute*
*Brigham and Women's Hospital*
*Boston, Massachusetts*

**Glen Chertow, MD, MPH**
*Instructor in Medicine*
*Instructor in Surgery*
*Harvard Medical School*
*Assistant Director of Dialysis, Renal Division*
*Metabolic Support Services*
*Brigham and Women's Hospital*
*Boston, Massachusetts*

# INTRODUCTION

*Harrison's Principles of Internal Medicine: PreTest Self-Assessment and Review* has been designed to provide physicians with a comprehensive, relevant, and convenient instrument for self-evaluation and review within the broad area of internal medicine. Although it should be particularly helpful for residents preparing for the American Board of Internal Medicine (ABIM) certification examination and for board-certified internists preparing for recertification, it should also be useful for internists, family practitioners, and other practicing physicans who are simply interested in maintaining a high level of competence in internal medicine. Study of this self-assessment and review book should help to (1) identify areas of relative weakness; (2) confirm areas of expertise; (3) assess knowledge of the sciences fundamental to internal medicine; (4) assess clinical judgment and problem-solving skills; and (5) introduce recent developments in general internal medicine.

This book consists of 823 multiple-choice questions that (1) are representative of the major areas covered in *Harrison's Principles of Internal Medicine,* 14th ed., and (2) parallel the format and degree of difficulty of the questions on the examination of the ABIM. Questions have been appropriately updated and chosen to reflect important recent developments in internal medicine, such as the increasing contributions of molecular biology to the understanding, diagnosis, and treatment of many disorders. Five experts in specific fields have contributed new and revised questions. Each question is accompanied by an answer, a paragraph-length explanation, and a reference to a specific chapter in *Harrison's.* In some cases references to more specialized textbooks and current journal articles are also given. A list of normal values used in the laboratory studies in this book can be found in the Appendix, followed by a Bibliography listing all the sources used for the questions. As in the current edition of *Harrison's,* the system of international units (SI) appears first in the text and the traditional units follow in parentheses. All color plates referred to in the text are found at the back of the book.

We have assumed that the time available to the reader is limited; therefore, this book has been designed to be used profitably a chapter at a time. By allowing no more than two and a half minutes to answer each question, you can simulate the time constraints of the actual board examinations. When you finish answering all the questions in a chapter, spend as much time as necessary verifying answers and carefully reading the accompanying explanations. If after reading the explanations for a given chapter, you feel a need for a more extensive and definitive discussion, consult the chapter in *Harrison's* or any of the other references listed.

Based on our testing experience, on most medical examinations, examinees who answer half the questions correctly would score around the 50th or 60th percentile. A score of 65 percent would place the examinee above the 80th percentile, whereas a score of 30 percent would rank him or her below the 15th percentile. In other words, if you answer fewer than 30 percent of the questions in a chapter correctly, you are relatively weak in that area. A score of 50 percent would be approximately average, and 70 percent or higher would probably be honors.

We have used three basic question types in accordance with the format of the ABIM certification and recertification examinations. In accordance with the changing format of these examinations, the number of matching and true/false questions has been reduced in this edition. Considerable editorial time has been spent trying to ensure that each question is clearly stated and discriminates between those physicians who are well prepared in the subject and those who are less knowledgeable.

This book is a teaching device that provides readers with the opportunity to evaluate and update their clinical expertise, their ability to interpret data, and their ability to diagnose and solve clinical problems.

# Harrison's
# PRINCIPLES OF
# INTERNAL MEDICINE

*PreTest® Self-Assessment and Review*

# I. INFECTIOUS DISEASES

## QUESTIONS

**DIRECTIONS:** Each question below contains five suggested responses. Choose the **one best** response to each question.

**I-1.** A 21-year-old female with relapsed acute lymphoblastic leukemia is treated with a five-drug induction regimen (cyclophosphamide, daunorubicin, vincristine, prednisone, and L-asparaginase). On the sixth day after the initiation of this therapy the patient develops a fever and is started on intravenous ceftazidime. The patient defervesces but develops another fever 5 days later and is started on amphotericin B. Ten days later the patient, still on oral steroids, remains febrile, neutropenic, and thrombocytopenic and is noted to have shortness of breath. Chest x-rays show a densely consolidated pulmonary infiltrate in the left lung zone. A sputum culture demonstrates normal oral flora and several colonies of *Aspergillus*. The most appropriate conclusion to draw is that

(A) the patient most likely has invasive pulmonary aspergilliosis
(B) the *Aspergillus* is a contaminant; the patient most likely has bacterial pneumonia
(C) biopsy is not required for a definitive diagnosis
(D) the patient most likely has viral pneumonitis
(E) the patient is colonized with *Aspergillus*, but the most likely etiology of the infiltrate is drug toxicity

**I-2.** A 28-year-old Egyptian farmer presents with left flank pain. Ultrasonography reveals enlargement of the left ureter and hydronephrosis of the left kidney. Cystoscopy reveals a mass extending from the left ureter into the bladder. Parasitic ova (150 by 50 mm) are noted in the urine and in a biopsy of the ureteral mass. Which of the following statements is correct?

(A) Renal failure is likely in the absence of treatment
(B) The lesion is not reversible by chemotherapy
(C) In the absence of treatment, the patient has an increased risk for transitional cell carcinoma of the bladder
(D) The patient is suffering from schistosomiasis
(E) The organism causing this problem is spread by fecal-oral contact

**I-3.** A 30-year-old homosexual male with known HIV infection and a CD4+ count of 200/μL presents for advice regarding an upcoming trip to Peru. Each of the following statements represents sound advice EXCEPT

(A) the patient should determine if Peru routinely denies entry to HIV-positive individuals
(B) the patient should receive pneumococcal polysaccharide and influenza vaccine
(C) the patient should not receive yellow fever vaccine
(D) no vaccines should be given because of the increased risk of HIV viremia after vaccination
(E) prophylaxis against traveler's diarrhea using bismuth subsalicylate is recommended

**I-4.** Which of the following patients would be most likely to harbor a *Helicobacter pylori* infection in the stomach?

(A) A 60-year-old middle-income American
(B) A 25-year-old American in a low-income group
(C) A 60-year-old Pakistani
(D) A 25-year-old Zairian
(E) A 70-year-old Dane

**I-5.** A 55-year-old woman from Oregon presents with diplopia 24 h after eating home-canned fruit. Within a few hours of presentation she is also noted to have dysphonia and arm weakness. Other symptoms include nausea, vomiting, dizziness, blurred vision, and dry mouth. The patient is afebrile, alert, and oriented. Which of the following is LEAST important in managing this patient's illness?

(A) Intravenous penicillin
(B) Spirometric monitoring
(C) Antitoxin therapy
(D) Laxatives
(E) Enema

**I-6.** Each of the following is a risk factor for the development of pneumonia in a hospitalized patient EXCEPT

(A) altered consciousness
(B) administration of ranitidine
(C) administration of sucralfate
(D) use of an endotracheal tube
(E) delayed gastric emptying

**I-7.** A 35-year-old male patient undergoing initial therapy for acute myeloid leukemia has tolerated the chemotherapy well. However, 6 days after the initiation of chemotherapy and approximately 10 days after the insertion of an indwelling transthoracic intravenous device (Hickman catheter), he develops a fever. Examination is negative except for erythema and tenderness at the insertion site and along the subcutaneous tunnel. Blood cultures and chest x-ray are negative. The most appropriate course of action at this point is to

(A) remove the line and insert a new one over a guidewire
(B) begin intravenous vancomycin
(C) begin intravenous vancomycin and gentamycin
(D) remove the line
(E) begin intravenous vancomycin, gentamycin, and amphotericin B

**I-8.** A 70-year-old male with a history of heavy smoking and moderately severe chronic obstructive pulmonary disease has been feeling poorly. He reports cough, chills, pleuritic chest pain, and low-grade fever. Chest x-ray reveals a small dense infiltrate in the right lower lobe. Gram's stain of the patient's sputum reveals numerous gram-negative cocci, many of which occur in pairs. The most appropriate therapy would be

(A) no antimicrobial therapy is required
(B) tetracycline
(C) ciprofloxacin
(D) trimethoprim-sulfamethoxazole
(E) penicillin-clavulanic acid

**I-9.** All the following statements regarding infection with *Shigella* are correct EXCEPT

(A) ingestion of significant numbers of *Shigella* is required for infection because of the relative inability of *Shigella* to survive the acidic conditions of the stomach
(B) examination of the stool from an infected patient will reveal polymorphonuclear leukocytes
(C) the hemolytic uremic syndrome may be associated with infection
(D) although the *Shigella* organisms are directly invasive, the colonic pathology also can be accounted for on the basis of toxin elaboration
(E) antibiotic treatment usually is unnecessary

A 35-year-old male with a history of abrasion of the right hand presents with acute pain in the right shoulder. His physical examination reveals a temperature of 103°F and rigor, and he appears to be quite ill. There is dusky erythema and edema of the right shoulder and right upper extremity with marked tenderness. Within a few hours the patient is unresponsive and is found to be hypotensive. Laboratory evaluation reveals an elevated serum creatinine, thrombocytopenia, and elevated hepatic transamenases. The soft tissues in the left upper extremity have begun to necrose. Blood culture, obtained at the time of initial presentation, has already turned positive.

**I-10.** The organism that is most likely to be responsible for this clinical syndrome is

(A) group A streptococci
(B) group D streptococci
(C) *Staphylococcus aureus*
(D) *Bacteroides fragilis*
(E) *Clostridium septicum*

**I-11.** The most appropriate therapy for this patient is
(A) penicillin G
(B) penicillin G–clavulanic acid
(C) erythromycin
(D) vancomycin
(E) surgery

**I-12.** Which of the following statements regarding cryptosporidiosis is correct?

(A) Symptomatic infection in immunocompetent hosts is unusual
(B) Serologic techniques are needed for the diagnosis
(C) While it is a common cause of diarrhea in patients with the acquired immune deficiency syndrome, severe manifestations, including weight loss and pain, are uncommon
(D) The disease is transmitted by the fecal-oral route
(E) The treatment of choice is praziquantel

**I-13.** Several weeks after eating a meal in rural France that included meat from locally bred horses and pigs, a 35-year-old female presents with muscle aches and swelling, particularly in both biceps and the neck. Physical examination reveals periorbital edema. Laboratory evaluation reveals eosinophilia, elevated serum IgE, and elevated creatinine phosphokinase levels. The most likely diagnosis is

(A) ocular larva migrans (*Toxocara canis* infection)
(B) trichinosis
(C) viral myositis
(D) polymyositis (autoimmune)
(E) typhoid fever

**I-14.** A 65-year-old alcoholic male is hospitalized with fever, hypotension, and a lobar infiltrate. A sputum culture obtained two days before admission is growing *Streptococcus pneumoniae*. Susceptibility testing will be available in 24 h. Which of the following is the most appropriate antibiotic choice for this patient?

(A) Erythromycin
(B) Penicillin G
(C) Vancomycin
(D) Cefotaxime
(E) Clindamycin

**I-15.** Which of the following is LEAST likely to yield a diagnosis that will detect the specific parasite?

(A) String test for duodenal sampling to detect *Cryptosporidium*
(B) Scotch tape technique on the perianal skin to detect beef tapeworm
(C) Aspiration of a liver abscess to detect *Entamoeba histolytica*
(D) Urine sediment examination to detect *Schistosoma haematobium*
(E) Silver stain on induced sputum to detect *Pneumocystis carinii*

**I-16.** All the following statements concerning predisposition to parasitic infections are correct EXCEPT

(A) depression of the CD4+ lymphocyte count predisposes to cryptosporidiosis
(B) patients infected with human T-lymphotropic virus type I are prone to infection with *Strongyloides*
(C) splenectomized patients are at risk for babesiosis
(D) patients with multiple myeloma may develop giardiasis
(E) Patients with cystic fibrosis are at a markedly increased risk for toxoplasmosis

**I-17.** Treatment strategies for patients with endemic trachoma include all the following EXCEPT

(A) single-dose oral tetracycline
(B) single-dose oral azithromycin
(C) topical ophthalmic tetracycline
(D) topical ophthalmic erythromycin
(E) surgical correction of inturned eyelids

**I-18.** Nonvenereal treponemal infections are best characterized by

(A) pulmonary infections with a tendency to form nodules
(B) biliary tract invasion
(C) infection of the genitourinary tract with episodes of hematuria and eventual renal failure
(D) primary cutaneous lesions that progress to include lymphadenopathy and bone destruction
(E) meningeal irritation with occasional parenchymal involvement

**I-19.** A 53-year-old black male who received a renal allograft seven months ago is now receiving azathioprine and prednisone. He presents to the hospital one week after developing fever, night sweats, and anorexia. He also complains of coughing and chest pain. Chest film reveals biapical infiltrates with an apparent cavity in the left upper lobe. Auramine-rhodamine staining reveals the presence of microorganisms consistent with tubercle bacilli. The patient's creatinine is 1.2 mg/dL. The treatment of choice at this time would be

(A) isoniazid, rifampin, and pyrazinamide
(B) isoniazid, rifampin, pyrazinamide, and ethembutol
(C) isoniazid and rifampin
(D) rifampin, pyrazinamide, and ethambutol
(E) isoniazid, rifampin, pyrazinamide, ethambutol, and streptomycin

**I-20.** A 43-year-old-sexually active female presents with low-grade fever, headache, malaise, dysuria, and vaginal discharge. Physical examination reveals several vesicular lesions on the labia bilaterally. She also has tender inguinal lymphadenopathy. All the following statements regarding the current situation are correct EXCEPT

   (A) oral acyclovir will be effective in speeding the resolution of her symptoms
   (B) if the patient has had prior HSV-1 infection, she will be less likely to have severe systemic symptoms
   (C) recurrent infection will be equally likely whether the patient is infected with HSV-1 or HSV-2
   (D) if her sexual partner uses a condom, transmission will be less likely
   (E) prolonged acyclovir use could reduce the likelihood of recurrent infection

**I-21.** A 55-year-old male with a history of seasonal allergic rhinitis develops a low-grade fever and cough. He complains to his physician that he is producing copious amounts of greenish sputum and coughing quite a bit. Since the patient is known to be allergic to penicillin, the physician prescribes erythromycin. The patient is also taking terfenadine because of his allergic symptoms. Which of the following is a potential complication in this clinical scenario?

   (A) Decreased bioavailability of erythromycin with failure to treat pulmonary infection
   (B) Congestive heart failure
   (C) Increased bleeding
   (D) Stevens-Johnson syndrome
   (E) A disulfiram-like reaction if ethanol is ingested

**I-22.** A 12-year-old girl presents with painful epitrochlear lymphadenopathy associated with low-grade fever and malaise. The patient has a cat and also gave a history of a papillary lesion in the left forearm about 1 week or ten days ago. The most likely etiologic agent in this situation is

   (A) *Bartonella henselae*
   (B) *Staphylococcus aureus*
   (C) Epstein-Barr virus
   (D) *Sporothrix schenkii*
   (E) *Yersinia pestis*

**I-23.** Which of the following statements concerning catheter-associated urinary tract infection is correct?

   (A) Most catheter-associated infections are symptomatic
   (B) Topical periurethral antibiotics should be applied
   (C) Routine antimicrobial prophylaxis is indicated
   (D) The majority of patients catheterized for longer than 2 weeks develop bacteriuria
   (E) Skin organisms such as *Staphylococcus* and *Streptococcus* are the most common cause of infections

**I-24.** Each of the following represents a reasonable hospital-wide strategy for reducing the incidence of *Aspergillus* infections EXCEPT

   (A) routine inspection of air-handling equipment
   (B) use of HEPA filters for air supply to rooms housing immunosuppressed patients
   (C) routine surveillance of air for the presence of *Aspergillus* spores
   (D) routine use of itraconazole in immunocompromised patients
   (E) extreme care in hospital renovations

**I-25.** A 23-year-old previously healthy female letter carrier works in a suburb in which the presence of rabid foxes and skunks has been documented. She is bitten by a bat, which then flies away. Initial examination reveals a clean break in the skin in the right upper forearm. She has no history of receiving treatment for rabies and is unsure about vaccination against tetanus. The physician should

   (A) clean the wound with a 20% soap solution
   (B) clean the wound with a 20% soap solution and administer tetanus toxoid
   (C) clean the wound with a 20% soap solution, administer tetanus toxoid, and administer human rabies immune globulin intramuscularly
   (D) clean the wound with a 20% soap solution, administer tetanus toxoid, administer human rabies immune globulin intramuscularly, and administer human diploid cell vaccine
   (E) clean the wound with a 20% soap solution and administer human diploid cell vaccine

**I-26.** During the summer, a previously healthy 10-year-old boy living in rural Louisiana presents with a brief illness characterized by 2 days of fever, headache, and vomiting that progresses to lethargy, disorientation, and most recently a grand mal seizure. Laboratory examination is remarkable for peripheral blood leukocytosis and a normal CSF examination except for the presence of 35 monocytes per microliter. An IgM enzyme–linked immunoassay for the LaCrosse virus returns positive. Anticonvulsive medicine has been administered. At this point the physician should

(A) tell the family that there is a high likelihood of improvement during the coming week and a good chance for discharge within 2 weeks
(B) order a brain biopsy to exclude herpes encephalitis
(C) administer empiric acyclovir
(D) administer empiric chloramphenicol and ampicillin
(E) share with the parents your concern that this illness, for which there is no specific therapy, is often fatal

**I-27.** The most common source of bacterial infection of intravenous cannulas is

(A) contamination of fluids during the manufacturing process
(B) contamination of fluids during insertion of the cannula
(C) contamination at the site of entry through the skin
(D) contamination during the injection of medications
(E) seeding from remote sites as a result of intermittent bacteremia

**I-28.** A 73-year-old previously healthy man is hospitalized because of the acute onset of dysuria, urinary frequency, fever, and shaking chills. His temperature is 39.5°C (103.1°F), blood pressure is 100/60 mmHg, pulse is 140 beats per minute, and respiratory rate is 30 breaths per minute. Which of the following interventions would be the most important in the treatment of this acute illness?

(A) Catheterization of the urinary bladder
(B) Initiation of antibiotic therapy
(C) Infusion of Ringer's lactate solution
(D) Infusion of dopamine hydrochloride
(E) Intravenous injection of methylprednisolone

**I-29.** Infection with *Pseudomonas* organisms is frequently associated with each of the following EXCEPT

(A) osteomyelitis after a nail puncture wound of the foot
(B) ecthyma gangrenosum
(C) both a mild form and an invasive form of otitis externa
(D) meningitis in neonatal infants
(E) endocarditis in drug addicts

**I-30.** A 65-year-old Greek woman visiting her children in New York City complains of upper abdominal pain. The patient is brought to the family physician, who notices icteric sclera and a mass in the right upper quadrant. CT reveals a 10-cm multiloculated cyst with mural calcification that is compressing the common bile duct. Which of the following statements is correct concerning this clinical situation?

(A) Treatment with the antiamebic agent chloroquine is indicated
(B) Treatment with an antiechinococcal agent such as albendazole is sufficient
(C) The adult parasite resides in the patient's intestine
(D) Infection was probably caused by exposure to infected dogs
(E) Surgery is contraindicated because of the risk of anaphylaxis from dissemination of infectious material

**I-31.** Diagnostic accuracy has been enhanced by the ability to detect specific DNA sequences in all the following infecting microorganisms EXCEPT

(A) cytomegalovirus (CMV)
(B) *Staphylococcus aureus*
(C) *Mycobacterium tuberculosis*
(D) *Legionella*
(E) human immunodeficiency virus (HIV)

**I-32.** The most common cause of "traveler's diarrhea" ("turista") in Americans traveling abroad is

(A) *Staphylococcus aureus*
(B) *Clostridium perfringens*
(C) *Escherichia coli*
(D) *Bacillus cereus*
(E) rotavirus

**I-33.** All the following vaccines are recommended for use in immunocompromised adults EXCEPT

(A) bacillus Calmette-Guerin (BCG) vaccine (against tuberculosis)
(B) inactivated influenza vaccine for current year
(C) 23-valent pnemococcal vaccine
(D) quadrivalent meningococcal vaccine
(E) inactivated polio vaccine

**I-34.** A 38-year-old homosexual male who is known to be infected with the HIV virus presents with a week of fever and tachypnea. Chest x-ray reveals bilateral alveolar infiltrates. Arterial blood gas determination reveals a $Pa_{O_2}$ of 55 mmHg on room air. Bronchoalveolar lavage is positive for methenamine silver staining material. Which of the following statements is correct concerning the current clinical situation?

(A) Transbronchial biopsy should be carried out to confirm the diagnosis
(B) Corticosteroids are contraindicated given the risk of other opportunistic infections in Kaposi's sarcoma
(C) Pentamidine therapy by the aerosolized route would be appropriate if the patient had a known allergy to sulfa drugs
(D) Trimethoprim-sulfamethoxazole and pentamidine should be administered in combination
(E) Trimethoprim-sulfamethoxazole alone should be administered

**I-35.** A 50-year-old woman emigrated from El Salvador approximately 10 years ago and currently resides in Washington, DC. She complains of shortness of breath. Chest x-ray reveals biventricular cardiac enlargement. An echocardiographic study shows biventricular enlargement, thin ventricular walls, and an apical aneurysm. The patient has no history of alcohol abuse, thyroid disease, risk factors for atherosclerotic heart disease, or family history of hemochromatosis. In considering a potential etiology for the patient's current problem, which of the following statements is correct?

(A) The etiologic agent can be demonstrated on Giemsa stain of the peripheral blood
(B) Other manifestations of infection could include involvement of the gastrointestinal tract
(C) The vector for the transmission of this disease is the tsetse fly
(D) Corticosteroids may be beneficial
(E) Given the progressive and ultimately fatal course, cardiac transplantation should be considered

**I-36.** Production of all the following factors contributes to the pathogenicity of staphylococci EXCEPT

(A) penicillinase
(B) coagulase
(C) enterotoxin
(D) exotoxin
(E) catalase

**I-37.** Which of the following organisms is most likely to cause infection of a shunt implanted for the treatment of hydrocephalus?

(A) *Staphylococcus epidermidis*
(B) *Staphylococcus aureus*
(C) *Corynebacterium diphtheriae*
(D) *Escherichia coli*
(E) *Bacteroides fragilis*

**I-38.** Meningococcal meningitis can be prevented by the administration of all the following preparations EXCEPT

(A) group A vaccine
(B) group B vaccine
(C) group C vaccine
(D) ciprofloxacin
(E) rifampin

**I-39.** A 25-year-old man who was recently admitted to a psychiatric hospital with the diagnosis of severe depression complicated by psychosis is brought to the emergency room because of worsening mental status and fever. The patient is unable to give a history because he is profoundly confused and claims to be on Mars. The psychiatrist informs you that the patient has been started recently on haloperidol and amitriptyline. Physical findings include a rectal temperature of 40.6°C (105°F), muscle rigidity, and dry skin. A cooling blanket is ordered, and you administer acetaminophen. Which of the following agents would be most appropriately ordered at this time?

(A) Bromocriptine
(B) Atropine
(C) Levarterenol
(D) Chlorpheniramine
(E) Methylprednisolone

**I-40.** A 60-year-old insulin-dependent man with diabetes mellitus has had purulent drainage from his left ear for 1 week. Suddenly, fever, increased pain, and vertigo develop. The most likely causative agent is

(A) *Aspergillus*
(B) *Mucor*
(C) *Pseudomonas*
(D) *Staphylococcus aureus*
(E) *Haemophilus influenzae*

**I-41.** Typhoid fever can be characterized by all the following statements EXCEPT

(A) the illness usually is acquired from ingestion of contaminated food, water, or milk
(B) leukopenia is more common than leukocytosis in acutely ill persons
(C) rose spots usually are present at the time when the fever begins
(D) chloramphenicol is not effective in preventing relapse
(E) fluoroquinolone antibiotics eradicate the organism even in the presence of gallstones

**I-42.** Exposure to which of the following mandates passive immunization with standard immune serum globulin?

(A) Rabies
(B) Hepatitis A
(C) Hepatitis B
(D) Tetanus
(E) Cytomegalovirus

**I-43.** *Haemophilus influenzae* infections occur with increased severity in association with all the following conditions EXCEPT

(A) alcoholism
(B) sickle cell disease
(C) splenectomy
(D) agammaglobulinemia
(E) chronic granulomatous disease

**I-44.** To determine whether a child with paroxysmal coughing and gasping has whooping cough, a physician should order

(A) white blood cell count and differential
(B) Gram stain of the sputum
(C) blood cultures
(D) chest x-ray
(E) lateral x-ray of the neck

**I-45.** Hypersensitivity reactions—such as erythema nodosum, erythema multiforme, arthritis, and arthralgias—are most frequently associated with which of the following infections?

(A) Histoplasmosis
(B) Cryptococcosis
(C) Aspergillosis
(D) Blastomycosis
(E) Coccidioidomycosis

**I-46.** Imipenem, a newer antibiotic with a broad antibacterial spectrum, is coadministered with cilastatin because

(A) the combination of these antibiotics is synergistic against *Pseudomonas* spp.
(B) cilastatin aids the gastrointestinal absorption of the active moiety, imipenem
(C) cilastatin inhibits a β-lactamase that destroys imipenem
(D) cilastatin inhibits an enzyme in the kidney that destroys imipenem
(E) cilastatin prevents the hypoprothrombinemic effect of imipenem

**I-47.** A 35-year-old man is seen 6 months after a cadaveric renal allograft. The patient has been on azathioprine and prednisone since that procedure. He has felt poorly for the past week with fever to 38.6°C (101.5°F), anorexia, and a cough productive of thick sputum. Chest x-ray reveals a left lower lobe (5 cm) nodule with central cavitation. Examination of the sputum reveals long, crooked, branching, beaded gram-positive filaments. The most appropriate initial therapy would include the administration of which of the following antibiotics?

(A) Penicillin
(B) Erythromycin
(C) Sulfisoxazole
(D) Ceftazidime
(E) Tobramycin

**I-48.** A previously healthy 28-year-old man describes several episodes of fever, myalgia, and headache that have been followed by abdominal pain and diarrhea. He has experienced up to 10 bowel movements per day. Physical examination is unremarkable. Laboratory findings are notable only for a slightly elevated leukocyte count and an elevated erythrocyte sedimentation rate. Wright's stain of a fecal sample reveals the presence of neutrophils. Colonoscopy reveals inflamed mucosa. Biopsy of an affected area discloses mucosal infiltration with neutrophils, monocytes, and eosinophils; epithelial damage, including loss of mucus; glandular degeneration; and crypt abscesses. The patient notes that several months ago he was at a church barbecue where several people contracted a diarrheal illness. While this patient could have inflammatory bowel disease, which of the following pathogens is most likely to be responsible for his illness?

(A) *Campylobacter*
(B) *S. aureus*
(C) *E. coli*
(D) *Salmonella*
(E) Norwalk agent

**I-49.** All the following are characteristic clinical features of chancroid EXCEPT

(A) initial presentation as a tender papule
(B) development of painful genital ulcers
(C) tender, enlarged inguinal lymph nodes
(D) *Haemophilus ducreyi* isolated from bacteriologic cultures
(E) response to ampicillin therapy

**I-50.** A 62-year-old gardener who has chronic lymphocytic leukemia develops lymphangitis and a painless, nodular lesion on his wrist. Subsequently, he becomes severely ill with cavitary right-upper-lobe pneumonia; *Sporothrix schenckii* is isolated. He should be treated with

(A) chloramphenicol
(B) potassium iodide
(C) penicillin
(D) amphotericin B
(E) flucytosine

**I-51.** An 86-year-old woman with a known history of rheumatic mitral valvular disease presents with a 2-week history of fevers and anorexia. She gives a history of dental work without prophylaxis approximately 3 weeks ago. Her laboratory examination is remarkable for an elevated erythrocyte sedimentation rate and microscopic hematuria. The patient is admitted to the hospital and treated with intravenous broad-spectrum antibiotics. Five days later blood cultures obtained before the start of antibiotics remain negative. Infection with all the following microorganisms could account for the patient's clinical endocarditis EXCEPT

(A) *Streptococcus viridans*
(B) *Haemophilus influenzae*
(C) *H. parainfluenzae*
(D) *H. aphrophilus*
(E) *Eikenella corrodens*

**I-52.** A 19-year-old woman visits the emergency room because of a swollen left knee. She has no past medical problems. She gives a history of several days of feeling feverish and having muscle and joint aches. Specifically, her hands and wrists were painful for a few days, but at this point she is bothered only by her knee. Physical examination is remarkable only for vesiculopustular skin lesions and a mildly swollen left knee. The procedure most likely to yield a diagnosis at this point would be

(A) cervical culture
(B) blood culture
(C) sinovial culture
(D) serum complement assay
(E) skin biopsy

**I-53.** Four days after he and his friends were killing muskrats along a rural creek, a boy becomes ill with headache, fever, and a macular rash. On examination, axillary adenopathy is noted, but otherwise the examination is normal. Which of the following tests would be most helpful in proving that this boy has tularemia?

(A) Blood culture
(B) Aspiration and culture of an axillary lymph node
(C) Determination of serum agglutinins for *Francisella tularensis*
(D) Bone marrow culture
(E) Examination of his friends

**I-54.** A 10-year-old boy is seen in a rural Arizona clinic because of prostration, fever of 40°C (104°F), and severe headache. Examination is negative for rash, stiff neck, joint tenderness, and chest and abdominal abnormalities. However, several tender, enlarged lymph nodes are palpated in the left axilla, which is very edematous. The test most likely to be of greatest help in the immediate management of this boy would be

(A) blood culture
(B) examination of a blood smear
(C) biopsy of an axillary lymph node
(D) aspiration and Gram stains of an axillary lymph node
(E) surgical excision of an axillary node

**I-55.** A 10-year-old boy presents with an abnormal appearing face. The boy lives in Rhode Island and has been playing outside a good deal this summer. He has been feeling poorly for a week with complaints of muscle aches and headache. His mother has noticed that her son has a low-grade fever and an oval rash on the back measuring about 10 cm in diameter. Physical examination reveals evidence of the oval erythema on the posterior thorax and evidence of right facial droop. Routine laboratory studies are unremarkable. A lumbar puncture reveals an opening pressure of 80 mmHg, total protein of 46 mg/dL, and glucose of 90 mg/dL with 10 white cells, all of which are lymphocytes. The most specific diagnostic study would be

(A) polymerase chain reaction–based DNA detection
(B) *Borrelia* serology
(C) blood culture for *Borrelia*
(D) cerebrospinal fluid culture for *Borrelia*
(E) western blot detection of *Borrelia* antigen in the cerebrospinal fluid

**I-56.** Intravenous acyclovir is indicated in each of the following situations EXCEPT

(A) a clinically severe initial episode of genital herpes simplex virus infection

(B) a clinically severe recurrent episode of herpes simplex virus infection

(C) oral herpes simplex 3 months after an allogeneic bone marrow transplant

(D) chickenpox in an adolescent female who is receiving steroids for lupus nephritis

(E) dermatomal herpes zoster infection in a middle-aged male being treated for large cell lymphoma

**I-57.** *Listeria monocytogenes* most frequently causes which of the following infections?

(A) Endocarditis
(B) Peritonitis
(C) Hepatitis
(D) Meningitis
(E) Conjunctivitis

**I-58.** Which of the following statements concerning infections with intestinal nematodes is correct?

(A) A relatively small number of organisms typically produce severe clinical symptoms

(B) *Ascaris* larvae enter the body via migration through dermal capillaries

(C) Hookworm infections result from the swallowing of hookworm eggs

(D) *Strongyloides* infection is associated with recurrent urticaria

(E) Pinworm infection is associated with iron deficiency anemia

**I-59.** Which of the following drugs would be LEAST likely to benefit a patient experiencing an acute attack of malaria?

(A) Quinine
(B) Chloroquine
(C) Primaquine
(D) Hydroxychloroquine
(E) Mefloquine

**I-60.** Which of the following food- or waterborne bacteria responsible for diarrheal illness has the LONGEST incubation period (time from ingestion to illness)?

(A) *Clostridium perfringens*
(B) *Staphylococcus aureus*
(C) *Bacillus cereus*
(D) *Campylobacter jejuni*
(E) *Vibrio parahaemolyticus*

**I-61.** A 22-year-old gay man from New Orleans presents with a 2-week history of fever, anorexia, and progressive diffuse lymphadenopathy. Physical findings reveal an emaciated young man who has several tongue ulcers. Hepatomegaly is noted. Laboratory examination reveals pancytopenia, an elevated alkaline phosphatase, and hyperkalemia. A chest radiograph reveals a miliary pattern of diffuse infiltration. A tongue biopsy reveals the presence of hyphae that bear both large and small spores. The correct diagnosis is

(A) histoplasmosis
(B) coccidioidomycosis
(C) cryptococcosis
(D) blastomycosis
(E) aspergillosis

**I-62.** A 45-year-old man with acute myeloid leukemia in second remission presents with cough, shortness of breath, and fever 3 months after an allogeneic bone marrow transplant. The patient was well before the transplant. At that time, serology revealed antibodies to cytomegalovirus (CMV). The graft was successful, but the patient has required the use of intermittent courses of corticosteroids to treat moderately severe graft-versus-host disease characterized by a diffusely erythematous skin rash and diarrhea.

On examination the patient appears mildly ill, has a temperature of 38.6°C (101.5°F), blood pressure of 130/80 mmHg, pulse of 110 beats per minute, and respiratory rate of 30 breaths per minute. Skin examination reveals a diffuse erythematous maculopapular rash, particularly on the arms and legs. Diffuse crackles are heard in both lungs. Chest x-ray demonstrates bilateral interstitial infiltrates, worse in the lower lobes. Examination of sputum fails to reveal a causative agent. Bronchoscopy is carried out, but the toludine blue stain, routine culture, and fungal stains are negative. Because the patient continues to have respiratory deterioration, he undergoes an open-lung biopsy. Examination of the lung tissue reveals the presence of cells that are several times larger than surrounding cells and contain a 10-μm inclusion placed centrally in the nucleus. There is also a plasmacytic and lymphocytic infiltrate in the lung. At this point, the best course of therapy would be to administer

(A) trimethroprim-sulfamethaxole
(B) acyclovir plus CMV immune globulin
(C) ganciclovir
(D) ganciclovir plus CMV immune globulin
(E) foscarnet

**I-63.** Which of the following samples of pleural fluid is most suggestive of tuberculous pleuritis?

| Fluid sample | Color | pH | Protein, g/L | Glucose, mmol/L | LDH, U/mL | WBC Total (per μL) | WBC % Lymphocytes |
|---|---|---|---|---|---|---|---|
| (A) | Clear yellow | 7.15 | 35 | 1.1 | 600 | 2,000 | 95 |
| (B) | Thick green | 7.00 | 40 | 1.1 | 600 | 10,000 | 50 |
| (C) | Clear yellow | 7.30 | 15 | 4.4 | 150 | 200 | 50 |
| (D) | Pink-tinged | 7.40 | 30 | 4.4 | 600 | 3,000 | 50 |
| (E) | Clear yellow | 7.30 | 35 | 3.3 | 150 | 2,000 | 95 |

LDH, lactate dehydrogenase; WBC, white blood cell count

**I-64.** A 10-year-old child has malaise, a low-grade fever, and submental lymphadenopathy. Biopsy of a cervical lymph node reveals granulomatous inflammation; the culture grows *Mycobacterium scrofulaceum*. The best treatment for this child would be

(A) excision of the infected nodes
(B) isoniazid and ethambutol
(C) streptomycin, isoniazid, and ethambutol
(D) rifampin, isoniazid, and ethambutol
(E) observation until the results of sensitivity studies are available

**I-65.** Which of the following statements concerning the use of fluoroquinolone antibiotics (e.g., ciprofloxacin, norfloxacin) is correct?

(A) Resistance can develop by bacterial plasmid-mediated expression of β-lactamase enzyme
(B) They are bacteriostatic rather than bactericidal
(C) They have activity against all known bacterial enteric pathogens
(D) They are excreted primarily by biliary clearance
(E) They are contraindicated in patients with fever and neutropenia because of their inability to eradicate *Pseudomonas* spp.

**I-66.** A 40-year-old Canadian who operates a tropical fish store sees his physician because of a nonhealing ulcer on his left arm. He is afebrile and gives no history of night sweats, weight loss, or other constitutional symptoms. Biopsy of the lesion shows granulomatous inflammation and rare acid-fast organisms. A tuberculin test is negative. This man most likely has an infection caused by

(A) *Mycobacterium tuberculosis*
(B) *Mycobacterium ulcerans*
(C) *Mycobacterium kansasii*
(D) *Mycobacterium marinum*
(E) *Mycobacterium fortuitum*

**I-67.** Which of the following statements concerning syphilis in HIV-infected persons is correct?

(A) Syphilis is as common in HIV-infected persons as it is in non-HIV-infected persons, though the course of the disease is more aggressive in the HIV-infected group
(B) Serologic testing cannot be used to confirm the diagnosis of syphilis in most patients with HIV infection
(C) Failure to respond to single-dose penicillin G therapy is more likely in patients infected with both HIV and syphilis than in those infected with syphilis alone
(D) Central nervous system syphilis is rare in HIV-infected patients
(E) Syphilis is not an independent risk factor for HIV infection

**I-68.** Legionnaire's disease is characterized by all the following statements EXCEPT

(A) the disease is not spread from person to person
(B) diarrhea, nausea, and vomiting often are prominent early symptoms
(C) chest x-ray usually shows few abnormalities, while chest examination usually is markedly abnormal
(D) fever usually is prolonged
(E) therapy with erythromycin is recommended

**I-69.** Which of the following statements concerning antifungal therapy is correct?

(A) Dose-related hepatotoxicity is a complication of ketoconazole treatment
(B) Clotrimazole is the preferred imidazole for the treatment of vaginal candidiasis
(C) Oral fluconazole may be used as primary therapy in patients with aspergillosis
(D) Flucytosine plus amphotericin B is useful in cases of refractory hepatic candidiasis
(E) The treatment of candidal hepatitis frequently requires 2 weeks of daily intravenous administration of amphotericin B

**I-70.** A 35-year-old HIV-infected homosexual man presents with fever, pain of the right upper quadrant, and a CT of the liver that shows a 10-cm, oval hypoechoic cyst in the right lobe. An ELISA assay detects the presence of antibodies to *Entamoeba histolytica*; cysts from the same organism are found in a stool specimen. Which of the following is the most appropriate next step in management?

(A) Administration of metronidazole
(B) Administration of chloroquine
(C) Drainage of the hepatic lesion for therapeutic purposes
(D) Aspiration of the hepatic lesion for diagnosis
(E) Hepatic resection

**I-71.** Which of the following statements concerning viral upper respiratory infections is correct?

(A) Risk factors for infection with rhinovirus include exposure to cold temperatures, fatigue, and sleep deprivation
(B) The incubation period for rhinoviral illness is approximately 1 week
(C) Infection with respiratory syncytial virus (RSV) is unusual in older children and adults
(D) Ribavirin given by aerosol is effective in treating infants with RSV
(E) Pentamidine is a useful prophylactic therapy against adenovirus infections

**I-72.** The characteristic "sulfur grains" of actinomycosis are composed chiefly of

(A) organisms
(B) neutrophils and monocytes
(C) monocytes and lymphocytes
(D) eosinophils
(E) calcified cellular debris

**I-73.** The best available therapy for disseminated *Mycobacterium avium-intracellulare* (MAI) infection in patients with AIDS is administration of

(A) isoniazid, rifampin, and ethambutol
(B) ciprofloxacin
(C) streptomycin and pyrazinamide
(D) clarithromycin
(E) clarithromycin and ethambutol

**I-74.** Antigen testing of blood and cerebrospinal fluid is most useful in the diagnosis of

(A) histoplasmosis
(B) blastomycosis
(C) cryptococcosis
(D) coccidioidomycosis
(E) sporotrichosis

**I-75.** A 55-year-old homeless man presents with fever and stiff neck several days after an upper respiratory infection. He also notes painful hands and hair loss. Physical examination reveals a disheveled male with a temperature of 40°C (104°F), blood pressure of 120/70, heart rate of 70, and respiratory rate of 20. The remainder of the physical examination is remarkable for an erythematous posterior pharynx, areas of alopecia on the head and body, swollen metacarpophalangeal joints, and a stiff neck. Laboratory evaluation is remarkable for a white blood cell count of 2300/μL with 25 percent neutrophils, 65 percent lymphocytes, and 10 percent monocytes; hematocrit is 42 percent, and platelet count is 55,000/μL. Other laboratory studies are unremarkable. Examination of the cerebrospinal fluid reveals normal opening pressure, total protein of 100 mg/dL, glucose of 20 mg/dL, and white count of 400/μL (80 percent lymphocytes and 20 percent neutrophils). Gram stain, acid-fast stain, and India ink stain are all negative. Which of the following statements about this patient is correct?

(A) Intravenous penicillin G is the treatment of choice
(B) The low CSF glucose is pathognomonic for bacterial meningitis
(C) A routine blood culture probably will establish the diagnosis
(D) The patient probably has come in contact with an infected rodent
(E) Alopecia is unrelated to the current infection

**I-76.** A 45-year-old man with acute myelogenous leukemia (AML) is seen 45 days after initial treatment with daunorubicin and cytosine arabinoside. After this therapy he sustained 22 days of neutropenia, during which time he became febrile and received broad-spectrum antibiotics. He was discharged feeling relatively well after a 28-day hospital course with a normal CBC and bone marrow. Within several days after hospital discharge, he developed a fever of 38.5°C (101.3°F) and mild abdominal pain, particularly in the right upper quadrant. Physical examination is unrevealing. His CBC is normal, as is the rest of his laboratory examination except for an elevated alkaline phosphatase. CT of the liver is nonspecifically abnormal. The most appropriate action at this point would be

(A) admission of the patient for administration of broad-spectrum antibacterial antibiotics
(B) magnetic resonance imaging (MRI) of the right upper quadrant
(C) abdominal ultrasonography
(D) bone marrow aspirate and biopsy
(E) liver biopsy

**I-77.** All the following antimicrobial agents inhibit the synthesis of bacterial cell walls EXCEPT

(A) bacitracin
(B) imipenem
(C) vancomycin
(D) clarithromycin
(E) ceftriaxone

**I-78.** Impaired immune competence is the predisposing factor in about half of all persons who develop

(A) histoplasmosis
(B) coccidioidomycosis
(C) blastomycosis
(D) cryptococcosis
(E) sporotrichosis

**I-79.** Which of the following agents, when administered to an intubated patient in an intensive care unit, is most likely to decrease the incidence of hospital-acquired pneumonia?

(A) Ranitidine
(B) Cimetidine
(C) Sucralfate
(D) Penicillin G
(E) Ciprofloxacin

**I-80.** The type of endocarditis most commonly found in patients who are intravenous drug abusers is

(A) *Staphylococcus aureus* infection of the tricuspid valve
(B) *S. aureus* infection of the mitral valve
(C) α-hemolytic streptococcal infection of the tricuspid valve
(D) α-hemolytic streptococcal infection of the mitral valve
(E) *Pseudomonas aeruginosa* infection of the pulmonic valve

**I-81.** A 28-year-old woman who works in a poultry processing factory develops an acute febrile illness. Which of the following signs and symptoms is LEAST suggestive of the diagnosis of psittacosis?

(A) Shaking chills with fever to 40.6°C (105°F)
(B) Severe headache
(C) Nonproductive cough
(D) Stiff back and neck
(E) Diarrhea

**I-82.** Which of the following is LEAST suggestive of infection with poliovirus?

(A) Low-grade fever and malaise with complete resolution in 2 to 3 days
(B) Biphasic illness with several days of fever, then meningeal symptoms and asymmetric flaccid paralysis 5 to 10 days later
(C) Descending symmetric motor paralysis with preservation of tendon reflexes and sensation
(D) Failure to isolate a virus from the cerebrospinal fluid in the presence of marked meningismus
(E) Recovery of function up to 6 months after initial paralysis

**I-83.** A 58-year-old schoolteacher is hospitalized after 10 days of a respiratory illness. For 2 days he has had a dramatically worsening cough and shortness of breath. He also has had severe malaise, myalgias, arthralgias, rhinorrhea, and pharyngitis and has lost 2.7 kg (6 lb). No sputum or respiratory secretions can be collected. Chest x-ray shows a diffuse bronchopneumonia. All the following antibiotics would be acceptable for the initial treatment of this man's illness EXCEPT

(A) penicillin G
(B) nafcillin
(C) vancomycin
(D) cephalothin
(E) clindamycin

**I-84.** Which of the following is LEAST likely to be a manifestation of late syphilis?

(A) Lymphadenopathy
(B) Aortitis
(C) Papulosquamous skin rash
(D) Hemiparesis
(E) Ataxic gait

**I-85.** Infection with *Mycobacterium tuberculosis* is common in HIV-infected patients. Which of the following statements concerning this problem is correct?

(A) Tuberculosis is a relatively rare presenting infection in a patient with AIDS
(B) Extrapulmonary tuberculosis is more common than pulmonary tuberculosis in HIV-infected patients
(C) HIV-infected patients with pulmonary tuberculosis need not be considered infectious
(D) Initial therapy for HIV-infected patients with tuberculosis should be the same as that for non-HIV-infected patients with tuberculosis (isoniazid, rifampin, and pyrazinamide)
(E) Isoniazid should not be administered to those with HIV infection and a positive tuberculin skin test until active infection is documented

I-86. A 35-year-old Jamaican emigrant develops diffuse lymphadenopathy, fever, lymphocytosis, hypercalcemia, and nodular skin infiltrates. Biopsy of a skin lesion reveals a monotonous population of lymphocytes that stain with antibody directed at CD4 (T4). Which infectious agent is associated with this disease?

(A) Human immunodeficiency virus 1 (HIV-1)
(B) HIV-2
(C) Human T-lymphotropic virus I (HTLV-I)
(D) HTLV-II
(E) Feline leukemia virus (FeLV)

I-87. There has been an outbreak of infections caused by methicillin-resistant *Staphylococcus aureus* in the surgical intensive care unit. The most effective means of limiting the spread is

(A) treatment with cephalosporins to which most strains are sensitive
(B) treatment with nafcillin and gentamicin, which have a synergistic effect
(C) use of high-dose nafcillin alone and isolation
(D) treatment with vancomycin
(E) minimization of the use of any antibiotics in affected patients because resistance will develop rapidly in other bacteria

I-88. A 40-year-old Filipino man has hypopigmented macular lesions and a palpably enlarged ulnar nerve. The diagnosis of leprosy can best be established by

(A) a positive lepromin skin test
(B) a culture of material obtained on skin biopsy
(C) the development of erythema and swelling of the lesions after a trial of dapsone therapy
(D) the demonstration of acid-fast organisms in skin or nerves
(E) none of the above; leprosy is a clinical diagnosis

I-89. A 35-year-old Samoan presents with recurrent fever, headache, photophobia, and painful lymphangitis in the left leg. The best way to diagnose filariasis caused by *Wuchereria bancrofti* is

(A) biopsy of any inflamed lymph nodes to demonstrate the adult worm
(B) serologic studies
(C) observation of intense itching after a single dose of diethylcarbamazine
(D) demonstration of microfilariae after injection of blood into mice
(E) demonstration of microfilariae in blood taken between 9 P.M. and 2 A.M.

I-90. All the following groups have an increased risk of infection with *Giardia lamblia* EXCEPT

(A) campers in mountainous areas
(B) patients receiving chemotherapy
(C) toddlers in day-care centers
(D) patients with IgA deficiency
(E) male homosexuals

**Questions 91–92**

An 18-year-old sexually active woman from the inner city presents with fever, pleuritic pain of the right upper quadrant, and lower abdominal pain. Pelvic examination reveals mucopurulent cervicitis and tenderness after the production of cervical motion. The right upper quadrant, uterine fundus, and adnexa are slightly tender. The white blood cell count and erythrocyte sedimentation rate are elevated, but the results of the remainder of the laboratory examination, including liver function tests, are normal.

I-91. Which of the following agents is the most likely cause of this clinical syndrome?

(A) Herpes simplex virus
(B) *Treponema pallidum*
(C) *Neisseria gonorrhoeae*
(D) *Chlamydia trachomatis*
(E) *Mycoplasma hominis*

I-92. Because the patient appears ill, she is hospitalized. Assuming that pregnancy and appendicitis are excluded, which of the following antibiotic regimens is the best choice?

(A) Doxycycline plus cefoxitin
(B) Doxycycline alone
(C) Acyclovir plus penicillin
(D) Penicillin alone
(E) Ceftriaxone

I-93. A 65-year-old retired banker who spends the summer on Nantucket Island off the Massachusetts coast returned to his home in Boston early in September. He noted the gradual onset of a febrile illness with chills, sweats, myalgias, and yellow eyes. His doctor palpated the spleen and noted a macrocytic anemia, hyperbilirubinemia, and a high serum level of lactic dehydrogenase on laboratory examination. Which of the following would be the most helpful diagnostic procedure at this point?

(A) Blood culture
(B) Examination of leukocytes on blood film
(C) Examination of erythrocytes on blood film
(D) Splenic biopsy
(E) Liver biopsy

**I-94.** All the following represent clinical syndromes produced by *Leishmania* EXCEPT

(A) fever, pancytopenia, and splenomegaly
(B) disfiguring facial ulcer
(C) diffuse skin lesions
(D) dysphagia, chest pain, and regurgitation
(E) nasal obstruction and epistaxis

**I-95.** In persons who have endocarditis, all the following factors would adversely affect the prognosis EXCEPT

(A) the presence of congestive heart failure
(B) abscess formation
(C) the isolation of organisms resistant to multiple antimicrobial agents
(D) the isolation of *Staphylococcus epidermidis* months (compared with days) after cardiac surgery
(E) drug addicts with *S. aureus* tricuspid valve infection

**I-96.** All the following conditions would warrant antibiotic prophylaxis against infective endocarditis in a patient experiencing invasive dental work EXCEPT

(A) atrial septal defect
(B) ventricular septal defect
(C) mitral stenosis
(D) mitral regulation without mitral valve prolapse
(E) mitral regurgitation associated with mitral valve prolapse

**I-97.** Which statement concerning *Acinetobacter* is correct?

(A) This organism often is confused with *Neisseria* on Gram stain
(B) This organism often is mistakenly identified as a diphtheroid on Gram stain
(C) This organism is a member of the Enterobacteriaceae family on the basis of its appearance on routine laboratory culture media
(D) This organism usually is sensitive to penicillin and ampicillin
(E) Organisms of the genus *Acinetobacter* are rarely isolated from normal patients

**I-98.** Correct statements concerning melioidosis include which of the following?

(A) Infection usually is caused by person-to-person transmission
(B) Patients with pneumonia usually have relatively few organisms in the sputum
(C) The diagnosis usually depends on serologic testing
(D) Cavitary lung lesions do not occur
(E) Therapy with a combination of two or three antibiotics is recommended for severely ill patients

**I-99.** Brucellosis can be described by all the following statements EXCEPT

(A) cattle are the most important source of human *Brucella* infections in the United States
(B) brucellosis is an important cause of abortion in cattle and pigs but not in humans
(C) brucellosis should be considered in the differential diagnosis of fever of unknown origin in the United States
(D) *brucella* cannot be grown in usual blood culture media
(E) a combination of tetracycline and streptomycin is the treatment of choice

**I-100.** Cholera can be characterized by all the following statements EXCEPT

(A) in endemic areas, it is predominantly a disease of children
(B) the most definitive means of diagnosis is by culture
(C) oral treatment must include replacement fluids containing glucose and sodium bicarbonate
(D) treatment with oral tetracycline shortens the duration of diarrhea
(E) vaccination affords good protection from infection

**I-101.** True statements about mucormycosis include all the following EXCEPT

(A) the organism is grown easily from most clinical specimens once an adequate tissue sample has been obtained
(B) a characteristic feature of *Mucor* is its tendency to invade blood vessels
(C) in persons with hematologic malignancies, the sinuses and lungs are the most common sites of infection
(D) diagnosis by serologic testing is not yet clinically practical
(E) the treatment of choice is amphotericin B and surgical debridement

**I-102.** True statements about Rocky Mountain spotted fever include all the following EXCEPT

(A) fleas are the characteristic vector of disease spread
(B) the disease is caused by the obligate intracellular organism *Rickettsia rickettsii*
(C) severe headache is a common early manifestation of infection
(D) the initial skin lesions usually appear on the extremities
(E) the treatment of choice consists of the early administration of chloramphenicol or doxycycline

**I-103.** Diphtherial infections are correctly characterized by which of the following statements?

(A) Human infection occurs only with strains that produce diphtheria toxin

(B) Serious disease can be prevented by mass immunization with diphtherial cell-wall poly-saccharide

(C) A pseudomembrane can be observed in both cutaneous and respiratory forms of infection

(D) A portion of the diphtheria toxin molecule is responsible for specificity; another part inflicts cellular damage by directly inhibiting DNA repair

(E) Cardiac disease is a rare complication of diphtherial pharyngitis

**I-104.** True statements concerning *Klebsiella* infections include all the following EXCEPT

(A) most clinical isolates are obtained from the urinary tract

(B) predisposing factors for Klebsiella pneumonia include alcoholism, diabetes mellitus, and chronic bronchopulmonary disease

(C) *Klebsiella* is closely related to *Enterobacter* and *Serratia*

(D) Detecting *Klebsiella* growth from a sputum culture obtained from an intubated patient mandates treatment with an aminoglycoside or a third-generation cephalosporin

(E) at least 2 weeks is often required to successfully treat an established *Klebsiella* infection

**I-105.** Toxoplasmosis can be described by all the following statements EXCEPT

(A) a pregnant woman who has acquired *Toxoplasma* any time before pregnancy is unlikely to deliver an infected infant

(B) a woman who develops acute toxoplasmosis during one pregnancy is more likely than are other women to give birth to an infected child in a subsequent pregnancy

(C) a woman who acquires toxoplasmosis during the last trimester of pregnancy is more likely to deliver an infected infant than she would be if she acquired the infection during the first trimester

(D) toxoplasmosis in a person with Hodgkin's disease probably is due to reactivation of a latent infection

(E) antibody response is not a reliable diagnostic indicator of toxoplasmosis in immunocompromised patients

**I-106.** A person with liver disease caused by *Schistosoma mansoni* would be most likely to have

(A) gynecomastia
(B) jaundice
(C) esophageal varices
(D) ascites
(E) spider nevi

**I-107.** Extrapulmonary tuberculosis can be characterized by all the following statements EXCEPT

(A) pleural effusions associated with tuberculosis usually occur in older patients, with reactivation disease developing after an insidious onset

(B) patients with laryngitis or bronchitis caused by tuberculosis are highly infectious

(C) Pott's disease, with extensive bony involvement of the midthoracic spine and paravertebral cold abscesses, usually responds well to chemotherapy alone

(D) cranial nerve findings frequently are associated with tuberculous meningitis because of basilar involvement by infection

(E) the terminal ileum is most likely to be involved in patients with gastrointestinal tuberculosis

**I-108.** True statements about influenza infection include all the following EXCEPT

(A) pandemics are caused by several simultaneous point mutations

(B) immunity is established by the development of antibodies to the hemaglutinin

(C) outbreaks of influenza B tend to be smaller than those of influenza A because the virus does not undergo extensive antigenic shift as it does in influenza A

(D) in a minority of patients, prolonged weakness and fatigue develop, but virions are no longer shed

(E) amantadine or rimantadine may be useful in prophylaxis of or therapy for influenza A if started within 48 h of infection

**DIRECTIONS:** Each question below contains five suggested responses. For each of the five responses listed with every question, you are to respond either YES (Y) or NO (N). In a given item all, some, or none of the alternatives may be correct.

**I-109.** Correct statements concerning the pathogenesis of fever include

(A) aspirin inhibits the production of endogenous pyrogens

(B) the major endogenous pyrogens in humans include interleukin 1 (IL-1) and tumor necrosis factor (TNF)

(C) endogenous pyrogens are produced by bacteria, protozoa, and fungi

(D) endogenous pyrogens raise body temperature through their effect on skeletal muscle beds

(E) endogenous pyrogens play a role in the cachexia of chronic infections

**I-110.** Correct statements concerning pneumococcal infection include which of the following?

(A) Pneumocococal bacteremia is prevalent in infants and the elderly

(B) Patients who have had a splenectomy for any reason should receive pneumococcal vaccine

(C) Pneumococcal pharyngitis is the most common precipitating event for pneumococcal meningitis in adults

(D) The occurrence of the "crisis" in pneumococcal pneumonia generally corresponds to the time of maximum leukocytosis

(E) Hypogammaglobulinemia is an important factor contributing to the unfavorable prognosis for pneumococcal pneumonia in alcoholic persons

**I-111.** True statements about the pathogenesis of streptococcal infections include which of the following?

(A) Streptococcal strains without M protein in the cell wall are nonpathogenic

(B) Manifestations of infection with group A streptococci are due primarily to direct invasion

(C) Penicillin significantly shortens the clinical course of the pharyngitis produced by group A streptococci

(D) Nonenterococcal group D streptococci cause endocarditis

(E) Streptococcal pyoderma does not lead to acute rheumatic fever

**I-112.** Leptospirosis may be characterized by which of the following statements?

(A) Fleas are the most important vector for the transmission of *Leptospira* to humans

(B) Leptospirosis usually begins with fever, headache, and myalgias

(C) Leptospiral hepatitis often causes marked hyperbilirubinemia with only moderate transaminasemia

(D) A normal glucose concentration and a moderately elevated white blood cell count (100 to 1000 cells/$\mu$L) are characteristic cerebrospinal fluid findings in leptospiral meningitis

(E) The best way to diagnose acute leptospirosis is by dark-field microscopic examination of blood smears

**I-113.** *Neisseria gonorrhoeae* infections can be described by which of the following statements?

(A) Gonococci with pili tend to be avirulent

(B) Strains of *N. gonorrhoeae* that produce $\beta$-lactamase are resistant to penicillin but usually are sensitive to "third-generation" cephalosporins such as ceftriaxone

(C) Gonococcemia frequently occurs during menstruation

(D) The skin lesions of gonococcemia usually appear first on the distal portions of the extremities

(E) Gonococcal arthritis usually is symmetric in distribution

**I-114.** True statements concerning infectious mononucleosis include which of the following?

(A) The most common symptom of infectious mononucleosis is sore throat

(B) In young adults, the incubation period for infectious mononucleosis is 30 to 50 days

(C) The atypical lymphocytes associated with infectious mononucleosis are T cells

(D) Heterophil antibody titers usually decline within 3 to 6 months from the onset of symptoms

(E) Antibodies to Epstein-Barr virus (EBV) generally persist longer in the circulation than do heterophil antibodies

**I-115.** True statements concerning malaria include

(A) malaria caused by each of the four plasmodial species can relapse after the initial illness
(B) red cells negative for the Duffy blood group antigen are resistant to *Plasmodium vivax*
(C) renal impairment is a grave prognostic sign in falciparum malaria
(D) *Plasmodium malariae* can cause immune-mediated nephropathy
(E) massive splenomegaly can result from repeated bouts of infection

**I-116.** Well-recognized complications of infection with Epstein-Barr virus include

(A) airway obstruction
(B) lymphoma
(C) thrombocytopenia
(D) hemolytic anemia
(E) hepatitis

**I-117.** Correct statements about clostridial infections include which of the following?

(A) Early antibiotic therapy is important after the isolation of clostridia from any wound to prevent more serious disease
(B) Alpha toxin, a lecithinase, is one of the major clostridial toxins
(C) *Clostridium perfringens* is one of the most common causes of food poisoning in the United States
(D) The diagnosis of clostridial myonecrosis can be difficult to make because few organisms are present in the skin lesions
(E) Septicemia with *C. septicum* has been associated with gastrointestinal malignancies

**I-118.** Anaerobic organisms should be considered as potential etiologic agents in which of the following patients?

(A) A previously healthy 18-year-old boy with sudden fever, cough, and right lower lobe infiltrate
(B) A 50-year-old man with alcoholism who has marked cellulitis, swelling, and pain in the left lower mandible
(C) A 40-year-old woman with a seizure disorder, low-grade fever, malaise, and a right lower lobe infiltrate
(D) A 50-year-old woman with fever, hypoxia, and pulmonary infiltrates 4 h after having general anesthesia for a cholecystectomy
(E) A 38-year-old man with a history of rheumatic fever and severe periodontitis in whom a low-grade fever, malaise, and a new heart murmur develop

**I-119.** True statements about varicella-zoster infection include which of the following?

(A) Once dermatomal herpes zoster develops in a patient, repeated recurrences are the rule
(B) Cerebellar ataxia is a serious complication of varicella in children
(C) Chickenpox is very contagious, with attack rates estimated at between 70 and 90 percent
(D) Varicella pneumonitis, the most serious complication of chickenpox, occurs more frequently in adults than in children
(E) Within 72 h of exposure, varicella-zoster immune globulin should be given, if applicable, to all patients to prevent the development of clinical disease

**I-120.** Cytomegalovirus (CMV) is accurately described by which of the following statements?

(A) Approximately 60 percent of infants who are breast-fed by seropositive mothers become infected; this represents the majority of cases of cytomegalic inclusion disease in newborn infants
(B) Although 1 percent of newborn infants may be infected with CMV in the United States, less than 0.05 percent have symptomatic disease
(C) CMV mononucleosis is the most common cause of heterophil-negative mononucleosis
(D) CMV pneumonia, a major cause of morbidity and mortality in bone marrow transplant patients, can be diagnosed only by viral cultures of sputum
(E) Cultures of CMV from urine, saliva, or buffy coat specimens confirm the presence of the virus but do not necessarily imply acute infection

**I-121.** Correct statements about viral gastroenteritis caused by rotavirus and Norwalk virus include which of the following?

(A) Both alter cyclic nucleotide levels and cause a secretory diarrhea
(B) Rotaviruses are the most important cause of severe diarrhea in infants
(C) Rotavirus infection can be diagnosed only retrospectively by serologic methods since isolation from stool is very difficult
(D) Norwalk virus has been associated with both food-borne and waterborne epidemics
(E) Both viruses cause a self-limited disease with vomiting and diarrhea

**I-122.** Tetanus is correctly characterized by which of the following statements?

(A) Neonatal tetanus develops after passage through a contaminated birth canal

(B) If given early enough after exposure, human tetanus immune globulin can modify the course of disease significantly

(C) Tetanus does not recur because lasting immunity develops

(D) Trismus is a common manifestation

(E) In a patient who is uncertain about his or her immunization status, both tetanus toxoid and immune globulin should be given for serious wounds

# I. INFECTIOUS DISEASES

## ANSWERS

**I-1. The answer is A.** (*Chap. 208*) *Aspergillus* spp. are commonly found in the environment, particularly on decaying vegetation. Thus, *Aspergillus* spores are ubiquitous, but invasive infection is rare except in patients subject to immunosuppression. Patients with granulocytopenia and/or lymphopenia resulting from corticosteroid or cyclosporin administration are at risk. Invasive *Aspergillus* infection is characterized by hyphal invasion of blood vessels with concomitant thrombosis. Invasive *Aspergillus* in an immunocompromised host usually presents as a densely consolidated pulmonary infiltrate that is rapidly progressive and is most common in those with prolonged neutropenia secondary to the treatment of acute leukemia and/or recipients of bone marrow transplants. A definitive diagnosis is difficult and requires biopsy; however, the isolation of even a single colony of *Aspergillus* from the sputum of a neutropenic patient with pneumonia, except for among patients who are smokers, suggests the diagnosis of invasive *Aspergillus*. While the fungus ball may be amenable to surgical resection, more typical invasive disease, such as that evidenced by this patient, requires prolonged therapy with amphotericin B. Itraconazole may play a role in less dramatic presentations. Unless the immunosuppression resolves rapidly, the chance for a cure with this type of infection is poor.

**I-2. The answer is D.** (*Chap. 224*) Schistosomiasis represents the clinical manifestation of infection with a trematode (fluke). The urinary tract disease noted in this patient is characteristic of *Schistosoma haematobium* infection, which is endemic in parts of Africa and the Middle East. The infective stage of this parasite, termed a *cercara*, penetrates the unbroken skin of a human who comes in contact with contaminated water. After several days the schistosomules (developing schistosomes) travel to the lungs and then to the portal vein, where they mate and migrate to the ureteral venules (for *S. haematobium*; *S. mansoni* and *S. japonicum* migrate to the venules of the mesentery). Eggs are deposited in the bladder and ureters, with mature ova being released into the water, where they hatch into a meracidium that infects the intermediate host, a snail, eventually releasing thousands of cercaria to renew the cycle. Eggs deposited in the ureters and bladder elicit an intense inflammatory and granulomatous response that may cause functional obstruction. These lesions are reversible with the use of antischistosomal chemotherapy such as praziquantel. As fibrosis ensues, chemotherapy is less effective. The diagnosis is based on the demonstration of the characteristic eggs in the tissues or urine. *S. haematobium* infection is a predisposing factor for the development of an unusual histologic variant of bladder cancer (squamous cell carcinoma).

**I-3. The answer is D.** (*Chap. 123*) Persons infected with human immunodeficiency virus (HIV) who wish to travel require specific advice if the CD4+ count is below 500/μL and especially if it is below 200/μL. Many countries detain those carrying anti-HIV drugs such as zidovudine at the border and refuse entry to such individuals. Routine immunizations for travel should be up to date in an HIV-infected individual; however, it must be recognized that the response to immunizations may be impaired if the CD4+ cell count is very low. While inactive pathogen or component vaccines such as pneumococcal polysaccharide, influenza, and polio vaccine have been shown to transiently increase HIV viremia, because of the potential severity of infection with these organisms in HIV-infected individuals and a lack of evidence that such viremia is detrimental, vaccination is recommended. The live oral polio vaccine should not be administered, although another live vaccine, the measles vaccine, may be given safely. It is also recommended that live yellow fever vaccine not be given to HIV-infected travelers; nonetheless, no reactions have been reported in those who have inadvertently received this agent. Traveler's diarrhea may be a particular problem because it tends to occur more frequently and be more severe in those with HIV infection. Pathogens such as *Salmonella, Shigella, Campylobacter, Cryptosporidium,* and *Isospora belli* are common organisms that produce diarrheal illness. Therefore, in addition to the consumption of only appropriately prepared fruits and vegetables, the use of a prophylactic agent such as bismuth subsalicylate is reasonable.

**I-4. The answer is C.** (*Chap. 156*) The most important risk factors for *H. pylori* infection include older age, low income, and residence in a developing country. It is believed that infection generally is acquired in childhood. Although humans are the major reservoir of *H. pylori,* the route of infection is unclear, with fecal-oral and oral-oral spread both being possible. *H. pylori* is endemic in only 30 percent of Americans, but prevalence rates are as high as 80 percent in developing countries. Infection with a related species, *H. heilmanii,* is about 1 percent as common as *H. pylori* infection.

**I-5. The correct answer is A.** (*Chap. 147*) Botulism is caused by protein neurotoxins elaborated by the *Clostridium botulinum* anaerobic gram-positive organism. These organisms form spores that are found in soils and marine environments throughout the world. Eight toxin types have been described; each can be inactivated by cooking at high temperatures. In the United States, toxin types A, B, and E usually are associated with food-borne botulism, often from home-canned food, particularly vegetables, fruit, and occasionally meat and fish.

The incubation period after the ingestion of food containing the toxin is usually 18 to 36 h but can vary. The disease usually is heralded by cranial neuropathies and then generally progresses to symmetric descending paralysis that is sometimes associated with nausea, vomiting, abdominal pain, dizziness, blurred vision, dry mouth, and dry sore throat. Although potentially anxious, patients are generally alert and oriented.

The diagnosis must be suspected clinically and should be distinguished from Guillian-Barré syndrome, Lambert-Eaton syndrome, polymyositis, tick paralysis, diphtheria, and chemical intoxication.

Treatment should include hospitalization and close monitoring for a potential decline in respiratory function, which should be treated with intubation and mechanical ventilation. Trivalent (including types A, B, and E) equine antitoxin should be administered immediately. Anaphylaxis and serum sickness may occur. In the absence of ileus, cathartics and enemas should be given to purge the toxin; gastric lavage will help only in cases where the time after ingestion is brief. Antimicrobial therapy plays no role in this situation, since the disease is not caused by a proliferation of bacteria but instead by previously elaborated toxins.

**I-6. The answer is C.** (*Chap. 13. Craven, Chest 108:1S, 1995.*) Nosocomial pneumonia, a pulmonary infection acquired during or as a result of hospitalization, is fairly common. Patients in an intensive care unit who have an endotracheal tube in place are at an increased risk from bacteria leaking around the cuff or contaminating humidifiers or the ventilator circuit condensate. Since an increased degree of colonization of the oropharynx or stomach is a very important factor in the development of nosocomial pneumonia, patients who have an increased propensity to aspirate because of a decreased gag reflex, depressed consciousness, poor gastric emptying, or the presence of a nasogastric tube are also at increased risk. Bacteria are more likely to colonize the stomach when the gastric pH is elevated, as is caused by $H_2$ histamine receptor antagonists such as ranitidine and other antacids. However, sucralfate heals ulcers without altering gastric pH and may produce less of a risk of gastric colonization and the subsequent development of nosocomial pneumonia.

I-7. **The answer is D.** (*Chap. 137*) Nosocomial bacteremia and infection of intravascular devices are common causes of morbidity related to hospitalization. Many times bacteria are cultured from a line without the clear presence of infection. The most common organisms causing such incidental bacteremias include coagulase-negative *Staphylococci*, *Candida* spp., *S. aureus*, and *Enterococci*. In the absence of physical findings compatible with infection in the skin, it may be possible to treat the patient with antibiotics while leaving the catheter in place, especially in the case of bacteremia caused by coagulase-negative *Staphylococci*. By contrast, a clinical line infection, manifested by fever and signs of cutaneous involvement such as erythema and induration at the insertion site or subcutaneous tunnel, should mandate blood cultures and removal of the line. Even though broad-spectrum antibacterial coverage could be administered, it is virtually impossible to eradicate these invasive infections around the plastic tubing with antibiotics alone, mandating line removal. Replacing an infected line over a guidewire may result in immediate contamination of the new line.

I-8. **The answer is E.** (*Chap. 111*) In addition to *H. influenzae* and *S. pneumoniae*, the gram-negative coccus *Moraxella (branhamella) catarhalis* is a common cause of exacerbations of chronic bronchitis and pneumonia in patients with moderately severe chronic obstructive pulmonary disease (COPD). The symptoms are typically modest in severity, although chills, pain, and malaise often are noted. Low-grade fevers and a lack of leukocytosis are also common. If the patient actually has pneumonia, the radiologic appearance is variable, and clinical parameters do not permit one to determine the organism causing illness in a heavy smoker with COPD. However, the Gram's stain in this case, which depicts the abundant presence of gram-negative cocci in pairs, is typical of *M. catarhalis*. Cephalosporins, tetracycline, erthyromycin, trimethoprim-sulfamethoxazole, and quinolones are all effective. However, since resistance to both trimethoprim-sulfamethoxazole and tetracycline has been reported, those with pneumonia require treatment with the most effective agent. Therefore, the most appropriate choice is the combination of ampicillin and clavulanic acid, which suppresses the *M. catarhalis* ß-lactamases.

I-9. **The answer is A.** (*Chap. 159*) The *Shigella* gram-negative bacilli are a potential cause of dysentry, typically manifested by watery or bloody diarrhea with or without fever. The clinical manifestations can be quite severe, especially in children from developing countries. As a result of both direct invasiveness and in some cases elaboration of *Shigella* toxins, the colonic mucosa reveals focal ulcerations, mucous discharge, and occasional hemorrhage. Extraintestinal manifestations of shigellosis are more common in developing countries but include the hemolytic uremic syndrome, which is more commonly caused in the United States by strains of *E. coli* that produce high levels of a *Shigella*-family toxin. Since culture results typically do not become available until the patient is better, there is usually little clinical need for antibiotic therapy. However, the use of agents such as ampicillin and trimethoprim-sulfamethoxazole can shorten the carriage period and reduce the duration of illness in severely infected patients. Unfortunately, the utility of these agents in developing countries is limited by the emergence of resistant strains. Infection occurs by the fecal-oral route; exposure to relatively few organisms may produce illness because of the relative insensitivity of these bacteria to acidic pH conditions, such as those found in the gastric mucosa.

I-10. **The answer is A.** (*Chap. 143*) This patient presents with the classic findings of necrotizing fasciitis, including systemic toxicity associated with minimal to marked skin changes. The site of inoculation, often resulting from simple trauma, usually is somewhat distant from the area of clinical involvement and may be due to simple trauma. Group A streptococci released during abdominal surgery also may cause this type of illness. While staphylococci, *Bacteroides* spp., or anaerobic streptococci also can cause a similar syndrome, group A streptococci account about 60 percent of these cases.

**I-11.    The answer is E.**    (*Chap. 243. Working Group on Severe Streptococcal Infection: Defining the Group A streptococcal toxic shock syndrome. JAMA 269:390, 1993.*)    As group A streptococcal necrotizing fasciitis progresses, the marked tenderness of involved skin may progress into anesthesia as a result of infarction of cutaneous nerves. Surgery is required for both diagnosis and therapy. The process usually extends beyond the area of clinical involvement, and therefore extensive debridement is required. Antibiotics are adjunctive therapy; penicillin G 2 to 4 million units IV every 4 h is recommended, although erythromycin 250 mg four times a day may be substituted in case of allergy. This patient also has group A streptococcal toxic shock-like syndrome, which, in contrast to *Staphylococcus aureus*–associated toxic shock syndrome, is associated with bacteremia. The mortality rate of this syndrome, which results from a pyrogenic exotoxin A produced by the bacteria, is approximately 30 percent.

**I-12.    The answer is D.**    (*Chap. 220. DuPont et al. N Engl J Med 332:855, 1995.*)    Cryptosporidiosis is transmitted by the fecal-oral route by animal-to-person or person-to-person contact. Waterborne transmission may occur since oocytes are hardy and resist killing by routine chlorination. Though symptomatic and asymptomatic infections can occur in an immunocompromised host, followed by a one-week incubation period, immunocompetent individuals typically develop watery nonbloody diarrhea with occasional pain, nausea, anorexia, and weight loss. In such individuals the illness usually subsides in 1 to 2 weeks; however, in those with acquired immune deficiency syndrome the disease can be more prolonged and much more severe. In addition to fluid and electrolyte depletion, weight loss, wasting, and severe abdominal pain may occur with ocassional biliary involvement. The diagnosis rests on stool examination to detect oocytes. Since the interpretation of routine smears is difficult, modified acid-fast and direct immunofluorescence stains have been employed to increase the sensitivity. Treatment is supportive, since no antibiotic has been shown to be definitively effective.

**I-13.    The answer is C.**    (*Chap. 221*)    *Trichinella* spp. are members of the nematode phylum (roundworms). Trichinosis occurs after eating meat containing *Trichinella* nematode oocytes. After the consumption of affected meat, the encysted larvae are released by the action of gastric acid and pepsin. The larvae penetrate the small interstitial mucosa and rapidly mature into adult worms. In one week, female worms release newborn larvae that travel via the circulation to striated muscle and then encyst. Clinical symptoms follow each of these phases. Initially gut invasion may be marked by abdominal pain, nausea, and constipation or diarrhea. Larval migration, which occurs during the second week after infection, produces a local and systemic hypersensitivity reaction manifested by fever, hypereosinophilia and periorbital and facial edema. Myocarditis, encephalitis, and pneumonitis are rare but potentially life-threatening complications that may occur during this phase. After larval encystment in muscle for 2 to 3 weeks, edema and symptoms of myositis, including muscle edema and weakness, develop. The symptoms subside gradually during what may be a prolonged convalescence. Antihelminthic drugs are ineffective against the encysted larvae. Trichinosis, which typically is associated with eosinophilia and an elevated IgE level, may be prevented by cooking pork until it is no longer pink or freezing it at −15°C for 3 weeks. Ocular larva migrans, another nematode infection, is caused by the invasion of *Toxocara* larvae into the eye, typically producing a granulomatous mass, usually in the posterior pole of the retina.

**I-14.    The answer is D.**    (*Chap. 141. Friedland, N Engl J Med 331:377, 1994.*)    The management of severe life-threatening pneumonia caused by *Streptococcus pneumoniae* demands an understanding that 15 to 20 percent of the strains isolated in the United States exhibit intermediate resistance to penicillin and 2 to 5 percent exhibit a high level of resistance to this antibiotic. Similarly, a varying proportion exhibit intermediate resistance to erythromycin, tetracyclines, trimethoprim-sulfamethoxazole, and clindamycin. However, the majority of strains still exhibit susceptibility to cefotaxime, ceftriaxone, and imipenem. Although almost all *S. pneumoniae* that have been isolated remain sus-

ry0

ceptible to vancomycin, the routine use of this antibiotic is discouraged because of the increased prevalence of vancomycin-resistant enterococci. For routine pneumonococcal pneumonia, empiric therapy with penicillin G is still advisable; however, any feature of life-threatening pneumococcal pneumonia requires treatment with a second-generation cephalosporin (assuming that the community does not have endemic resistance to these agents). For patients with life-threatening infections who are known to be severely allergic to ß-lactam antibiotics, vancomycin is the most appropriate choice.

**I-15.**    **The answer is C.**   (*Chap. 213*)   After taking a thorough history in the setting of a suspected parasitic infection, the clinician must have a fairly good idea of the parasite with which infection is likely so that the appropriate diagnostic test can be ordered. Since many helminths and protozoa exit the body in the fecal stream, examination of the stool is critical in many parasitic infestations. Microscopic examination of the stool can, if a motile tapeworm is noted, help make a diagnosis of *Taenia saginata*. This organism also could be readily detected by the Scotch tape technique applied to the perianal skin, sometimes revealing the ovae even if the motile segments have disintegrated. *Giardia lamblia, Cryptosporidium,* and *Stronglyoides* often infect the duodenum, and therefore a string test in which the contents of this organism can be examined may be necessary to make the diagnosis. *Entamoeba histolytica* has been difficult to diagnose in the setting of a presumed liver abscess because the organism grows primarily in the cavity wall. Aspirated fluid is frequently negative for the organism. The diagnosis of *Pneumocystis carinii* is routinely made by examination of a silver-stained induced sputum specimen. *Schistosoma haematobium*, a common cause of hematuria (and sometimes cancer) in third world patients, can be detected easily by examination of the stool for characteristic forms.

**I-16.**    **The answer is E.**   (*Chap. 212. Mannheimer, Infect Dis Clin North Am. 8:43, 1994.*) The approach to a patient with potential parasitic infestation must include a detailed travel and dietary history as well as an understanding of whether any behaviors have predisposed the patient to exposure, such as wading or swimming in fresh water (relevant to the acquisition of schistosomiasis). Residents in institutional settings or child care centers where fecal-oral hygeine may be substandard not infrequently develop giardiasis, cryptosporidiosis, or pinworm infestations. Immune status also determines predisposition to parasitic infection. For example, individuals infected with the human immunodeficiency virus type I, especially those with depressed CD4+ lymphocyte counts, may develop infections with *Toxoplasmosis, Isospora, Cyclospora,* cryptosporidia, *Leishmania,* American trypanosomes, and free-living amoebae. Patients infected with the retrovirus human T-lymphotropic type retrovirus type I are likely to be infected with *Strongyloides*. Persons with asplenism, either anatomic or functional (as in patients with sickle cell anemia), are at risk for developing florid infection from intraerythrocytic protozoa such as malaria and babesiosis. Those with cystic fibrosis or hypogammaglobulinemia (e.g., multiple myeloma or CLL) may develop major infestation with giardiasis.

**I-17.**    **The answer is A.**   (*Chap. 181*)   Endemic trachoma represents a chronic conjunctivitis caused by repetitive infection with certain serotypes of *Chlamydia trachomatis*. Blindness is caused by recurrent infections that lead to repeat episodes of conjunctivitis, including corneal vascularization (pannus formation). The conjunctival scarring can be so severe that the eyelids turn inward with subsequent abrasion of the cornea by the inturned lashes, requiring surgical correction. Destruction of the lacrimal gland with ensuing "dry eye" syndrome may lead to further corneal abrasions. Treatment consists of topical tetracycline or erythromycin or single-dose azithromycin.

**I-18.**    **The answer is D.**   (*Chap. 175*)   Nonvenereal treponematoses occur in less developed areas of the world and include yaws, pinta, and endemic syphilis, each caused by *Treponema pallidum*. These conditions may be distinguished epidemiologically and clinically from venereal syphilis. Pinta involves the skin alone, whereas yaws affects the skin and bones; endemic syphilis involves the skin, bones, and mucus membranes. Yaws is

characterized by the development of one or more initial skin lesions followed by relapsing nondestructive secondary lesions of the skin and bones, but with ultimate destruction
occurring in the late stages. A manifestation of endemic syphilis is usually an intraoral
mucous lesion, resembling what is seen in secondary syphilis. Pinta may begin with a
small papule that may coalesce with adjacent satellite papules and produce seasonal lymphadenopathy. Treatment for all the endemic treponematoses consists of the intramuscular administration of 2.4 units of benzathine penicillin G.

**I-19.**    **The answer is B.**    (*Chaps. 170, 171. American Thoracic Society and Centers for Disease
Control, Am J Respir Crit Care Med 149:1359, 1994.*)    Isoniazid, rifampin, pyrazinamide,
ethambutol, and streptomycin are considered first-line agents for antituberculous treatment.
All except streptomycin are given orally and are well absorbed. They are all bactericidal
and are associated with a low rate of drug resistance induction. Multiple second-line drugs
are useful in patients who have drug resistance or intolerance to the first-line agents. Such
drugs include ofloxacin, cycloserine, and *p*-aminosalicylic acid as well as the injectable
agents kanamycin, amikacin, and capriomycin. The backbone of the initial treatment regimen, which is designed to produce maximal antimycobacterial kill, is two months of treatment with isoniazid, rifampin, pyrazinamide, and, except for those who seem to have a low
likelihood of harboring a drug-resistant strain on epidemiologic grounds, ethambutol. Once
the sputum culture reveals drug-sensitive tuberculosis, ethambutol can be dropped from the
regimen for the remaining two months. Pyridoxine should be added to the regimen to prevent isoniazid-associated neuropathy, which is more common in those at high risk of vitamin deficiency, such as alcoholics, and those with conditions in which neuropathy is likely,
such as chronic renal failure, diabetes, and AIDS. It is also important that patients be super-
vised during the period of drug treatment to ensure compliance. After the initial two-month
treatment phase, a continuation phase of four months is recommended during which treatment with isoniazid and rifampin should be sufficient to eradicate the organism.

**I-20.**    **The answer is C.**    (*Chap. 184. Benedetti, Ann Intern Med 121:847, 1994.*)    Herpes
simplex viruses types I and II are double-stranded DNA viruses. Sequence homology
between the two strains is about 50 percent. HSV-1 and HSV-2 are the causes of symptomatic genital and perianal infections, corneal infections, encephalitis, and disseminated
disease in immunocompromised individuals. The first episode of primary genital herpes
may be manifested by a systemic illness with fever, headache, and malaise in conjunction with local symptoms such as pain, itching, dysuria, and vaginal discharge. The systemic illness may be mitigated somewhat if the patient has had a prior HSV-1 infection.
Lesions in the perineal area, particularly on the labia, may include vesicles, pustules, and
painful ulcers. Recurrence rates are highly variable but approach 90 percent for those
with HSV-2 infection, and are only 50 percent for those with HSV-1 infection. Recurrence rates can be decreased somewhat by means of chronic oral acyclovir therapy. Acyclovir and related compounds can speed the healing and resolution of symptoms in first
and recurrent episodes of genital HSV-1 and HSV-2 infections. Oral acyclovir is well
tolerated; however, acyclovir-resistant strains of HSV are being isolated with increasing
frequency. Prevention of recurrent HSV disease is also very important; barrier forms of
contraception such as condoms decrease but do not eliminate the likelihood of transmission of HSV infection, especially if obvious skin lesions are present.

**I-21.**    **The answer is B.**    (*Chap. 140*)    Although antibiotics typically have a very high therapeutic index, they may interact with other drugs that are being ingested by the patient,
with a potential for deleterious consequences. For example, erythromycin and other
macrolide antibiotics that are well tolerated as single agents (except for frequent gastrointestinal toxicity) can inhibit the hepatic metabolism of many concurrently administered drugs, such as theophylline, terfenadine, warfarin, and ergot alkyloids. In any of
these cases, the non-antibiotic drug may cause toxicity as a result of increased serum
concentrations. Decreased metabolism of terfenadine can lead to severe cardiac dysfunction. Erythromycin can inhibit the metabolism of cyclosporine, consequently leading to a

higher likelihood of cyclosporine-induced complications such as renal failure. Clarithromycin has a greater effect on hepatic metablism than does azithromycin.

**I-22.  The answer is A.**  *(Chap. 165. Zangill, N Engl J Med 329:8, 1993.)*  This patient exhibits the typical manifestation of cat-scratch disease, which is a painful regional lymphadenopathy that persists for several weeks or months after a cat scratch. Before the development of the lymphadenopathy, a localized papule or pustule that eventually crusts develops within a few days after the scratch. Since scratches most often occur on the hand or face in children, youngsters account for 60 percent of cases. The epitrochlear, axillary, pectoral, and cervical lymph nodes are commonly involved. Systemic symptoms and even severe manifestations such as encephalitis, seizures, and coma may occur. Most cases are self-limited and can be diagnosed by microscopic examination of a lymph node biopsy specimen. The cat-scratch disease skin test is no longer used because of fear of the transmission of viral agents. Serologic tests can confirm that the causative organism is the gram-negative bacillus, *Bartonella henselae*. Bacillary angiomatosis, also caused by *Bartonella henselae*, causes skin lesions resembling Kaposi's sarcoma, and occurs in patients with immunocompromised states such as an HIV infection. The Wharthin-Starry silver stain can detect the *Bartonella* spp. in both conditions; it appears that ciprofloxin and doxycycline have activity in *Bartonella* infections.

**I-23.  The answer is D.**  [*Chap. 131. Stamm, Am J Med (Suppl 3B):655, 1991.*]  Bacteruria is a common problem in institutionalized patients with urethral catheters. Since the risk of infection is about 3 to 5 percent per day of catheterization, most patients who have a catheter in for longer than 2 weeks eventually develop bacteria in the urine. Infections generally result from migration through the column of urine in the catheter lumen or from organisms moving up the mucous sheath outside the catheter. In either case, the most common organisms causing such infections are *Proteus, Pseudomonas, Klebsiella, E. coli,* and *Serratia.* Other important factors are female sex, severe underlying illness, disconnection of the catheter and drainage tube, and lack of systemic antimicrobial therapy. Despite these facts, prevention with short courses of systemic antimicrobial therapy, topical application of periurethral ointments and the addition of antimicrobials to the drainage bag is not recommended for general use. Though most catheter-associated infections cause minimal symptoms, gram-negative bacteremia is a complication that may occur in 1 to 2 percent of those who have catheter-associated bacteruria. In fact, the most common cause of gram-negative bacteremia in hospitalized patients is a catheterized urinary tract. The best treatment, if possible, is removal of the catheter in conjunction with a short course of antibiotics to which the organism is susceptible. However, if the catheter must be left in place, antibiotic therapy usually engenders resistance and should probably be cause for ignoring the bacteruria as long as it remains asymptomatic.

**I-24.  The answer is D.**  *(Chap. 138)*  Since *Aspergillus* spores are common in the environment, particularly in dusty areas such as construction sites, any hospital renovation must be carried out carefully if immunocompromised patients are nearby. Routine surveillance of bone marrow transplant patients and other neutropenic patients for infections with filamentous fungi may be indicated. All air-handling equipment, ideally HEPA filters, should be inspected on a routine schedule. There is no role for the routine use of prophylactic antibiotics for this very resistant fungal infection.

**I-25.  The answer is D.**  *(Chap. 199. Fishbein, Robinson, N Engl J Med 329:1632, 1993.)*  The patient in question has been bitten by a member of a species known to carry rabies in an area in which rabies is endemic. Based on the animal vector and the facts that the skin was broken and that saliva possibly containing the rabies virus was present, postexposure rabies prophylaxis should be administered. If an animal involved in an unprovoked bite can be captured, it should be humanely killed and the head should be sent immediately to an appropriate laboratory for rabies examination by the technique of fluorescent antibody staining for viral antigen. If a healthy dog or cat bites a person in an endemic area, the animal should be captured, confined, and observed for 10 days. If the animal remains healthy for this period of time, the bite is highly unlikely to have transmitted rabies. Postexposure prophylactic therapy includes vigorous cleaning of the wound with a 20% soap solution to remove any virus particles that may be present. Tetanus toxoid and antibiotics also should be administered. Passive immunization with antirabies antiserum in the form of human rabies immune globulin (rather than the corresponding equine antiserum because of the risk of serum sickness) is indicated at a dose of 10 units/kg into the wound and 10 units/kg intramuscularly into the gluteal region. Second, one should actively immunize with an antirabies vaccine [either human diploid cell vaccine or rabies vaccine absorbed (RVA)] in five 1-mL doses given intramuscularly, preferably in the deltoid or anterior lateral thigh area. The five doses are given over a 28-day period. The administration of either passive or active immunization without the other modality results in a higher failure rate than does the combination therapy.

**I-26.**   **The answer is A.**   *(Chap. 200)*   The presence of IgM antibodies in either the serum or the CSF that are reactive with the LaCrosse (California) arbovirus is highly suggestive of acute infection with this agent. Moreover, the patient resides in an endemic area (the North Central states, New York, wooded areas of eastern Texas and Louisiana, and along the eastern seaboard). The virus is present in the woodland mosquito, *Aedes triseratus*; chipmunks and squirrels serve as amplifier hosts. Human infections occur most often during the summer months, when the mosquito is active, and usually involve 5- to 10-year-old boys who live in rural areas. The clinical presentation may be the abrupt epileptic type, as in this patient, or the more lethargic form. While EEGs are typically abnormal and imaging studies of the brain also may reveal abnormalities in the temporal lobe, the presence of the specific antibody obviates the need for brain biopsy to exclude herpes encephalitis, which is also typically localized in the temporal lobes. Despite the abrupt clinical onset and severity, there is progressive improvement beginning about the fourth day, with almost all patients becoming afebrile, seizure-free, and able to leave the hospital within several weeks. The mortality is under 2 percent; however, about 15 percent of affected persons may develop short- or long-term sequelae, including personality and behavioral changes.

**I-27.**   **The answer is C.**   *(Chap. 137)*   Infection of cannulas occurs most commonly by contamination during insertion or manipulation. Although the daily application of an antibacterial ointment is recommended by some authorities, the best way to prevent these infections is to change the cannula periodically, no less frequently than every 2 or 3 days. An exception is the use of cuffed catheters, which are inserted surgically into the subclavian vein and can be used for many weeks. Infections of such devices with relatively nonpathogenic organisms, such as coagulase-negative staphylococci, may be treated with intravenous antibiotics; however, gram-negative rod and candidal infections usually mandate removal of the indwelling catheter. Infections of cannulas occur much less frequently as a result of the other factors listed in the question.

**I-28.**   **The answer is B.**   *(Chap. 124. Lynn, Clin Infect Dis 20:143, 1995.)*   In the case presented, the history and physical examination strongly suggest gram-negative sepsis stemming from a urinary-tract infection. In older men, obstruction resulting from prostatic hypertrophy is usually the cause. Prompt initiation of appropriate antibiotic therapy is most important. The choice of antibiotics can be guided by the history and microscopic examination of a Gram-stained urine specimen. In the absence of definitive laboratory information, initial treatment with maximal doses of broad-spectrum antibiotics, such as gentamicin or tobramycin plus ampicillin or a cephalosporin, is indicated. Bladder catheterization may be necessary to relieve the obstruction or monitor urine flow. Intravenous infusion of bicarbonate solutions and Ringer's lactate or dextrose-in-saline solutions is needed acutely to correct acidosis, restore vascular volume, and maintain renal perfusion. Corticosteroids may protect against the lethal effects of endotoxin in experimental animals, but recent placebo-controlled trials have failed to support their use in most clinical situations. Antiendotoxin antibodies and agents that interfere with the action of cytokines (e.g., TNFα and IL-1β) that mediate the manifestations of septic shock are under investigation.

**I-29.   The answer is D.**   *(Chap. 157)*   Primary *Pseudomonas* osteomyelitis is very unusual except in intravenous drug addicts, but it should be considered in a nail puncture wound that does not respond to local or oral antibiotic therapy. Ecthyma gangrenosum, an indurated black area approximately 1 cm in diameter with an ulcerated center and surrounding erythema, is highly suggestive of *Pseudomonas* bacteremia. *Pseudomonas* is the most common cause of chronic otitis externa, which usually responds to local measures. In diabetics, however, a rapidly invasive form may develop and require aggressive debridement and antibiotic therapy. *Escherichia coli* is the most common cause of gram-negative meningitis in neonatal infants. The development of *Pseudomonas* meningitis usually occurs only after introduction by surgery, trauma, or foreign objects such as shunts. *Pseudomonas* endocarditis may affect intravenous drug users or patients undergoing open-heart surgery.

**I-30.   The answer is D.**   *(Chap. 225. Gil-Grande et al., Randomized controlled trial of efficacy of albendezole in intra-abdominal hydatid disease. Lancet 342:1269, 1993.)*   This patient hails from an area where echinococcal infection is endemic. It is prevalent in areas where livestock is raised in association with dogs. Dogs, which are the definitive hosts, harbor the adult *E. granulosus* worm and pass eggs in their feces, which can then be ingested by the intermediate hosts, including sheep, cattle, and humans. After ingestion of the eggs, the hatched embryos enter the portal circulation and frequently travel to the liver or lungs. The larvae develop into fluid-filled hydatid cysts from which secondary cysts develop. A slowly enlarging mass ultimately develops. After 5 to 20 years the mass may enlarge to the point where it may cause symptoms, such as those resulting from compression of the bile duct. Leakage of cyst fluid into the biliary tree also can mimic recurrent chole-lithiasis; episodic leakage from the cyst can produce a syndrome of fever, pruritus, and urticaria or possibly even fatal anaphylaxis. The presence of daughter cysts within larger cysts and eggshell calcification in the wall of the cyst is essentially pathognomonic for *E. granulosus* infection and suggests that carcinoma, bacterial or amebic liver abscess, and hemangioma are less likely. Aspiration of the cyst may be conducted carefully for diagnostic purposes. Serology is not specific. Albendazole is not sufficiently effective to be used as monotherapy. Surgery is indicated for such a space-occupying lesion, although the risks of anaphylaxis and dissemination of infectious scolices may be minimized by instilling ethanol into the cyst cavity.

**I-31.   The answer is B.**   *(Chap. 121. Tompkins, N Engl J Med 327:1290–1297, 1992.)*   Recombinant DNA technology has made it possible to identify specific microbial DNA sequences in clinical material. Although specific, this technique, which does not depend on variability, may be too sensitive in some cases and thus may blur the distinction between infection and colonization. Probes have been developed for a wide variety of microorganisms, including CMV, EBV, hepatitis B virus, and HIV, as well as mycoplasma, chlamydia, legionella, group A streptococci, *Gardnerella vaginalis*, and gonococci. These probes become even more sensitive with the use of the polymerase chain reaction to amplify specific sequences.

**I-32.   The answer is C.**   *(Chap. 128. Dupont, N Engl J Med 328:1821, 1993.)*   Toxigenic *Escherichia coli* is the major cause of diarrhea ("turista") for Americans abroad. *Staphylococcus aureus, Clostridium perfringens*, and *Bacillus cereus* cause various types of acute food poisoning owing to bacterial proliferation and elaboration of toxins in improperly stored food. Children throughout the developing world suffer acute diarrhea, similar to traveler's diarrhea, caused by rotavirus infection. All five of these agents cause watery diarrhea that generally is without blood, mucus, or fecal leukocytes, as opposed to illness caused by *Shigella, Salmonella,* or *Campylobacter,* which produces a more invasive, dysenteric type of disease.

**I-33. The answer is A.** *(Chap. 122)* Since BCG is a live attenuated organism and has been reported to cause disseminated infection in immunocompromised patients, it should not be administered to those with HIV infection or those with suspected immunodeficiency. Though patients with immune dysfunction often do not mount a good response to an administered vaccine, they should still receive certain preparations. Patients about to undergo splenectomy or cancer chemotherapy should, when possible, be vaccinated before therapy. Influenza vaccine should be given in autumn to those with any chronic medical illness in addition to those with an obvious immune deficiency. The chronically ill, the immunosuppressed, and those at risk for infection with encapsulated microorganisms (e.g., anatomic or functional asplenia, multiple myeloma) should receive pneumococcal vaccine. The last group plus those with terminal complement component deficiencies should receive the quadrivalent meningococcal vaccine. Patients with HIV infection, especially those who are potential household contacts of children receiving the oral polio vaccine (attenuated live virus), should receive three doses of the inactivated polio vaccine.

**I-34. The answer is E.** *(Chap. 211. Maser, N Engl J Med 323:1500, 1990.)* Patients with AIDS, premature malnourished infants, children with primary immunodeficiency diseases, and patients receiving immunosuppressive therapy (particularly corticosteroids for cancer or organ transplantation) are at risk for developing *Pneumocystis carinii* pneumonia. Although infection usually is confined to the lungs, disseminated infection can occur in up to 3 percent of patients. In this patient, sputum obtained at bronchoalveolar lavage has yielded diagnostic material. Toludine blue, which also selectively stains the wall of the pneumocystis cyst, would have been appropriate, as would immunofluorescent or immunoperoxidase staining. Further diagnostic studies are not required in this setting, and treatment should be undertaken. For patients with severe hypoxemia, corticosteroids may be effective in mitigating immune-mediated lung damage. Steroids should be administered in conjunction with appropriate antimicrobial therapy, which includes either intravenous trimethoprim-sulfamethoxazole or intravenous pentamidine. Therapy should continue for 21 days in patients with AIDS. Aerosolized pentamidine is effective as prophylaxis but is not indicated in primary infections. Combination therapy with trimethoprim-sulfamethoxazole and pentamidine has not been shown to be more effective than either agent alone.

**I-35. The answer is B.** *(Chap. 218. Kirchoff, N Engl J Med 329:639–644, 1993.)* This patient formerly resided in an area endemic for the protozoan parasite *Trypanosoma cruzi.* So-called American trypanosomiasis, or Chagas' disease, is found in almost all Latin American countries. Given the increased number of immigrants from these countries to the United States, the domestic prevalence of the infection is increasing. Transmission occurs through the bite of blood-sucking insects known as reduviid bugs, in contrast to African trypanosomiasis (sleeping sickness), which is transmitted to humans by tsetse flies. The acute infection is self-limited and is characterized by a mild febrile illness often associated with lymphadenopathy. Years or even decades later an estimated 10 to 30 percent of infected patients will be afflicted with symptomatic Chagas' disease. The heart is most commonly affected; manifestations include dilated biventricular cardiomyopathy, conduction disturbances, arrhythmias, and the development of mural thrombi complicated by thromboembolic phenomena. Dilation of the esophagus or colon also can be seen. The diagnosis is made by serology; active parasitic forms cannot be found in the peripheral blood. Treatment is supportive. Corticosteroids or the immunosuppression required for heart transplantation is contraindicated because of the possibility of reactivation and subsequent development of acute Chagas' disease. Prophylactic treatment with antitrypanosomal drugs such as benznidazole and nifurtimox is not effective enough to provide protection against acute infections.

**I-36.** **The answer is A.** *(Chap. 142)* The pathogenicity of staphylococci is related to a number of biologic properties, including the production of coagulase, catalase, exotoxin, and enterotoxin. Coagulase and catalase are thought to protect staphylococci within a host from being destroyed by phagocytes. Some staphylococcal strains produce exotoxins that can cause intraepidermal cleavage and bullae formation as well as toxic shock syndrome. Other strains elaborate an enterotoxin that produces gastrointestinal disease. The production of penicillinase, though rendering a pathogenic organism harder to destroy pharmacologically, does not contribute to pathogenicity.

**I-37.** **The answer is A.** *(Chaps. 142, 377)* Probably because of its ubiquity and ability to stick to foreign surfaces, *Staphylococcus epidermidis* is the most common cause of infections of central nervous system shunts as well as an important cause of infection on artificial heart valves and orthopedic prostheses. *Corynebacterium* spp. (diphtheroids), just like *S. epidermidis*, colonize the skin. When these organisms are isolated from cultures of shunts, it is often difficult to be sure if they are the cause of disease or simply contaminants. Leukocytosis in cerebrospinal fluid, consistent isolation of the same organism, and the character of a patient's symptoms all are helpful in deciding whether treatment for infection is indicated.

**I-38.** **The answer is B.** *(Chap. 149)* Vaccines prepared from high-molecular-weight antigens of *Neisseria meningitidis*, serotypes A and C, have proved effective, but an effective group B vaccine is not available. Chemoprophylaxis is appropriate for intimate contracts in the household or a day care center and for those with oral contact. Useful regimens include refempin, a fluoroguinolone, or IM ceptriexone (especially for pregnant females).

**I-39.** **The answer is A.** *(Chap. 17. Caroff, Med Clin North Am 77:185, 1993.)* This patient is suffering from the neuroleptic malignant syndrome, which is characterized by muscle rigidity, autonomic dysregulation, and hyperthermia. The patient probably has been exposed to phenothiazines for the first time, given his relatively recent admission to the psychiatric facility. This syndrome represents an idiosyncratic reaction to inhibition of central dopamine receptors that results in increased heat production and failure of heat dissipation. In addition to rapid physical cooling and administration of an antipyretic or acetaminophen (but not aspirin), the use of the dopamine agonist bromocriptine or dantrolene should be strongly considered. Dantrolene reverses the hypothalamic dysfunction caused by major tranquilizers.

**I-40.** **The answer is C.** *(Chap. 157)* *Pseudomonas* organisms can cause a rapidly invasive infection of the external ear that results in extensive bony erosion in diabetics. Aggressive surgical debridement and parenteral administration of antibiotics are required. *Aspergillus* organisms can be isolated frequently from external ear swabs but do not cause invasive disease. Mucormycosis must be considered in any seriously ill diabetic patient with sinus or ocular involvement. Infection usually spreads from the nasal cavity and does not involve the ears. Insulin-dependent diabetics are likely to have their skin colonized by *S. aureus*, but this is not associated with external otitis. *H. influenzae* is a frequent cause of otitis media, especially in children, but not of otitis externa.

**I-41.** **The answer is C.** *(Chap. 158. Cherubin, Rev Infect Dis 13:343–344, 1991.)* *Salmonella typhi* survives well in food and water and generally causes infection by penetrating the intestinal mucosa and entering the bloodstream. Usually at the time when affected persons present with fever and other signs of an acute illness, the white blood cell count is depressed. In contrast, rose spots usually do not occur until the second week of illness. Therapy with chloramphenicol does not prevent relapses but does alter the course of the acute illness. A chronic carrier state can develop, in large part because of the propensity of *S. typhi* to seed and inhabit the gallbladder, especially in adults with gallstones. The fluoroquinolones are becoming the treatment of choice to eradicate the chronic carrier state.

**I-42.** **The answer is B.** *(Chap. 122)* Passive immunization can be used to provide temporary immunity in a person who is exposed to an infectious disease and has not been previously actively immunized. Standard human immune serum globulin does not contain known antibody content for a specific agent, unlike special immune serum globulins that exist for the treatment of susceptible patients exposed to hepatitis B, varicella (which is indicated for postexposure prophylaxis of susceptible immunocompromised persons, susceptible pregnant women, and exposed newborn infants), rabies, tetanus, and cytomegalovirus (used in bone marrow and kidney transplant recipients). Intramuscular immune globulin can be used for hepatitis A pre- and postexposure prophylaxis as well as hepatitis non-A, non-B (C) postexposure prophylaxis; it is of questionable efficacy in postexposure prophylaxis for hepatitis B and rubella but may play a role in postexposure prophylaxis for immunocompromised persons exposed to measles.

**I-43.** **The answer is E.** *(Chap 152. Farley, Ann Intern Med 116:806–812, 1992.)* Persons who have sickle cell disease or agammaglobulinemia and those who have been splenectomized have immune systems that poorly opsonize encapsulated bacteria such as *Haemophilus influenzae*. *Haemophilus influenzae* infections also are more common in alcoholic persons, in part because of abnormal cellular defense mechanisms. Persons who have chronic granulomatous disease have problems combating infection with *Staphylococcus aureus*, *Salmonella*, and *Serratia* but not *H. influenzae*. Other important risk factors for *H. influenzae* include pregnancy, steroid therapy, diabetes, and malignancy (with or without chemotherapy).

**I-44.** **The answer is A.** *(Chap. 154)* Because a marked lymphocytosis characteristically is observed in children (less commonly in older persons) who have *Bordetella pertussis* infection (whooping cough) and is rare in patients with other respiratory illnesses, a white blood cell count with differential would be useful in making the diagnosis. Blood cultures would be negative, and Gram stain of the sputum and chest and neck x-rays would show nonspecific changes unless a lobar pneumonia superinfection had occurred. The diagnosis of pertussis is confirmed in most cases by nasopharyngeal culture, though ELISA and DNA-based detection methods are alternative diagnostic procedures. Supportive care and the administration of erythromycin are the mainstays.

**I-45.** **The answer is E.** *(Chap. 204. Stevens, N Engl J Med 332:1077, 1995.)* Coccidioidomycosis, caused by the inhalation of *Coccidioides immitis*, may present clinically with manifestations of hypersensitivity reactions. Arthralgias and frank arthritis (so-called desert rheumatism) as well as skin reactions such as erythema nodosum and erythema multiforme are associated far more frequently with coccidioidomycosis than with the other mycoses listed in the question. Delayed hypersensitivity to *C. immitis* antigens tends to be a good prognostic sign.

**I-46.** **The answer is D.** *(Chap. 140)* Imipenem is a novel β-lactam antibiotic in the carbapenem class with activity against most gram-positive organisms, including those which produce β-lactamase. Imipenem's antibacterial spectrum is quite broad and extends to all pathogens except xanthomonas, resistant *Pseudomonas* spp., methicillin-resistant staphyloccoci, and *Enterococcus faecium*. This drug must be given intravenously because of its instability in gastric acid. Since imipenem is hydrolyzed in the renal tubule by dihydropeptidase I, the coadministration of cilastatin, an inhibitor of this enzyme, serves to markedly boost levels of this broad-spectrum antibiotic. Clavulanate is a β-lactamase inhibitor used with partial success when combined with amoxicillin (Augmentin) for the treatment of resistant otitis and urinary tract infections.

**I-47.** **The answer is C.** *(Chap. 167)* This patient is chronically immunosuppressed from his antirejection prophylactic regimen, which includes both corticosteroids and azathioprine. However, the finding of a cavitary lesion on chest x-ray considerably narrows the possibilities and increases the likelihood of nocardial infection. The other clinical findings, including production of profuse thick sputum, fever, and constitutional symptoms, are also quite common in patients who have pulmonary nocardiosis. The Gram stain, which demonstrates filamentous branching gram-positive organisms, is characteristic. Most species of *Nocardia* are acid-fast if a weak acid is used for decolorization (e.g., modified Kinyoun method). These organisms also can be visualized by silver staining. They grow slowly in culture, and the laboratory must be alerted to the possibility of their presence on submitted specimens. Once the diagnosis, which may require an invasive approach, is made, sulfonamides are the drugs of choice. Sulfadiazine or sulfisoxazole from 6 to 8 g/d in four divided doses is generally administered, but doses up to 12 g/d have been given. The combination of sulfamethoxazole and trimethoprim also has been used, as have the oral alternatives minocycline and ampicillin and intravenous amikacin. There is little experience with the newer β-lactam antibiotics, including the third-generation cephalosporins and imipenem. Erythromycin alone is not effective, though it has been given successfully along with ampicillin. In addition to appropriate antibiotic therapy, the possibility of disseminated nocardiosis must be considered; sites include brain, skin, kidneys, bone, and muscle.

**I-48. The answer is A.** *(Chap. 160)* Campylobacters are motile, curved gram-negative rods. The principal diarrheal pathogen is *C. jejuni*. This organism is found within the gastrointestinal tract of many animals used for food production and usually is transmitted to humans in raw or undercooked food products or through direct contact with infected animals. Over half the cases are due to insufficiently cooked contaminated poultry. *Campylobacter* is a common cause of diarrheal disease in the United States. The illness usually occurs within 2 to 4 days after exposure to the organism in food or water. Biopsy of an affected patient's jejunum, ileum, or colon reveals findings indistinguishable from those of Crohn's disease and ulcerative colitis. While the diarrheal illness is usually self-limited, it may be associated with constitutional symptoms, lasts more than 1 week, and recurs in 5 to 10 percent of untreated patients. Complications include pancreatitis, cystitis, arthritis, meningitis, and Guillain-Barré syndrome. The symptoms of *Campylobacter* enteritis are similar to those resulting from infection with *Salmonella*, *Shigella*, and *Yersinia*; all these agents cause fever and the presence of fecal leukocytes. The diagnosis is made by isolating *Campylobacter* from the stool, which requires selective media. *E. coli* (enterotoxogenic) is not generally associated with the finding of fecal leukocytes, nor is the Norwalk agent. *Campylobacter* is a far more common cause of a recurrent relapsing diarrheal illness that could be pathologically confused with inflammatory bowel disease than are *Yersinia*, *Salmonella*, *Shigella*, and enteropathogenic *E. coli*.

**I-49. The answer is E.** *(Chap. 152)* *Haemophilus ducreyi* causes painful genital ulcers that begin as small tender papules. In contrast, syphilitic ulcers are usually painless, and the initial lesions of genital herpes simplex infections are usually vesicular. The organism causing the chancroid can be isolated from both the ulcers and the affected lymph nodes; in fact, culturing the lymph nodes may produce a pure culture of this organism. Unlike infection with other members of the genus *Haemophilus*, chancroid is not effectively treated with ampicillin. Trimethoprim-sulfamethoxazole and erythromycin are the antibiotic agents of choice.

**I-50. The answer is D.** *(Chap. 210)* Patients who have localized sporotrichosis can be treated successfully with potassium iodide. However, systemic infections, particularly pneumonia in immunocompromised persons, should be treated with amphotericin B. Untreated persons can develop chronic sporotrichosis. Itraconazole also may be effective in treating this condition.

**I-51. The answer is B.** *(Chaps. 126, 152)* The classic organisms responsible for subacute bacterial endocarditis after a dental procedure are viridans streptococci. However, certain *Haemophilus* spp. as well as other members of the so-called HACEK group, fastidious organisms that require incubation in an atmosphere containing carbon dioxide, also may account for infective endocarditis in patients with underlying valvular disease or prosthetic valves and those who have used intravenous drugs. Vegetations may be large, and embolization is not uncommon. Therapy should be based on antibiotic sensitivity, though initial treatment with ampicillin and an immunoglycoside in combination is recommended. Blood cultures must be observed for at least 7 days because of the slow growth of these organisms. The HACEK group includes *Haemophilus aphrophilus*, *H. paraphrophilus*, *H. parainfluenzae*, *Actinobacillus actinomycetemcomitans*, *Cardiobacterium hominis*, *Eikenella corrodens*, and *Kingella kingae*.

**I-52.** **The answer is A.** *(Chap. 150)* One of the most common causes of infectious arthritis in young adults, particularly in urban medical centers, is gonococcal infection. Entry occurs via sites of sexual contact: the genitourinary tract, oropharynx, or rectum. Infection at one of these sites, particularly in menstruating females, pregnant women, and those with complement deficiencies, may lead to dissemination. Such an occurrence produces a biphasic illness that is first manifested by constitutional symptoms, migratory arthritis (particularly in the knee, shoulder, wrists, and interphalangeal joints of the hand), tenosynovitis, and vesiculopustular skin lesions. While these symptoms may abate, joint involvement may progress to a purulent mono- or polyarticular arthritis. Synovial culture and Gram stain are usually negative early in the course of the illness but may be positive at later stages. Blood cultures may be positive, but only in the early stage of the illness. Complement deficiencies are present only in patients who have congenital hypocomplementemia. Gonococci are demonstrable by Gram stain in the skin lesions in about two-thirds of cases. However, diagnosis is best made by observing the intracellular gram-negative diplococci in leukocytes from Gram-stained smears of urethral or endocervical exudates. Because of the presence of other gram-negative diplococci in normal oral flora, Gram stains of pharyngeal smears are not specific. Selective media, such as Thayer-Martin, should be used to culture gonococcus from the urethra, endocervix, pharynx, or rectum. The endocervical culture is positive in 80 to 90 percent of women with gonorrhea. Treatment for disseminated gonococcal infection includes hospitalization and the administration of ceftriaxone, ceftizoxime, or cefotaxime. If the patient is proved to have gonorrhea, a serologic test for syphilis and confidential testing for HIV infection also should be undertaken.

**I-53.** **The answer is B.** *(Chap. 163)* Aspiration and culture of an enlarged axillary lymph node would be most helpful in yielding a diagnosis of tularemia in the case described in the question; however, culture is positive in only 10 percent of cases. Agglutinin reactions ordinarily are not positive for a least 1 week after infection but are specific. A wide variety of animals and insects can transmit tularemia to humans.

**I-54.** **The answer is D.** *(Chap. 164)* In the case presented, the diagnosis of plague (*Yersinia pestis* infection) must be considered. To make this diagnosis, affected lymph nodes should be aspirated and the contents should be Gram-stained. In most cases of bubonic plague, lymph-node aspirates teem with pleomorphic gram-negative bacilli, which can be definitively identified by immunofluorescent staining of the specimen. Blood culture, bone marrow examination, and lymph-node biopsy may be used to diagnose plague, but with undue delay. In this situation, great care should be exercised in handling the infected materials, as there is a significant risk of infection for the laboratory workers.

**I-55.** **The answer is C.** *(Chap. 178. Spach, N Engl J Med 329:936–947, 1993.)* Ninety percent of cases of Lyme disease (Lyme borreliosis) have occurred in the northeastern coastal states. The principal vectors for the causative agent of this disease, *Borrelia burgdorferi*, are *Ixodes* ticks. Less than half of patients with Lyme disease recall receiving a tick bite. Most infections occur during the months of May to August, when human outdoor activities are maximal, and coincide with the time when nymphal *Ixodes* ticks are most active. Like syphilis, another spirochete-mediated disease, the affliction occurs in stages. The initial localized stage frequently is characterized by a macular dermatitis, erythema migrans, which develops at the site of the tick bite. The incubation period is 7 to 10 days and frequently is accompanied by constitutional symptoms. Erythema migrans is typically oval, well demarcated, and more than 5 cm in diameter. Within a few days to weeks after the initial infection, dissemination occurs. The most frequent neurologic manifestation of early disseminated Lyme disease is cranial neuritis, especially facial palsy. Peripheral neuropathy or lymphocytic meningitis also may occur. Nonneurologic manifestations of Lyme disease include atrioventricular block, myopericarditis, and chronic arthritis. The diagnosis generally is made on clinical grounds; however, the most specific diagnostic test for Lyme disease is isolation of the causative organism from blood or erythematous lesions; culture from the CSF is very difficult. An ELISA-based antibody test is frequently plagued by false-positive and false-negative results. Detection of the presence of the organism by a DNA-based method (polymerase chain reaction) remains experimental.

**I-56.  The answer is B.**  *(Chap. 183. Whitley, N Engl J Med 327:782–789, 1992.)*  Acyclovir is one of the most important antiviral agents currently available. It is converted by herpes virus–encoded thymidine kinase to acyclovir monophosphate and then subsequently to the triphosphate form. This process does not occur in uninfected mammalian cells. Acyclovir triphosphate inhibits viral DNA synthesis much more specifically than it does cellular DNA polymerase. The drug is active against herpes simplex virus type I, herpes simplex virus type II, and varicella-zoster virus. Intravenous acyclovir is highly effective for the first episode of genital herpes and will result in a significant reduction in the duration of viral shedding and in the length of time needed to complete healing. However, because of the requirement for hospitalization, such therapy should be reserved for patients who are severely affected. In contrast, recurrent genital herpes, even when severe, is only slightly improved after the administration of oral acyclovir, and there is no known role for intravenous acyclovir. Most patients with allogeneic bone marrow transplants currently receive acyclovir prophylaxis. However, in patients who develop mucocutaneous herpes in the peritransplant period, intravenous acyclovir should be administered. Oral acyclovir will reduce the duration of new lesions in patients with chickenpox and does improve constitutional symptoms. Intravenous use is certainly not appropriate for the average youngster who develops chickenpox, but intravenous acyclovir has been shown to improve the outcome in immunocompromised children with chickenpox. The increased frequency of morbidity in immunocompromised adults who develop herpes zoster, even dermatomal, suggests that intravenous acyclovir therapy is indicated. Severely immunocompromised patients, such as those receiving combination chemotherapy, including steroids, for large cell lymphoma, and marrow transplant recipients should be treated with intravenous acyclovir even in cases where dissemination is not apparent.

**I-57.  The answer is D.**  *(Chap. 145)*  *Listeria monocytogenes* is a gram-positive motile bacillus that tends to infect infants as well as persons over age 55 years. Major illnesses in both groups are meningitis and other forms of central nervous system infection. Many of the older patients are immunosuppressed because of disease (e.g., cancer), immunosuppressive drug therapy, or both. Endocarditis, peritonitis, hepatitis, and conjunctivitis also can be caused by *Listeria* infection.

**I-58.  The answer is D.**  *(Chap. 222)*  Infection with intestinal nematodes is extraordinarily common worldwide, particularly in tropical developing countries. Usually, large worm burdens are required to elicit clinical manifestations of disease. However, in the case of *Ascaris lumbricoides*, single worms (reaching up to 40 cm in length) can cause biliary obstruction or cholecystitis. *Ascaris* is transmitted by the hand-to-mouth fecal carriage route, with subsequent larval development followed by hematogenous migration to the lungs [possibly resulting in eosinophilic pneumonitis (Loeffler's syndrome)]. By contrast, hookworm larvae are hatched in the soil, where, after a 1-week development period, the infectious filariform larvae penetrate the skin and reach the lungs by way of the bloodstream. They are then swallowed and may reach the small intestine, where they produce epigastric pain, diarrhea, and iron deficiency if the worm burden is high enough. Unlike other nematodes, *Strongyloides* replicates in humans, and this permits many cycles of autoinfection with intestinal production of larvae. These infections can persist for decades. As is the case for hookworms, *Strongyloides* larvae hatch in the soil, penetrate the skin or mucous membranes, and ultimately reach the small intestine. Migrating larvae may elicit a pathognomonic serpiginous eruption, which can cause intense pruritus and may be recurrent over a period of many years. Nausea, diarrhea, bleeding, colitis, and weight loss may also be seen with high-burden *Strongyloides* infection. Many American schoolchildren are infected with pinworm *(Enterobius vermicularis)*. Eggs are released only in the perianal region and may be transmitted by hand to mouth to complete the life cycle. Perianal pruritus is the most typical clinical symptom. The diagnosis may be made by applying clear cellulose tape to the perianal region in the morning and transferring the tape to a microscopic slide where the characteristic pinworm eggs may be demonstrated.

**I-59.   The answer is C.**   *(Chaps. 214, 216)*   Most antimalarial drugs—including quinine, 4-aminoquinolines (e.g., chloroquine, hydroxychloroquine), and 4-quinoline-methanols (e.g., mefloquine)—concentrate in erythrocytes and thus destroy the intracellular schizonts responsible for the acute manifestations of malarial illness. However, these drugs do not readily concentrate in the liver and therefore allow survival of hepatic schizonts and reinfection at a later date. In contrast, primaquine, an 8-aminoquinoline, can eradicate hepatic parasites but is not effective in acute illness.

**I-60.   The answer is D.**   *(Chap. 128)*   Bacteria that cause diarrhea via elaboration of toxins generally are associated with a shorter time from ingestion to illness than are invasive strains. For example, enterotoxigenic *E. coli* (the most common cause of traveler's diarrhea), *C. perfringens* (associated with poorly cooked meat or poultry), *S. aureus* (associated with improperly refrigerated dairy foods), and *B. cereus* (associated with grossly contaminated uncooked rice) all have incubation periods of 24 h or less. Even though the pathogenesis may depend on direct mucosal damage, *V. parahaemolyticus*, which is present in inadequately cooked seafood, can cause a diarrheal illness within 6 to 48 h after consumption of a contaminated food. Ingestion of water contaminated with the intestinal flora of wild or domestic animals may cause infection with *C. jejuni*, a common cause of acute, sometimes bloody diarrhea. The incubation period for this invasive bacterium is 2 to 6 days, longer than that associated with other pathogens. Therapy is usually supportive, though erythromycin will shorten the duration of illness.

**I-61.   The answer is A.**   *(Chap. 203. Wheat, Am J Med 98:336, 1995.)*   The patient in question is presumably an HIV-infected man with acute disseminated histoplasmosis, often mistaken for miliary tuberculosis because of its similar pattern of constitutional findings and diffuse chest x-ray abnormalities. Indurated ulcers of the mouth, tongue, nose, or larynx also occur in about 25 percent of patients with acute disseminated histoplasmosis. Addison's disease, granulomatous hepatitis, gastrointestinal ulcerations, endocarditis, and chronic meningitis also may be seen. Since patients with HIV infection may present with febrile syndromes on the basis of multiple organisms and since serologic tests for histoplasmosis are plagued by frequent false-negative and false-positive results, a definitive diagnosis requires demonstration of the organism by culture or histology. The classic morphology of hyphae that bear large and small spores in this clinical setting is diagnostic. Treatment requires initial administration of amphotericin B, followed by prolonged administration of itraconazole.

**I-62.   The answer is D.**   *(Chap. 187)*   Cytomegalovirus (CMV), a double-stranded herpes virus, is transmitted by intimate contact. Once infected, a patient carries the virus for life with actual disease occurring only in the setting of immunosuppression. However, congenital CMV infections may result in significant psychomotor, hearing, ocular, or developmental abnormalities. Second, the most common clinical manifestation of CMV infection, CMV mononucleosis, occurs in normal hosts and resembles the mononucleosis syndrome caused by Epstein-Barr virus, although pharyngitis and lymphadenopathy are much less common with CMV infection. The bone marrow transplant recipient described in the question is clearly at increased risk for CMV-associated syndromes, which may include fever and leukopenia, hepatitis, pneumonitis, esophagitis, gastritis, colitis, and retinitis. Risk factors for infection in transplant patients include the presence of graft-versus-host disease, older age, and known CMV seropositivity in the recipient. Pneumonitis is often manifested by tachypnea, hypoxia, and nonproductive cough. Chest x-ray may reveal bilateral interstitial or reticulonodular infiltrates, particularly beginning in the lower lobes. Since the number of organisms that cause such diffuse pulmonary changes in the posttransplant setting is large, it is important to determine the specific diagnosis. Virus isolation from the specimen obtained at bronchoscopy would be the ideal way to make the diagnosis, but cultures may be falsely negative and results may take several days to return. Cytomegalic cells, demonstrated at open-lung biopsy, are the pathologic hallmark of CMV infection. Cytomegalic cells are characterized by large size and the presence of an 8- to 10-$\mu$m intranuclear inclusion that is centrally placed and sometimes surrounded by a clear halo ("owl's eye" appearance). Cytoplasmic inclusions also may be found. The use of blood from seronegative donors, deglycerolized packed red blood cells, and leukoreduced transfusions may all reduce the risk of transfusion-associated CMV in the posttransplant period. Other prophylactic measures include the use of acyclovir (in high doses) and the use of immunoglobulin. The best results for an active infection have been obtained with the use of ganciclovir, a drug similar in structure to acyclovir, but with more activity against CMV than the parent compound. While ganciclovir alone has been most effective for the treatment of CMV retinitis or colitis, in bone marrow transplant patients who develop CMV pneumonia, ganciclovir is more effective when combined with CMV immunoglobulin. Prolonged therapy may be required. Foscarnet inhibits viral DNA polymerase and may be effective in ganciclovir-resistant CMV infections. Foscarnet is considerably more toxic than is ganciclovir; side effects include renal failure, electrolyte wasting, seizures, and fever.

**I-63. The answer is A.** *(Chap. 171)* The diagnosis of a tuberculous pleural effusion is suggested by the following set of pleural-fluid findings: color, clear yellow; pH, < 7.20; protein, > 30 g/L; glucose, < 1.2 mmol/L (25 mg/dL); lactate dehydrogenase (LDH), > 450 U/mL; and a lymphocytosis. Tubercle bacilli rarely are identified on a smear of infected pleural fluid, and cultures are positive in no more than one-quarter of cases. Antituberculous treatment should begin as soon as the diagnosis is suspected.

**I-64. The answer is A.** *(Chap. 173)* Two of the lesser-known species of *Mycobacterium, M. scrofulaceum* and *M. avium-intracellulare*, cause lymphadenitis in children. Lymph nodes that drain the buccal mucosa usually are affected. Both *M. scrofulaceum* and *M. avium-intracellulare* respond poorly to chemotherapy. The treatment of choice, therefore, is prompt lymph-node excision before rupture has occurred.

**I-65. The answer is C.** *(Chap. 140. Hooper, N Engl J Med 324:384–394, 1991.)* The fluoroquinolones are an important new class of antimicrobial agents with excellent bioavailability. They are renally excreted, and their concentrations increase in chronic renal failure, but generally not to toxic levels. Adverse effects are rare; gastrointestinal symptoms, headache, sleep disturbances, and allergic reactions occur in less than 4 percent of these patients. Theophylline clearance is inhibited by these agents, and care must be taken if coadministration is necessary. Their mechanism of action is novel: they appear to inhibit bacterial topoisomerase II (also known as DNA gyrase), an enzyme involved in the uncoiling of DNA. Their spectrum of activity includes most Enterobacteriaceae, *H. influenzae, Neisseria* spp., *Pseudomonas aeruginosa*, and *Staphylococcus aureus* (including the penicillin-resistant variety). In addition, activity against *Chlamydia, Mycoplasma*, and *Legionella* spp. has been demonstrated. They are bactericidal and play a wide range of potential roles, but they may be preferred in complicated urinary tract infections (because of their excellent concentration in the urine with activity against many otherwise difficult to treat species), chronic *Salmonella* carriage, exacerbation of cystic fibrosis (because of excellent activity against *Pseudomonas aeruginosa*), gram-negative osteomyelitis, and malignant otitis externa. Finally, fluoroquinolone antibiotics may be the treatment of choice for patients with bacterial gastroenteritis who are ill enough to require treatment. These agents are effective against enterotoxigenic *E. coli*, which often causes traveler's diarrhea, as well as *Shigella*. Unfortunately, resistant *Staphylococci* and *Pseudomonas* spp. have been noted.

**I-66.  The answer is D.**  *(Chap. 173)*  *Mycobacterium marinum* is known as the "swimming pool" or "fishtank" bacillus because ulcerative cutaneous infections can be acquired from contact with contaminated swimming pools and aquariums. *M. ulcerans* also causes ulcerative skin lesions but characteristically is confined to tropical regions. Other "atypical" mycobacteria that cause cutaneous infections in humans include *M. avium-intracellulare*, *M. scrofulaceum*, *M. kansasii*, and *M. fortuitum*.

**I-67.  The answer is C.**  *(Chap. 174. Hook, N Engl J Med 326:1060-1069, 1992.)*  Syphilis, like other diseases associated with genital ulcers, is more common in HIV-infected patients, probably because of the increased efficiency of HIV inoculation via the ulcer itself. It is unclear, however, whether syphilis in patients coinfected with HIV actually follows an accelerated clinical course. Though the serologic analysis of syphilis in patients with HIV infection is altered, accurate information is still provided for most patients with HIV infection. Significantly higher serum antitreponemal titers have been reported in patients with HIV compared with those not infected with the virus. Patients with documented secondary syphilis may fail to exhibit positive serology. False-positive serologic studies are also possible in HIV-infected patients who may exhibit polyclonal B-cell activation early in the course of their infection. It has been shown consistently that single-dose penicillin therapy for early syphilis is more prone to failure in HIV-infected patients than in those who are not infected with the virus. It is particularly troubling that the central nervous system may be a sanctuary from penicillin.

**I-68.  The answer is C.**  *(Chap. 153)*  Person-to-person spread of *Legionella pneumophila* has not been documented. Gastrointestinal symptoms that precede pneumonia are sometimes a clue to the diagnosis. In many cases, chest x-ray shows dense infiltrates despite a paucity of physical signs, such as rales or rhonchi; in this regard, the disease resembles *Mycoplasma* pneumonia. Although *L. pneumophila* has been found in vitro to be sensitive to several drugs, erythromycin is the treatment of choice.

**I-69.  The answer is D.**  *(Chap. 202)*  Successful treatment of antifungal infections is not as straightforward as that for bacterial infections. The topical imidazoles that are available for the treatment of vaginal candidiasis include miconazole, clotrimazole, and butoconazole; the triazole terconazole is also available. No substantial difference in efficacy or toxicity among these agents has been noted. Ketoconazole therapy is useful in the treatment of several fungal infections, including esophageal candidiasis, but is associated with several dose-related toxicities, including anorexia and inhibition of steroidogenesis in the adrenal cortex or gonads; hepatotoxicity is idiosyncratic. Fluconazole is an orally administered triazole that may have activity in candidal infection and is useful in a prophylactic role in allogeneic bone marrow transplant patients. Amphotericin B itself is a difficult drug to administer because of frequent toxicities, including azotemia, anemia, hypokalemia, nausea, anorexia, weight loss, phlebitis, and hypomagnesemia. Nonetheless, amphotericin B is indicated for the treatment of invasive infections such as candidal hepatitis. Given a daily dose of about 0.5 mg/kg and the requirement that at least 2 g of the drug should be given in this situation, prolonged therapy is required. Flucytosine, a synthetic oral drug converted to the antimetabolite 5-FU in the fungal cell, may aid in the treatment of refractory invasive candidal disease that is not responsive to amphotericin B alone. Flucytosine is not substituted for, but instead is added to, amphotericin B. Patients on flucytosine should be monitored carefully, since this drug may be myelosuppressive.

**I-70.   The answer is A.**   *(Chap. 215. Reed, Am J Med 90:269, 1991.)*   AIDS patients, particularly homosexual men, have a significant incidence of infection with *Entamoeba* spp., though they are frequently asymptomatic. The most common amebic-related syndrome is that of colitis. Extraintestinal infection by the organism *E. histolytica* usually involves the liver. While the symptoms (fever, pain in the right upper quadrant, and pleural effusion) and the radiologic findings (hypoechoic hepatic cysts) are nonspecific and also can be seen in bacterial abscesses and cancer, such symptoms in a patient with positive serology are quite helpful in making the diagnosis of invasive amebiasis. For that reason, no further diagnostic studies are indicated in the patient. Except in patients with threatened imminent rupture of the cyst or failure to respond to medical therapy, drainage or aggressive aspiration is not necessary. The drug of choice is metronidazole, though the less effective agent chloroquine also may be considered.

**I-71.   The answer is D.**   *(Chap. 191)*   While the clinical syndromes induced by viruses that cause upper respiratory illness are not sufficiently distinct to delineate which virus is the cause of a given clinical syndrome, knowledge of the epidemiologic setting does aid in diagnosis. Rhinoviruses are a common cause of the common cold. They are spread by direct contact with infected secretions and are transmitted efficiently by hand-to-hand contact. Rhinoviral infections are generally uncomplicated; the incubation period is about 2 days. Respiratory syncytial virus (RSV) infections are a major cause of lower respiratory disease in infants, but the virus also may infect older children and adults. Reinfection with this agent is common. Though most patients recover in a week or two, occasionally more severe illness may develop and require admission to an intensive care unit. The diagnosis of RSV infection can be made by culturing the agent from nasal swabs or respiratory secretions or by demonstrating the preserved anti-RSV antibodies. While therapy for RSV infection is mainly symptomatic, aerosolized ribavirin will speed resolution in affected infants. Adenoviruses are also a common cause of upper respiratory infection in infants, children, and adults, especially in military personnel. There is no active therapy available for this infection; however, live viral vaccines, which have been administered to military recruits, may be useful.

**I-72.   The answer is A.**   *(Chap. 168)*   In the examination of purulent material from persons suspected of having actinomyosis, it is important to search the material for the characteristic "sulfur grains" and then examine the grains for organisms. Actinomycetes are gram-positive, branching organisms. If they are detected in a patient who presents with a suggestive clinical picture, such as a chronic draining sinus in the oropharyngeal area, gastrointestinal tract, or pelvic area, the diagnosis of actinomycosis is confirmed. A prolonged treatment course with intravenous penicillin is indicated.

**I-73.   The answer is E.**   *(Chaps. 170, 173)*   MAI infections often are considered to be rapidly fatal in patients with AIDS. Until recently there was no effective treatment. However, the new macrolide antibiotic clarithromycin (6-*O*-methylerythromycin) appears to be the best available drug for disseminated MAI infections in those with AIDS. It is similar to erythromycin in its mechanism of action but does not cause the gastrointestinal distress seen after exposure to the parent compound. Because the MAI organism may acquire resistance to clarithromycin, it should be combined with other antimycobacterial agents, such as ethambutol or rifampin or both. The standard dose of clarithromycin is 500 mg twice daily. Standard triple-drug therapy with isoniazid, rifampin, and ethambutol may be useful in the treatment of MAI lung disease in HIV-negative patients.

**I-74.   The answer is C.**   *(Chap. 206)*   The initial diagnosis of cryptococcal meningitis usually is based on finding encapsulated yeast on an India ink preparation. This test, however, is positive in only about half the cases in which the diagnosis is eventually made. Testing of serum and cerebrospinal fluid for cryptococcal antigen is a very helpful adjunctive test because antigen is found in about 90 percent of cases. In pulmonary cryptococcosis, only about one-third of affected persons are antigen-positive.

**I-75.** **The answer is D.** *(Chap. 201)* Lymphocytic choriomeningitis (LCM) virus is an RNA virus associated both with an influenza-like illness manifested by rash, arthritis, or orchitis and with aseptic meningitis. These two syndromes may occur simultaneously or consecutively. Mice and other rodents are the major natural hosts for LCM infection. Human infections generally are due to residence in a rodent-infested house, but laboratory animals and pets also may be vectors. The mode of entry is the respiratory tract with subsequent penetration of the blood-brain barrier. An influenza-like illness may resolve but be followed by arthralgias (particularly in the hands), hair loss, testicular pain or orchitis, bradycardia, pharyngeal injection, and occasionally axillary adenopathy. Most patients recover within 1 to 4 weeks, though those who develop encephalitis have a significant risk of long-term neurologic sequelae. Laboratory findings include leukopenia and thrombocytopenia (during the first week of the illness). In those with meningeal signs, examination of the CSF reveals lymphocytosis (up to 1000 lymphocytes/$\mu$L), as well as elevated CSF protein and a normal or low glucose, a finding unusual in nonbacterial infections. Culturing the virus from blood or the spinal fluid requires a biosafety level 3 facility; antibody detection methods are available. Since there is no specific treatment available, supportive care is the optimum approach.

**I-76.** **The answer is E.** *(Chap. 207. Thaler, Ann Intern Med 198:88, 1988.)* This patient represents a classic case of hepatic candidiasis, which might be better termed *disseminated candidiasis* because in addition to hepatic involvement the disease often involves other tissues, such as the kidneys. Prolonged neutropenia with concomitant administration of broad-spectrum antibacterial antibiotics, especially during induction therapy for acute myeloid leukemia, is an important risk factor for the development of invasive candidiasis. A fever that develops around the time of neutrophil recovery, especially if it is associated with pain in the right upper quadrant or elevated alkaline phosphatase (which should be proved to be of hepatic origin), is strongly suggestive of hepatic candidiasis. The definitive diagnosis depends on documentation of yeast or pseudohyphae in a granulomatous lesion obtained from infected tissue. Empiric amphotericin B may be indicated. While CT or MRI may reveal "bull's-eye" lesions, a tissue diagnosis is required. If the liver biopsy was nonspecific and failed to reveal organisms and the patient was persistently febrile, especially if his alkaline phosphatase value continued to rise, a more aggressive attempt at diagnosis, possibly even including an open biopsy, would be required. Prolonged administration of amphotericin B often is needed (up to 2 to 4 g) to effect an improvement in the clinical and laboratory findings.

**I-77.** **The answer is D.** *(Chap. 140)* Since mammalian cells do not possess a cell wall, antibiotics that target the synthesis of bacterial cell walls have intrinsic selectivity. Both gram-positive and gram-negative bacteria possess a peptidoglycan cell wall; gram-negative bacteria also possess another membrane external to the aforementioned layer. The classic cell wall–specific antibiotics include $\beta$-lactam-ring agents such as the penicillins, cephalosporins, carbapenems, and monobactams. These drugs prevent the cross-linking reaction that forms peptide cross-bridges (resulting from the cleavage of a terminal D-alanine residue) in the cell wall. The target enzyme, a transpeptidase, actively binds $\beta$-lactam antibiotics. Preventing cell wall synthesis in this fashion not only results in loss of cell wall integrity but also induces the bacteria's own cell wall–remodeling enzymes (autolysins), which may actually cause the microorganisms' "self-destruction." The glycopeptide vancomycin binds to the terminal D-alanine component of the bacterial cell wall peptide and thus inhibits the addition of subunits to the peptidoglycan backbone. Bacitracin prevents the generation of an active lipid carrier that moves the peptidoglycan subunits through the cell membrane to the cell wall. The macrolide antibiotics erythromycin and clarithromycin bind specifically to a 50S portion of the bacterial ribosome and thus inhibit peptide chain elongation. Bacteria frequently develop resistance to β-lactam antibiotics, often by elaborating antibiotic-destroying enzymes known as β-lactamases, which hydrolyze the antibiotic's critical ring. One strategy to deal with this problem is to combine the antibiotic with a molecule, such as clavulanic acid or sulbactam, that inhibits β-lactamases.

**I-78.  The answer is D.**  *(Chap. 206)*  Fungal and yeast infections, predominantly candidiasis, aspergillosis, and mucormycosis, occur frequently in severely immunosuppressed patients, particularly those who have received broad-spectrum antibiotics for a prolonged period. A number of other types of fungal infection occur in these patients. About 75 percent of all cases of *Cryptococcus neoformans* infection occur in persons who have AIDS or lymphoma, are taking glucocorticosteroids, or are otherwise immunocompromised. The association of cryptococcal meningitis and Hodgkin's disease is important clinically.

**I-79.  The answer is C.**  *(Chap. 137)*  Nosocomial (hospital-acquired) pneumonias are common in intubated patients. Other patients at risk include those with altered levels of consciousness, those with nasogastric tubes, elderly persons, patients with chronic obstructive lung disease, and postoperative patients. It was noted recently that oropharyngeal and subsequent gastric colonization with potentially pathogenic organisms is quite common in such patients. Aspiration of these colonized gastrointestinal contents occurs frequently in patients with nasogastric tubes or decreased gag reflexes. Bacterial colonization of the stomach is increased in the presence of decreased acidity caused by $H_2$ blockers or antacids. Sucralfate heals ulcers but does not alter gastric pH; it is an ideal medicine for ICU use if the goal of preventing nosocomial pneumonias is paramount. Neither of the two antibiotics listed in the question would be appropriate prophylactic agents, since penicillin G would not cover the gram-negative rod organisms that are common pathogens in this setting and ciprofloxacin would be relatively ineffective for *Staphylococcus aureus*, which is also a common cause of nosocomial pneumonia.

**I-80.  The answer is A.**  *(Chaps. 126, 134)*  *S. aureus* accounts for well over half of all endocarditis infections in intravenous drug users. Unfortunately, a substantial proportion of such infections are due to methicillin-resistant strains, which are now isolated frequently from skin sites of such persons. *S. aureus* frequently is found in association with right-sided lesions, particularly those on the tricuspid valve, which could be a function of its bombardment with injected particulate matter. Tricuspid valve endocarditis is associated with a high fever and frequent pulmonary involvement. There have been epidemics of *Pseudomonas* endocarditis in drug users, but such infections are much less common than are those due to staphylococci. The least pathogenic organisms, such as viridans streptococci and enterococci, are much less common and tend to infect previously damaged or diseased left-sided valves. Diagnosis involves obtaining a positive blood culture. Treatment consists of the administration of the appropriate antibiotic for 4 weeks.

**I-81.  The answer is E.**  *(Chap. 181)*  Fever, chills, headache, cough, and myalgias are the typical presenting signs and symptoms of psittacosis. Gastrointestinal symptoms also may occur but are much less common. The diagnosis of psittacosis usually depends on serologic tests or cultures of respiratory secretions but often is made clinically on the basis of an appropriate history and nonspecific radiographic findings. A low-titer positive complement fixation antibody test in conjunction with the clinical setting described would strongly suggest the diagnosis of psittacosis and warrant the use of tetracycline.

**I-82.  The answer is C.**  *(Chap. 195)*  Up to 90 percent of patients with poliovirus are asymptomatic or have only a self-limited febrile illness. Paralytic polio is characterized by an initial febrile illness that resolves and is followed by the development of aseptic meningitis and asymmetric paralysis. In contrast to polio, the Guillain-Barré syndrome is characterized by symmetric muscle weakness with frequent paresthesia but normal reflexes. Motor neurons are primarily affected by poliovirus infection with the resultant loss of reflexes and flaccid paralysis. Return of neuronal function may be possible for up to 6 months after infection.

**I-83.   The answer is A.**   *(Chap. 193)*   The man described in the question has symptoms that suggest influenza complicated by bacterial pneumonia. Pneumococci, *Haemophilus influenzae*, and staphylococci are the leading pathogens that cause secondary bacterial infection in this situation, and effective therapy would include drugs that act against penicillinase-producing staphylococci. The agent of choice is nafcillin or another semi-synthetic penicillinase-resistant penicillin; penicillin G would be an ill-advised choice. Other acceptable alternative therapies include vancomycin, clindamycin, and cephalothin.

**I-84.   The answer is A.**   *(Chap. 174)*   Lymphadenopathy and a papulosquamous rash that includes the palms and soles characteristically accompany secondary syphilis, which appears about 8 weeks after the healing of the primary chancre. Lymphadenopathy is not a well-recognized manifestation of late syphilis. The inflammatory lesions of late syphilis are diverse and range from asymptomatic neurosyphilis, which is characterized only by pleocytosis or elevated protein on CSF examination, to the complex intellectual and functional disturbances caused by parenchymal damage of brain tissue (general paresis). Meningovascular syphilis can lead to middle cerebral artery strokes, which produce hemiparesis and dysphasia. Demyelinization of the posterior columns leads to the ataxic gait and destroyed joints from loss of position sense characteristic of tabes dorsalis. About 10 percent of patients with late untreated syphilis experience cardiovascular complications, usually in the form of aneurysms of the ascending aorta. Gummas are nodules of granulomatous inflammation that involve the skin and skeleton. Gummas of the skin may take the form of nodules, a papulosquamous eruption, or ulcers.

**I-85.   The answer is D.**   *(Chap. 171. Antonucci, JAMA 274:143, 1995.)*   The resurgence of tuberculosis in the United States may well be due to the increase in the number of HIV-infected patients and the frequent occurrence of tuberculosis in this risk group. Tuberculosis usually occurs in HIV-infected patients without preexisting AIDS, probably because *M. tuberculosis* is more virulent than are other HIV-associated pathogens that occur at a stage of disease when the T4 count is more profoundly affected. Extrapulmonary tuberculosis is quite common in patients with HIV infection, but pulmonary involvement occurs in 74 to 100 percent of such patients. Therefore, tuberculosis remains a critical diagnostic consideration in those with abnormal chest roentgenograms. Hilar adenopathy, pleural effusions, and cavitation are most useful diagnostically, since they are rarely seen in other common causes of pneumonia in HIV-infected patients. Although more prolonged treatment is recommended in those with HIV infection compared with non-HIV-infected patients, the initial drug treatment strategy is identical and appears to be effective. This treatment involves the use of three drugs: isoniazid, rifampin, and pyrazinamide. Those with pulmonary tuberculosis are highly infective because of the generally high titers of organisms present in these immunocompromised patients. Although false-negative skin tests are not uncommon, the newly positive intradermal reaction against tuberculosis bacilli should mandate a prophylactic year of antituberculosis therapy, just as it would in a non-HIV-infected patient.

**I-86.   The answer is C.**   *(Chap. 192. Hollsberg, N Engl J Med 328:1173, 1995.)*   Retroviruses contain an RNA genome that requires reverse transcription into DNA after entrance to the host cell. The DNA copy of the viral genome may then integrate into the host genome, which allows viral gene transcription and ultimately leads to complete viral replication. AIDS, the best known human retroviral disease, is caused by human immunodeficiency virus 1 (HIV-1), which attaches to CD4 molecules on lymphocytes and monocytes and produces lymphopenic immunodeficiency. HIV-2, isolated in Africa, appears to be an uncommon cause of AIDS. The two retroviruses associated with transformation of human cells are human T-lymphotropic viruses I and II (HTLV-I and HTLV-II). The role of HTLV-II in human disease is unclear, although the virus was originally isolated from a patient with a T-cell variant of hairy cell leukemia. One to three percent of those infected with HTLV-I develop a fulminant and refractory malignancy of CD4-positive lymphocytes called adult T-cell leukemia/lymphoma, which is characterized by lymphocytosis, leukemic skin infiltrates, bone lesions, and hypercalcemia. Increased numbers of interleukin 2 (IL-2) receptors can be found on the surface of the malignant cells. A demyelinating disorder termed tropical spastic paraparesis and a chronic T-cell leukemia represent other diseases associated with HTLV-I infection. Feline leukemia virus (FeLV), which is responsible for tumors in cats, does not cause human disease.

**I-87.   The answer is D.**   *(Chap. 142)*   Methicillin-resistant *Staphylococcus aureus* has become a major source of morbidity and mortality. In vitro sensitivity testing may demonstrate sensitivity to cephalosporins, but these tests are unreliable and all strains are resistant in vivo. These strains have an altered penicillin-binding protein and are resistant to all penicillinase-resistant penicillins, alone or in combination with an aminoglycoside. Resistance is not plasmid-mediated, and there is no risk of spread to other bacteria. Administration of vancomycin is the most effective treatment.

**I-88.   The answer is D.**   *(Chap. 172)*   A papular reaction usually develops in patients with tuberculoid leprosy a month after the injection of killed suspensions of *Mycobacterium leprae*, but it is not diagnostic since positive reactions occur in nearly all adults. Culture of *M. leprae* is exceedingly difficult and can be accomplished only in mice and armadillos. A minimum of 6 months usually is required before the results are available; therefore, cultures are not practical for diagnosis. Erythema of existing skin lesions with dapsone therapy is not diagnostic. Demonstration of the organism on microscopic examination of a biopsy specimen is the only definitive way to make the diagnosis of leprosy. A sensitive serologic assay that is effective in diagnosing lepromatous disease recently was developed.

**I-89.   The answer is E.**   *(Chap. 223)*   Adult worms reside in lymph nodes, but biopsy is relatively insensitive and problematic because of the potential to exacerbate lymphatic drainage. Serologic testing is available at specialized centers with indirect hemagglutination, but cross-reactions with other filariae are common. Intense pruritus and a rash after the administration of diethylcarbamazine (Mazzotti test) suggest dermal microfilariae; this reaction typically occurs in patients with onchocerciasis. Maintenance of filariae in cultures or animals is extremely difficult. The best animal model is cats, but this technique plays no role in clinical diagnosis. Diagnosis is best made by demonstrating microfilariae on a Giemsa stain of blood after special techniques to concentrate the parasites. *W. bancrofti* microfilariae usually maintain a nocturnal periodicity and are found in the bloodstream in greatest numbers at night. The exact reason for the periodicity is not known, but it may be related to oxygen tension in the pulmonary vessels.

**I-90.   The answer is B.**   *(Chap. 220. Lengerich et al, Severe giardiasis in the United States. Clin Infect Dis 18:760, 1994.)*   The infective cysts of *G. lamblia* can survive for several months in cold water and have been responsible for large epidemics in communities such as Vail, Colorado. Immunity to *Giardia* is not well understood, but there is no increased incidence in granulocytopenic patients. Intestinal IgA may be important, as deficient patients appear to be at increased risk of infection. Transmission occurs primarily by the fecal-oral route, resulting in a higher incidence in male homosexuals, retarded patients in institutions, and children in day-care centers.

**I-91.   The answer is C.**   *(Chap. 130)*   The findings on pelvic examination, coupled with the elevated sedimentation rate in this setting, strongly suggest acute pelvic inflammatory disease (PID). About 5 percent of women with PID have associated perihepatitis, termed the *Fitz-Hugh–Curtis syndrome*, manifested by pleuritic pain of the right upper quadrant and tenderness on palpation, along with normal liver function tests and ultrasound of the right upper quadrant. *N. gonorrhoeae* is the primary pathogen in this condition, but chlamydial salpingitis is increasing in incidence, particularly in higher socioeconomic groups. Organisms typically found in the vagina, such as peptostreptococci, *E. coli*, and group B streptococci also may play a primary or secondary role in PID.

**I-92. The answer is A.** *(Chap. 130. Walker, J Infect Dis 168:969, 1993.)* It is important to pick a well-tolerated regimen with good activity against both *N. gonorrhoeae* (including penicillinase-producing strains) and *C. trachomatis* for the treatment of patients with severe pelvic inflammatory disease (PID). Activity against vaginal anaerobes and members of the Enterobacteriaceae family, which also may play a role in the pathogenesis of this disorder, would also be desirable. A combination of doxycycline and cefoxitin offers the broad-spectrum coverage required for optimal treatment. Clindamycin plus gentamicin acutely, plus a 2-week course of doxycycline, to definitively treat *C. trachomatis* is an acceptable alternative regimen. Ceftriaxone lacks adequate coverage against *Chlamydia*. Sexual partners also must be examined and treated.

**I-93. The answer is C.** *(Chap. 216)* This patient was in the right location and has the typical clinical features of a patient infected with *Babesia*, tick-borne protozoa that multiply in red blood cells. The clinical manifestations can be more severe in splenectomized persons. The best way to make the diagnosis is to demonstrate the parasite's presence in erythrocytes in Giemsa-stained peripheral blood smears. Serologic confirmation also can be helpful. The combination of quinine and clindamycin constitutes the most effective treatment.

**I-94. The answer is D.** *(Chap. 217)* The four major clinical syndromes of leishmaniasis— visceral (kala azar), cutaneous, diffuse cutaneous, and mucocutaneous—represent sandfly-borne disease caused by members of the protozoal genus *Leishmania*. Kala azar is manifested by fever, cough, diarrhea, splenomegaly, and pancytopenia and may be diagnosed by buffy coat examination. A number of species in each hemisphere account for the various cutaneous syndromes. In the Middle East and in the Republic of Georgia, *L. tropica* causes ulcerating facial lesions. Mucocutaneous leishmaniasis, or espundia, is caused by *L. braziliensis*, which can produce (after a long initial quiescent period) excessive destruction of facial soft tissue, including nasal obstruction and epistaxis, as well as systemic signs and symptoms. Massive dissemination of skin lesions without visceral involvement also can occur. This form is refractory to therapy, which usually consists of antimony. Esophageal dysfunction is seen in Chagas' disease, a trypanosomal-mediated infestation.

**I-95. The answer is D.** *(Chap. 126)* Subacute bacterial endocarditis can be treated quite successfully. However, for persons in whom the offending organisms are highly resistant to β-lactam antibiotics, such as fungi and gram-negative bacteria, the prognosis is less favorable. Cure rates are high (79 percent) for *S. aureus* tricuspid valve endocarditis in IV drug abusers but are much lower in patients with aortic involvement for any reason. The development of congestive heart failure is a most ominous sign. Endocarditis resulting from *Staphylococcus epidermidis* carries a poor prognosis if it is acquired at the time of cardiac surgery or is complicated by the adverse factors mentioned above. Valve ring or myocardial abscess also indicates a failure of medical therapy.

**I-96. The answer is A.** *(Chap. 126. Kaye, Ann Intern Med 114:803–804, 1991.)* After transient bacteremia, subacute endocarditis may develop at endocardial sites at which a jet of blood flows from a high-pressure area to a low-pressure area. Such lesions include ventricular septal defects, all valve stenoses, and mitral regurgitation. Blood flow velocity across an isolated atrial septal defect is much lower, and endocarditis is extremely uncommon in this condition. Similarly, long-standing permanent pacemakers and coronary bypass grafts very rarely result in the degree of turbulent blood flow necessary to incite endocardial infection. The degree of mitral insufficiency associated with mitral valve prolapse that requires prophylaxis is not clear. A reasonable approach consists of mandatory prophylaxis only in the setting of holosystolic murmur and prolapse.

**I-97.**    **The answer is A.**  *(Chap. 155)*  *Acinetobacter* is a ubiquitous commensal organism that is an important cause of bacteremia, pneumonia, and other serious infections. It is a gram-negative rod when grown in broth that can be confused with other members of the Neisseriaceae family (*Moraxella, Neisseria,* and *Kingella*) on Gram stain because of its pleomorphic appearance, particularly when it is grown in agar. It is also confused with Enterobacteriaceae species in cultures because of its simple growth requirements. Unlike the Neisseriaceae, it is resistant to penicillin and ampicillin but sensitive to gentamicin and tobramycin; this difference in antibiotic sensitivity makes it very important to distinguish this organism from Neisseriaceae in clinical isolates from patients with serious illnesses.

**I-98.**    **The correct answer is E.**  *(Chap. 157)*  Melioidosis is caused by *Pseudomonas pseudomallei*, a gram-negative bacillus that is ubiquitous in many tropical areas of Asia and Africa. Infection occurs from contact with contaminated soil. Pulmonary infections are the most common; in patients acutely ill with pneumonia, many organisms can be detected in sputum. The organisms can be grown on routine culture media. Serologic tests are used largely for epidemiologic studies. Melioidosis, particularly the chronic form, may be mistaken for tuberculosis; granulomas may develop, but calcification of cavitary lung lesions does not occur. In acute melioidosis, therapy with tetracycline and chloramphenicol or ceftazidime plus trimethoprim-sulfamethoxazole is recommended. Although the organism usually is sensitive to each of these agents, the high fatality rate of this disease (over 50 percent) has led to the use of a multiple antibiotic regimen.

**I-99.**    **The answer is D.**  *(Chap. 162)*  Brucellosis is an important veterinary disease in the parts of the world from which it has not been eradicated. It is still a problem in cattle-raising areas of the United States. The disease can have protean manifestations but usually presents with low-grade fever and constitutional symptoms; affected persons have lymphadenopathy, splenomegaly, and sometimes hepatomegaly. During the early bacteremic phase of the illness, *Brucella* can be isolated using routine cultures, provided that they are kept long enough (i.e., up to 4 weeks). The diagnosis also is made by using agglutination tests. The optimal therapy consists of a combination of an aminoglycoside and doxycycline.

**I-100.**    **The correct answer is E.**  *(Chap. 161)*  *Vibrio cholerae* enterotoxin causes a diffuse noninflammatory secretion of isotonic intestinal fluid without injury to the absorptive surface. Early diagnosis is aided by dark-field microscopy or immobilization of organisms with type-specific antisera; a definitive diagnosis, however, depends on culturing the organisms. Oral therapy with solutions that contain sodium bicarbonate and either glucose or sucrose is recommended. This therapy usually is begun on the basis of a presumptive diagnosis in endemic areas. Oral tetracycline also is useful because it can shorten the symptomatic period, but it is not recommended for children under age 8. Infection confers some immunity, so that in endemic areas children are usually the ones affected. Cholera vaccine is not particularly effective and is not ordinarily recommended by U.S. authorities for travelers to endemic areas.

**I-101.**    **The correct answer is A.**  *(Chap. 209. Teddler et al, Ann Thorac Surg 57:1044, 1994.)*  The mold species *Rhizomucor* and *Rhizopus*, the main causes of mucormycosis, are more often seen in than grown from pathologic specimens. The reasons they are so hard to grow have not been identified. Fungal hyphae tend to invade blood vessels, leading to hemorrhagic necrosis. Sinusitis is the predominant illness in infected persons who have diabetes mellitus; in persons with hematologic malignancies, pulmonary disease is also common. Diagnosis is best accomplished by biopsy and histologic examination. Amphotericin is the only known nonsurgical treatment of mucormycosis.

**I-102.**    **The correct answer is A.**    *(Chap. 179)*    Rocky Mountain spotted fever is a tick-borne disease caused by *Rickettsia rickettsii*, an obligate intracellular organism. The disease is associated with severe headache, myalgias, and arthralgias but not with frank arthritis. The characteristic rash is at first macular and confined to the extremities; after several days, the rash spreads to involve the buttocks, trunk, axilla, neck, and face and becomes maculopapular, then hemorrhagic, and finally ulcerative. Treatment with doxycycline or chloramphenical, each of which is a rickettsiostatic agent, is most effective if it is begun before the rash has become hemorrhagic. Ticks found on household pets should be removed carefully with tweezers, not by hand, to prevent infection through minor skin abrasions.

**I-103.**    **The correct answer is C.**    *(Chap. 144)*    The gram-positive rod *Corynebacterium diphtheriae* may produce human disease after infection of skin or mucous membranes. Specific viruses, termed *corynephages*, must infect *C. diphtheriae* to convert the bacterium to a toxin-producing strain. Disease can occur as a result of infection with toxin-producing or toxin-negative strains, but the serious manifestations of carditis and neuritis occur as a result of toxins. The toxin, which is elaborated as a single polypeptide chain by the lysogenized bacteria, is proteolytically cleaved into an A portion, which binds to cell membranes, and a B portion, which catalyzes the adenosine diphosphate ribosylation and inactivation of elongation factor 2, a vital element in ribosome-mediated protein synthesis. Most unimmunized patients with diphtherial pharyngitis experience myocardial abnormalities with manifestations ranging from an abnormal electrocardiogram to congestive heart failure (in about 10 to 25 percent) and ventricular fibrillation. Formaldehyde-treated diphtheria toxin creates toxoid, a vaccine component that can provide 10 years of protection against serious disease. Pharyngeal and cutaneous infections with toxigenic strains produce edema, hyperemia, and a dense fibrinopurulent exudate (termed a pseudomembrane) teeming with *C. diphtheriae*. Formation of the pseudomembrane can lead to obstruction of the upper airway. Administration of antitoxin is the primary specific modality of treatment for those with suspected infections.

**I-104.**    **The correct answer is D.**    *(Chap. 155)*    *Klebsiella* and the related *Serratia* and *Enterobacter* are the most important enteric organisms other than *E. coli* to infect humans. Although respiratory disease is important (*Klebsiella* accounts for 1 percent or less of community-acquired pneumonia), most clinical isolates now come from the urinary tract. All three genera are important pulmonary nosocomial pathogens. However, merely finding these organisms growing in the sputum of a very ill hospitalized patient does not necessarily implicate the bacteria as pathogenic in that particular circumstance and may indicate colonization rather than infection. Clinical context and procurement of the sample in a sterile fashion (transtracheal aspiration, bronchoscopy) will aid in the diagnosis. Chronic alcoholics, diabetics, and those with chronic lung disease are at increased risk for *Klebsiella* pneumonia, a difficult disease to treat because of the frequency of suppurative complications (empyema and abscess) with the associated requirement for prolonged (more than 2 weeks) therapy.

**I-105.**    **The correct answer is B.**    *(Chap. 219)*    Toxoplasmosis is a relatively common infection; serologic data indicate that up to two-thirds of the U.S. adult population may have had some form of the infection. The most serious manifestations appear to arise when the disease is acquired during pregnancy. Infection during the first trimester can result in spontaneous abortion, stillbirth, prematurity, or severe disease in any of several organ systems; infection during the third trimester most commonly leads to neonatal infection, which, however, tends to be asymptomatic. Infections acquired before pregnancy generally are of little consequence to the offspring. Immunocompromised persons usually have recrudescent disease. Diagnosis in these patients is often difficult to make, in part because the serologic responses are blunted by the underlying disease process. Serologic screening of asymptomatic immunocompromised patients may be helpful for recognizing toxoplasmosis at a later date.

**I-106.  The answer is C.** *(Chap. 224)* *Schistosoma mansoni* infection of the liver causes cirrhosis from vascular obstruction caused by periportal fibrosis but relatively little hepatocellular injury. Hepatosplenomegaly, hypersplenism, and esophageal varices develop quite commonly, and schistosomiasis usually is associated with eosinophilia. Spider nevi, gynecomastia, jaundice, and ascites are less commonly observed than they are in alcoholic and postnecrotic fibrosis.

**I-107.  The answer is A.** *(Chap. 171)* Pleural effusions occur most frequently in young patients with primary infection associated with an abrupt onset of symptoms. Effusions are being noted more frequently in older patients with reactivation disease, but they still account for less than one-third of patients in North America with pleurisy. Laryngeal and bronchitic tuberculosis are very infectious because the bacilli are readily aerosolized. The response to therapy is usually good. In the absence of neurologic abnormalities, extensive bony involvement by tuberculosis usually requires chemotherapy alone. Involvement of the basilar meninges is very common in meningeal tuberculosis and results in cranial nerve abnormalities. Gastrointestinal infection usually occurs in association with cavitary disease with large numbers of organisms. The terminal ileum and cecum are the most common sites, resulting in disease that can be difficult to differentiate from Crohn's disease. The stomach is very resistant to infection.

**I-108.  The answer is A.** *[Chap. 193. CDC, MMWR 44(RR-3):1, 1995.]* Major epidemics are associated only with influenza A and have been attributed to "antigenic shifts" or reassortment of genomic segments, possibly with animal strains. Between pandemics, minor antigenic variations ("drifts") occur through point mutations. Antibodies against the hemagglutinin are most important, presumably because they prevent viral attachment. Influenza B tends to cause smaller outbreaks, with less severe disease, because there is no animal reservoir and because major antigenic shifts do not occur. Prolonged fatigue or "postinfluenzal asthenia" may occur, but the etiology is not known. Viral shedding usually stops 2 to 5 days after symptoms in uncomplicated influenza. Both amantadine and rimantadine can prevent or attenuate infection with influenza A. In major outbreaks, therapy may be useful until immunity can be established by means of immunization.

**I-109.  The answer is A-N, B-Y, C-N, D-N, E-Y.** *(Chap. 17. Dinarello, Rev Infect Dis 10:168, 1988.)* A host of stimuli, including infection with virtually any microorganism, cause macrophages, lymphocytes, fibroblasts, and other cells to elaborate the key mediators of fever production, such as TNFα, TNFβ (lymphotoxin), interferon α, and the interleukins, which are 17-kilodalton (kDa) glycoproteins that promote the synthesis of E series prostaglandins in the hypothalamus and thus reset the central thermostat at a higher level. Aspirin and nonsteroidal anti-inflammatory agents act by inhibiting cyclooxygenase activity so that prostaglandin $E_2$ ($PGE_2$) cannot be synthesized; they do not act by reducing TNF and IL-1 production. Glucocorticoids suppress fever by both interfering with arachidonic acid metabolism and down-regulating the production of endogenous pyrogens. TNF and IL-1 also possess diverse effects, including the induction of cachexia by TNF.

**I-110.  The answer is A-Y, B-Y, C-N, D-N, E-N.** *(Chap. 141. Shapiro, N Engl J Med 325:1453, 1991.)* The incidence of pneumonococal bacteremia drops after 2 years of age but rises again in those over age 55. All splenectomized patients, even those without underlying disease, should receive pneumococcal vaccine. The "crisis" in pneumococcal pneumonia ordinarily corresponds to the appearance of type-specific antibodies, not maximum leukocytosis. Alcoholic persons who develop pneumococcal pneumonia have a poor prognosis for several reasons: their tendency to aspirate pharyngeal flora, poor functioning of bronchial clearance mechanisms, and impaired leukocyte response (hypogammaglobulinemia generally is not a contributing factor). Pneumococcal pneumonia frequently precedes pneumococcal meningitis. Pneumococci cause pharyngitis extremely rarely.

**I-111.** **The answer is A-Y, B-N, C-N, D-Y, E-Y.** *(Chap. 143)* Streptococcal M protein is the factor most strongly associated with virulence; strains rich in M protein resist phagocytosis. Streptococcal pyoderma may lead to acute glomerulonephritis but not to acute rheumatic fever. The reason for this phenomenon is not understood. Group A streptococci elaborate a host of toxins important in infections: membrane-damaging streptolysins, DNAses, proteases, and pyrogenic exotoxins A, B, and C. Penicillin therapy for streptococcal pharyngitis decreases the incidence of suppurative and nonsuppurative complications but does not alter the duration of the sore throat. Nonenterococcal group D streptococci, such as *S. bovis*, are quite pathogenic and tend to cause endocarditis in patients with colonic neoplasms.

**I-112.** **The answer is A-N, B-Y, C-Y, D-Y, E-N.** *(Chap. 176)* Leptospirosis can be transferred from infected animals directly to humans who have contact with contaminated tissue or urine. Leptospirosis often is confused with influenza because of its initial manifestations: fever, headache, and myalgias. It causes hepatitis that often is associated with very elevated serum bilirubin levels, probably as a result of both intravascular hemolysis and impaired bilirubin excretion. Leptospiral meningitis resembles a viral, or aseptic, meningitis; cerebrospinal fluid has a normal glucose concentration, and although a few neutrophils may be present, lymphocytes are the predominant cell type observed. The diagnosis of acute leptospirosis is made best by blood cultures; dark-field microscopy too often gives false-positive or false-negative results.

**I-113.** **The answer is A-N, B-Y, C-Y, D-Y, E-N.** *(Chap. 150)* Gonococcemia tends to be a problem of menstruating women, although men also are affected. The characteristic skin lesions are small pustules that usually occur first on the fingers and feet. The arthritis associated with gonococcemia is rarely symmetric, a clinical finding that often is helpful in making the diagnosis. Gonococci that produce β-lactamase are resistant to penicillin and ampicillin but are sensitive to the newer cephalosporins, such as ceftriaxone. Treatment with spectinomycin is also effective; this agent usually is recommended as the first choice for treatment failures attributed to penicillinase production by the organism. Gonococci with pili are more virulent than are gonococci without pili (pili may help the organism stick to epithelial cells to initiate infection), but the latter type may facilitate spread.

**I-114.** **The answer is A-Y, B-Y, C-Y, D-Y, E-Y.** *(Chap. 186)* The most common features of infectious mononucleosis are fever, sore throat, and lymphadenopathy. Sore throat, the most commonly described symptom, is observed in about 80 percent of young adults with this infection. Atypical lymphocytes, identified as T cells with suppressor-cytotoxic action responding to EBV-infected B lymphocytes, appear in the peripheral blood during the first week of illness. Heterophil antibodies, which are sheep red-cell agglutinins associated with the immunoglobulin M serum fraction, usually persist in the serum for a few months. By contrast, antibodies to Epstein-Barr virus, especially to EBV nuclear antigens, often can be detected for years in the serum of persons who have had infectious mononucleosis. The incubation period in young adults is thought to be 30 to 50 days; in children, the incubation period is much shorter.

**I-115.** **The answer is A-N, B-Y, C-N, D-Y, E-Y.** *(Chap. 216)* Only in *P. vivax* and *P. ovale* infections may relapses occur because a portion of the intrahepatic forms remain dormant. *P. vivax* depends on the Duffy antigen to enter red cells; patients who lack this antigen are resistant. *P. falciparum* produces a form of disease that can lead to coma and death. Seizures and hypoglycemia, which are grave prognostic signs, also may be present. Renal failure in falciparum malaria seems to occur on the basis of tubular sequestration of parasitized erythrocytes and tends to abate. Renal failure with *P. malariae* infection may be due to deposition of soluble immune complexes in glomeruli. Repeated malarial infections can result in massive splenomegaly.

**I-116.** **The answer is A-Y, B-Y, C-Y, D-Y, E-Y.** *(Chap. 186)* Serious complications of infectious mononucleosis (IM) caused by infection with Epstein-Barr virus (EBV) are uncommon. Mild hepatitis occurs in 90 percent of these patients. Airway obstruction, which is sensitive to glucocorticoid therapy, sometimes results from the massive pharyngeal adenopathy that accompanies IM. IgM antibodies elicited by EBV may be directed against the i antigen on red blood cell membranes, and this causes a transient autoimmune hemolytic anemia. Mild antibody-mediated thrombocytopenia is common, but a serious drop in the platelet count is unusual. Some patients develop cranial nerve palsies and encephalitis as a result of EBV infection. There is growing recognition of the association between EBV infection and B-cell lymphoproliferative disorders in immunocompromised patients.

**I-117.** **The answer is A-N, B-Y, C-Y, D-N, E-Y.** *(Chap. 148)* *Clostridium* spp. are present in high numbers in normal intestinal flora and soil, and it is not surprising that they are common isolates from wound cultures. The presence of necrotic tissue and a low oxidation reduction potential are necessary to establish severe disease. Treatment is based on the clinical setting, and a culture positive for clostridia alone does not warrant therapy. *Clostridium perfringens* produces at least 12 toxins, one of the most important of which is the alpha toxin. It has been associated with hemolysis and capillary and platelet damage. *C. perfringens* is a common cause of food poisoning associated with contaminated meats and poultry. The serous discharge from the overlying skin in a patient with gas gangrene has many gram-positive rods but few inflammatory cells, and this emphasizes the importance of an early Gram stain when the diagnosis is suspected. More than 70 percent of cases of *C. septicum* septicemia reported in the literature are associated with malignant neoplasms, especially of the gastrointestinal tract.

**I-118.** **The answer is A-N, B-Y, C-Y, D-N, E-N.** *(Chap. 169)* Anaerobic pulmonary infections most often develop in the setting of aspiration. The sudden development of a bacterial pneumonia in a healthy teenager would most likely be caused by *Streptococcus pneumoniae*. Both anaerobic and aerobic organisms are implicated in Ludwig's angina, an infection that originates in the third molar and can spread rapidly through soft tissues of the mandible and pharynx. Pharyngeal anaerobic bacteria, including *Bacteroides melaninogenicus*, *Fusobacterium* sp., and anaerobic cocci, cause bacterial aspiration pneumonia in a patient who has a diminished gag reflex, such as occurs with a seizure disorder. It is important to differentiate bacterial aspiration, which requires antibiotic therapy, from aspiration of stomach contents, which usually occurs after general anesthesia and resolves with symptomatic therapy. Anaerobic bacteria are a very unusual cause of endocarditis, which, as is the case with aerobic gram-negative organisms, may in part be explained by a failure to adhere to damaged valves.

**I-119.** **The answer is A-N, B-Y, C-Y, D-Y, E-N.** *(Chap. 185)* Less than 5 percent of patients will have a second recurrence of herpes zoster unless they are immunosuppressed. Acute cerebellar ataxia is the most common form of neurologic involvement in children. This benign condition usually develops 3 weeks after the rash and resolves spontaneously. Chickenpox is one of the most contagious diseases; it infects up to 90 percent of seronegative persons, presumably via the respiratory route. Varicella pneumonia can cause fever and severe hypoxia and thus can complicate the course of chickenpox infection in up to 20 percent of adults. Varicella-zoster immune globulin is recommended only for immunodeficient patients under age 15 years who have been exposed to varicella.

**I-120.**   **The answer is A-N, B-Y, C-Y, D-N, E-Y.**  *(Chap. 187)*   Perinatal transmission of CMV occurs by passage through an infected birth canal or through the breast milk of a seropositive mother. Although such transmission is very common, symptomatic infection is distinctly unusual except in premature infants in whom interstitial pneumonitis may develop. Congenital infection with CMV occurs in approximately 1 percent of births in the United States, but detectable disease develops in less than 0.05 percent of births, almost exclusively in association with primary maternal infections. CMV produces a syndrome very similar to mononucleosis associated with EBV. Cervical lymphadenopathy and exudative pharyngitis usually are not present, however, and heterophil antibodies are absent. CMV pneumonia can prove fatal in more than 80 percent of bone marrow transplant patients. Salivary excretion of the virus or positive sputum cultures do not implicate CMV as the cause of pulmonary infiltrates. The definitive diagnosis rests on the demonstration of the characteristic pathologic finding—intranuclear inclusions in enlarged, epithelial cells—on lung biopsy. The diagnosis of CMV infection rests on characteristic pathologic findings, a fourfold rise in serology titer, or culture of CMV, usually from urine, saliva, or buffy coat. Because viral excretion can continue for weeks to months, isolation of CMV does not always indicate acute infection.

**I-121.**   **The answer is A-N, B-Y, C-N, D-Y, E-Y.**  *(Chap. 194)*   Both Norwalk virus and rotavirus infect the small intestinal epithelium and cause malabsorption and osmotic diarrhea. Worldwide, rotavirus is the most important cause of dehydrating diarrhea in infants. Rotavirus is shed in large quantities in the stool, allowing for easy diagnosis by culture or immunoassays to detect viral antigens. Norwalk virus presumably is spread by the fecal-oral route and also has been implicated in food-borne and waterborne epidemics. The clinical manifestations of infection by both viruses are characterized by vomiting, diarrhea, and occasionally low-grade fever. Rotavirus is a major cause of diarrhea in children under 3 years of age, while Norwalk virus causes disease more often in older children and adults.

**I-122.**   **The answer is A-N, B-Y, C-N, D-Y, E-Y.**  *(Chap. 146)*   Neonatal tetanus is associated with a mortality rate above 60 percent. It is caused by infections of the umbilical stump. In third-world countries the infection often is associated with practices of applying dirt or feces to the umbilical stump to speed sloughing. Human immune globulin cannot affect tetanus toxin that is already bound in the central nervous system, but it can be helpful if given early to bind any free toxin. Such small amounts of tetanospasmin are present that no immunity develops and active immunization must be initiated. Trismus, or lockjaw, is the most common manifestation of tetanus; it is caused by neuromuscular blockade and central disinhibition of motor neurons. Immune globulin provides protective antibody levels for up to 4 weeks and should be given along with toxoid for serious wounds if fewer than two previous doses of toxoid have been given.

# II. DISORDERS OF THE HEART AND VASCULAR SYSTEM

## QUESTIONS

*DIRECTIONS:* Each question below contains five suggested responses. Choose the **one best** response to each question.

**II-1.** A 48-year-old man is admitted to the coronary care unit with an acute inferior myocardial infarction. Two hours after admission, his blood pressure is 86/52 mmHg; his heart rate is 40 beats per minute with sinus rhythm. Which of the following would be the most appropriate initial therapy?

(A) Immediate insertion of a temporary trans-venous pacemaker
(B) Intravenous administration of atropine sulfate, 0.6 mg
(C) Administration of normal saline, 300 mL over 15 min
(D) Intravenous administration of dobutamine, 0.35 mg/min
(E) Intravenous administration of isoproterenol, 5.0 μg/min

**II-2.** A 68-year-old man with a history of hypertension, diabetes, and urinary retention awoke feeling nauseated and light-headed. He did not respond to questions from his wife. When the emergency medical technicians arrived, his blood pressure was 60 by palpation. IV fluids and oxygen were administered. Vital signs obtained in the ER were blood pressure 60, heart rate 120 and regular, temperature 38.9°C (102°F), and respiratory rate 30. A brief physical examination revealed coarse rales approximately halfway up in the chest bilaterally and inaudible heart sounds. An indwelling urinary catheter was placed with drainage of 10 to 20 mL of dark urine. Chest x-ray revealed bilateral interstitial infiltrates; ECG was unremarkable except for sinus tachycardia. Antibiotics were administered, and the patient was transferred to the ICU, where a right heart catheterization was performed. Pulmonary capillary wedge pressure was 28 mmHg. Cardiac output was 1.9 L/min. Right atrial mean pressure was 10 mmHg. The most likely cause of this man's hypotension was

(A) left ventricular dysfunction
(B) right ventricular infarction
(C) gram-negative sepsis
(D) gastrointestinal bleeding
(E) pulmonary emboli

**II-3.** A middle-aged man who suddenly collapsed on the golf course is brought to the emergency department. The emergency medical technicians diagnosed cardio-respiratory arrest, performed CPR, applied a 200-joule shock to the patient's chest, and inserted an endo-tracheal tube and an intravenous line. At the time of arrival in the emergency room, the patient has no spontaneous pulse or respiration. After viewing the rhythm strip shown below, you order additional defibrillatory shocks: first 200 joules, then 300 joules, and finally 360 joules. CPR is continued. Which of the following is the most appropriate drug to administer at this time?

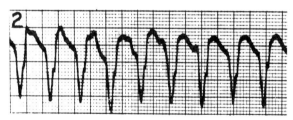

From Schlant, et al: *Hurst's The Heart,* 8/e. New York, McGraw-Hill, 1994, with permission.

(A) Procainamide
(B) Bretylium tosylate
(C) Epinephrine
(D) Lidocaine
(E) Sodium bicarbonate

**II-4.** All the following are features of captopril **EXCEPT** that it

(A) decreases plasma renin activity
(B) retards the degradation of circulating bradykinin
(C) inhibits the formation of angiotensin II
(D) can be used safely in combination with a beta blocking agent
(E) is contraindicated in patients with bilateral renal artery stenosis

**II-5.** Which of the following physical findings is associated with the chest x-ray shown below?

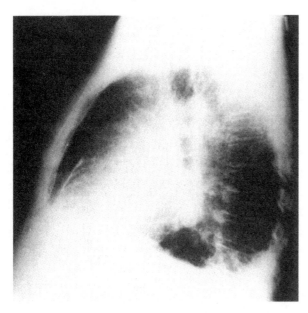

(A) Wide splitting of the second heart sound
(B) Opening snap and diastolic rumble
(C) Pericardial knock
(D) Late-peaking systolic ejection murmur
(E) Central cyanosis

**II-6.** A 55-year-old man with known coronary heart disease develops recurrent anginal symptoms 2 months after undergoing an apparently successful percutaneous transluminal coronary angioplasty (PTCA) procedure. The original PTCA procedure was performed because of angina unresponsive to medical therapy in the setting of two proximal 90 percent occlusions (one in the right coronary artery and the other in the left circumflex). Cardiac catheterization reveals that the left circumflex lesion has reoccluded. Which of the following statements concerning the patient's current condition is correct?

(A) The patient probably will require coronary artery bypass surgery
(B) If the patient had been treated with aspirin daily from the time of his initial PTCA, this problem would have been less likely

(C) A cholesterol-lowering agent would have been useful in preventing this problem
(D) The administration of warfarin therapy for 6 months after PTCA is indicated to prevent this problem
(E) Coronary artery smooth muscle hyperplasia probably played a role in the current problem

**II-7.** A 67-year-old man who has experienced recurrent episodes of dizziness over the last several months is admitted to the hospital because of a fainting episode. No evidence of acute myocardial infarction is documented. On the evening of admission, the patient tells his nurse that approximately 10 min earlier he experienced several minutes of dizziness. His current rhythm appears to be normal sinus; however, a monitoring strip obtained at the time of this episode reveals absent QRS complexes every third beat. The PR interval, while slightly prolonged, is constant from beat to beat. P waves are present at regular intervals. Which of the following is the most appropriate therapeutic action?

(A) Insertion of permanent cardiac pacemaker
(B) Insertion of temporary cardiac pacemaker followed by insertion of permanent cardiac pacemaker
(C) Administration of atropine, 2 mg IV
(D) Administration of isoproterenol, 2 mg/min IV
(E) No specific therapy is required for this benign arrhythmia

**II-8.** A 42-year-old woman has bilateral ankle edema of recent onset. On examination, her jugular venous pulse is 5 cmH$_2$O and the hepatojugular reflux is negative. All the following should be considered in the differential diagnosis of the woman's ankle edema **EXCEPT**

(A) pelvic thrombophlebitis
(B) venous varicosities
(C) cyclic edema
(D) hypoalbuminemia
(E) right heart failure

**II-9.** Examination of the carotid pulse reveals two impulses or peaks during ventricular systole. Which of the following physical findings probably would be associated with this finding?

(A) Diastolic murmur beginning after an opening snap
(B) Decrease in systolic arterial pressure during inspiration
(C) Systolic murmur increasing during the Valsalva maneuver
(D) Right-sided third heart sound
(E) Left-sided third heart sound

**II-10.** The electrocardiogram shown below is consistent with which of the following clinical situations?

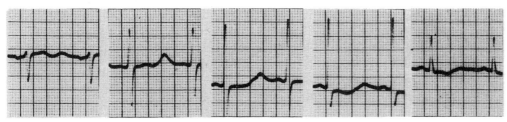

From Schlant, et al: *Hurst's The Heart*, 8/e. New York, McGraw-Hill, 1994, with permission.

(A) A 55-year-old man complaining of crushing substernal chest pain

(B) A 25-year-old woman with acute renal failure resulting from lupus nephritis

(C) A 27-year-old man with prolonged neutropenia after induction therapy for acute myeloid leukemia who is receiving amphotericin B

(D) A 57-year-old woman with metastatic breast cancer receiving etidronate

(E) A 72-year-old woman receiving digitalis therapy for chronic congestive heart failure

**II-11.** Digitalis glycosides enhance myocardial contractility primarily by which of the following mechanisms?

(A) Opening of calcium channels

(B) Release of calcium from the sarcoplasmic reticulum

(C) Stimulation of myosin ATPase

(D) Stimulation of membrane phospholipase C

(E) Inhibition of membrane $Na^+$, $K^+$-ATPase

**II-12.** A 65-year-old man with a long history of untreated hypertension complains of recurrent shortness of breath on minimal exertion. Examination of the cardiovascular system is normal except for a prominent precordial impulse. Chest x-ray is normal except for a prominent left ventricular shadow. An exercise tolerance test with thallium scanning reveals no evidence of myocardial ischemia. Two-dimensional echocardiography reveals left ventricular hypertrophy. Radionuclide ventriculography reveals normal right and left ventricular ejection fractions. What is the most likely explanation for the patient's symptoms?

(A) Chronic obstructive pulmonary disease

(B) Reactive airways disease

(C) Systolic congestive heart failure

(D) Diastolic congestive heart failure

(E) Myocardial ischemia

**II-13.** Clues to the presence of atrioventricular nodal block (as opposed to trifascicular block) would include all the following EXCEPT

(A) clinical evidence of inferior myocardial infarction

(B) Wenckebach periodicity to conduction

(C) escape-focus rate faster than 50 beats per minute

(D) a narrow QRS complex at the escape focus

(E) unresponsiveness of the escape focus to atropine

**II-14.** Which of the following agents has been shown to reduce mortality in patients with congestive heart failure?

(A) Digitalis

(B) Furosemide

(C) Enalapril   *and β. Blockers*

(D) Procainamide

(E) Aspirin

**II-15.** A 68-year-old Haitian man presents with a chronic nonproductive cough, dyspnea on exertion, and chronic nonexertional chest pain. The patient notes a loss of 10 pounds over the past 6 months, decreased appetite, and swelling of the ankles. Physical findings reveal an ill-appearing man with decreased skeletal mass. Blood pressure is 100/70 without a significant inspiratory decrease in systolic pressure. Heart rate is 110; respiratory rate is 25; temperature is 37.2°C (99.0°F) orally. Significant physical findings include the absence of rales on chest examination and the presence of jugular venous distention with a decline during inspiration. The apical cardiac pulse is reduced. The heart sounds are distant; an early third heart sound occurs very shortly after aortic valve closure; there are no murmurs. Both the liver and the spleen are enlarged, and there is a fluid wave on abdominal examination. Electrocardiography displays low QRS voltage but is otherwise unremarkable. Chest x-ray reveals clear lungs and an enlarged cardiac silhouette. Which of the following findings is most likely to appear on echocardiographic examination?

(A) Enlarged right ventricular size
(B) Pericardial effusion
(C) Thickened myocardium
(D) Thickened pericardium
(E) Right ventricular diastolic collapse

**II-16.** A 60-year-old man is admitted to a hospital because of respiratory failure and tachycardia. Rectal temperature is 38.3°C (101°F), respiratory rate is 32 breaths per minute, and blood pressure is 100/60 mmHg. His admission electrocardiogram is shown below. Which of the following measures would constitute the most appropriate management for this man?

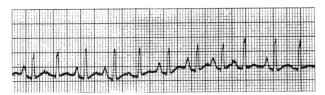

(A) Electrical cardioversion after the blood pressure is raised
(B) Supplemental oxygenation or mechanical ventilation
(C) Administration of digitalis
(D) Administration of quinidine
(E) Administration of verapamil

**II-17.** Each of the following patients was noted to have an abnormally high serum cholesterol and was placed on a reduced calorie, cholesterol, and fat diet for the past 3 months. None has any history of ischemic heart disease. In which of the following patients would it be most appropriate to recommend lipid-lowering drug therapy at this time?

(A) A 52-year-old smoker and diabetic with an LDL cholesterol value of 3.2 mmol/L (120 mg/dL)
(B) A 60-year-old hypertensive woman with an LDL cholesterol value of 3.5 mmol/L (140 mg/dL)
(C) A 50-year-old man with cholesterol of 6 mmol/L (230 mg/dL)
(D) A 45-year-old man with LDL cholesterol of 5 mmol/L (200 mg/dL)
(E) A 58-year-old male smoker with cholesterol of 5.5 mmol/L (220 mg/dL) and LDL cholesterol of 4 mmol/L (150 mg/dL)

**II-18.** All the following statements regarding secundum atrial septal defect are true EXCEPT

(A) surgical correction is advisable when the pulmonary-to-systemic flow ratio has reached 2.0
(B) affected persons are usually asymptomatic in childhood
(C) electrocardiography shows a leftward axis
(D) echocardiography shows abnormal ventricular septal motion
(E) atrial arrhythmias are common

**II-19** A 75-year-old man presents with recurrent episodes of shortness of breath on minimal exertion. He has no prior significant past medical history. Physical examination reveals blood pressure of 110/70 without pulsus paradoxus, heart rate of 110, respiratory rate of 25, and temperature of 37°C (98.6°F) orally. Jugular veins are distended and the heart sounds are distant, but there are third and fourth extra heart sounds. The liver is enlarged, and pedal edema is present. The electrocardiogram shows nonspecific ST-T wave changes and occasional premature ventricular contractions. The chest x-ray reveals clear lung fields and a mildly dilated cardiac silhouette. Echocardiography reveals normal systolic function and thickened ventricular walls with a "speckled" appearance. Which of the following conditions is most consistent with the patient's clinical presentation?

(A) Alcoholic cardiomyopathy
(B) Hemochromatosis
(C) Amyloidosis
(D) Viral myocarditis
(E) Tuberculosis

**II-20.** The chest x-rays below probably would have been taken of which of the following persons?

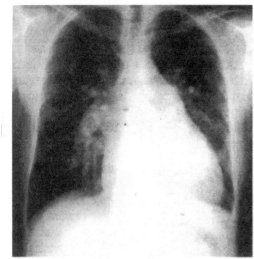

A

B

*rupture brandud veins*

(A) A 38-year-old woman who has hemoptysis, dyspnea on exertion, and fatigability *- Pulmonary HT*

MS *A(C) Atrial*

(B) A 36-year-old woman who has a heart murmur but is asymptomatic *ASD?*

(C) A 32-year-old woman who has a continuous murmur, widened systemic pulse pressure, and dyspnea on exertion *PDA*

(D) A 40-year-old woman who has a loud first heart sound, a diastolic rumble, a large *v* wave in her jugular pulse, and ascites *Tricuspid Regurgitation*

(E) None of the above

*Roth's spot (Retinal Vasculitis)*

*Fever    splenomegly    Janeway lesions*

*Hepatomegly                → palmar lesions*

*Splenomegly - Murmurs*

*• Infective Endocarditis    Osler's nodes*

*α viri. Sp Viridans 35-50%    → painful lesions on finger pulps*

**II-21.** A 20-year-old woman has mild pulmonic stenosis (transvalvular gradient is 20 mmHg). All the following statements regarding this situation are true EXCEPT

(A) heart size on chest x-ray is likely to be normal

(B) electrocardiogram is likely to be normal

(C) her jugular *a* wave is likely to be prominent

(D) compared to other valvular defects, the risk of endocarditis is relatively low

(E) frequent monitoring for progression of the stenosis is indicated

**II-22.** All the following findings would be expected in a person with coarctation of the aorta EXCEPT

(A) a systolic murmur across the anterior chest and back and a high-pitched diastolic murmur along the left sternal border

(B) a higher blood pressure in the right arm than in the left arm

(C) inability to augment cardiac output with exercise

(D) rib notching on chest x-ray

(E) persistent hypertension despite complete surgical repair

**II-23.** A 15-year-old boy residing with his parents on a military base presents with a fever of 38.6°C (101.5°F) and complains of lower back, knee, and wrist pain. The arthritis is not localized to any one joint. He gives a history of a severe sore throat several weeks earlier. Physical examination of the skin reveals pea-sized swellings over the elbows and wrists. He also has two serpiginous, erythematous pink areas on the anterior trunk, each about 5 cm in diameter. Laboratory investigation includes negative blood cultures, negative throat culture, normal CBC, and an erythrocyte sedimentation rate (ESR) of 100. An antistreptolysin-O (ASO) titer is elevated. At this point, appropriate therapy would consist of

(A) supportive care alone

(B) parenteral penicillin

(C) parenteral penicillin and glucocorticoids

(D) parenteral penicillin and aspirin

(E) parenteral penicillin, aspirin, and diazepam

*• Rheumatic fever - Group A β. Haemolytic → Pyogenes.*

*• Acute GMN*

*MR AR Carey Coombs    • Group B → Dgalactiae*

*Sleeping 7g    Major Criteria    Minor Criteria*

*Changing murmurs*

*Pericardial rub → Carditis 45-70%    • Raised ESR - C-RP*

*HF - Dmegaly    • Migratory polyarthritis 75%    • Arthralgia*

*Conduction problems    • Sydenham's Chorea 10% >♀ (Halogen)    • Fever*

*• Subcutaneous nodules 2-20%    • Hx of previous RF or RHD*

*• Erythema Marginatum Trunk 2-10%    • Prolonged PR interval*

*Suggestive RF by: Recent Scarlet fever (>1)*

*+ve growth from throat*

*& ASOT >200 U/mL*

*Dx: 1 Suggestive + 2 major*

*Revised Jones Crit.    + 1 > and 2 <*

**II-24.** A 62-year-old woman was started on a regimen of quinidine sulfate because of asymptomatic ventricular couplets. One week later, she was admitted to the hospital after a syncopal episode. Serum electrolyte concentrations were normal. The arrhythmia shown below appeared transiently on her cardiac monitor. The recommended course at this time is to

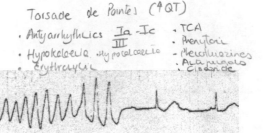

Torsade de Pointes (↑QT)
· Antyarrhythmics Ia -Ic    · TCA
                III          · Phenytoin
· Hypokalaemia ·Hypocalaemia  - Phenothiazines
· Erythromycin                · Antifungals
                              · Cisapride

(A) increase the quinidine dose
(B) discontinue the administration of quinidine and observe
(C) begin the intravenous administration of procainamide 2 mg/min
(D) administer sodium bicarbonate, 70 meq, intravenously
(E) administer potassium chloride, 10 meq, intravenously over 1 h

**II-25.** Each patient below is alert and oriented and has a blood pressure of 110/60. In which patient would adenosine constitute appropriate initial therapy?

(A) A 65-year-old man with no ischemic heart disease and wide complex tachycardia - VT
(B) A 65-year-old woman with known ischemic disease and narrow complex tachycardia
(C) A 25-year-old woman with known preexcitation WPW syndrome and narrow complex tachycardia   verapamil
(D) A 28-year-old man with known preexcitation WPW syndrome and wide complex tachycardia — SVT + BBB
(E) A 44-year-old man with atrial fibrillation — VT (rect os without a prior history of heart disease   Lignocaine
                                                    Digoxin

**II-26.** Factors accounting for the pedal edema associated with congestive heart failure include all the following EXCEPT

(A) increased secretion of aldosterone
(B) increased effective arterial blood volume
(C) increased level of plasma renin
(D) renal vasoconstriction
(E) sympathetic nervous system–mediated renal vasoconstriction

**II-27.** Aspirin has been shown to reduce the risk of myocardial infarction in all the following groups EXCEPT

(A) patients with chronic stable angina
(B) patients who have survived unstable angina
(C) patients who have survived myocardial infarction
(D) patients experiencing unstable angina
(E) patients with ischemic cardiomyopathy

**II-28.** Which of the following statements best describes long-acting nitrate preparations?

(A) Tolerance often develops
(B) Their effect can be blocked by high doses of beta$_2$ selective inhibitors
(C) Transdermal patches are more likely to be associated with headaches than are sublingual nitrates
(D) Oral preparations are more effective than sublingual ones
(E) Oral administration of isosorbide should not exceed 15 mg every 3 to 4 h

**II-29.** A 70-year-old retired banker with no past medical history presents to the emergency department 4 h after the onset of severe substernal crushing chest pain with radiation to the left arm and neck. Electrocardiography reveals significant ST-segment elevation in leads I, L, V$_5$, and V$_6$. The patient has no clear-cut medical contraindications to anticoagulation. Which of the following would be the optimal management strategy at this time?

(A) Intravenous tissue plasminogen activator alone
(B) Intravenous tissue plasminogen activator and aspirin
(C) Intravenous tissue plasminogen activator and heparin
(D) Intravenous tissue plasminogen activator, heparin, and aspirin
(E) Thrombolytic therapy is contraindicated because of the patient's age

**II-30.** This two-dimensional echocardiogram most likely was recorded in which of the following patients?

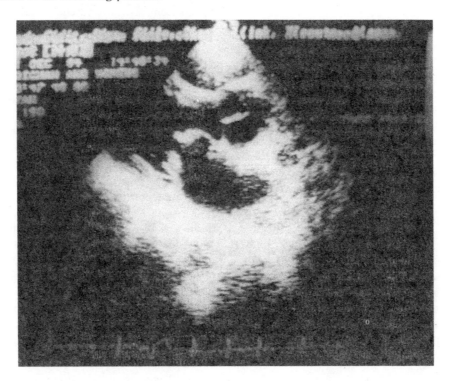

(A) A 54-year-old man with syncopal episodes when bending forward

(B) A previously healthy 68-year-old man with sudden onset of pulmonary edema and a new holosystolic murmur

(C) A 17-year-old girl with atypical chest pain and a midsystolic click

(D) A 42-year-old woman with palpitations, exertional dyspnea, and episodes of hemoptysis

(E) An asymptomatic 32-year-old cardiologist

**II-31.** All the following statements regarding myocardial hypertrophy are true EXCEPT

(A) norepinephrine induces the synthesis of fetal myosin forms

(B) the proto-oncogenes c-*sis*, c-*myc*, c-*ras*, and c-*fos* are all induced in myocardial tissue during hypertrophy

(C) a gene responsible for familial hypertrophic cardiomyopathy has been mapped to chromosome 14

(D) angiotensin II can stimulate hypertrophy by direct effects on smooth muscle

(E) hypertrophy caused by hemodynamic overload is accompanied by a similar synthetic induction of fetal myosin forms to that observed in the hypertrophy associated with hyperthyroidism

**II-32.** A previously healthy 58-year-old man is admitted to the hospital because of an acute inferior myocardial infarction. Within several hours, he becomes oliguric and hypotensive (blood pressure is 90/60 mmHg). Insertion of a pulmonary artery (Swan-Ganz) catheter reveals the following pressures: pulmonary capillary wedge, 4 mmHg; pulmonary artery, 22/4 mmHg; and mean right atrial, 11 mmHg. This man would best be treated with

(A) fluids

(B) digoxin

(C) norepinephrine

(D) dopamine

(E) intraaortic balloon counterpulsation

**II-33**   A 63-year-old black woman with a long history of hypertension and diabetes is brought to the emergency department by relatives because she has become incoherent over the past 24 h. Physical examination reveals a disoriented woman whose blood pressure is 230/160, respiratory rate is 25, and pulse is 110. The patient is afebrile. The chest reveals bibasilar rales. Cardiac examination is remarkable only for the presence of an $S_4$. There is no organomegaly or focal neurologic findings. The patient is oriented to person only.

The family revealed that the patient has not been taking her antihypertensive medicines in the past several weeks. The patient is placed on a cardiac monitor, and both intravenous and intraarterial lines are placed. An emergent CT scan reveals no evidence of hemorrhage or mass lesion. The most appropriate next step in management would be to

(A)  observe the patient in a quiet room for 1 h before administering therapy
(B)  wait for laboratory values to return before deciding on specific therapy
(C)  administer sodium nitroprusside
(D)  administer diazoxide
(E)  administer intravenous nicardipine

**II-34.**   All the following statements regarding physiologic maneuvers used to distinguish one cardiac condition from another are true EXCEPT

(A)  the Valsalva maneuver results in decreased length and intensity for most systolic murmurs, except those caused by mitral valve prolapse and hypertrophic cardiomyopathy
(B)  in the case of mitral valve prolapse, squatting results in increased intensity of the systolic murmur
(C)  handgrip exercise increases the intensity of the murmurs of mitral stenosis and mitral regurgitation
(D)  murmurs of tricuspid regurgitation and tricuspid stenosis increase during inspiration
(E)  the murmur of aortic stenosis increases after a ventricular premature beat

**II-35.**   Which of the following patients should undergo operative excision of an abdominal aortic aneurysm and replacement with a vascular graft?

(A)  A 58-year-old man with an 8-cm abdominal aneurysm who sustained a myocardial infarction 3 months ago
(B)  A 65-year-old man with a 7-cm aneurysm who sustained a myocardial infarction 1 year ago
(C)  A 65-year-old woman with a 4-cm aneurysm and no prior history of heart or lung disease
(D)  A 58-year-old man with a 7-cm aneurysm and $FEV_1$ of 0.8 L
(E)  A 67-year-old man with an 8-cm aneurysm and creatinine 3.2 mg/dL

**II-36.**   A 68-year-old man who has had a recent syncopal episode is hospitalized with congestive heart failure. His blood pressure is 160/80 mmHg, his pulse rate is 80 beats per minute, and there is a grade III/VI harsh systolic murmur. An echocardiogram shows a disproportionately thickened ventricular septum and systolic anterior motion of the mitral valve. Which of the following findings would most likely be present in this man?

(A)  Radiation of the murmur to the carotid arteries
(B)  Decrease of the murmur with handgrip
(C)  Delayed carotid upstroke
(D)  Reduced left ventricular ejection fraction
(E)  Signs of mitral stenosis

**II-37.**   Which factor accounts for the prolonged QRS complex depicted in this figure?

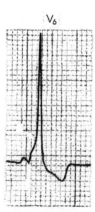

(A)  Left ventricular hypertrophy
(B)  Accessory conducting fibers parallel to the AV junction
(C)  Right ventricular infarction
(D)  Left bundle branch block
(E)  Right bundle branch block

**II-38.** Each of the following techniques can detect non-viable myocardium EXCEPT

(A) positron emission tomography (PET)
(B) thallium 210 scintigraphy
(C) technetium 99m stannous pyrophosphate scintigraphy
(D) standard computed tomography (CT)
(E) echocardiography

**II-39.** For the last 6 h, a 33-year-old man has had sharp, pleuritic substernal chest pain that is relieved when he sits upright. His electrocardiogram shows diffuse ST-segment elevation. Which of the following observations would LEAST support a diagnosis of acute pericarditis?

(A) Frequent atrial premature beats
(B) PR-segment depression
(C) Diffuse T-wave inversion with ST-segment elevation
(D) Twice-normal serum creatine phosphokinase concentration
(E) No rub

**II-40.** All the following electrocardiographic findings may represent manifestations of digitalis intoxication EXCEPT

(A) bigeminy
(B) junctional tachycardia
(C) atrial flutter
(D) atrial tachycardia with variable block
(E) sinus arrest

**II-41.** All the following are indications for surgical intervention in the treatment of dissection of the aorta EXCEPT

(A) compromised femoral pulse
(B) new murmur of aortic regurgitation
(C) persistent chest pain
(D) involvement of the ascending aorta
(E) involvement of the descending aorta

**II-42.** All the following congenital cardiac disorders will lead to a left-to-right shunt, generally without cyanosis, EXCEPT

(A) anomalous origin of the left coronary artery from the pulmonary trunk
(B) patent ductus arteriosus without pulmonary hypertension
(C) total anomalous pulmonary venous connection
(D) ventricular septal defect
(E) sinus venosus atrial septal defect

**II-43.** Clear contraindications to the use of thrombolytic agents in the setting of an acute anterior myocardial infarction include all the following EXCEPT

(A) left carotid artery occlusion with hemiparesis 1 month ago
(B) transurethral resection of the prostate 1 week ago
(C) diastolic blood pressure of 110 mmHg during chest pain
(D) patient age greater than 70
(E) epigastric pain and melena 1 week ago treated with histamine receptor antagonists

**II-44.** Which of the following situations in the peri-infarction period would suggest the presence of ventricular septal perforation?

(A) Systolic murmur, large *v* waves in pulmonary capillary wedge tracing; $P_{O_2}$ in right atrium equals that in right ventricle
(B) Systolic murmur, large *v* waves in pulmonary capillary wedge tracing; $P_{O_2}$ in the right atrium is greater than that in the right ventricle
(C) Systolic murmur, large *v* waves in pulmonary capillary wedge tracing; $P_{O_2}$ in the right atrium is less than that in the right ventricle
(D) Diastolic murmur, large *v* waves in the pulmonary capillary wedge tracing; $P_{O_2}$ in the right atrium is less than that in the right ventricle
(E) Diastolic murmur, large *v* waves in the pulmonary capillary wedge tracing; $P_{O_2}$ in the right atrium is greater than that in the right ventricle

**II-45.** A 50-year-old man with a history of smoking, hypertension, and chronic exertional angina develops several daily episodes of chest pain at rest compatible with cardiac ischemia. The patient is hospitalized. All the following would be part of an appropriate management plan EXCEPT

(A) intravenous heparin
(B) aspirin
(C) intravenous nitroglycerin
(D) lidocaine by bolus infusion
(E) diltiazem

**II-46.**   All the following patients are at increased risk for the development of deep venous thrombosis EXCEPT

(A)  a 35-year-old woman with systemic lupus erythematosus and a prolonged partial thromboplastin time

(B)  a 75-year-old woman with a Colles fracture of the wrist

(C)  a normotensive 18-year-old woman taking an oral contraceptive

(D)  a 55-year-old man 3 days after an uncomplicated inferior myocardial infarction

(E)  a 55-year-old man 5 days after complete resection of a squamous cell carcinoma 2 cm in diameter in the periphery of the right lung

**II-47.**   This figure most likely represents the pulmonary capillary wedge and left ventricular pressure tracing from which of the following patients?

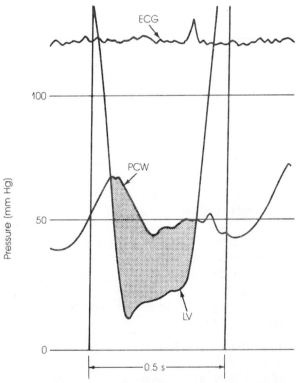

From Grossman W (ed): *Cardiac Catheterization and Angiography*, 3d ed. Philadelphia, Lea & Febiger, 1986, with permission.

(A)  A 40-year-old woman with a history of rheumatic fever, orthopnea, and hemoptysis

(B)  A 24-year-old intravenous drug abuser with fever, a holosystolic murmur, and large mitral valve vegetation

(C)  A 26-year-old man with long arms, abnormal lenses, and a diastolic murmur

(D)  A 72-year-old man with left ventricular hypertrophy, syncope, and a systolic murmur

(E)  A 35-year-old woman with elevated neck veins and a large mediastinal mass caused by non-Hodgkin's lymphoma

**II-48.**   A 22-year-old Michigan woman presents to her local emergency room complaining of dizziness over the past several days, including two syncope episodes followed in each case by unresponsiveness for several minutes. She has always been in excellent health, having played varsity soccer in college. Her last illness occurred 4 months ago, when she developed fever, chills, and generalized weakness; those symptoms cut short a 2-week camping trip to the Cape Cod National Seashore. She uses oral contraceptives but no other prescription medications. She admits to inhaling cocaine over the last 4 months. Physical examination reveals blood pressure of 100/62 and pulse of 30 but is otherwise unremarkable. Chest x-ray and serum chemistries are unremarkable. ECG demonstrates complete heart block with nonspecific ST- and T-wave changes. There is no evidence of prior myocardial infarction. The most likely cause of her complete heart block is

(A)  myocardial infarction from cocaine use

(B)  myocardial infarction caused by a coronary artery embolus

(C)  infection resulting from *Ixodes damini*

(D)  infection caused by *Borrelia burgdorfei*

(E)  infection caused by HIV

**II-49.**   A 70-year-old man is admitted to the hospital with chest pain of 8 h duration. ECG demonstrates anterior ST elevation, for which he is given tissue plasminogen activator, heparin, and intravenous nitroglycerin. His symptoms resolve, and serum chemistries reveal a peak CPK of 1400 and a CK-MB fraction of 80. He is eventually started on oral medications and transferred out of the cardiac intensive care unit. His subsequent hospital course is uneventful until day 4, when he develops severe shortness of breath. Blood pressure is 110/70, and pulse is 120. Examination reveals a new systolic murmur. The most appropriate therapeutic intervention would be

(A)  emergent cardiac surgery consultation and transfer to the operating room

(B)  IV heparin

(C)  IV heparin and streptokinase

(D)  IV heparin and furosemide

(E)  IV sodium nitroprusside

**II-50.** All the following are known clinical markers for acute myocardial infarction EXCEPT

(A) CK-MB2
(B) CK-MB1
(C) cardiac-specific troponin I
(D) cardiac-specific troponin T
(E) cardiac-specific tropomyosin I

**II-51.** A 68-year-old man with known aortic sclerosis was admitted with chest pain and ruled out for myocardial infarction but had recurrent symptoms during weaning from IV heparin and nitroglycerin over the ensuing 5 days. Cardiac catheterization revealed three-vessel disease with a normal ejection fraction, and he underwent coronary bypass grafting. On postoperative day 3, he complained of pain in the right arm and was found to have an absent right brachial pulse and a cold distal right arm. Laboratory work revealed a hematocrit of 38 percent, platelets 32,000, prothrombin time 15 INR 1.4, and partial thromboplastin time 65. What is the most likely explanation for this patient's absent brachial pulse?

(A) Left ventricular thrombus caused by a myocardial infarction with a subsequent brachial artery embolus
(B) Embolization from aortic sclerosis
(C) Embolization from paradoxical emboli through a patent foramen ovale from a DVT arising postoperatively
(D) Thrombosis in situ caused by postoperative hypercoagulability
(E) Heparin-induced thrombocytopenia

**II-52.** A 60-year-old man without a significant medical history presents for his annual physical. An electrocardiogram demonstrates two ventricular premature complexes (VPCs) within the 12-lead tracing. All the following statements are true EXCEPT

(A) sixty percent of all males have VPCs on 24-h Holter monitoring
(B) this patient's VPCs predict a higher incidence of cardiac mortality
(C) VPCs such as those documented in this patient can cause symptoms
(D) both the frequency and the nature of VPCs can be correlated with increased mortality in patients with known coronary artery disease
(E) the frequency of isolated VPCs increases with age

**II-53.** Echocardiography can be used successfully to aid in the diagnosis or management of all the following situations EXCEPT

(A) determining left ventricular function after a myocardial infarction
(B) estimating the mitral valve area in a patient with mitral valve stenosis
(C) establishing the presence of an atrial septal defect
(D) excluding the presence of pericarditis
(E) assisting with pericardiocentesis

**II-54.** All the following statements regarding the activation of cardiac myocytes are true EXCEPT

(A) a cardiac cell is polarized at rest
(B) in a resting cardiac cell, the intracellular concentration of sodium is low while the extracellular concentration is high
(C) the rise in intracellular sodium is the triggering event in myocyte contraction
(D) calcium binds to troponin C and releases cells from the inhibitory influence of this repressor
(E) ATP provides the source of the energy that drives myocyte contraction

**II-55.** A 72-year-old female with a prior history of hypertension is receiving low-dose atenolol, an unknown diuretic, and long-acting diltiazem. She has no other significant cardiac history. The patient is brought to the emergency room after having passed out while getting up to go to the bathroom at 6 A.M. this morning. She is seen by the surgical service, which finds her to have an orbital fracture from when she struck the sink. Internal medicine consultation is requested when an ECG reveals sinus bradycardia at 40 with occasional sinus arrest with pauses of 2 to 3 s but no other abnormalities. She remains somewhat light-headed. Blood pressure is 90/50. Physical examination is otherwise benign. She has been without oral intake since the previous evening. The next steps in treating this patient's arrhythmia would consist of

(A) placement of a temporary wire; implant permanent pacer this afternoon
(B) placement of a temporary wire; discontinue diltiazem and atenolol and follow
(C) placement of external pacing pads; implant permanent pacer this afternoon
(D) discontinue diltiazem and admit
(E) proceed directly to permanent pacer implantation

**II-56.** A 52-year-old male with significant obstructive pulmonary disease on the basis of tobacco use presents with shortness of breath for 2 days and palpitations for the last 2 h. On examination, he is found to have diffuse expiratory wheezing and an irregular heart rate. ECG demonstrates rapid atrial fibrillation at a rate of 170 and nonspecific ST- and T-wave changes. All the following could be used to treat the patient's trial fibrillation EXCEPT

(A) digoxin
(B) metoprolol
(C) verapamil
(D) diltiazem
(E) cardioversion

**II-57.** A 64-year-old man with known allergies to penicillin and lobster undergoes a left hip replacement. Recovery is uneventful until the day before discharge, when he begins experiencing palpitations. ECG reveals his baseline right bundle branch block and new atrial flutter at a rate of 110 to 120. He is otherwise asymptomatic. Heparin is started. He remains in atrial fibrillation over the next 2 days while a workup demonstrates normal potassium, magnesium, thyroid-stimulating hormone, and chest x-ray. The decision is made to proceed with chemical cardioversion. He is given intravenous procainamide. Halfway though the infusion, the telemetry suddenly reveals a rate of 240 with narrow QRS complexes. He is found to be pulseless, CPR is begun, and he is defibrillated with 100 joules, which restores sinus rhythm that degenerates into atrial fibrillation. This reaction could have been prevented if

(A) the patient's allergy to procainamide had been known
(B) the infusion of procainamide had been administered more slowly
(C) pretreatment before procainamide had been undertaken with digoxin, propranolol, or verapamil
(D) quinidine had been used instead of procainamide
(E) his QTc had been followed more carefully at periodic points during the procainamide infusion

**II-58.** The following are all risk factors for increased mortality from cardiac catheterization EXCEPT

(A) class IV congestive heart failure
(B) combination of severe valvular disease and coronary artery disease
(C) unstable angina
(D) insulin-dependent diabetes mellitus
(E) ejection fraction below 30 percent

**II-59.** All the following statements regarding cardiac imaging are correct EXCEPT

(A) Sestamibi imaging can be readily used to identify hibernating myocardium
(B) thallium can be readily used to identify hibernating myocardium
(C) dipyridamole stress testing should not be performed in patients with significant COPD
(D) the effects of dipyridamole can be reversed with intravenous theophylline
(E) Sestamibi can be injected during chest pain to distinguish cardiac from noncardiac chest pain

**II-60.** All the following may be a manifestation of digitalis toxicity EXCEPT

(A) headaches
(B) diplopia
(C) yellow vision
(D) gingival hyperplasia
(E) nausea and vomiting

**II-61.** Cystic medial necrosis is prevalent in all the following EXCEPT

(A) Marfan syndrome
(B) Ehlers-Danlos syndrome type IV
(C) pregnancy
(D) hypertension
(E) temporal arteritis

**II-62.** A 68-year-old man complaining of chest pain radiating to his back is brought to the emergency room. Blood pressure is 160/80 in the right arm and 150/80 in the left; the pulse is 64. No diastolic murmur is heard. ECG does not show ischemia. Aortic dissection is suspected. All the following would be appropriate to confirm the diagnosis EXCEPT

(A) aortography
(B) MRI
(C) transesophageal echocardiography
(D) positron emission tomography
(E) transthoracic echocardiography

**II-63.** A 16-year-old male is referred by his high school coach for a physical examination before joining the football team. His older brother died suddenly during football practice; no autopsy was obtained. The patient has a loud systolic murmur. All the following would be consistent with hypertrophic cardiomyopathy EXCEPT

(A a crescendo-decrescendo systolic murmur
(B) radiation into the neck
(C) brisk carotid upstrokes
(D) increase in the murmur on Valsalva or standing
(E) decrease with passive leg raising

**II-64.** All the following are recognized causes of pulmonary edema not solely on the basis of increased pulmonary venous pressure EXCEPT

(A) exposure to high altitude
(B) heroin overdose
(C) central nervous system disorders
(D) sarcoidosis
(E) gram-negative septicemia

**II-65.** In patients with established coronary artery disease and elevated LDL levels, all the following statements regarding HMG coreductase inhibitors are true EXCEPT

(A) treatment is associated with a significant decrease in mortality from cardiovascular events
(B) treatment is associated with a significant decrease in total mortality
(C) treatment is associated with a decrease in the number of invasive cardiac procedures, both angioplasty and coronary bypass
(D) the average LDL lowering of these agents is approximately 20 to 40 percent
(E) patients with homozygous familial hypercholesterolemia, typically with markedly elevated LDL levels, are particularly responsive to the LDL-lowering effect of all HMG coreductase inhibitors

**II-66.** All the following are currently accepted cardiac risk factors EXCEPT

(A) male gender
(B) cigarette smoking
(C) family history of coronary artery disease in any first-degree relative
(D) peripheral vascular disease
(E) HDL level < 35 mg/dL

**II-67.** All the following statements regarding the vascular biology of the atherosclerotic process are true EXCEPT

(A) the fatty streak is the initial lesion of atherosclerosis
(B) cellular hallmarks of lesions that may lead to myocardial infarction include large necrotic lipid cores, thin fibrous caps, and large numbers of macrophages
(C) the clinical benefit of lipid-lowering therapy with HMG coreductase inhibitors does not appear to stem from a significant decrease in the extent of coronary stenosis
(D) adhesion molecules such as VCAM-1 are expressed by endothelial cells and act as receptors for circulating lymphocytes and monocytes
(E) early atherosclerotic lesions encroach on the vessel lumen but do not create significant limitations of flow, explaining the greater clinical significance of severe occlusive coronary disease seen on cardiac catheterization

**II-68.** A 54-year-old female presents to the office asking for a second opinion regarding her shortness of breath. She has a history of cigarette smoking for many years but stopped two years ago, when she was found to have breast cancer. She underwent a modified radical mastectomy but received no additional therapy. She also has a history of hypertension previously controlled with hydrochlorothiazide (HCTZ). Approximately 6 months ago, she saw her internist because of mild shortness of breath unresponsive to an increase in the HCTZ dose or a subsequent change to furosemide. She developed ankle swelling, worsened shortness of breath, and orthopnea. Blood pressure is 130/100 without pulsus paradoxus, and pulse is 110. She appears to be in moderate respiratory distress. Chest examination reveals faint bibasilar crackles. Heart sounds are decreased but unremarkable. The abdomen is benign. There is 2+ pitting edema. Chest x-ray reveals moderate cardiomegaly and bilateral pleural effusions. ECG demonstrates low voltage but no evidence of right ventricular strain. Which of the following statements are true?

(A) The increasing doses of diuretics have helped her remain at home and free of worsening dyspnea

(B) The patient probably has direct myocardial invasion by a tumor

(C) An echocardiogram would offer absolute proof of the diagnosis

(D) The lack of pulsus paradoxus could suggest the presence of an atrial septal defect

(E) Heparin and IV nitroglycerin should be instituted until Doppler ultrasound of the lower extremities is obtained and she is ruled out for myocardial infarction

**II-69.** Amiodarone (True or False)

(A) is an effective therapy for atrial fibrillation

(B) is an effective therapy for ventricular tachycardia

(C) can be given intravenously or orally

(D) requires careful vigilance regarding the doses of beta blockers and warfarin a patient is taking

(E) although side effects are significantly reduced with low-dose therapy, complications can include hypothyroidism, pulmonary disease, and skin discoloration

*DIRECTIONS:* Each question below contains five suggested responses. For **each** of the five responses listed with each question, you are to respond either YES (Y) or NO (N). In a given item **all, some, or none** of the responses may be correct.

**II-70.** A 62-year-old man loses consciousness in the street, and resuscitative efforts are undertaken. In the emergency room an electrocardiogram is obtained, part of which is shown below. Which of the following disorders could account for this man's presentation?

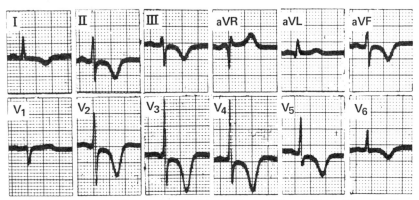

From Marriott HJL: *Practical Electrocardiography*, 7th ed. Baltimore, Williams & Wilkins, 1983, p 400, with permission.

(A) Subendocardial infarction
(B) Hyperkalemia
(C) Intracerebral hemorrhage
(D) Myocardial ischemia
(E) Hypocalcemic tetany

**II-71.** Acute hyperkalemia is associated with which of the following electrocardiographic changes?

(A) QRS widening
(B) Prolongation of the ST segment
(C) Decrease in the P wave
(D) Prominent U waves
(E) Peaked T waves

**II-72.** True statements regarding exercise tolerance tests include which of the following?

(A) Requiring ≥ 2.0 mm of ST depression to define a test as positive enhances the sensitivity of the test compared with a situation in which only 0.5 mm of ST depression is required to count as positive
(B) Given a specificity of 90 percent and a sensitivity of 80 percent, a positive test in a patient whose prior probability of having coronary artery disease (based on clinical factors) is 10 percent suggests a greater than 80 percent likelihood that the patient actually has coronary artery disease
(C) Thallium 201 exercise scanning increases both the sensitivity and the specificity for detecting ischemic heart disease
(D) A thallium 201 scan done at peak exercise that reveals a nonperfused area of myocardium indicates that the patient has suffered a prior myocardial infarction
(E) A marked increase in blood pressure during the test suggests poor conditioning and probably will cause the test to be nondiagnostic

**II-73.** The rhythm shown on the electrocardiogram below can be associated with

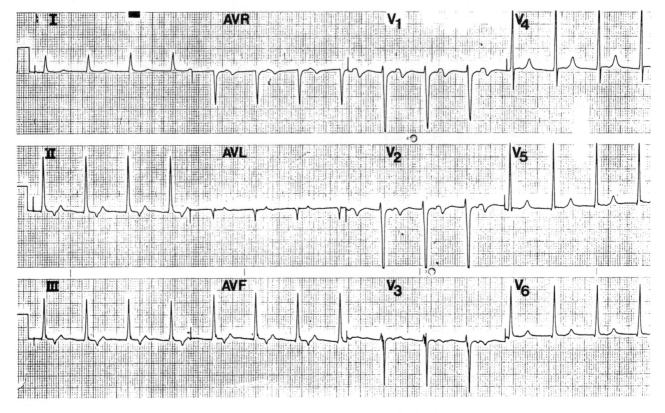

(A) digitalis toxicity
(B) acute myocarditis
(C) anterior myocardial infarction

(D) mitral valve surgery
(E) hypercalcemia

**II-74.** Mild heart failure resulting from left ventricular dysfunction is accurately described by which of the following statements?

(A) Cardiac output would be depressed at rest
(B) Plasma norepinephrine levels would be higher than those in normal controls during exercise
(C) Myocardial norepinephrine content would be high
(D) Left ventricular end-diastolic pressure would rise more during exercise than it does in normal controls
(E) Cardiac output would fail to rise appropriately when oxygen consumption was increased during exercise

**II-75.** Drugs that would antagonize the interaction of catecholamines with adrenergic receptors include

(A) prazosin
(B) clonidine
(C) phenylephrine
(D) yohimbine
(E) isoproterenol

**II-76.** A 37-year-old man with Wolff-Parkinson-White syndrome develops a broad-complex irregular tachycardia at a rate of 200 beats per minute. He appears comfortable and has little hemodynamic impairment. Useful treatment at this point might include

(A) digoxin
(B) quinidine
(C) propranolol
(D) verapamil
(E) direct-current cardioversion

**II-77.** Sudden cardiac death is accurately described by which of the following statements?

(A) Ventricular tachycardia or ventricular fibrillation during the convalescent phase (3 days to 8 weeks) after a myocardial infarction is a risk factor for subsequent sudden cardiac death

(B) A patient convalescing from a myocardial infarction and displaying a salvo of three ventricular premature beats is at greater risk than is a similar patient who has 35 unifocal premature beats per hour

(C) If only one person is present to provide basic life support, chest compressions should be performed at a rate of 80 per minute, and breaths twice in succession every 15 s

(D) Assuming there is no spontaneous pulse, a 400-joule shock should be delivered immediately upon recognition of ventricular tachycardia or ventricular fibrillation

(E) Intravenous sodium bicarbonate should be given approximately every 5 min during cardiac arrest

**II-78.** A 17-year-old girl has an atrial septal defect of the sinus venosus type, with a 3:1 pulmonary-to-systemic blood flow ratio. True statements concerning her condition include which of the following?

(A) She is probably asymptomatic

(B) She probably has partial anomalous connection of the pulmonary veins

(C) The magnitude of the shunt is a function of the amount of total blood flow

(D) A systolic murmur probably would be due to flow across the defect

(E) A diastolic rumble would strongly suggest the coexistence of mitral stenosis (Lutembacher's syndrome)

**II-79.** The initial positive deflection in the jugular venous pulse (*a* wave) can be accentuated in which of the following conditions?

(A) Junctional rhythm
(B) Tricuspid stenosis
(C) Atrial fibrillation
(D) Multiple pulmonary emboli
(E) Complete heart block

**II-80.** For which of the following patients would cardiac surgery be appropriately recommended?

(A) An asymptomatic 18-year-old woman who has an atrial septal defect with a 2:1 pulmonary-to-systemic flow ratio

(B) An asymptomatic 19-year-old man who has a loud murmur and a ventricular septal defect with a 1.5:1 pulmonary-to-systemic flow ratio

(C) A 33-year-old man who has chest pain, fatigue, cyanosis, a large ventricular septal defect, a 2:1 right-to-left shunt, and a normal pulmonary outflow tract and pulmonic valve

(D) A 52-year-old man who has chronic mitral regurgitation and has recently developed pulmonary edema associated with the onset of rapid atrial fibrillation

(E) A 54-year-old man who has aortic stenosis and has chest pain on moderate to strenuous exertion

**II-81.** True statements regarding balloon valvuloplasty include

(A) balloon dilatation of a stenotic pulmonary valve is not feasible because of the danger of rupture of the thin-walled pulmonary artery

(B) mitral valvuloplasty increases the effective diastolic valve area to normal size

(C) balloon aortic valvuloplasty is contraindicated in calcific aortic stenosis because the fracture of calcium deposits on the leaflets leads to cerebral emboli

(D) restenosis after aortic valvuloplasty is a significant problem

(E) aortic valvuloplasty results in symptomatic improvement for most patients

**II-82.** True statements regarding hemodynamic changes occurring during exercise include which of the following?

(A) Venous return is augmented by the pumping action of skeletal muscles

(B) The increased adrenergic nerve impulses to the heart as well as an increased concentration of circulating catecholamines help augment the contractile state of the myocardium

(C) Venoconstriction in exercising muscles as well as increased cardiac output leads to marked increases in systemic blood pressure

(D) End-diastolic volume increases in a failing heart during exercise

(E) Stroke volume and heart rate increase

**II-83.** A 34-year-old woman is bothered by palpitations and chest pain. On auscultation, the first heart sound is normal, but there is a midsystolic click and a late systolic murmur. Her electrocardiogram shows T-wave inversions in leads II, III, and aVF. True statements concerning her condition include which of the following?

(A) An exercise stress test would most likely be positive

(B) An echocardiogram may show abrupt posterior displacement of both mitral leaflets

(C) The woman's chest pain could be due to excessive stress on the papillary muscles

(D) The click and murmur would be expected to occur later in systole when the woman stands

(E) Prophylactic measures should be taken to prevent subacute bacterial endocarditis

**II-84.** A permanent atrioventricular sequential pacemaker (DDD) would be preferred to a standard ventricular pacemaker (VVI) in which of the following patients?

(A) A 64-year-old woman with atrial fibrillation and a ventricular rate of 40 beats per minute

(B) A 56-year-old man with complete heart block and a global left ventricular ejection fraction of 36 percent

(C) An active 46-year-old man with high-grade atrioventricular block

(D) An 80-year-old woman with symptomatic brady-arrhythmias and normal left ventricular function

(E) A 50-year-old man with hypertrophic cardio-myopathy and infranodal second-degree atrio-ventricular block

**II-85.** A 58-year-old man with a history of severe hypertension, three prior myocardial infarctions, and a left ventricular ejection fraction of 15 percent presents with a 30-pound weight loss. A workup for malignancy is negative. Which of the following factors could explain the patient's cachexia and weight loss?

(A) Digitalis intoxication

(B) Protein loss in the gastrointestinal tract as a result of high right-sided pressures

(C) Elevation of the metabolic rate

(D) Malabsorption of nutrients

(E) Incomplete gastric filling

**II-86.** Correct statements regarding cardiac transplantation include

(A) the 5-year survival is 25 to 50 percent

(B) two P waves are typically evident on the electrocardiogram of patients with a transplanted heart

(C) risk factors for accelerated coronary vascular disease include the number of rejection episodes and hyperlipidemia

(D) coronary disease accounts for the majority of late (>1 year after transplant) deaths

(E) immunosuppressive drugs can be discontinued after 5 years, since the risk of rejection after that point is extremely low

**II-87.** A 50-year-old woman with a history of hypertension (but taking no medication currently) presents to the emergency ward with a complaint of sudden palpitations and faintness. Her pulse is 120, and the 12-lead ECG discloses a wide-complex tachycardia. Which of the following characteristics would suggest a ventricular origin for her tachycardia rather than supraventricular tachycardia with aberrant conduction?

(A) A QRS complex of 0.12 s

(B) A QRS complex of 0.22 s

(C) Very irregular rhythm

(D) Atrioventricular dissociation

(E) A Q wave in lead $V_6$ and a broad R wave in $V_1$

**II-88.** A 23-year-old man has had recent onset of exertional dyspnea. A grade III/VI systolic murmur is heard at the left sternal border. Electrocardiography shows apical and lateral Q waves and left ventricular hypertrophy. Echocardiography reveals asymmetric septal hypertrophy without evidence of obstruction. Correct statements regarding this clinical situation include which of the following?

(A) The man's dyspnea is best explained by lateral wall infarction

(B) First-degree relatives should be evaluated

(C) The risk of sudden death is low

(D) Calcium channel blockers may relieve the symptoms

(E) The man's heart is normal histologically aside from changes of infarction

**II-89.** Aortic regurgitation is accurately characterized by which of the following statements?

(A) Most cases of aortic regurgitation (with or without associated lesions) are due to congenital (including Marfan's syndrome), syphilitic, or spondylitic causes

(B) *Quincke's pulse* refers to the pistol-shot sound audible over the femoral arteries

(C) The Graham Steell murmur of pulmonary regurgitation is frequently associated

(D) The echocardiogram frequently reveals fluttering of the anterior leaflet of the mitral valve

(E) Surgical correction can be delayed if the patient is asymptomatic and retains normal left ventricular function

**II-90.** Which of the following findings probably would be present in a patient who sustained recurrent pulmonary emboli?

(A) Decreased lung volumes on spirometric testing

(B) Enlarged P waves on electrocardiographic examination

(C) Tricuspid regurgitant flow on Doppler echocardiography

(D) Positive right ventricular uptake on thallium 201 scintigraphy

(E) Prominent *a* waves on physical examination of jugular venous pulsation

**II-91.** True statements regarding the effect of alcohol on the heart include which of the following?

(A) Chronic ingestion of alcohol will lead to a restrictive cardiomyopathy

(B) Once heart failure develops, discontinuing the consumption of alcohol will not appreciably affect the natural history of the disease

(C) If thiamine deficiency is present in an alcoholic, high output failure is noted

(D) If a patient with heart failure caused by ethanol continues to drink, he or she is unlikely to be alive in 3 years

(E) The most common arrhythmia associated with a drinking binge is ventricular tachycardia

**II-92.** True statements regarding cardiac neoplasms include

(A) lymphoma is the most common malignant neoplasm that primarily involves the heart

(B) the most common site for a myxoma is the left atrium

(C) myxomas may arise as part of a familial syndrome that also includes pigmented skin lesions and endocrine abnormalities

(D) a midsystolic "plop" typically indicates the presence of a cardiac myxoma

(E) weight loss and fever are frequent presenting manifestations of cardiac myxoma

**II-93.** For the purpose of diagnosing secondary causes of high blood pressure, which of the following patients with hypertension should have a workup beyond routine laboratory studies (blood urea nitrogen, glucose, creatinine, calcium, uric acid, potassium, cholesterol, triglycerides, electrocardiogram, and chest x-ray)?

(A) A 35-year-old man with a prior history of normotension who presents with a blood pressure of 160/105 but an otherwise normal physical examination

(B) A 35-year-old woman with a prior history of normotension who presents with a blood pressure of 160/105 and an abdominal bruit

(C) A 60-year-old man with a prior history of normotension who presents with a blood pressure of 160/100

(D) A 40-year-old woman with a prior history of normotension who presents with a blood pressure of 160/105 unresponsive to enalapril and hydrochlorothiazide

(E) A 45-year-old man with an unknown prior history who presents with a blood pressure of 160/100 and left ventricular heave on physical examination

*DIRECTIONS:* The group of questions below consists of lettered headings followed by a set of numbered items. For each numbered item select the **one** lettered heading with which it is **most** closely associated. Each lettered heading may be used **once, more than once, or not at all.**

*Questions II-94–II-97.*

Match each of the causes of right heart failure below with the most characteristic set of hemodynamic measurements.

|  | Right Atrial Pressure, mmHg | Pulmonary Arterial Pressure, mmHg | Pulmonary Capillary Wedge Pressure, mmHg |
|---|---|---|---|
| (A) | 16 | 75/30 | 11 |
| (B) | 16 | 35/17 | 16 |
| (C) | 16 | 100/30 | 28 |
| (D) | 16 | 45/22 | 20 |
| (E) | 16 | 22/12 | 10 |
| Normal values | 0–5 | 12–28/3–13 | 3–11 |

**II-94.**    Right ventricular infarction

**II-95.**    Cor pulmonale from bronchitis

**II-96.**    Mitral stenosis

**II-97.**    Constrictive pericarditis

# II. DISORDERS OF THE HEART AND VASCULAR SYSTEM

## ANSWERS

**II-1. The answer is B.** *(Chap. 243)* The combination of hypotension and bradycardia suggests a vagal response in the setting of an acute myocardial infarction. Administration of the anticholinergic agent atropine is the treatment of choice. If the bradyarrhythmia and hypotension persist after 2.0 mg of atropine has been administered in divided doses, the insertion of a temporary pacemaker is indicated. Isoproterenol should be avoided in patients with acute myocardial infarction, since it may greatly increase myocardial oxygen consumption and thus intensify ischemia. Volume replacement or inotropic support may be required if hypotension persists after correction of the bradyarrhythmia, but they are not indicated as initial therapies.

**II-2. The answer is A.** *(Chaps. 38, 243)* A patient presenting with hypotension and oliguria is critically ill and requires urgent definition of the etiology of this condition. The clinical presentation with shock, fever, and pulmonary infiltrates is consistent with either noncardiogenic or cardiogenic pulmonary edema. The elevated pulmonary capillary wedge pressure strongly suggests failure of left ventricular output as a result of primary myocardial dysfunction or obstruction caused by pericardial tamponade. Pulmonary emboli, septic shock, and hypovolemia from gastrointestinal blood loss would all cause the pulmonary capillary wedge pressure to be decreased. Although pericardial tamponade could produce elevated pulmonary capillary wedge pressure, the obstruction to right ventricular inflow should be associated with equally abnormal right atrial mean, right ventricular end-diastolic, and pulmonary artery end-diastolic pressures. Therefore, this patient is suffering from cardiogenic shock caused by left ventricular myocardial dysfunction on the basis of myocardial infarction, severe cardiomyopathy, or myocarditis. Given the relatively normal electrocardiogram and the fever, the last condition is a distinct possibility.

**II-3. The answer is D.** *[Chap. 39. Standards and guidelines for cardiopulmonary resuscitation (CPR) in emergency cardiac care (ECC). JAMA 255:2905, 1986]* The successful resuscitation of a patient with cardiac arrest depends on the rapidity of the initiation of resuscitative efforts, the clinical status of the patient before the arrest, and the mechanism of the event. In this case the patient has a reasonable chance of recovery because of his good initial performance status (the event occurred while he was golfing), rapid institution of CPR by trained personnel, and sustained ventricular tachycardia (VT) as the mechanism for the event. The most appropriate management of cardiac arrest induced by VT is an initial 200-joule defibrillation. Additional shocks at higher energies, up to a maximum of 360 joules, should be attempted in the event of an initial failure to abolish the VT. Whether the initial defibrillation attempt is successful or not, lidocaine should be given intravenously as a 1 mg/kg bolus, to be followed in 2 min by the same dose if the arrhythmia is persistent. Second-line drugs that can be used in the event of lidocaine failure include intravenous procainamide and bretylium. If persistent ventricular fibrillation (VF) is the cause of the event, epinephrine may be administered every 5 min. Intravenous sodium bicarbonate and calcium are no longer considered safe or necessary for routine administration. Intravenous calcium gluconate would be indicated in the setting of hyperkalemia as the triggering event for resistant VF, in the presence of known hypocalcemia, and in those who have received high doses of calcium channel antagonists.

**II-4.   The answer is A.**   *(Chap. 246. Williams, N Engl J Med 319:1517, 1989)*   Captopril is an inhibitor of angiotensin converting enzyme and thus impairs the production of angiotensin II, a potent vasoconstrictor. Through removal of feedback inhibition, renin secretion is increased. Additional antihypertensive effects of captopril result from reduction of bradykinin degradation and stimulation of vasodilating prostaglandin production. Converting-enzyme inhibitors can be added to a regimen of beta blockade to achieve an additional antihypertensive effect. Captopril is contraindicated in patients with bilateral renal artery stenosis, since a reduction in systemic arterial pressure may lead to progressive renal hypoperfusion.

**II-5.   The answer is C.**   *(Chap. 240)*   The lateral-view chest film demonstrates calcification of the anterior pericardium, consistent with constrictive pericarditis. This pattern is seen in approximately one-half of patients with long-standing constriction, and pericardial thickening often can be confirmed by echocardiography. In patients with this disease, a pericardial knock is often heard 0.06 to 0.12 s after aortic valve closure, corresponding to the sudden cessation of ventricular filling. Murmurs are typically absent.

**II-6.   The answer is E.**   *(Chap. 245)*   PTCA to reduce one or more coronary stenoses in the treatment of chronic angina unresponsive to medical therapy, unstable angina, or acute myocardial infarction has been employed with increasing frequency. The risks and benefits of PTCA compare favorably with those of conventional surgery. Given the decreased cost and recovery and hospitalization time, PTCA is preferred whenever possible. While the current PTCA success rate exceeds 90 percent, a return of cardiac ischemia within 6 months strongly suggests restenosis of the dilated segment. Such restenosis appears to result from excessive local smooth muscle cell hyperplasia triggered by platelet adhesion on the balloon-damaged surface. While the use of nitrates, calcium channel antagonists, heparin, and aspirin just before and up to 6 months after the procedure helps prevent an acute closure resulting from spasm and thrombus formation, no anatomic or pharmacologic strategy has substantially reduced the restenosis rate. When recurrent ischemia develops more than 6 months after a PTCA, progression of disease at another site is more likely than restenosis. However, repeat PTCA is quite successful in treating patients with restenosis; bypass surgery is required in 10 percent or fewer of such patients.

**II-7.   The answer is A.**   *(Chap. 230)*   The electrocardiogram discloses sudden failure of atrial ventricular conduction without a preceding change in the PR interval, termed Mobitz type II second-degree AV block, which usually reflects significant disease of the conduction system. It may occur after a significant anterior myocardial infarction or in Lev's disease, which involves calcification and sclerosis of the fibrous cardiac skeleton (frequently involving the aortic and mitral valves), or Lenegre's disease, which involves only the conducting system. Mobitz type II block is inherently unstable and tends to progress to complete heart block with a slow, lower escape pacemaker. Therefore, pacemaker implantation is necessary in this condition, particularly if the patient is symptomatic, as in this case.

**II-8.   The answer is E.**   *(Chaps. 37, 233)*   Many persons who have ankle edema are inappropriately diagnosed as having heart failure. In particular, the diagnosis of right heart failure should not be made in the absence of jugular venous distention. Venous varicosities, cyclic edema, thrombophlebitis, and hypoalbuminemia all cause ankle edema and should be considered in the differential diagnosis.

**II-9.   The answer is C.**   *(Chaps. 227, 239)*   Assessment of the central aortic pulse wave is best carried out by examination of the carotid pulsations. Normally, the carotid pulse is characterized by a fairly rapid rise to a somewhat rounded peak. If two such peaks are found, diagnostic considerations include aortic regurgitation and hypertrophic cardiomyopathy. In the latter condition, obstruction to outflow usually occurs in midsystole. Moreover, obstruction is more manifest during reduced left ventricular size, such as after a Valsalva maneuver with subsequent decreased venous return. A brief decline in pressure follows the sudden decrease in the rate of left ventricular ejection during midsystole because of the development of obstruction. The second peak is caused by a smaller positive pulse wave produced by the remainder of ventricular ejection and by reflected waves from peripheral sources. The so-called bisferiens pulse should be distinguished from pulsus alternans, in which there is a regular alteration of the pressure pulse amplitude from beat to beat, usually associated with severe impairment of left ventricular function and therefore occurring in the setting of a third heart sound. Pulsus paradoxus, which is found in pericardial tamponade, severe airway disease, and superior vena cava obstruction, reflects an exaggerated decrease in systolic arterial pressure during inspiration.

*>10 mmHg*

**II-10.  The answer is C.**  *(Chap. 228)*   This ECG reveals an abnormal increase in the amplitude of the U wave, a small deflection following the T wave that usually has the same polarity as the T wave. Recognition of a pronounced U wave is important, for it may represent increased susceptibility to a torsades de pointes type of ventricular tachycardia. Prominent U waves are most commonly seen after the use of antiarrhythmic drugs such as quinidine, procainamide, and disopyramide or are due to hypokalemia. The latter condition would be typical of a patient receiving amphotericin B, which typically produces severe renal potassium wasting as a result of renal tubular damage. A patient with acute renal failure and hyperkalemia would display peaked T waves or an increased QRS duration on the ECG. Hypercalcemia, such as occurs in patients with metastatic breast cancer, and digitalis intoxication tend to produce short QT intervals. Inverted U waves are sometimes a subtle sign of myocardial ischemia.

**II-11.  The answer is E.**  *(Chap. 233)*   Digitalis glycosides augment contractility of the heart and slow atrioventricular condition and heart rate. The primary mechanism of action is inhibition of $Na^+$, $K^+$-ATPase, which is located in the sarcolemmal membrane. This action leads to intracellular accumulation of sodium and subsequently calcium by way of a sodium-calcium exchange mechanism.

**II-12.  The answer is D.**  *(Chap. 233. Grossman, N Engl J Med 325:1557–1564, 1991)*   Despite the fact that this patient's ejection fraction is normal, the presence of left ventricular hypertrophy, suggested by physical examination and confirmed by noninvasive testing, implicates the heart as the source of the problem. The patient has no evidence of either ischemic heart disease or lung disease, yet his ejection fraction is normal. However, it is increasingly recognized that increased resistance to filling of one or more cardiac ventricles, so-called diastolic heart failure, can produce increased pulmonary capillary wedge pressures with resultant respiratory complaints. In conditions such as advanced myocardial hypertrophy, impaired diastolic relaxation occurs. While hypertrophic heart disease is probably the best recognized cause of diastolic dysfunction, resistance to filling also can be seen in a diverse spectrum of conditions, including aortic valve stenosis, constrictive pericarditis, dilated cardiomyopathy, and even the "stunned" myocardium seen in ischemic heart disease. Treatment with beta blockers and calcium channel blockers may provide some degree of relief of symptoms related to diastolic dysfunction.

**II-13.  The answer is E.**  *(Chap. 230)*   The escape focus in atrioventricular nodal block is relatively high in the conduction system in an area of vagal innervation. Thus, a beneficial response to vagolytic drugs such as atropine is usually apparent. The rate at the escape focus is relatively rapid, and the QRS complex is narrow. Unless complete heart block persists, some Wenckebach periodicity can be observed. Inferior myocardial infarction, mitral valve surgery, and digitalis toxicity can lead to atrioventricular nodal block.

**II-14.  The answer is C.**  *(Chap. 233. SOLVD Investigators, N Engl J Med 325:293–302, 1991)*   The agents most typically used in the treatment of congestive heart failure—diuretics and cardiac glycosides—have never been formally shown to prolong survival. However, there have been at least four trials that have demonstrated benefit in the use of afterload reduction in the treatment of heart failure. Vasodilators, including angiotensin converting enzyme inhibitors and hydralazine, reduce left ventricular afterload; in the case of angiotensin inhibitors such as enalapril, anti-ischemic properties also may play a role by inhibiting the formation of angiotensin II in the coronary artery wall. There is no role for procainamide or other antiarrhythmics in treating patients with congestive heart failure unless the presence of ventricular tachycardia has been documented. Aspirin is indicated only for those with known coronary artery disease and a history of myocardial infarction or angina.

**II-15.   The answer is D.**   *(Chap. 240. Fowler, JAMA 266:99–103, 1991)*   Obstruction to cardiac filling and concomitant elevated right-sided pressures that produce elevated neck veins, congestive organomegaly, and pedal edema may be found in several conditions. It often is difficult to distinguish between pericardial tamponade, constrictive pericarditis, restrictive cardiomyopathy, and right ventricular myocardial infarction. In cardiac tamponade, accumulation of fluid in the pericardium is sufficient to cause significant obstruction to the inflow of blood to the ventricles. There is an elevation of intracardiac pressures, a limitation to diastolic filling, and florid cardiac failure. An important physical finding in tamponade is a paradoxical pulse, which is an exaggeration of the normal inspiratory augmentation of right ventricular volume, and a reciprocal reduction in left ventricular volume manifested by a significant inspiratory decrease in systolic arterial pressure. Paradoxical pulse is rare in constrictive pericarditis, restrictive cardiomyopathy, and right ventricular infarction. Right ventricular infarction usually is distinguishable by the absence of low electrocardiographic voltage and frequently can be distinguished by the presence of an injury current on the acute electrocardiogram. The distinction between constrictive pericarditis and restrictive cardiomyopathy is more difficult. In constrictive pericarditis, which results from the healing of a former acute pericarditis or a chronic pericardial effusion with obliteration of the pericardial cavity, filling is reduced abruptly when the elastic limit of the pericardium is reached, unlike tamponade, in which filling is impeded throughout diastole. Patients with constrictive pericarditis often appear to have a chronic illness. Venous pressures decline during inspiration (Kussmaul's), and congestive organomegaly is common, as is ascites. The apical pulse is reduced, and heart sounds are typically distant. An early heart sound, or pericardial knock, may occur 0.06 to 0.12 s after aortic valve closure, earlier than the third heart sound associated with ventricular failure. The electrocardiogram frequently displays low QRS voltage. Restrictive cardiomyopathy (e.g., resulting from amyloidosis, hemochromatosis, sarcoidosis, or scleroderma) can be distinguished from chronic constrictive pericarditis by the presence of a well-defined apical beat, frequent attacks of acute left ventricular failure, left ventricular hypertrophy, true S3, bundle branch block, and occasional Q waves on the electrocardiogram in the latter condition. In acute pericardial tamponade, diastolic right ventricular collapse is characteristic. In restrictive cardiomyopathy, myocardial thickness is frequently increased and abnormalities of the pericardium are absent. Right ventricular size is typically enlarged in right ventricular myocardial infarction. Echocardiographic findings consistent with constrictive pericarditis include the presence of a thickened pericardium (which is often calcified) in the absence of other findings. The patient in question may have tuberculous pericarditis that has progressed from the original acute stage to a chronic condition with obliteration of the pericardial space and loss of pericardial elasticity.

**II-16.   The answer is B.**   *(Chap. 231)*   The rhythm demonstrated in the electrocardiogram presented is multifocal atrial tachycardia, which is characterized by variable P-wave morphology and PR and RR intervals. Control of multifocal atrial tachycardia, which usually is associated with severe pulmonary disease, comes with improved ventilation and oxygenation. Carotid sinus massage, electrical cardioversion, and the administration of digitalis, verapamil, or quinidine are of little benefit, although verapamil may temporarily slow the ventricular rate.

**II-17.  The answer is D.**  *(Chap. 242)*   Given the clearly defined benefits of lipid lowering in patients at risk for ischemic heart disease, screening measurement of blood cholesterol levels (nonfasting) is recommended for all adult patients, especially young patients with a family history of premature heart disease. If hyperlipidemia is detected, secondary causes such as hypothyroidism, nephrotic syndrome, and uremia should be considered, along with stopping drugs that can aggravate the condition, including oral contraceptives, estrogens, thiazides, and beta blockers. Once these effects are considered, the primary step is attention to diet. Attempts should be made to bring the patient to normal weight and encourage the patient to undergo dietary therapy with reduced intake of calories, cholesterol, and saturated fat. However, patients who remain at high risk after 3 months of an intensive regimen of dietary therapy should be strongly considered for lipid-lowering drug therapy. Such therapy is recommended for any adult patient whose LDL cholesterol remains greater than 4.9 mmol/L (190 mg/dL) or greater than 4.1 mmol/L (160 mg/dL) in the presence of two or more risk factors. A more aggressive approach is recommended for patients with a prior history of ischemic heart disease. Other risk factors for early atherosclerosis include diabetes mellitus, hypertension, familial hyperlipidemias, hypothyroidism, systemic lupus, and homocysteinemia. Drugs that act to lower LDL cholesterol include bile acid-binding resins such as cholestyramine, nicotinic acid, and hydroxymethylglutaryl coenzyme A (HMG-CoA) reductase inhibitors.

**II-18.  The answer is C.**  *(Chap. 235)*   Atrial septal defect (ASD) is usually asymptomatic in childhood. Clinical presentation occurs in the third or fourth decade of life and results from atrial arrhythmias and pulmonary hypertension. A common cause of symptoms and of right heart failure is coexistent left ventricular dysfunction; even mild left atrial pressure is not tolerated well when transmitted into the systemic venous circulation. Secundum atrial septal defect is associated with a rightward axis on electrocardiography; the axis is leftward in primum defects. Echocardiography also reveals evidence of right ventricular volume overload, including abnormal motion of the ventricular septum (i.e., right-to-left movement) during diastole. Though small shunts are well tolerated, operative repair usually is indicated when the pulmonary flow is at least 1.5 times the systemic flow.

**II-19.  The answer is C.**  *(Chaps. 239, 240)*   The restrictive cardiomyopathies are characterized pathophysiologically by an impairment to ventricular filling. The cardiac silhouette is usually mildly, if at all, enlarged. Electrocardiography typically displays low-voltage QRS complexes, atrioventricular conduction defects, and a host of nonspecific arrhythmias. Echocardiography frequently reveals normal systolic and increased left ventricular wall thickness. In amyloidosis, the left ventricular wall appears to be "speckled." While primary cardiac amyloidosis typically produces diastolic dysfunction or restrictive cardiomyopathy as in this question, systolic dysfunction, arrhythmias, and orthostatic hypotension may be alternative presentations. Hemochromatosis also may cause a restrictive picture, but the speckled appearance noted in the echocardiogram would be absent. Alcoholism and viral infections typically cause dilated cardiomyopathies. Chronic tuberculous pericarditis can manifest clinical symptoms similar to those seen in restrictive cardiomyopathy. Patients with constrictive pericarditis have clinical presentations similar to those of patients with restrictive cardiomyopathy but tend to have normal ventricular wall thickness on echocardiography, pericardial calcification, and the absence of third or fourth heart sounds on chest auscultation.

**II-20.  The answer is B.**  *(Chaps. 235, 237)*   The chest x-rays presented in the question show enlargement of the right ventricle and main pulmonary artery and pulmonary vascular plethora, or "shunt" vasculature—classic findings for an atrial septal defect, which could well be asymptomatic in a 36-year-old woman. The chest x-ray of a patient with mitral stenosis and hemoptysis and dyspnea would show left atrial enlargement and, in the presence of primary or secondary tricuspid regurgitation, ascites and a large jugular venous v wave. Continuous murmur, widened systemic pulse pressure, and dyspnea on exertion in combination suggest patent ductus arteriosus, which would produce x-ray evidence of left ventricular and perhaps left atrial enlargement and shunt vasculature without right ventricular enlargement.

**II-21.   The answer is E.**   *(Chap. 235)*   Adults with mild pulmonic stenosis are generally asymptomatic. Unlike congenital aortic stenosis, this condition usually does not progress; thus, follow-up need not be frequent. The risk of endocarditis is somewhat lower for pulmonic valves than for the other heart valves, whether normal or stenotic. Clinical signs of mild pulmonic stenosis include a prominent *a* wave on jugular venous pulse, a normal electrocardiogram, and normal cardiac size on chest x-ray.

**II-22.   The answer is C.**   *(Chap. 235)*   Coarctation of the aorta usually occurs just distal to the origin of the left subclavian artery; if it arises above the left subclavian, blood pressure elevation may be evident only in the right arm. The associated murmur is continuous only if obstruction is severe; otherwise, a systolic ejection murmur is heard anteriorly and over the back. Coarctation of the aorta commonly is accompanied by a bicuspid aortic valve, which can produce the diastolic murmur of aortic regurgitation. X-ray findings include the "3" sign, caused by aortic dilation just proximal and distal to the area of stenosis, and rib notching, caused by increased collateral circulation through dilated intercostal arteries. Hypertension is the major clinical problem and may persist even after complete surgical correction. Unless hypertension is very severe or left ventricular failure has ensued, cardiac output responds normally to exercise.

**II-23.   The answer is D.**   *(Chap. 236)*   Acute rheumatic fever is a nonsuppurative complication of infection with group A streptococci. While the incidence of rheumatic fever has been declining, there have been recent domestic outbreaks on military bases. In such outbreaks the attack rate of rheumatic fever after streptococcal pharyngitis may be as high as 3 percent. The diagnosis of rheumatic fever requires two of the following major manifestations of the illness: carditis, migratory polyarthritis, chorea, erythema marginatum, and subcutaneous nodules. The patient in question has three such features. In addition to fever, he has evidence of a recent history of streptococcal infection by virtue of an elevated ASO titer. Even if streptococci cannot be isolated, it is preferable to administer a therapeutic course of parenteral penicillin (a single injection of 1.2 million units of benzathine penicillin IM for 10 days). Prophylactic therapy with penicillin should be administered indefinitely to prevent recurrent attacks. Glucocorticoid therapy is probably unnecessary, especially in patients without carditis. Arthritis can be managed entirely with salicylates. Prophylactic therapy for the associated movement disorder is unnecessary.

**II-24.   The answer is B.**   *(Chap. 231)*   The rhythm strip shows polymorphic ventricular tachycardia characteristic of torsades de pointes ("twisting of the points"). This life-threatening rhythm is associated with prolongation of the QT interval, resulting in this case from the administration of quinidine. The appropriate therapy is to discontinue the offending agent and withhold other agents that prolong the QT interval, such as procainamide. Hypokalemia can prolong the QT interval and result in this rhythm; however, this patient had normal serum electrolyte concentrations.

**II-25.   The answer is B.**   *(Chap. 231. Oates, N Engl J Med 325:1621–1629, 1991)*   Adenosine is currently approved for the termination of paroxysmal supraventricular tachycardias at doses of 6 mg and, if 6 mg fails, 12 mg. The primary mechanism of adenosine is to decrease conduction velocity through the AV node. As such, it is an ideal drug for acute termination of regular reentrant supraventricular tachycardia involving the AV node. Side effects may include chest discomfort and transient hypotension. The half-life is extremely short, and the side effects tend to be brief. Patients with wide complex tachycardia suggestive of ventricular tachycardia or known preexcitation syndrome should be treated with agents that decrease automaticity, such as quinidine and procainamide. However, in patients with apparent ventricular tachycardia who have neither a history of ischemic heart disease nor preexcitation syndrome, adenosine may be a useful diagnostic agent to determine whether a patient has a reentrant tachycardia, in which case the drug may terminate it; an atrial tachycardia, in which case the atrial activity may be unmasked; or a true, preexcited tachycardia, in which case adenosine will have no effect. While adenosine is not the recommended primary therapy for patients with wide complex tachyarrhythmia, patients with junctional tachycardia who have evidence of poor ventricular function or concomitant beta-adrenergic blockade may be reasonable candidates for its use.

**II-26.   The answer is B.**   *(Chap. 37)*   A fall in cardiac output from any cause leads to a decrease in effective arterial blood volume. Increased release of renin from juxtaglomerular cells in the kidney leads to the release of angiotensin I from its hepatically synthesized substrate, angiotensinogen. The decapeptide angiotensin I is proteolytically cleaved to angiotensin II, a vasoconstrictor and secretagogue for aldosterone. After release from the adrenal gland, aldosterone leads to renal proximal tubular salt and water retention. Renal vasoconstriction, which also causes proximal sodium absorption by increasing the filtration fraction, is also caused by the augmented sympathetic nervous system activity associated with diminished cardiac output. A fall in the glomerular filtration rate and the associated renal vasoconstriction furthers the edematous state.

**II-27.   The answer is E.**   *(Chap. 244. Willard, N Engl J Med 327:175–181, 1992)*   Management of patients with angina pectoris involves improving the ratio of oxygen delivery to oxygen utilization. Therfore, some degree of altered lifestyle may be necessary. Standard antianginal drugs include nitrates, beta-adrenergic blockers, and calcium-channel antagonists. Aspirin, an irreversible inhibitor of platelet cyclooxygenase, interferes with platelet activation and therefore may reduce the risk of coronary thrombosis at sites of atherosclerotic plaques. Administration of aspirin should be considered in all patients who have coronary artery disease but do not have aspirin allergy or risk factors for bleeding. Low-dose chronic aspirin therapy (100 to 325 mg orally every day or every other day) has been shown to decrease the likelihood of myocardial infarction in asymptomatic adult men, patients with asymptomatic ischemia after myocardial infarction, patients with chronic stable angina, and patients who have survived unstable angina and myocardial infarction. Aspirin is an important part of the therapeutic strategy for patients in the middle of a myocardial infarction who require thrombolytic therapy as well as for those with unstable angina.

**II-28.   The answer is A.**   *(Chap. 244)*   Nitrates are generalized smooth-muscle dilators whose direct effect on the vasculature cannot be blocked by any currently available agents. Long-acting preparations of nitroglycerin may be completely degraded by the liver in some patients and thus are generally less effective than sublingual forms. Because individual variability in metabolism is considerable, doses should be titrated against side effects and should not conform to a rigidly standardized regimen. Tolerance is common and must be considered if a patient fails to respond to a previously efficacious dose. Long-acting preparations such as transdermal patches are less likely to produce the nitrate-associated side effects of headaches and dizziness than are the more rapidly acting sublingual forms.

**II-29.   The answer is D.**   *(Chap. 236. Anderson, N Engl J Med 329:703–709, 1993)*   It is now recognized that most cases of acute myocardial infarction occur because of thrombus formation at the site of an atherosclerotic plaque, with resultant sudden coronary artery obstruction. The ability to lyse such clots by means of intravenous administration of plasminogen-activating agents has resulted in the reduction of mortality from early postmyocardial infarction. A problem with the use of thrombolytic therapy has been reocclusion of the reperfused arteries. Administration of adjunctive agents may reduce this risk. Aspirin has such an activity based on interference with platelet aggregation. Heparin forms a complex with antithrombin 3, blocking the action of several protease procoagulants, including thrombin. When given in association with tissue plasminogen activator, heparin reduces mortality to a greater degree than occurs when tissue plasminogen activator is given alone. Thrombolytic therapy including adjunctive heparin and aspirin is beneficial in patients at least up to 75 years of age. Absolute contraindications to the use of such thrombolytic therapy include major surgery or trauma within the past 6 weeks, gastrointestinal or genitourinary bleeding within 6 months, a known history of bleeding diathesis, and the presence of aortic dissection or pericarditis. Additional risks include the presence of a known intracranial tumor, neurosurgery, stroke, and head trauma within the past 6 months. This patient meets the required electrocardiographic criteria for an acute Q-wave infarction in evolution and is seen early enough in the event to be expected to receive a significant benefit from thrombolytic therapy. Even patients who are seen between 6 and 12 h after the onset of symptoms may experience some improvement from the initiation of thrombolytic therapy.

**II-30.** **The answer is D.** *(Chap. 237)* The echocardiogram shows that the left atrium is enlarged, and there is calcification and thickening of the mitral valve and chordal apparatus. The mitral leaflets show diastolic doming resulting from fusion of the valve commissures. These are the typical findings of rheumatic mitral stenosis, as exemplified by this 42-year-old woman. The aortic leaflets are also mildly thickened, consistent with rheumatic disease. The symptoms of the patient described in option A are suggestive of a left atrial myxoma. The patient in option B has acute mitral regurgitation. The patient in option C has mitral valve prolapse.

**II-31.** **The answer is E.** *(Chap. 205. Jarcho, N Engl J Med 321:1372, 1989)* Thyroid hormone acts directly via nuclear receptors to regulate myosin heavy chain gene transcription, thus increasing the level of myosin enzyme $V_1$ (fast myosin), whereas in response to pressure load on the heart, fetal forms of myosin such as $V_3$ (slow myosin) are induced. The c-*sis* proto-oncogene, which encodes for the B chain of platelet-derived growth factor; c-*myc* and c-*fos*, which encode for nuclear proteins involved in the regulation of the cell cycle; and c-*ras*, which encodes for guanosine-binding proteins, are all induced in myocardial tissue undergoing hypertrophy. Lineage analysis through the use of restriction fragment length polymorphisms has allowed the mapping of a gene (now known to be the adult myosin heavy chain gene) associated with familial hypertrophic cardiomyopathy to chromosome 14. Angiotensin II and beta agonists augment proto-oncogene expression, stimulate protein synthesis, and induce the synthesis of fetal forms of actin and myosin, leading to hypertrophy of smooth muscle.

**II-32.** **The answer is A.** *(Chap. 243)* The man described in the question probably has a right ventricular infarction complicating his inferior myocardial infarction because right atrial pressure is elevated out of proportion to left atrial (pulmonary capillary wedge) pressure. Cardiac output is depressed on the basis of an insufficient left heart filling pressure. The best treatment consists of the administration of fluids.

**II-33.** **The answer is C.** *(Chap. 246. Calhoun, N Engl J Med 323:1177–1183, 1991)* A hypertensive emergency is defined by the presence of end-organ damage in the setting of a severe elevation in blood pressure, usually with a diastolic pressure above 130 mmHg. Syndromes qualifying as a hypertensive emergency include hypertensive encephalopathy as in this patient, cerebral infarction, intracerebral hemorrhage, myocardial ischemia or infarction, pulmonary edema, aortic dissection, eclampsia, acute renal insufficiency, severe ophthalmoscopic changes, and severe microangiopathic hemolytic anemia. Those with a severe elevation of blood pressure but without evidence of end-organ injury can be managed in a more gradual fashion with attempts to lower the blood pressure over a period of 24 to 48 h. However, for those with true hypertensive emergencies, immediate therapy, even before the results of all laboratory tests are available, should be undertaken. Hypertensive emergencies require immediate but not precipitous lowering of the mean arterial pressure by approximately 25 percent with an attempt to reduce the diastolic blood pressure to 100 to 110 mmHg over a period of minutes to hours. Sodium nitroprusside is the drug of choice because it allows for titratable blood pressure reduction. However, the administration of this agent by continuous intravenous infusion requires continuous monitoring of the arterial blood pressure, which has been provided for in this patient. Diazoxide can be used in situations where arterial monitoring is not immediately available. However, the use of diazoxide may be complicated by hypotension and tachycardia (thereby exacerbating myocardial ischemia). Intravenous labetolol, a titratable beta blocker, and intravenous nicardipine, a calcium channel antagonist, may prove to be acceptable alternatives. The symptoms of hypertensive encephalopathy may include headache, nausea, vomiting, visual disturbances, confusion, and generalized weakness. Focal neurologic signs such as asymptomatic reflexes also may be seen.

**II-34.   The answer is B.**   *(Chaps. 227, 237)*   Inspiration, which augments systemic venous return because of negative intrathoracic pressure, causes accentuation of right-sided murmurs. Prolonged expiratory pressure against a closed glottis (Valsalva maneuver) reduces the intensity of most murmurs by diminishing both right and left ventricular filling. With reduced filling and thus reduced chamber size, the murmurs of hypertrophic cardiomyopathy and mitral valve prolapse increase. The cycle after a premature ventricular beat will have a larger stroke volume, and so the gradient across an obstructed semilunar valve (aortic or pulmonary) will increase, leading to a louder murmur. Squatting, which increases both venous return and chamber size as well as systemic arterial resistance, increases most murmurs, except those caused by hypertrophic cardiomyopathy and mitral valve prolapse. Sustained handgrip, which increases heart rate and systemic arterial pressure, often accentuates the murmurs of mitral stenosis and mitral regurgitation by impeding outflow and decreasing diastolic filling.

**II-35.   The answer is B.**   *(Chap. 247. Ernst, N Engl J Med 328:1167–1172, 1993)*   The vast majority of aortic aneurysms are due to atherosclerosis; 75 percent of such aneurysms are located in the distal aorta below the renal arteries. Although these aneurysms are typically asymptomatic, rupture may occur with devastating consequences. The prognosis is related to the size of the aneurysm as well as the presence of coexistent vascular diseases. Patients with aneurysms exceeding 6 cm who are not treated surgically have 50 percent mortality in 1 year, while those with lesions between 4 and 6 cm have 25 percent mortality during the first year. Surgical excision and replacement with a prosthetic graft are indicated for patients with aneurysms greater than 6 cm in diameter as well as in symptomatic patients or those with rapidly enlarging aneurysms regardless of the absolute diameter. Depending on the degree of operative risk, surgery also may be recommended in those with aneurysms with diameters between 5 and 6 cm. Contraindications to elective reconstruction include myocardial infarction within the past 6 months, intractable congestive heart failure, ongoing severe angina pectoris, severe obstructive lung disease, severe chronic renal failure, history of stroke with residual neurologic deficits, and life expectancy less than 2 years. An extensive preoperative evaluation including assessment of coronary disease, renal failure, and pulmonary function studies should be carried out, and if abnormalities are found, they should be ameliorated when possible. For patients in whom the diameter of the aneurysm is less than 6 cm or in whom there is significant operative risk, serial ultrasound may be helpful in defining a group that more urgently requires surgical intervention based on expansion of 0.5 cm or more over time.

**II-36.   The answer is B.**   *(Chap. 239)*   Echocardiographic evidence of a disproportionately thickened ventricular septum and systolic anterior motion of the mitral valve strongly suggests idiopathic hypertrophic subaortic stenosis (IHSS). The typical harsh systolic murmur usually does not radiate to the carotid arteries and decreases when ventricular volume enlarges with isometric exercise (e.g., handgrip). The carotid upstroke is brisk, and often bifid. Congestive failure often occurs because of reduced ventricular compliance despite normal ventricular systolic function. Malposition of the mitral apparatus, a result of the distorted septum, often leads to some degree of mitral regurgitation.

**II-37.   The answer is B.**   *(Chap. 228)*   A delta wave or slowed QRS upstroke is depicted. This finding occurs in the Wolff-Parkinson-White syndrome, in which accessory Kent bundles result in an apparently short PR interval caused by the bypassed AV node and early onset of the QRS complex. Left bundle branch block could result in marked initial delay, whereas right bundle branch block results in late delay. Left ventricular hypertrophy causes minor uniform QRS prolongation. Right ventricular infarction has little effect on QRS duration in the absence of right bundle branch block.

**II-38.   The answer is D.**   *(Chap. 194)*   Lack of motion (akinesis) in a segment of myocardium visualized by echo indicates tissue death, as does an area of reduced thallium accumulation during exercise that does not "fill in" at rest. Since pyrophosphate appears to bind calcium and macromolecules in irreversibly damaged myocardial cells, an area of increased uptake indicates myocardial infarction if the injection is performed between 48 and 72 h after a suspected transmural infarction. Using a combination of $[^{13}N]H_3$ (blood flow marker) and $[^{18}F]$deoxyglucose (glucose uptake), PET can identify nonviable myocardium if there is a defect in the uptake of both isotopes. Standard CT cannot detect global or regional left ventricular function, although fast, or cine, CT may be able to detect infarction by monitoring changes in ventricular volume and wall thickness.

**II-39.   The answer is C.**   *(Chap. 240)*   Acute pericarditis is associated with ST-segment elevation and frequently PR-segment depression. Usually reciprocal ST-segment depression is not present. T waves begin to invert only after the ST segment becomes isoelectric. Elevations in serum creatine phosphokinase levels to twice normal may be associated with uncomplicated pericarditis.

**II-40.   The answer is C.**   *(Chap. 233)*   Digitalis glycosides are effective in increasing myocardial contractility and in the treatment of certain atrial tachyarrhythmias. However, digoxin actually increases myocardial automaticity (increase in premature beats) and facilitates reentry (atrial tachycardias). Digoxin also slows conduction through AV nodal tissue and has central effects that can mimic vagal influence on the heart and thus may produce sinus arrest. Paroxysmal atrial tachycardia with variable block represents the classic rhythm of digitalis intoxication. Digoxin is profibrillatory, but its administration should not lead to atrial flutter.

**II-41.   The answer is E.**   *(Chap. 247)*   Complications of dissection of the aorta include loss of a major pulse, dissection into the pericardial or pleural space, and acute aortic regurgitation. When these events occur, surgical intervention is required. Because the risk of these complications is higher in persons with dissection of the ascending aorta, these persons usually are treated surgically. In contrast, persons with dissection of the descending aorta often can be treated medically. Persistence of pain, which suggests that dissection is continuing, is another indication for surgery.

**II-42.   The answer is C.**   *(Chap. 235)*   Left-to-right shunts occur in all types of atrial and ventricular septal defects but generally do not result in cyanosis, whereas large right-to-left shunts frequently do. The magnitude of the shunt depends on the size of the defect, the diastolic properties of both ventricles, and the relative impedance of the pulmonary and systemic circulations. Defects of the sinus venosus type occur high in the atrial septum near the entry of the superior vena cava or lower near the orifice of the inferior vena cava and may be associated with anomalous connection of the right inferior pulmonary vein to the right atrium. In the case of anomalous origin of the left coronary artery from the pulmonary artery, as pulmonary vascular resistance declines immediately after birth, perfusion of the left coronary artery from the pulmonary trunk ceases and the direction of flow in the anomalous vessel reverses. Twenty percent of patients with this defect can survive to adulthood because of myocardial blood supply flowing totally through the right coronary artery. In the absence of pulmonary hypertension, blood will flow from the aorta to the pulmonary artery throughout the cardiac cycle, resulting in a "continuous" murmur at the left sternal border. In total anomalous pulmonary venous connection, all the venous blood returns to the right atrium; therefore, an interatrial communication is required and right-to-left shunts with cyanosis are common.

**II-43.** **The answer is D.** *(Chap. 243)* While prompt initiation of thrombolytic therapy during an acute myocardial the infarction is associated with improvement in mortality and limitation of the size of the infarct, all thrombolytic agents, including tissue plasminogen activator, are associated with an increased risk of major bleeding. These agents should not be given if there is a history of a cerebrovascular accident, a surgical procedure within the past 2 weeks, active peptic ulcer disease, or marked hypertension during acute presentation (systolic pressure greater than 180 or diastolic pressure greater than 100 mmHg). Other situations in which the risk of bleeding may be higher, such as advanced age, are not absolute contraindications, but the potential benefit from the administration of thrombolytic therapy should be considered carefully in each case.

**II-44.** **The answer is C.** *(Chap. 243)* Apical systolic murmurs associated with a myocardial infarction may represent either mitral regurgitation (on the basis of papillary muscle rupture or newly dilated heart size) or ventricular septal defect. In both conditions, large *v* waves may be recorded in the pulmonary capillary wedge position. In the case of a ventricular septal defect but not mitral regurgitation, there will be an increase in the partial pressure of oxygen as a catheter is advanced from the right atrium to the right ventricle.

**II-45.** **The answer is D.** *(Chap. 244. Fuster, N Engl J Med 326:242, 310, 1992)* Any patient with recent onset of severe and frequent angina, accelerating angina, or angina at rest is considered to have unstable angina. Such patients are likely to have one or more stenoses in major coronary arteries and require emergent management. Hospitalization with identification and treatment of predisposing conditions (e.g., heart failure, fever, thyrotoxicosis) is indicated. Since thrombus formation frequently complicates this condition, intravenous heparin followed by oral aspirin should be given. Beta blockers and calcium channel blocking drugs should be administered if possible. Antiarrhythmics are required only in the presence of specific arrhythmias. Intravenous nitroglycerin is effective but requires continuous blood pressure monitoring. If evidence of ischemia, based on clinical symptoms or electrocardiographic findings, does not abate within 24 to 48 h of aggressive medical management, diagnostic cardiac catheterization should be performed.

**II-46.** **The answer is B.** *(Chap. 248)* Conditions associated with stasis, vascular damage, or hypercoagulability lead to an increased risk for deep venous thrombosis. This risk is increased by any condition leading to immobility, such as recuperation after a myocardial infarction (of any severity), a major thoracic resection (even if the cancer was completely resected), and trauma or an operation involving the hip or leg. A wrist fracture in an elderly woman probably would not lead to any increased risk if her baseline mobility was present. Hypercoagulable states include systemic cancers; pregnancy; exogenous or endogenous estrogens; deficiencies of antithrombin III, protein C, and protein S; circulating lupus anticoagulant (manifested by elevated partial thromboplastin time); and myeloproliferative disease.

**II-47.** **The answer is A.** *(Chap. 229)* A gradient between the left atrium (as measured by the pulmonary capillary wedge tracing) and the left ventricle in diastole indicates mitral stenosis as exemplified by the woman with a history of rheumatic fever and hemoptysis. The intravenous drug abuser with mitral regurgitation caused by mitral valve vegetation would exhibit large *v* waves on the pulmonary capillary wedge tracing. The aortic regurgitation associated with Marfan's syndrome would cause an equilibration between left ventricular and peripheral pressures. A feature of severe aortic regurgitation that occurs when left ventricular pressure exceeds pulmonary capillary wedge (i.e., left atrial) pressure during early diastole may result in premature mitral valve closure. In aortic stenosis, as exemplified by the elderly man with left ventricular hypertrophy, the left ventricular pressure is higher than the aortic pressure during systole. In pericardial tamponade, as might be seen in the patient with lymphoma, there is equalization of right and left diastolic pressures.

**II-48.   The answer is D.**   *(Chap. 178. McAlister et al, Ann Intern Med 110:339–345, 1989)* This patient's clinical scenario is consistent with secondary manifestations of Lyme disease, which is caused by the spirochete *Borrelia burgdorferi*. Her exposure presumably occurred on Cape Cod, a high-risk area of New England. Lyme disease occurs in three stages: the initial infection shortly after the tick bite, manifested by a skin rash (erythema chronica migrans) and often flu like symptoms; a secondary stage with cardiac and/or neurologic signs and symptoms; and a tertiary stage with arthritis.

Lyme carditis most often is manifested by AV nodal conduction disturbances, including first-, second-, or third-degree heart block. Antibiotic therapy, typically high-dose penicillin, usually leads to resolution of the heart block without the need for permanent pacing, although a temporary pacemaker may be necessary. Spirochetes can be detected within cardiac tissue, suggesting that the carditis is due to the presence of the organism. Other cardiac manifestations include nonspecific ECG changes, myocardial inflammation, and left ventricular dysfunction.

Cocaine can result in myocardial ischemia and infarction, but this would more likely be an acute complication, making the timing incorrect in this case. *Ixodes dammini* is the deer tick whose bite transmits the infection to humans. This patient's presentation is inconsistent with an acute coronary embolus. Complete heart block is not commonly seen with HIV carditis.

**II-49.   The answer is E.**   *(Chap. 243)*   This patient is most likely having a ventricular septal rupture and a subsequent defect, a not uncommon complication of myocardial infarction (MI) that explains the need to auscultate the heart on a daily basis during the early period after a myocardial infarction. Myocardial rupture after an MI can occur either in the free wall, with bleeding into the pericardium, tamponade, and a high incidence of fatality, or in the ventricular septum, with a greater potential for successful therapy despite the fact that this is a critical complication. Therapy is geared toward decreasing afterload and systemic vascular resistance. Interventions to be considered include IV nitrogylcerin, IV sodium nitroprusside, and/or *intraaortic* balloon counterpulsation. Often cardiac surgery with septal repair is the only viable long-term intervention; however, this is best undertaken when the patient has stabilized and ideally once the infarction has healed. In many cases, the patient does not stabilize, at which point acute surgical intervention is indicated.

**II-50.   The answer is D.**   *(Chap. 243)*   Creatinine phosphokinase (CK) increases within 4 to 8 h after a myocardial infarction (MI), returning to normal by 72 h. The MB isoenzyme has more specificity than does total CK for myocardial tissue. MB1 is produced by cleavage of CK-MB2; a ratio of CK-MB2 to CK-MB1 greater than 1.5 is highly sensitive for the diagnosis of an MI. The cardiac-specific troponins were recently demonstrated to be cardiac-specific markers, based on the development of antibodies that distinguish the amino acid differences between the cardiac and skeletal forms of troponin. Troponin is more sensitive than CK-MB for the detection of myocardial damage, allowing the diagnosis of "microinfarction" that is seen sometimes in unstable angina. In addition, both cardiac troponin T and cardiac troponin I remain elevated for over 1 week, allowing the diagnosis of MIs occurring more than 48 h before presentation. Troponin I and troponin T are the tests of choice rather than the previously used LDH and its isoenzymes. Myoglobin rises within hours after an MI but also declines rapidly. Tropomyosin has not been used clinically.

**II-51.   The answer is E.**   *(Chap. 119. King et al., Ann Intern Med:8:325–332, 1980)* Heparininduced thrombocytopenia (HIT) syndrome occurs in 1 to 5 percent of patients treated with heparin and probably is due to platelet aggregation caused by heparin- induced antibodies. Therapy usually consists of discontinuation of the heparin, and the use of other anticoagulants, in particular warfarin, with several days of overlap if possible. If the platelet count falls beneath approximately 50,000/μL, heparin should be discontinued. If proximal deep venous thrombosis is present, consideration may have to be given to the placement of an inferior vena caval filter. Arterial thrombosis also may be a manifestation of the HIT syndrome and represents a separate indication for the discontinuation of heparin. The thrombosis is thought to be due to antibody-mediated platelet activation, which can lead to platelet aggregation.

**II-52.** **The answer is B.** *(Chap. 231)* VPCs are a common finding seen in approximately 60 percent of men who undergo Holter monitoring; in the absence of known coronary artery disease (CAD), they are not of particular significance. They can cause symptoms such as palpitations, perhaps as a result of the cannon *a* waves that can result from contraction of the ventricle while the mitral valve is still open. Symptoms also may stem from the fact that stroke volume often is decreased by decreased overall ventricular filling. Rarely, frequent VPCs can result in syncopal symptoms on this basis. In patients with known CAD, the incidence (80 percent), frequency, and significance of VPCs rise. Both the frequency (>10/h), and the complexity (couplets or greater) have been associated with increased mortality in this patient population. Epidemiologic evidence suggests an increase in the frequency of VPCs with advancing age.

**II-53.** **The answer is D.** *(Chap. 226)* Echocardiography is a valuable tool in a variety of clinical settings. It provides an estimate of left ventricular function and can help localize regional wall motion abnormalities. When Doppler signals are used, the continuity equation can be applied to the flow across a stenotic valve to derive an estimated valve area. With intravenous administration of a contrast agent, most often agitated saline, the right atrium and right ventricle can be opacified. Most of these bubbles are trapped by the pulmonary circulation. Therefore, the appearance of bubbles in the left atrium establishes the presence of an atrial septal defect. Often echocardiographic images also can specify the type of atrial septal defect (secundum, primum, sinus venosus, or coronary sinus). An echocardiogram may demonstrate a thickened or "shaggy" pericardium, suggesting pericarditis; however, its sensitivity and specificity are not particularly high.

**II-54.** **The answer is C.** *(Chap. 232)* A resting cardiac cell has low intracellullar sodium, but higher potassium, as opposed to the extracellular compartment which has high sodium but lower potassium. These differences, which are maintained by the ATP- dependent $Na^+$-$K^+$ pump, result in the resting potential seen in myocytes. A slow inward current of $Ca^{2+}$ occurs during the plateau phase of the action potential, ultimately leading to a larger release of calcium from the sarcoplasmic reticulum, and myocyte contraction after calcium complexes with troponin C and removes this repression of contraction. Repolarization consists of the regaining of calcium by the sarcoplasmic reticulum by pumping against a concentration gradient.

**II-55.** **The answer is B.** *(Chaps. 230, 246)* This elderly patient has developed significant symptomatic sinus bradycardia and sinus arrest while on a beta blocker. She is receiving the beta blocker as therapy for hypertension, not as an antianginal medication. Some patients, particularly elderly ones, can be quite sensitive to AV nodal blocking agents such as beta blockers and calcium channel blockers such as diltiazem, particularly when used in combination. Therefore, one would want to establish the continued need for a permanent pacemaker in this patient when she was not on an AV nodal agent. Her ongoing symptoms, borderline vital signs, and acute fracture all argue for stabilizing her rhythm status through a temporary pacer insertion.

**II-56.** **The answer is B.** *(Chap. 231)* Beta blockers, even selective ones, carry a risk of stimulating beta$_2$ receptors and worsening bronchospasm. Any of the other medications or alternatives listed could be used more safely in this patient. Digoxin requires time to load and to establish a reasonable therapeutic level. Both verapamil and diltiazem have a rapid onset of action and can be administered intravenously. The well-documented onset of symptoms in this case most likely corresponds to the onset of atrial fibrillation, and would allow one to proceed with electrical cardioversion with a low risk for embolism. However, a more reasonable treatment plan might be to establish rate control and complete the evaluation before cardioversion. In this process, one might have the opportunity to correct electrolytes such as magnesium and potassium, improve the pulmonary status, and treat pneumonia, all of which might be factors that could result in recurrent atrial fibrillation after a successful electrical cardioversion.

**II-57.   The answer is C.**   *(Chap. 231)*   This patient did not suffer an allergic reaction to procainamide. Torsades de pointes on the basis of a prolonged QT interval would have caused an unstable complex. The most likely explanation for his rhythm was one-to-one conduction of atrial flutter through the AV node. This could have been prevented through an adequate AV nodal blockade before the administration of procainamide. Quinidine, which could have resulted in the same response, also requires adequate AV nodal blockade before its administration. Both quinidine and procainamide actually speed conduction through the AV node and must be used cautiously, ideally after the adequate administration of a nodal agent.

**II-58.   The answer is C.**   *[Chap. 229. Baim DS, Grossman W (eds), Cardiac Catheterization, Angiography and Intervention, 5th ed. Williams & Wilkins, 1996]*   Coronary catheterization is an important diagnostic tool that is used routinely on a daily basis in scores of hospitals nationally. The frequency of its uncomplicated use is tempered by the potential risk for significant morbidity and a finite possibility of mortality. Older patients (over 80 years) appear to be at higher risk for mortality. Class IV CHF, left main disease, and a low ejection fraction (below 30 percent) are all associated with a a 10-fold greater chance for mortality than is the case in patients without these conditions. In addition, severe valvular abnormalities, especially when combined with significant coronary disease, renal insufficiency, and advanced cerebrovascular and peripheral vascular disease, carry an increased risk of death or serious complications from cardiac catheterization.

**II-59.   The answer is A.**   *(Chap. 244)*   Technetium 99m sestamibi differs from thallium 201 in that sestamibi does not redistribute as well as thallium does in hibernating myocardium. Positron emission tomography is the "gold standard" for detecting myocardial viability but is not routinely available. Thallium, which is dependent on the Na$^+$-, K$^+$-ATPase pump for uptake, can be used to assess the viability of myocardial tissue. Dipyrimadole is an inhibitor of adenosine metabolism and can result in bronchospasm. Therefore, caution must be used in patients with severe (FEV$_1$ below 40 percent of predicted) obstructive pulmonary disease. Injection of sestamibi can be done safely during chest pain. Normal perfusion during pain, as well as hypoperfusion that fails to reverse with the resolution of symptoms, suggests that the symptoms do not stem from inadequate myocardial perfusion.

**II-60.   The answer is D.**   *(Chaps. 230, 231)*   Digitalis intoxication is a potentially life-threatening complication of digitalis therapy. Both cardiac and noncardiac manifestations of digitalis toxicity may be seen. Virtually every type of cardiac arrhythmia has been described. Noncardiac manifestations include disturbances such as blurred vision and a sensation of a halo surrounding lights. Gastrointestinal complaints are also common among patients suffering from digitalis intoxication. Gingival hyperplasia is a complication of nifedipine and other calcium channel antagonists but is not secondary to digitalis use.

**II-61.   The answer is E.**   *(Chap. 247)*   Cystic medial necrosis is a descriptive term for pathologic changes seen in the aorta. This entity consists of degeneration of collagen and elastin fibers in the tunica media of the aorta as well as cell loss in the medial layer. A mucoid material replaces the space occupied by the degenerated cells. This abnormality typically is seen in the proximal aorta and the sinuses of Valsalva, leading to weakness and aneursym formation. Cystic medial necrosis is a risk factor for aortic dissection.

**II-62. The answer is D.** *(Chap. 247. Nienaber et al, N Engl J Med 328:1, 1993)* Confirmation of aortic dissection can be achieved through a variety of imaging techniques. Aortography can establish the diagnosis as well as the entry point of the dissection, the false and true lumen, and the intimal flap. However, this dye study is an invasive procedure and may be difficult to obtain. Transthoracic echocardiography can be performed easily and rapidly with a sensitivity of 60 to 85 percent, and perhaps even higher for proximal ascending aortic dissections. Transesophageal echocardiography is very sensitive and specific (98 percent) for ascending and descending aortic dissections; however, this technique is somewhat limited in detecting arch dissections. CT or MRI yields the greatest degree of information, including the site of the intimal flap, the extent of dissection, the presence of intramural hemorrhage, and antegrade versus retrograde flow. The limitations include local unavailability and a lack of experts and inability to obtain the study on an emergent basis.

**II-63. The answer is B.** *(Chaps. 227, 239)* The murmur of hypertrophic cardiomyopathy is caused by the turbulence created by flow past the intracavitary obstruction in the left ventricle. Therefore, all maneuvers that increase left ventricular blood volume will "move" the muscular obstruction protruding into the outflow track away from the opposite wall, decreasing the obstruction and the murmur. Ventricular volume-expanding maneuvers include squatting and passive leg raising. Conversely, maneuvers that decrease left ventricle size increase the outflow obstruction and the intensity of the murmur. Such maneuvers include the Valsalva maneuver (decreased venous return to the right ventricle), standing, and the inhalation of amyl nitrate, which is no longer routinely used.

**II-64. The answer is D.** *(Chaps. 226, 233)* Pulmonary edema can be categorized as either cardiogenic or noncardiogenic. In cardiogenic pulmonary edema, an increase in pulmonary venous pressure is antecedent to the interstitial edema that progressses to frank alveolar edema. Pulmonary edema is influenced by the counterbalancing Starling forces. Pulmonary edema occurring without a preceding increase in pulmonary venous pressure but still resulting from an imbalance of Starling forces is known as noncardiogenic pulmonary edema. Examples of this condition include shock (e.g., hemorrhagic pancreatitis, gram-negative septicemia, postcardiopulmonary bypass), aspiration, and widespread pulmonary infections. At least three forms of pulmonary edema that are not due to increases in vessel permeability, decreased lymphatic flow, or other alterations in Starling forces have been identified: narcotic overdose, high-altitude exposure in unconditioned individuals, and neurogenic pulmonary edema. Sarcoidosis can cause cardiogenic pulmonary edema from cardiomyopathy or dyspnea from diffuse lung disease.

**II-65. The answer is F.** *(Chaps. 242, 391. National Cholesterol Education Program, Adult Treatment Panel II, National Institute of Health, Pub 93-3095, 9/1993. Scandinavian Simvastatin Survival Study Group. Lancet 344:1383–1389, 1994)* Several large-scale, randomized, placebo-controlled studies have demonstrated the benefits of HMG coreductase inhibitors in both patients with known coronary artery disease and patients at significant risk for cardiac events without a prior known myocardial infarction. These studies have documented a statistically significant decrease in cardiac events and the need for invasive cardiac procedures in both patients with coronary disease and those at significant risk for cardiac disease. Importantly, the 4S trial demonstrated decreased total mortality in patients treated with this type of agent, helping to diminish prior concerns about the lack of an overall benefit in regard to total mortality in patients treated with lipid-lowering agents. HMG coreductase inhibitors are the most potent medications for lowering LDL. Their mechanism of action is due to inhibition of the key steps in cholesterol biosynthesis, leading to an up-regulation of LDL receptors and increased clearance of LDL from the circulation. Patients with known homozygous familial hypercholesterolemia have various genotypes that lead to a complete absence or functional absence of the LDL receptor; therefore, they may have a minimal response to these agents because of their inability to up-regulate LDL receptors.

**II-66.   The answer is C.**   *[Chap. 242. National Cholesterol Education Program, Adult Treatment Panel II, National Institute of Health, Pub 93-3095, 9/1993. Davies MJ, Woolf N., Br Heart J 69(Suppl):6–11, 1993]*   The Adult Treatment Panel (ATP) II report released in 1993 based its conclusions on large amounts of previous epidemiologic evidence, and generated an updated consensus on cardiovascular risk factors. Tobacco smoke promotes atherosclerosis in a multifactorial fashion: promoting thrombosis, injuring endothelial cells, adversely affecting the lipid profile, stimulating catecholamine, and even possibly causing mutagenesis and clonal expansion of vascular smooth muscle cells. ATP II confirmed that male gender and low HDL associated with increased cardiac events and recognized the protective benefits of elevated HDL levels (> 45 mg/dL). The presence of peripheral vascular disease should raise the suspicion of coexistent coronary artery disease. Patients with vascular disease may be free of angina because of their limited ability to ambulate. The eliciting of a family history of coronary artery disease is aimed at uncovering an underlying genetic component for cardiac risk. This genetic component reflects a history of premature coronary disease, which is defined as disease evident before age 55 years in a male relative or 65 in a female relative. The incidence of coronary disease in the West is so high that coronary disease in older first-degree relatives has fewer implications for a given patient than does evidence of familial premature disease.

**II-67.   The answer is E.**   *(Chap. 242. Libby, Circulation 91:2844, 1995)*   The fatty streak is the initial lesion of atherosclerosis, resulting from lipid deposition in the arterial wall and subsequent recruitment of monoyctes and lymphocytes via endothelial attachment to adhesion molecules such as VCAM-1 and ICAM-1 and other receptors, such as members of the selectin family. Inflammation and mitogenesis play significant roles in atherosclerosis through leukocytes and elaboration of mediators such as cytokines (e.g., TNFα, interleukins, and growth factors, such as PDGF). Early atherosclerosis occurs in an abluminal direction, with lesions not being apparent on a routine coronary angiography, since only the lumen is defined. Nevertheless, these non-flow-limiting-lesions are often responsible for myocardial infarction resulting from plaque rupture. Risk factor modification may decrease the likelihood of plaque formation and rupture. For example, lipid-lowering agents have caused only minimal changes in the frequency of coronary stenoses measured by angiography, yet a major clinical benefit has been noted.

**II-68.   The answer is D.**   *(Chap. 240)*   This patient has a history and physical examination consistent with pericardial effusion and possibly hemodynamically significant tamponade. Her history of breast cancer raises the possibility of malignant pericardial effusion. Empiric treatment with escalating doses of diuretics may in fact have worsened her status by decreasing her ventricular volume and pressure, thus decreasing the difference between the intrapericardial pressure and the intraventricular pressure and worsening the effects of the tamponade. On examination, the narrow pulse pressure is one element that suggests the possibility of tamponade. No pulsus paradoxus is seen in approximately 10 percent of patients with tamponade and can reflect either an atrial septal defect or, perhaps more likely in this clinical scenario, preexisting increased diastolic pressure. Typically, the neck veins would be elevated. Bronchial breath sounds at the inferior border of the left scapula constitute Ewart's sign and are suggestive of pericardial effusion. ECG changes associated with pericardial effusion include low voltage and electrical alternans as the heart swings within the pericardial fluid. An echocardiogram would be very helpful in this clinical situation to establish the pericardial fluid volume and diagnose tamponade. The definitive diagnosis of tamponade is made by measuring intrapericardial pressure with simultaneous hemodynamic monitoring. The intrapericardial pressure should fall after pericardiocentesis. Cytology from the fluid in this case returned positive for recurrent breast carcinoma; metastatic deposits are frequently found on the pericardial surface but less commonly in the myocardium.

**II-69.   The answers are A, True; B, True; C, True; D, True; E, True.**

**II-70.   The answer is A-Y, B-N, C-Y, D-Y, E-N.** *(Chap. 228)* The electrocardiographic T wave represents myocardial repolarization, and its configuration can be altered nonspecifically by metabolic abnormalities, drugs, neural activity, and ischemia through a dispersion effect on the activation or repolarization of action potentials. Although myocardial ischemia and subendocardial infarction can produce deep, symmetric T-wave inversions which would result in tachyarrhythmias and syncope, noncardiac phenomena such as intracerebral hemorrhage can similarly affect ventricular repolarization. Hyperkalemia is manifested by tall, peaked T waves, not inverted ones. Hypocalcemia is manifested by prolonged QT intervals.

**II-71.   The answer is A-Y, B-N, C-Y, D-N, E-Y.** *(Chap. 228)* Hyperkalemia leads to partial depolarization of cardiac cells. As a result, there is slowing of the upstroke of the action potential as well as reduced duration of repolarization. The T wave becomes peaked, the RS complex widens and may merge with the T wave (giving a sine-wave appearance), and the P wave becomes shallow or disappears. Prominent U waves are associated with hypokalemia; ST-segment prolongation is associated with hypocalcemia.

**II-72.   The answer is A-N, B-N, C-Y, D-N, E-N.** *(Chaps. 2, 244)* Making a test's cutoff point for positivity more stringent (i.e., > 2.0 mm of ST depression rather than 0.5 mm) will enhance specificity (there will be fewer false positives) at the expense of sensitivity (there will be more false negatives). Bayesian analysis dictates that low prior probability (e.g., 10 percent—odds 1:9) can be enhanced only to a 50 percent posttest (or posterior) probability for a test with the given operating characteristics [1:9 × sensitivity / (1 − specificity)], where sensitivity is defined as the probability of a positive test result in a patient with the disease and specificity is defined as the probability of a negative test result in a patient without the disease. Thallium scans can increase the sensitivity for detecting coronary artery disease by about 20 percent and can increase specificity by 10 percent. Such scans are most useful in patients with an uninterpretable or nondiagnostic electrocardiogram resulting from failure to achieve 85 percent of the predicted maximal heart rate, left ventricular hypertrophy, left bundle branch block, or drug effects. A prior myocardial infarction can be inferred if a defect on thallium scintigraphy noted during exercise also fails to be perfused at rest. Blood pressure and heart rate should rise during a normal exercise tolerance test. Failure of the blood pressure to rise or an actual decrease may suggest global left ventricular dysfunction.

**II-73.   The answer is A-Y, B-Y, C-N, D-Y, E-N.** *(Chaps. 228, 231)* The electrocardiogram presented in the question demonstrates nonparoxysmal junctional tachycardia. The junctional rhythm is at a rate of 82 beats per minute, which is faster than the usual escape nodal rhythm. Retrograde P waves can be seen. This rhythm can occur after mitral valve surgery and in association with digitalis toxicity, acute myocarditis, and inferior myocardial infarction. These processes all can irritate the atrioventricular node and accelerate its action.

**II-74.   The answer is A-N, B-Y, C-N, D-Y, E-Y.** *(Chap. 232. Cohn, N Engl J Med 311:819, 1984)* Stroke volume and cardiac output at rest are not sensitive indexes of myocardial dysfunction. Stroke volume is often normal, though at the expense of higher end-diastolic volume (Frank-Starling mechanism). Even when stroke volume begins to diminish, cardiac output can be maintained by increases in heart rate. However, when the heart is stressed by exercise, cardiac output does not rise proportionately to oxygen consumption and left ventricular end-diastolic pressure rises more than it does in normal controls. Although plasma norepinephrine levels are elevated in persons with left ventricular dysfunction, myocardial levels are typically low.

**II-75. The answer is A-Y, B-N, C-N, D-Y, E-N.** *(Chap. 70)* The antihypertensive agent prazosin blocks alpha$_1$ receptors that mediate vasoconstriction. Clonidine is also an antihypertensive agent but works by stimulating alpha$_2$ receptors in the brainstem, thereby reducing sympathetic outflow. Phenylephrine, an alpha$_1$ agonist with pressor effects, is frequently employed in over-the-counter nasal decongestants. By antagonizing presynaptic alpha$_2$ receptors, yohimbine increases parasympathetic activity that may augment penile blood flow and may be useful in the treatment of erectile impotence. Isoproterenol stimulates beta$_1$ and beta$_2$ receptors and can increase chronotropy in the setting of heart block.

**II-76. The answer is A-N, B-Y, C-N, D-N, E-Y.** *(Chap. 231)* Persons who have Wolff-Parkinson-White syndrome are predisposed to develop two major types of atrial tachyarrhythmias. The first, which resembles paroxysmal supraventricular tachycardia (SVT) with reentry, involves the atrioventricular node in anterograde conduction and the bypass tract in retrograde conduction. This tachycardia typically has a narrow QRS complex and can be treated similarly to other forms of SVT. The other, more dangerous tachyarrhythmia (present in the man described in the question) is atrial fibrillation, which usually is conducted anterograde down the bypass tract and has a wide QRS configuration. The ventricular rate in such a situation is quite rapid, and cardiovascular collapse or ventricular fibrillation may result. The usual treatment is direct-current cardioversion, though quinidine may slow conduction through the bypass tract. Verapamil and propranolol have little effect on the bypass tract and may further depress ventricular function, which already is compromised by the rapid rate. Digoxin may accelerate conduction down the bypass tract and lead to ventricular fibrillation.

**II-77. The answer is A-Y, B-Y, C-Y, D-N, E-N.** *(Chap. 39)* Frequent premature ventricular complexes (defined as >30 per minute), salvos or nonsustained ventricular tachycardia, and a low ejection fraction (<20 percent) are associated with an increased risk of sudden cardiac death. Advanced forms (triplets or longer) are more predictive of risk than is even a high density of unifocal premature beats. It is unclear whether suppressing ectopic activity can reduce risk. Conventional techniques of cardiopulmonary resuscitation require lung inflation every 15 s and chest compressions 80 times per minute if only one provider is present. In the case of ventricular fibrillation or ventricular tachycardia in a pulseless patient, the first shock should be delivered at 200 joules, followed by additional higher-energy shocks (up to 360 joules in the absence of a response). Intravenous sodium bicarbonate, formerly recommended, is no longer considered routinely necessary and may be dangerous (unless pH monitoring indicates profound acidosis).

**II-78. The answer is A-Y, B-Y, C-N, D-N, E-N.** *(Chap. 235)* Atrial septal defects (ASDs) of the sinus venous type are located high in the atrial septum and commonly are associated with anomalous pulmonary venous return. The magnitude of the shunt depends on defect size, relative ventricular compliance, and the relative resistances in the pulmonary and systemic circuits but not on total blood flow. The systolic ejection murmur associated with ASD arises from increased flow across the pulmonic valve; a diastolic rumble resulting from increased flow across the tricuspid valve is common and should not necessarily be attributed to mitral stenosis, which is associated with ASD in a disorder known as Lutembacher's syndrome. Most persons with a large ASD are asymptomatic until late in adult life.

**II-79. The answer is A-Y, B-Y, C-N, D-Y, E-Y.** *(Chap. 227)* Large *a* waves indicate contraction of the right atrium against increased resistance, as might occur with obstruction at the tricuspid valve (tricuspid stenosis) or more commonly with increased resistance to right ventricular filling. Right ventricular filling could be impaired in pulmonary stenosis or in any condition that causes pulmonary hypertension, such as multiple pulmonary emboli. The *a* wave also will be pronounced if the right atrium contracts while the tricuspid valve is closed by right ventricular systole, as would be the case in atrioventricular dissociation, complete heart block, or junctional rhythm. The *a* wave is absent in patients with atrial fibrillation, since no organized atrial contraction occurs.

**II-80.** **The answer is A-Y, B-N, C-N, D-N, E-Y.** *(Chaps. 235, 237)* The risks of cardiac surgery always must be weighed against the potential benefits. The risk is extremely low in the correction of atrial septal defects, and surgery may prevent the development of atrial arrhythmia and pulmonary hypertension, complications that can arise later in life. Small ventricular septal defects, in constrast, almost never cause hemodynamic problems later in life. The presence of Eisenmenger's reaction—cyanosis and a right-to-left shunt from pulmonary hypertension—is a contraindication to surgery regardless of the underlying lesion. Persons with symptomatic aortic stenosis warrant consideration for surgery because hemodynamic deterioration can ensue quickly. Chronic mitral regurgitation, however, is far more indolent, and mild symptoms or acute decompensation from a correctable cause does not necessarily require surgical intervention.

**II-81.** **The answer is A-N, B-N, C-N, D-Y, E-Y.** *(Chap. 245. Kuntz, N Engl J Med 325:17, 1991)* Safe and effective (it reduces gradients from 75 to 15 mmHg), balloon valvuloplasty is the preferred treatment for pulmonary stenosis. Rheumatic mitral stenosis secondary to commissural fusion with associated leaflet thickening is the mitral lesion most amenable to treatment with balloon dilatation. Such dilatation can increase valve size to 2.0 cm$^2$ or more but usually not to the normal 3.5 to 5.0 cm$^2$. The indications for balloon aortic valvuloplasty in patients who are poor operative risks include congenital, rheumatic, and acquired calcific aortic stenosis. In the last group, valvuloplasty fractures leaflet calcium and provides new hinge points along which leaflets may open. Surprisingly, stroke is an uncommon complication of this procedure, and most patients experience a reduction in symptoms. The best results are obtained in patients with preserved left ventricular function before the procedure. Restenosis is common but can be treated with repeat aortic valvuloplasty.

**II-82.** **The answer is A-Y, B-Y, C-N, D-Y, E-Y.** *(Chap. 232)* The cardiac output must increase during exercise, since oxygen demand is greater. This increase is accomplished by a physiologic augmentation in stroke volume and heart rate. The pumping action of hyperventilation increases ventricular filling, and therefore stroke volume rises. Catecholamine synthesis and secretion increase, leading to a faster heart rate and greater stroke volume through augmented myocardial contractility. Since blood pressure is determined by cardiac output and resistance, once cardiac output increases, blood pressure also tends to rise. However, vasodilation in muscle beds counteracts this tendency somewhat. In a normal heart, catecholamine-mediated changes in the force-volume curve lead to decreased or similar end-diastolic volumes (filling pressure) during exercise; heart failure is characterized by marked and sometimes dangerous rises in end-diastolic volume, possibly even to the point of pulmonary edema.

**II-83.** **The answer is A-N, B-Y, C-Y, D-N, E-Y.** *(Chap. 237. Marks, N Engl J Med 320:1031, 1989)* The systolic click-murmur syndrome is associated with mitral valve prolapse, which can place excessive stress on the papillary muscles and lead to ischemia and chest pain. Although often associated with inferior T-wave changes, the systolic click-murmur syndrome only occasionally results in an ischemic response to exercise. On standing or during the Valsalva maneuver, as ventricular volume gets smaller, the click and murmur move earlier in systole. Echocardiography reveals midsystolic prolapse of the posterior mitral leaflet or, on occasion, both mitral leaflets into the left atrium. Persons with mitral regurgitation from prolapse are at risk of developing subacute bacterial endocarditis and should be treated accordingly.

**II-84.** **The answer is A-N, B-Y, C-Y, D-N, E-Y.** *(Chap. 230)* The choice of a permanent pacemaker type depends on the underlying conduction disease and the patient's clinical profile. DDD pacing preserves the normal relationship between atrial and ventricular contraction, and physiologic atrial sensing with ventricular pacing improves exercise tolerance in young, active persons. As this form of pacing preserves the normal atrial contribution to cardiac output, it is desirable in patients with decreased left ventricular function or hypertrophied ("stiff") left ventricular chambers. DDD pacing is contraindicated in atrial fibrillation or flutter, since the ventricular rate response is unpredictable.

**II-85.   The answer is A-Y, B-Y, C-Y, D-Y, E-Y.**   *(Chap. 230)*   With severe chronic heart failure from any cause there may be severe weight loss as a result of (1) elevation of the metabolic rate, which results from extra respiratory muscle work, (2) anorexia, nausea, and vomiting caused by central causes, digitalis intoxication, or congestive hepatomegaly and abdominal fullness (including ascites with impairment of gastric filling and early satiety), (3) impaired intestinal absorption resulting from intestinal venular congestion, and (4) a protein-losing enteropathy.

**II-86.   The answer is A-N, B-Y, C-Y, D-Y, E-N.**   *(Chap. 234)*   A 5-year survival rate of 70 percent suggests that cardiac transplantation is the therapy of choice for patients with end-stage heart disease. Because the posterior walls of the host's atria are left in place at the time of transplantation, the recipient's sinus node remains innervated and under the influence of the autonomic nervous system, but the donor sinus node controls the rate of the transplanted heart (and has a regular PR interval, in contrast to the dissociated P waves generated by the residual host atria). Accelerated coronary vascular disease (chronic rejection) is the major factor limiting long-term survival. The vascular disease, which may be ameliorated somewhat by early posttransplant use of diltiazem, is a consequence of fibrointimal hyperplasia brought on by injury during rejection episodes and high serum lipids. The high serum lipids are a side effect of the immunosuppressive medicines that must be administered. Immunosuppression must continue for a lifetime. Neoplasms, particularly Epstein-Barr virus–associated lymphomas, represent another class of late complications.

**II-87.   The answer is A-N, B-N, C-N, D-Y, E-Y.**   *(Chap. 231)*   Ventricular tachycardia (VT) generally accompanies some form of structural heart disease, most commonly chronic ischemic heart disease associated with a prior myocardial infarction. The ECG diagnosis of VT is suggested by a wide-complex tachycardia at a rate exceeding 100 beats per minute. It is important, however, to differentiate supraventricular tachycardia with aberration of intraventricular conduction from VT, since the clinical implications and management of these two entities are so different. A very irregular rhythm suggests atrial fibrillation (AF) with conduction via a bypass tract (WPW syndrome). If a tracing previously obtained during sinus rhythm demonstrates a bundle branch block pattern with the same morphologic features as those which occur during the tachycardia, a supraventricular origin is favored. Characteristics of the 12-lead ECG during the arrhythmia that suggest a ventricular origin are (1) a QRS complex >0.14 s in the absence of antiarrhythmic therapy (although a QRS complex >0.20 s suggests a preexcitation syndrome), (2) AV dissociation or variable retrograde conduction, (3) a superior QRS axis in the presence of a right bundle block pattern, (4) concordance of the QRS pattern in all precordial leads, and (5) other QRS patterns that are inconsistent with typical bundle branch block patterns. Intracardiac electrical recordings would be required to confirm this important distinction.

**II-88.   The answer is A-N, B-Y, C-N, D-Y, E-N.**   *(Chap. 239)*   The symptoms of dyspnea in persons with asymmetric septal hypertrophy are related as much to decreased left ventricular (diastolic) compliance as to the degree of obstruction. The use of calcium channel blockers often relieves dyspnea by decreasing left ventricular stiffness. Sudden death in affected persons does not correlate with the degree of obstruction and is thought to be due to arrhythmias. On electrocardiography, Q waves commonly are seen and do not imply a coexistent infarction. Histologic abnormalities consist of disorganized arrangements of myocytes in the ventricular septum. As many as 50 percent of these cases have familial predisposition, often resulting from one of several mutations in the beta cardiac myosin heavy chain gene on chromosome 14.

**II-89.** **The answer is A-N, B-N, C-N, D-Y, E-Y.** *(Chap. 237)*  In approximately two-thirds of patients with aortic regurgitation (AR), the disease is rheumatic in origin, although this etiology is less common in those with isolated AR. Manifestations of the rapidly falling arterial pressure during late systole and diastole include Corrigan's "water-hammer" pulse, capillary pulsations visible at the root of nails (Quincke's pulse), a pistol-shot (Traube's) sound over the femoral arteries, and a to-and-fro murmur (Duroziez's sign) audible over a lightly compressed femoral artery. In addition to a midsystolic ejection murmur, a second associated murmur may be the Austin Flint murmur, a low-pitched, rumbling diastolic bruit. Such a murmur is produced by the anterior displacement of the anterior leaflet of the mitral valve by the aortic regurgitant stream (characteristically seen on echocardiography). Close follow-up by means of echocardiography is necessary to ensure that an operation is performed before irreversible left ventricular dysfunction occurs.

**II-90.** **The answer is A-N, B-Y, C-Y, D-Y, E-Y.** *(Chap. 238)*  Pulmonary hypertension resulting from chronic pulmonary vascular disease such as that produced by multiple pulmonary emboli produces characteristic findings on physical examination, including a loud pulmonary second heart sound, a prominent *a* wave in the jugular venous pulse, and the systolic murmur of tricuspid regurgitation (the abnormal jet of blood flow is easily detectable on Doppler echocardiography). Pulmonary function testing may reveal an enlarged dead space, but there usually are no abnormalities on spirometry. The usual findings on ECG include P pulmonale (tall, peaked P waves) and right axis deviation. The hypertrophied right ventricle can be imaged on thallium 201 scintigraphy, whereas this chamber normally remains invisible because of the marked uptake of the left ventricle.

**II-91.** **The answer is A-N, B-N, C-N, D-Y, E-N.** *(Chap. 239)*  Chronic alcoholics may develop a clinical picture virtually identical to that of idiopathic dilated cardiomyopathy. Ceasing the consumption of alcohol may result in halting the progression of heart disease. With continued alcohol abuse, however, 75 percent of afflicted persons will die within 3 years. While beriberi heart disease leads to high output failure, alcoholic cardiomyopathy is associated with a low cardiac output. Atrial arrhythmias, particularly fibrillation, are the most common electrical disorder seen in what is termed "holiday heart syndrome."

**II-92.** **The answer is A-N, B-Y, C-Y, D-N, E-Y.** *(Chap. 241)*  The most common type of primary cardiac tumor is the benign myxoma, which most frequently arises in the left atrium. Auscultation may reveal a "tumor plop" in diastole as the tumor hits the ventricular wall. Although most myxomas are sporadic, some are familial with autosomal dominant inheritance. Features of the familial syndromes associated with cardiac myxomas include pigmented nevi, nodular disease of the adrenal cortex, mammary fibroadenomas, and testicular and pituitary tumors. Systemic symptoms that are typically confused with those of endocarditis, noncardiac malignancy, or collagen vascular disease may be associated with myxomas. Sarcoma is the most common primary malignant cardiac tumor.

**II-93.** **The answer is A-N, B-Y, C-Y, D-Y, E-N.** *(Chap. 246)*  The abrupt onset of severe hypertension or the onset of high blood pressure of any severity in a person under age 25 or after age 50 years should lead to additional tests to exclude renovascular hypertension and pheochromocytoma. The presence of an abdominal bruit (though not a very sensitive screening test) should prompt a workup for renovascular hypertension. Any patient whose hypertension is not controlled by a two-drug regimen such as an angiotensin converting enzyme inhibitor and a diuretic at adequate doses should undergo a further workup. While evidence for left ventricular hypertrophy on physical examination or electrocardiography suggests long-standing hypertension, such a finding does not necessarily imply the presence of Cushing's syndrome, pheochromocytoma, or a renovascular disease.

**II-94–II-97. The answers are 94-E, 95-A, 96-C, 97-B.**  *(Chaps. 237, 238, 240)*   Right heart failure, or elevated right-heart filling pressure, can develop from many causes. Right heart failure most commonly occurs as a result of pulmonary artery hypertension. Pulmonary artery hypertension in turn arises either from increased pulmonary vascular resistance with lung disease, in which case the pulmonary capillary wedge pressure (left atrial pressure) is not elevated, or from left-sided failure or valvular disease, in which case left atrial pressure is increased. Massive right ventricular infarction can cause the right side of the heart to fail at low systolic pressures. With primary myocardial disease, both left and right atrial pressures are elevated; however, when diastolic pressures are equal in the left and right cardiac chambers, external compression, such as constrictive pericarditis, must be the suspected cause.

# III. DISORDERS OF THE KIDNEY AND URINARY TRACT

## QUESTIONS

**DIRECTIONS:** Each question below contains five suggested responses. Choose the one best response to each question.

**III-1.** A patient with lymphoma who is known to excrete 1.5 g urinary protein per day has a negative dipstick evaluation for urinary protein. The reason for the seeming inconsistency is

(A) the size of the excreted protein is too small to be picked up by the test strip
(B) the urine is not concentrated enough
(C) only heavy chain sequences are recognized by the test strip
(D) Tamm-Horsfall protein blocks the reaction between the secreted protein and the test strip
(E) dipsticks preferentially detect albumin compared with immunoglobulin because albumin is negatively charged

**III-2.** A 75-year-old female nursing home resident is brought to the emergency department because of increasing obtundation. She is found to communicate poorly. Brief physical examination reveals diminished skin turgor. Blood pressure is 100/60, pulse 120, respiratory rate 20, and temperature 37°C (98.6°F). Blood tests reveal the following serum electrolytes: sodium 160 mmol/L, potassium 5.0 mmol/L, bicarbonate 30 mmol/L, chloride 110 mmol/L. The most appropriate management at this time would include administration of 5% dextrose in

(A) normal saline, 100 mL/h
(B) normal saline solution, 250 mL/h
(C) half normal saline, 100 mL/h
(D) half normal saline, 200 mL/h
(E) water, 150 mL/h

**III-3.** Laboratory evaluation of a 19-year-old man being worked up for polyuria and polydipsia yields the following results:

Serum electrolytes (mmol/L): $Na^+$ 144; $K^+$ 4.0;
$\quad Cl^-$ 107; $HCO_3^-$ 25
BUN: 6.4 mmol/L (18 mg/dL)
Blood glucose: 5.7 mmol/L (102 mg/dL)
Urine electrolytes (mmol/L): $Na^+$ 28; $K^+$ 32
Urine osmolality: 195 mosmol/kg water

After 12 h of fluid deprivation, body weight has fallen by 5 percent. Laboratory testing now reveals the following:

Serum electrolytes (mmol/L): $Na^+$ 150; $K^+$ 4.1;
$\quad Cl^-$ 109; $HCO_3^-$ 25
BUN: 7.1 mmol/L (20 mg/dL)
Blood glucose: 5.4 mmol/L (98 mg/dL)
Urine electrolytes (mmol/L): $Na^+$ 24; $K^+$ 35
Urine osmolality: 200 mosmol/kg water

One hour after the subcutaneous administration of 5 units of arginine vasopressin, urine values are as follows:

Urine electrolytes (mmol/L): $Na^+$ 30; $K^+$ 30
Urine osmolality: 199 mosmol/kg water

The likely diagnosis in this case is

(A) nephrogenic diabetes insipidus
(B) osmotic diuresis
(C) salt-losing nephropathy
(D) psychogenic polydipsia
(E) none of the above

**III-4.** A 70-year-old man with diabetes mellitus and hypertension has the following serum chemistries:

Electrolytes (mmol/L): $Na^+$ 138; $K^+$ 5.0; $Cl^-$ 106; $HCO_3^-$ 20
Glucose: 11 mmol/L (200 mg/dL)
Creatinine: 176 μmol/L (2.0 mg/dL)

All the following may contribute to worsening hyperkalemia EXCEPT

(A) propranolol
(B) indomethacin
(C) captopril
(D) digitalis
(E) carbenicillin

**III-5.** A 40-year-old alcoholic male presents with a 6-day history of binge drinking. Serum chemistry tests reveal the following:

Electrolytes (mmol/L): $Na^+$ 145; $K^+$ 5.0; $Cl^-$ 105; $HCO_3^-$ 15
BUN: 7.1 mmol/L (20 mg/dL)
Creatinine: 133 μg/L (1.5 mg/dL)
Glucose: 9.6 mmol/L (172 mg/dL)

The nitroprusside (Acetest) agent gives a minimally positive result. Optimal therapy to ameliorate the patient's acid-base disorder would include 5% dextrose in

(A) water
(B) normal saline
(C) normal saline, insulin, and sodium bicarbonate
(D) half normal saline and insulin
(E) half normal saline, insulin, and sodium bicarbonate

**III-6.** A 45-year-old woman who has had slowly progressive renal failure begins to complain of increasing numbness and prickling sensations in her legs. Examination reveals loss of pinprick and vibration sensation below the knees, absent ankle jerks, and impaired pinprick sensation in the hands. Serum creatinine concentration, checked during her most recent clinic visit, is 790 μmol/L (8.9 mg/dL). The woman's physician should now recommend

(A) a therapeutic trial of phenytoin
(B) a therapeutic trial of pyridoxine (vitamin B[6])
(C) a therapeutic trial of cyanocobalamin (vitamin B[12])
(D) initiation of renal replacement therapy
(E) neurologic referral for nerve conduction studies

**III-7.** In patients with chronic renal failure, all the following are important contributors to bone disease EXCEPT

(A) impaired renal production of 1,25-dihydroxy-vitamin $D_3$
(B) hyperphosphatemia
(C) aluminum-containing antacids
(D) loss of vitamin D and calcium via dialysis
(E) metabolic acidosis

**III-8.** A 50-year-old man is hospitalized for treatment of enterococcal endocarditis. He has been receiving ampicillin and gentamicin for the past 2 weeks but is persistently febrile. Laboratory results are as follows:

Serum electrolytes (mmol/L): $Na^+$ 145; $K^+$ 5.0; $Cl^-$ 110; $HCO_3^-$ 20
BUN: 14.2 mmol/L (40 mg/dL)
Serum creatinine: 300 μmol/L (3.5 mg/dL)
Urine sodium: 20 mmol/L
Urine creatinine: 3000 mmol/L (35 mg/dL)

Which of the following is the most likely cause of this patient's acute renal failure?

(A) Tubular necrosis
(B) Insensible skin losses
(C) Renal artery embolism
(D) Cardiac failure
(E) Nausea and vomiting

**III-9.** A 23-year-old man has recurrent episodes of hematuria over the past year. Each of the episodes seems to be associated with an upper respiratory infection. Physical examination currently is normal. Urinalysis reveals a relatively bland sediment; dipstick is positive for both protein and blood. Renal biopsy most likely will reveal

(A) extensive extracapillary proliferation on light microscopy
(B) diffuse mesangial proliferation on light microscopy
(C) autosomal dominant polycystic kidney disease
(D) diffuse mesangial deposition of IgA on immunofluorescence
(E) deposition of C3 in capillary walls on immunofluorescence

**III-10.** The condition of a 50-year-old obese woman with a 5-year history of mild hypertension controlled by a thiazide diuretic is being evaluated because proteinuria was noted during her routine yearly medical visit. Physical examination disclosed a height of 167.6 cm (66 in.), weight 91 kg (202 lb), blood pressure 130/80 mmHg, and trace pedal edema. Laboratory values are as follows:

Serum creatinine: 106 μmol/L (1.2 mg/dL)
BUN: 6.4 mmol/L (18 mg/dL)
Creatinine clearance: 87 mL/min
Urinalysis: pH 5.0; specific gravity 1.018; protein 3+;
    no glucose; occasional coarse granular cast
Urine protein excretion: 5.9 g/d

The results of a renal biopsy are shown below. Sixty percent of the glomeruli appeared as shown (by light microscopy); the remainder were unremarkable.

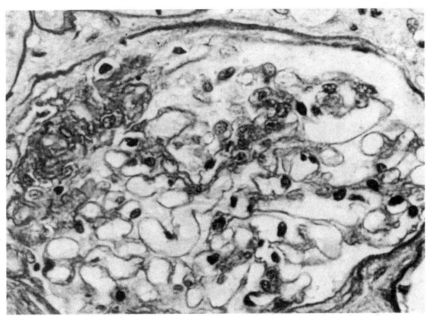

The most likely diagnosis is

(A) hypertensive nephrosclerosis
(B) focal and segmental sclerosis
(C) minimal-change (nil) disease

(D) membranous glomerulopathy
(E) crescentic glomerulonephritis

**III-11.** In a person who has carcinoma of the lung and the depicted urinalysis, renal biopsy most likely will show

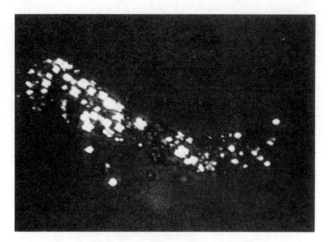

(A) minimal-change disease
(B) diffuse proliferative glomerulonephritis
(C) membranoproliferative glomerulonephritis
(D) membranous glomerulopathy
(E) focal glomerulosclerosis

**III-12.** Which of the following case histories would most likely be associated with the urinary sediment depicted?

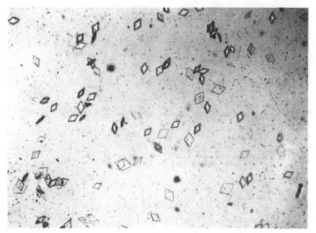

(A) A 23-year-old man with newly diagnosed lymphoblastic lymphoma who is found to have a rising creatinine level 2 days after the administration of combination chemotherapy
(B) A 23-year-old woman 1 year after surgery performed because of morbid obesity
(C) A 45-year-old woman with a history of multiple urinary tract infections with urea-splitting organisms
(D) A 40-year-old man with edema, hypoalbuminemia, and proteinuria
(E) An 18-year-old man with flank pain, hematuria, and a positive family history for renal stones in youth

**III-13.** A 72-year-old woman with rheumatic heart disease is being treated with ampicillin and gentamicin for enterococcal endocarditis. One week into the course she develops a morbilliform skin rash and fever. Laboratory evaluation is remarkable for a doubling of serum creatinine and blood urea nitrogen from their baseline values. Urinalysis dipstick is positive for blood, protein, and white cells. Ultrasonography reveals bilaterally enlarged kidneys. Based on the available data, the most likely cause of the patient's azotemia is

(A) tubular necrosis caused by aminoglycoside
(B) membranous nephropathy resulting from endocarditis
(C) enterococcal pyelonephritis
(D) cystitis
(E) hypersensitivity reaction to ampicillin

**III-14.** A 40-year-old woman who has never had significant respiratory disease is hospitalized for evaluation of hemoptysis. Urinalysis reveals 2+ proteinuria and microscopic hematuria. BUN concentration is 7.1 mmol/L (20 mg/dL), and serum creatinine concentration is 177 μmol/L (2.0 mg/dL). Serologic findings include normal complement levels and a negative assay for fluorescent antinuclear antibodies. Renal biopsy reveals granulomatous necrotizing vasculitis with scattered immunoglobulin and complement deposits. The most likely diagnosis in this case is

(A) mesangial lupus glomerulonephritis
(B) Henoch-Schönlein purpura
(C) microscopic polyarteritis
(D) Wegener's granulomatosis
(E) Goodpasture's syndrome

**III-15.** Which of the following patients is LEAST likely to develop destruction of renal papillae with concomitant tubulointerstitial damage?

(A) A middle-aged man who has consumed "moonshine" alcohol distilled in automobile radiators
(B) An older man with repetitive episodes of acute urinary retention resulting from prostatic hypertrophy
(C) A young adult woman with sickle cell anemia
(D) An older woman who uses analgesics for chronic headaches
(E) A middle-aged woman with a history of multiple urinary tract infections associated with pyuria, flank pain, fever, and poor response to short courses of oral antibiotics

**III-16.** A 45-year-old woman with long-standing systemic lupus erythematosus who has had intermittent bouts of acute renal failure over the last 6 years presents with anorexia. Physical examination is noncontributory. Laboratory evaluation includes hematocrit 29 percent, white count 5000 with a normal differential, and platelet count 27,500/μL. Renal biopsy shows sclerosis of 14/15 glomeruli, tubular atrophy, and interstitial fibrosis. The following values are also found:

Serum electrolytes (mmol/L): $Na^+$ 136; $K^+$ 6; $Cl^-$ 90;
    $HCO_3^-$ 20
BUN: 35.5 mmol/L (100 mg/dL)
Serum creatinine: 665 μmol/L (7.5 mg/dL)

Anti-double-strand DNA and C3 levels have been stable. Renal biopsy shows obliterative sclerosing glomerular lesions. The most appropriate management strategy would be

(A) high-dose intravenous methylprednisolone
(B) high-dose intravenous methylprednisolone and azathioprine
(C) high-dose intravenous methylprednisolone and intravenous cyclophosphamide (500 mg/m$^2$)
(D) intravenous cyclophosphamide (500 mg/m$^2$) plus low-dose prednisone
(E) dialysis

**III-17.** A 30-year-old woman with diabetic nephropathy received a cadaveric renal allograft. On the third postoperative day her serum creatinine concentration was 160 μmol/L (1.8 mg/dL). She is being treated with cyclosporine and prednisone. On the sixth postoperative day she experiences a decrease in urine output from 1500 mL/d to 1000 mL/d; the serum creatinine concentration increases to 194 μmol/L (2.2 mg/dL). Her blood pressure remains stable at 170/90 mmHg, and her temperature is 37.2°C (99°F). The best initial step in management would be to

(A) decrease the dose of cyclosporine
(B) obtain ultrasonography of the renal allograft
(C) obtain a biopsy of the renal allograft
(D) administer pulsed steroid therapy
(E) administer an intravenous bolus of furosemide

**III-18.** A 55-year-old man undergoes intravenous pyelography (IVP) as part of a workup for hypertension. A 3-cm solitary radiolucent mass is noted in the left kidney; the study otherwise is normal. The man complains of no symptoms referable to the urinary tract, and examination of urinary sediment is within normal limits. Which of the following studies should be performed next?

(A) Repeat intravenous pyelography in 6 months
(B) Early-morning urine collections for cytology (three samples)
(C) Selective renal arteriography
(D) Renal ultrasonography
(E) CT scanning (with contrast enhancement) of the left kidney

**III-19.** Risk factors for carcinoma of the bladder include all of the following EXCEPT

(A) exposure to cigarette smoke
(B) use of cyclophosphamide
(C) exposure to dyes
(D) positive family history
(E) schistosomal infestation

**III-20.** A 10-year-old girl complaining of profound weakness, occasional difficulty walking, and polyuria is brought to the pediatrician. Her mother is sure the girl has not been vomiting frequently. The girl takes no medicines. She is normotensive, and no focal neurologic abnormalities are found. Serum chemistries include sodium 142 mmol/L, potassium 2.5 mmol/L, bicarbonate 32 mmol/L, and chloride 100 mmol/L. A 24-h urine collection on a normal diet reveals sodium 200 mmol/d, potassium 50 mmol/d, and chloride 30 mmol/d. Renal ultrasound demonstrates symmetrically enlarged kidneys without hydronephrosis. A stool phenolphthalein test and a urine screen for diuretics are negative. Plasma renin levels are found to be elevated. Which of the following conditions is most consistent with the above data?

(A) Conn's syndrome
(B) Chronic ingestion of licorice
(C) Bartter's syndrome
(D) Wilms' tumor
(E) Proximal renal tubular acidosis

**III-21.** A previously healthy 45-year-old man who developed weight gain, fatigue, and vomiting within the past week presents to his physician. He had been seen 3 months earlier for a routine checkup, at which time a physical examination, complete blood count, and serum chemistries were all normal. Relevant physical findings now include blood pressure of 155/110 mmHg and periorbital edema. Serum studies reveal a BUN of 30 mmol/L (85 mg/dL) and a creatinine of 796 μmol/L (9 mg/dL). Urinalysis reveals 2+ proteinuria and the sediment findings depicted below. Which of the following statements is LEAST likely to be correct?

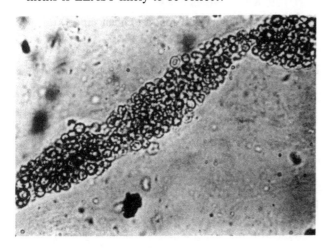

(A) Renal biopsy is indicated
(B) Poststreptococcal glomerulonephritis is an important diagnostic consideration
(C) Extracapillary proliferation is probable
(D) Spontaneous resolution of the renal disease is likely
(E) A trial of high-dose glucocorticoids is indicated

**III-22.** Complications of long-term dialysis include all the following EXCEPT

(A) increased risk of gastrointestinal malignancy
(B) myocardial infarction
(C) carpal tunnel syndrome
(D) protein-calorie malnutrition
(E) high-output congestive heart failure

**III-23.** Low serum complement levels would be seen in patients with hematuria, proteinuria, and hypertension resulting from all of the following EXCEPT

(A) mixed essential cryoglobulinemia
(B) hepatitis C–associated membranoproliferative glomerulonephritis
(C) diffuse proliferative lupus nephritis
(D) Henoch-Schönlein purpura
(E) poststreptococcal (or postinfectious) glomerulonephritis

**III-24.** In acute renal failure, dietary protein should be restricted in which of the following?

(A) All patients
(B) All patients with BUN >100
(C) All patients with creatinine >10
(D) Only in patients who are well nourished on hospital admission
(E) If azotemia is advanced and dialysis is not an option

**III-25.** A 37-year-old man is admitted with confusion. Physical examination shows a blood pressure of 140/70 with no orthostasis, normal jugular venous pressure, and no edema. Serum chemistries are notable for sodium 120 mmol/L, $K^+$ 4.2 mmol/L, bicarbonate 24 mmol/L, and uric acid 0.177 mmol/L (2 mg/dL). The most likely diagnosis is

(A) hepatic cirrhosis
(B) cerebral toxoplasmosis with SIADH
(C) Addison's disease
(D) significant gastrointestinal fluid loss
(E) congestive heart failure

**III-26.** Nephrotic syndrome is the hallmark of all the following primary kidney diseases EXCEPT

(A) membranous glomerulopathy
(B) focal segmental glomerulosclerosis
(C) minimal-change disease
(D) IgA nephropathy (Berger's disease)
(E) HIV-associated nephropathy with or without glomerular collapse

**III-27.** A 56-year-old diabetic woman with end-stage renal disease (ESRD) has been treated with peritoneal dialysis (prescription of four, 2 L exchanges per day) for 6 years. She is 5 ft. 6 in. tall and weighs 70 kg (154 lb). The patient complains of anorexia, abdominal discomfort, fatigue, and insomnia. Medications include erythropoietin, calcium carbonate, metoprolol, and a water-soluble vitamin supplement. Laboratory studies are notable for hematocrit 38 percent, BUN 56 mg/dL, bicarbonate 14 meq/L, calcium 10.4 mg/dL, and phosphate 2.3 mg/dL.

The most likely diagnosis is

(A) mycobacterial peritonitis
(B) dialysis disequilibrium
(C) uremia
(D) peritoneal carcinomatosis
(E) diabetic ketoacidosis

**III-28.** Hyperammonemia can be reduced by all the following maneuvers EXCEPT

(A) protein restriction
(B) a branched-chain amino acid–enriched protein mixture
(C) neomycin
(D) lactulose
(E) loop diuretics

**III-29.** Nephrocalcinosis can be associated with

(A) the routine use of calcium-based phosphate binders
(B) the routine use of aluminum-based phosphate binders
(C) calcitonin-related peptide
(D) secondary hyperparathyroidism
(E) Crohn's disease

**III-30.** Obesity is associated with all the following EXCEPT

(A) focal segmental glomerulosclerosis
(B) membranoproliferative glomerulonephritis
(C) peritoneal dialysis
(D) renal transplantation
(E) diabetes mellitus

**III-31.** A 60-year-old man with alcoholism presents to the emergency department with severe confusion, vomiting, and tachycardia. Blood pressure is 90/60, heart rate is 110, and respiratory rate is 32. Laboratory studies are remarkable for the following (mmol/L): $Na^+$ 128, $K^+$ 3.9, $Cl^-$ 90, bicarbonate 6. BUN was 12 mg/dL, and creatinine was 2.9 mg/dL. Acetest is negative. Urinalysis shows 4+ calcium oxalate crystals. The most likely diagnosis is

(A) alcoholic rhabdomyolysis with acute tubular necrosis
(B) alcoholic ketoacidosis
(C) renal tubular acidosis type 1
(D) ingestion of ethylene glycol
(E) alcoholic hepatitis with pancreatitis and multiple organ dysfunction

**III-32.** A 72-year-old man develops acute renal failure after cardiac catheterization. Physical examination is notable for diminished peripheral pulses, livedo reticularis, epigastric tenderness, and confusion. Laboratory studies include (mg/dL) BUN 131, creatinine 5.2, and phosphate 9.5. Urinalysis shows 10 to 15 WBC, 5 to 10 RBC, and one hyaline cast per HPF. The most likely diagnosis is

(A) acute interstitial nephritis caused by drugs
(B) rhabdomyolysis with acute tubular necrosis
(C) acute tubular necrosis secondary to radiocontrast exposure
(D) cholesterol embolization
(E) renal arterial dissection with prerenal azotemia

**III-33.** The hyperlipidemia of nephrotic syndrome is characterized by

(A) elevation of all plasma lipids but no increase in atherogenesis
(B) elevation of total cholesterol but no increase in atherogenesis
(C) selective elevation of LDL cholesterol with increased atherogenesis
(D) no response to HMG-CoA reductase inhibitors
(E) myositis in 20 percent of patients treated with lipid-lowering agents

**III-34.** Inhibitors of angiotensin converting enzyme would be expected to slow the progression of renal insufficiency in all the following conditions EXCEPT

(A) diabetes mellitus type I
(B) diabetes mellitus type II
(C) chronic glomerulonephritis with more than 1 g daily proteinuria
(D) autosomal dominant polycystic kidney disease (ADPKD)
(E) IgA nephropathy

**DIRECTIONS:** Each question below contains five suggested responses. For **each** of the five responses listed with each item, you are to respond either YES (Y) or NO (N). In a given item **all, some, or none** of the alternatives may be correct.

**III-35.** A 43-year-old construction worker is noted to be anuric after a crush injury to the lower extremities. Serum electrolytes (mmol/L) obtained 8 h after admission are $Na^+$ 138, $K^+$ 8.8, $Cl^-$ 100, and $HCO_3^-$ 19. Electrocardiography reveals peaked T waves, prolongation of the PR interval, and widening of the QRS complex. Which of the following measures would rapidly lower serum potassium concentration in the man described?

(A) Intravenous infusion of 10 mL of a 10% calcium gluconate solution

(B) Intravenous infusion of 10 mL of a 10% magnesium sulfate solution

(C) Intravenous infusion of 50 mL of a 50% glucose solution with 10 units of regular insulin

(D) Intravenous infusion of 2 ampules of sodium bicarbonate

(E) Administration by nasogastric tube of 60 mL of a potassium-binding resin

**III-36.** Rhabdomyolysis or acute myoglobinuric renal failure can develop as a result of

(A) strenuous muscular exercise

(B) cocaine overdose

(C) ethanol ingestion

(D) hypophosphatemia

(E) volume depletion

**III-37.** Patients in whom the mechanism leading to urinary incontinence puts them at risk for hydronephrosis include those with

(A) Alzheimer's dementia

(B) Guillain-Barré syndrome

(C) normal-pressure hydrocephalus

(D) diabetes mellitus

(E) hypothyroidism

**III-38.** Metabolic abnormalities associated with the nephrotic syndrome include

(A) increased serum lipid levels

(B) increased serum thyroxine levels

(C) reduced serum calcium levels

(D) reduced serum zinc levels

(E) increased serum antithrombin III (heparin cofactor) levels

**III-39.** True statements about acute poststreptococcal glomerulonephritis (PSGN) include which of the following?

(A) The latent period appears to be longer when PSGN is associated with cutaneous rather than pharyngeal infections

(B) Serologic evidence of a streptococcal infection may not be forthcoming if antimicrobial therapy is begun early

(C) Antimicrobial therapy for streptococcal infection is without value once the presence of renal disease is established

(D) Long-term antistreptococcal prophylaxis is indicated after documented cases of PSGN

(E) Lasting and progressive deterioration in renal function is more common in adults than in children with PSGN

**III-40.** The inheritance of a tendency to develop adult polycystic kidney disease is correctly described by which of the following?

(A) A mutation on the short arm of chromosome 16 has been linked to the disease

(B) A polymorphic locus near the alpha-globin gene cluster has been linked to the disease

(C) Most cases are due to new mutations

(D) Adult polycystic kidney disease displays autosomal recessive inheritance

(E) A person found to be homozygous at the polymorphic locus linked to the disease cannot be analyzed for predisposition to the disease

**III-41.** Which of the following patients could be appropriately matched with the urine sediment depicted?

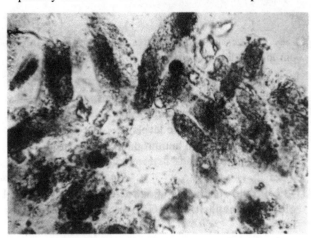

(A) A 75-year-old man 1 day after complicated surgery for the repair of an abdominal aortic aneurysm

(B) A 75-year-old man with a porcine aortic valve prosthesis, malaise, fever, and positive blood cultures

(C) A 50-year-old man with a history of chronic alcoholism who presents with stupor and a history of having been found on the street with multiple bruises

(D) A 75-year-old man with known benign prostatic hypertrophy and inability to void who presents with an enlarged bladder and a creatinine level of 220 μmol/L (2.5 mg/dL)

(E) A 35-year-old woman with idiopathic dilated cardiomyopathy and an ejection fraction of 15 percent who is awaiting cardiac transplantation

**III-42.** A 45-year-old black woman on chronic hemodialysis for renal failure caused by uncontrolled hypertension has a hematocrit of 22 percent with a mean red cell volume (MCV) of 89. Correct statements about her condition include which of the following?

(A) A trial of erythropoietin is unlikely to improve her hematocrit because erythropoiesis is relatively unresponsive to this hormone in the face of chronic uremia

(B) The patient may be experiencing chronic blood loss because of the use of heparin with dialysis or the abnormal hemostasis associated with chronic renal failure

(C) Folic acid deficiency is possible, even though the anemia is normocytic

(D) Multiple blood transfusions could lead to direct heart damage

(E) If the patient requires surgery, vasopressin or cryoprecipitate could be used to ameliorate the bleeding tendency

**III-43.** A 48-year-old woman is hospitalized for elective knee surgery. Routine preoperative laboratory evaluation reveals the following:

Serum electrolytes (mmol/L): $Na^+$ 138; $K^+$ 3.5; $Cl^-$ 110; $HCO_3^-$ 20
Blood glucose: 5.2 mmol/L (95 mg/dL)
Serum creatinine: 160 μmol/L (1.8 mg/dL)
BUN: 7.1 mmol/L (20 mg/dL)
Urinalysis: pH 5.2; specific gravity 1.005; protein 1+; glucose 2+; 3 to 5 white blood cells per high-power field

This woman says she voids several times during the night but is unaware of any problem with her kidneys. Disorders associated with the findings in this case would include

(A) multiple myeloma

(B) diabetic nephropathy

(C) Sjögren's syndrome

(D) penicillamine-induced nephropathy

(E) analgesic abuse

**III-44.** A 45-year-old woman presents with the third episode of nephrolithiasis. Laboratory studies disclose the following:

Serum electrolytes (mmol/L): $Na^+$ 134; $K^+$ 2.5;
  $Cl^-$ 106; $HCO_3^-$ 18
Serum chemistries: creatinine 97 $\mu$mol/L (1.1 mg/dL);
  calcium 2.4 mmol/L (9.5 mg/dL); albumin 40 g/L
  (4.0 g/dL)
Arterial blood gas values: $P_{CO_2}$ 4 kPa (30 mmHg); $P_{O_2}$
  14 kPa (108 mmHg); pH 7.30
Urine pH: 7.2

A plain film of the abdomen is shown below. Correct statements about this clinical picture include which of the following?

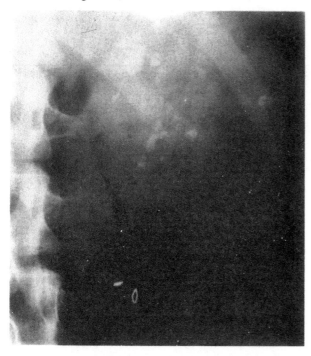

(A) The findings are consistent with the presence of multiple myeloma
(B) The findings are consistent with the presence of medullary sponge kidney
(C) There is evidence of type I distal renal tubular acidosis (RTA)
(D) Family members should be screened for electrolyte disorders
(E) Intravenous pyelography would provide further useful information

**III-45.** Correct statements regarding renal allografting include which of the following?

(A) A potential living donor who does not share the same blood type as the recipient cannot be considered even if the tissue types are HLA-identical
(B) The degree of HLA mismatch with cadaveric donor kidneys is a determinant of long-term graft survival
(C) Progressive renal failure in a transplant recipient, termed chronic rejection, is associated with renal vascular damage
(D) Allopurinol must be coadministered with azathioprine to prevent urate nephropathy associated with drug-induced cell turnover
(E) Cyclosporine inhibits IL-2 production by helper T cells

**III-46.** A 42-year-old man with a history of hypertension presents to the emergency room with the third episode of severe right flank pain over the past 5 years. Correct statements include which of the following?

(A) It is likely that a scout film of the abdomen will be positive
(B) If the pain is due to a renal stone and does not remit, direct removal will be necessary
(C) The patient should be asked about a history of bowel surgery
(D) After resolution of the acute episode, urine calcium, creatinine, uric acid, citrate, and oxalate should be measured
(E) If the patient is found to have calcium stones, thiazide diuretics should be avoided

**DIRECTIONS:** The group of questions below consists of lettered headings followed by a set of numbered items. For each numbered item select the **one** lettered heading with which it is **most** closely associated. Each lettered heading may be used **once, more than once, or not at all**.

*Questions III-47–III-49*

   For each case history that follows, select the set of laboratory values with which it is most likely to be associated.

| | $Na^+$ | $K^+$ | $Cl^-$ | $HCO_3^-$ | Serum Creatinine | pH | |
| | | | | | [$\mu$mol/L (mg/dL)] | | |
| | (Serum, mmol/L) | | | | | Arterial Blood | Urine |
|---|---|---|---|---|---|---|---|
| (A) | 143 | 4.8 | 100 | 10 | 265 (3.0) | 7.25 | 5.0 |
| (B) | 135 | 4.5 | 107 | 21 | 265 (3.0) | 7.37 | 5.0 |
| (C) | 140 | 2.5 | 114 | 14 | 265 (3.0) | 7.30 | 6.2 |
| (D) | 139 | 5.1 | 104 | 21 | 265 (3.0) | 7.37 | 5.0 |
| (E) | 139 | 6.3 | 108 | 19 | 265 (3.0) | 7.35 | 5.0 |

**III-47.**   A 28-year-old man, comatose, is believed to have been drinking ethylene glycol

**III-48.**   A 48-year-old woman has been given amphotericin B for the treatment of disseminated coccidioidomycosis

**III-49.**   A 19-year-old man is recovering from acute poststreptococcal glomerulonephritis

# III. DISORDERS OF THE KIDNEY AND URINARY TRACT

## ANSWERS

**III-1. The answer is E.** *(Chap. 47)* Up to 150 mg/d of protein may be excreted by a normal person. The bulk of normal daily excretion is made up of the Tamm-Horsfall mucoprotein. Urine dipsticks may register a trace result in response to as little as 50 mg protein per liter and are definitively positive once the urine protein exceeds 300 mg/L. A false negative may occur if the proteinuria is due to immunoglobulins, which are positively charged. If proteinuria is suspected or documented, a 24-h urine collection should be undertaken to measure the absolute protein excretion. Urine immunoelectrophoresis also may identify the particular immunoglobulin that is produced in excess.

**III-2. The answer is E.** *(Chap. 49)* Because of the powerful effect of ADH secretion in the setting of hypertonicity, severe persistent hypernatremia is possible only in patients who cannot respond to thirst by ingesting water. A nursing home patient with a fever may lose significant amounts of body fluid, which can result in dangerous levels of hypernatremia. Manifestations of hypernatremia include central nervous system dysfunction such as neuromuscular irritability, seizures, obtundation, or coma. Calculation of water replacement needs is based on total body water, since water loss occurs from both intracellular and extracellular sites. In this case, a 60-kg woman has a plasma sodium of 160 mmol/L, which one would like to lower to 140 mmol/L. Total body water is roughly 60 percent of weight (36 L). To reduce the plasma sodium, this volume must be increased to 160/140 times 36 L, or about 41 L. Thus, a positive water balance of 5 L (41 − 36) is needed. This deficit is best corrected fairly slowly, with the aim being to replace about half the water deficit in the first day. If correction is done in this conservative fashion with close monitoring of electrolytes, progressive central nervous system dysfunction is not likely. If the patient had signs of circulatory collapse indicating an associated sodium deficiency, treatment would begin with normal saline to provide intracellular volume. In certain situations, such as hyperosmolar diabetic coma, the plasma osmolarity is elevated because of hyperglycemia as well as hypernatremia. Therefore, initial treatment should consist of normal saline to ensure circulatory integrity and insulin to lower plasma glucose and partially reduce intracellular osmolarity. Finally, half normal saline could be used to slowly replace the remaining water and salt deficits.

**III-3. The answer is A.** *(Chaps. 47, 330)* Failure to concentrate urine despite substantial hypertonic dehydration suggests a diagnosis of diabetes insipidus. A nephrogenic origin will be postulated if there is no increase in urine concentration after exogenous vasopressin. The only useful mode of therapy is a low-salt diet and use of a thiazide or amiloride, a potassium-sparing distal diuretic agent. The resultant volume contraction presumably enhances proximal reabsorption and thereby reduces urine flow.

**III-4. The answer is E.** *(Chaps. 47, 332)* This man's electrolyte pattern is consistent with the "syndrome of hyporeninemic hypoaldosteronism," or type IV renal tubular acidosis. The defect is believed to be due to an insufficiency of both angiotensin (because of impaired renin release) and adrenal mineralocorticoid secreting capacity. Inhibition of the renin-angiotensin system by nonsteroidal anti-inflammatory agents, converting-enzyme inhibitors, and beta$_2$-adrenergic blockade can contribute to hyperkalemia. Beta blockade also can interfere with intracellular potassium uptake. Potassium can leak out of cells owing to the digitalis-induced poisoning of the $Na^+$, $K^+$-ATPase. Use of carbenicillin can lead to hypokalemia, since this drug acts as an unresorbed anion, promoting the potassium loss associated with distal tubular secretion.

**III-5.   The answer is B.**  *(Chap. 50. Wrenn, Am J Med 91:119, 1991.)*   A reasonable way to approach the diagnosis of metabolic acidosis is to separate patients into those with an increased anion gap and those with a normal anion gap (hyperchloremic acidosis). A calculation of these unmeasured anions consists of the sum of plasma bicarbonate and chloride minus the plasma sodium concentration (the normal value is 8 to 16 mmol/L). Reasons for increased acid production include diabetic ketoacidosis, alcoholic ketoacidosis (as in this patient), starvation, lactic acidosis caused by circulatory failure, certain drugs and toxins, and poisoning resulting from salicylates, ethylene glycol, or methanol. Finally, renal failure increases the anion gap because sulfate, phosphate, and organic acid ions are not excreted normally. Normal anion gap acidosis is due to renal tubular dysfunction or colonic losses. Since the ratio of beta-hydroxybutyrate to acetoacetate is high in alcoholic ketoacidosis, ketonemia can be missed by the routinely employed nitroprusside (Acetest) reagent, which detects acetoacetate but not beta-hydroxybutyrate. Patients suffering from alcoholic ketoacidosis do well on infusions of glucose and saline. Neither insulin nor alkali is required in these situations unless the acidosis is extreme (bicarbonate less than 6 to 8 mmol/L).

**III-6.   The answer is D.**  *(Chap. 271)*   Development of advancing peripheral neuropathy is an indication for dialysis. Delaying dialysis could allow the development of irreversible motor deficits, such as foot drop. Prompt institution of dialysis, by contrast, usually prevents the progression of uremic peripheral neuropathy and may ameliorate early sensory defects. No pharmacologic agent would be of significant benefit in the clinical situation described.

**III-7.   The answer is D.**  *(Chap. 271)*   Impaired renal production of 1,25-dihydroxyvitamin $D_3$ leads to decreased calcium absorption from the gut. Impaired renal phosphate excretion leads to hyperphosphatemia, which initiates hyperparathyroidism. Hyperparathyroidism is worsened by hypocalcemia, which is present because of hyperphosphatemia and decreased enzymatic conversion of 25(OH)D to 1,25(OH)D, leading to decreased gut absorption of calcium. Finally, 1,25(OH)D deficiency worsens hyperparathyroidism, as 1,25(OH)D is a direct inhibitor of PTH secretion into bone. The resultant decreased serum calcium concentration leads to secondary hyperparathyroidism. Chronic metabolic acidosis leads to dissolution of bone buffers and decalcification. Aluminum administered in long-term therapy, although useful in controlling hyperphosphatemia and thereby hypocalcemia, can be taken up by bone and contribute to altered bone matrix. There is *no* significant loss of vitamin D or calcium associated with currently employed dialysis techniques.

**III-8.   The answer is A.**  *(Chap. 50)*   To offer optimal management to patients with acute renal failure, it is helpful to distinguish prerenal azotemia (generally managed with volume replacement or amelioration of cardiac dysfunction) from intrinsic renal dysfunction. Sodium reabsorption, which is quite avid in prerenal azotemia, is impaired in intrinsic renal disease. However, creatinine is reabsorbed less efficiently than sodium in both conditions. Therefore, the fractional excretion of sodium is very helpful in distinguishing between these two etiologies of renal failure. The fractional excretion of sodium is calculated by multiplying the urine sodium by the plasma creatinine, dividing this by the plasma sodium times the urine creatinine, and multiplying by 100. In this case the result is approximately 1.4, which suggests that impaired reabsorption of sodium is ongoing and that intrinsic renal failure is occurring. Only about 15 percent of patients receiving nephrotoxins such as aminoglycosides or radiocontrast agents have renal failure associated with a fractional excretion of sodium of less than 1 percent, and so an elevated value in this case points in the direction of nephrotoxic injury. The other causes of acute renal failure listed here are all associated with prerenal azotemia and therefore with a more avid reabsorption of sodium than that described.

**III-9.** **The answer is D.** *(Chap. 274)* One of the more common forms of asymptomatic urinary abnormalities is Berger's disease, which may be a cause of recurrent hematuria of glomerular origin. Such episodes of macroscopic hematuria may be associated with minor flulike illnesses or vigorous exercise. Skin rash, arthritis, and abdominal pain usually are absent, which tends to distinguish this entity from Henoch-Schönlein purpura. Occasionally patients develop a nephrotic or nephritic syndrome. Serum IgA levels are increased in about 50 percent of all cases, though serum complement is normal. Renal biopsy in these situations may reveal a spectrum of changes, though diffuse mesangial proliferation or focal and segmental proliferative glomerulonephritis is most common. The essential feature of Berger's disease is the finding of diffuse mesangial deposition of IgA on immunofluorescence microscopy. IgG, C3, and properdin, but not C1q or C4, also may be found on this study. Although the disease progresses slowly, about 50 percent of patients develop end-stage renal failure within 25 years of the original presentation. Men with hypertension and proteinemia (> 1 g/d) are most likely to progress. Except for a recent report suggesting that omega-3 fatty acids may play a role, specific therapy has not been useful. However, glucocorticoids or antibiotics may reduce the frequency of episodic gross hematuria. IgA deposition in the kidney and recurrent renal failure may occur in about 35 percent of those who receive a renal allograft. Fortunately, such recurrent pathologic findings usually are not associated with loss of renal function.

**III-10.** **The answer is B.** *(Chap. 274)* The characteristic pattern of focal (not all glomeruli) and segmental (not the entire glomerulus) glomerular scarring is shown. The history and laboratory features are also consistent with this lesion: some associated hypertension, diminution in creatinine clearance, and a relatively inactive urine sediment. The "nephropathy of obesity" may be associated with this lesion secondary to hyperfiltration; this condition may be more likely in obese patients with hypoxemia, obstructive sleep apnea, and right-sided heart failure. Hypertensive nephrosclerosis exhibits more prominent vascular changes and patchy, ischemic, totally sclerosed glomeruli. In addition, nephrosclerosis seldom is associated with nephrotic-range proteinuria. Minimal-change disease usually is associated with symptomatic edema and normal-appearing glomeruli as demonstrated by light microscopy. This patient's presentation is consistent with that of membranous nephropathy, but the biopsy is not. With membranous glomerular nephritis all glomeruli are uniformly involved with subepithelial dense deposits. There are no features of crescentic glomerulonephritis present.

**III-11.** **The answer is D.** *(Chap. 274)* Persons who have solid tumors and develop nephrotic syndrome usually have membranous glomerulopathy. Diagnosis of the nephrotic syndrome may precede recognition of the primary tumor. In several cases, tumor antigens have been discovered in the glomerular deposits; the nephrotic syndrome may remit after effective tumor therapy. Patients with Hodgkin's disease may develop nephrotic syndrome on the basis of minimal-change disease (diffuse epithelial foot process effacement on ultrastructural examination).

**III-12.** **The answer is A.** *(Chaps. 276, 279)* Cystine crystals appear as flat hexagonal plates and are found in association with cystine stones, which are caused by a hereditary deficiency in tubular cystine transport. Struvite stones result from chronic urinary tract infection with *Proteus* spp. These bacteria degrade urea to carbon dioxide and ammonia, which alkalinizes the urine, thereby favoring the formation of the insoluble triple salt $MgNH_4PO_4$. Struvite crystals can appear in the urine as rectangular prisms. Patients with proteinuria resulting from albuminuria exhibit a sediment characteristic of the nephrotic syndrome with oval fat bodies. Patients with intestinal malabsorption with concomitant steatorrhea, as in the case of a jejunoileal bypass done for obesity, may hyperabsorb oxalate and form calcium oxalate renal stones. Calcium oxalate crystals appear bipyramidal or as biconcave ovals. The sediment depicted here displays flat, square plates, which represent one of the several forms uric acid crystals manifest. Hyperuricemia may accompany rapid cell turnover (as occurs in the rapid lysis of lymphomas with large tumor burdens after chemotherapy). In such settings aggressive hydration, the use of allopurinol, and urinary alkalinization may provide effective prophylaxis against uric acid nephropathy.

**III-13. The answer is E.** *(Chap. 276)* A number of drugs may elicit an acute interstitial nephritis. The classic offender is methicillin, although ampicillin, penicillin, cephalothin, thiazides, furosemide, and nonsteroidal anti-inflammatory drugs also have been associated with this problem. Hematuria, fever, and skin rash may occur within 1 to 2 weeks of exposure to the drug. Urinalysis reveals protein, pyuria, and eosinophiluria. Ultrasonography discloses enlarged kidneys. A biopsy (usually not necessary, since withdrawal of the offending drug leads to complete resolution) will reveal normal glomeruli but infiltration of the interstitium with polymorphonuclear leukocytes, lymphocytes, plasma cells, and eosinophils.

**III-14. The answer is D.** *(Chap. 275)* A variety of diseases involve both pulmonary and renal (and often dermal) microvasculature and may present with either prominent pulmonary or renal manifestations. When a firm diagnosis cannot be made serologically or by biopsy of skin or lesions of the upper respiratory tract, renal biopsy may be necessary. In the case described in this question, the serologic findings, though not specific, are typical of Wegener's granulomatosis, a diagnosis established by the renal biopsy report. Granulomas are an uncommon microscopic finding in polyarteritis as well as in lupus nephritis and Henoch-Schönlein purpura, though a spectrum of pathologic abnormalities may be seen in the latter two conditions. Antineutrophil antibodies in the serum are highly suggestive of Wegener's granulomatosis and other systemic vasculitides. The renal biopsy in Goodpasture's syndrome usually reveals linear immunoglobulin deposits.

**III-15. The answer is A.** *(Chap. 276. Bennet, N Engl J Med 320:1269, 1989.)* Patients with damage to renal papillae may be unable to excrete maximally concentrated urine owing to chronic tubular damage. Moreover, the necrosed papillae can lead to the gradual development of renal failure. Although renal papillary necrosis classically has been associated with long-term abuse of analgesics (phenacetin or acetaminophen), such a finding also can be present in those with sickle cell anemia, diabetic nephropathy, or obstructive uropathy (as in the man with prostate disease) or after many episodes of pyelonephritis caused by urinary tract infections. Aspirin can potentiate the deleterious effects of chronic analgesic abuse by inhibiting the production of renal vasodilatory prostaglandins. Ingestion of lead, such as that caused by lead leaching out from an unusual distilling apparatus, can lead to a nephropathy manifested by tubular atrophy and fibrosis of small renal arteries.

**III-16. The answer is E.** *(Chap. 275)* The pathophysiology of nephrotoxic involvement by systemic lupus erythematosus (SLE) is thought to be immune complex deposition. Renal disease in SLE can range from mild abnormalities of the urinalysis to a fulminant inflammatory process that leads to progressive renal failure. Renal biopsy findings in patients with SLE who have worsening renal function can range from minimal glomerular lesions to diffuse proliferative lupus glomerulonephritis and membranous lupus glomerulonephritis. Patients with membranous lupus glomerulonephritis may be managed conservatively with therapy directed toward extrarenal manifestations. By contrast, those with more extensive or proliferative glomerular lesions require a more aggressive approach using corticosteroids (with or without another immunosuppressive agent, such as azathioprine or cyclophosphamide). However, little is gained by using immunosuppressant therapy in patients with advanced renal failure characterized by obliterative sclerosing lesions of the glomeruli. If such patients have other indications for dialysis, such as systemic symptoms and hyperkalemia, they are best managed with dialysis followed by renal transplantation. Measurement of serologic evidence of disease (e.g., double-stranded DNA autoantibodies or a decrease in serum complement components) may be helpful. Patients with end-stage lupus nephritis can be managed successfully with hemodialysis. Moreover, patients with SLE who have undergone renal allografting rarely experience recurrence of disease in the new kidney.

**III-17. The answer is B.** *(Chap. 272)* In the first week after renal transplantation the differential diagnosis of graft dysfunction includes early rejection, hypovolemia, cyclosporine intoxication, acute tubular necrosis, urinary obstruction, and renal artery thrombosis. Cyclosporine can mask many of the classic signs of rejection, such as fever and graft tenderness; renal biopsy often is needed to make the diagnosis. However, renal ultrasonography should precede any manipulation to rule out mechanical outflow obstruction, as it should in any patient with acute deterioration of renal function.

**III-18. The answer is D.** *(Chap. 96)* The most important differential diagnosis in the case presented is between a renal cell carcinoma and a benign cystic lesion. Urinalysis may be normal in the presence of renal cell carcinoma, and urinary cytology is unfortunately of little value in the diagnosis of this lesion. Ultrasonography will reveal whether the lesion is cystic. If the lesion fulfills the criteria for a simple cyst (lack of internal echoes, smooth borders, through transmission) and the patient does not have hematuria, the cyst can be considered benign with a diagnostic accuracy of 97 percent. If greater assurance is required or if there are changes on follow-up radiologic studies, needle aspiration should be carried out. If the ultrasound appearance is not consistent with a simple cyst, contrast-enhanced CT scanning, the optimal test for the diagnosis and staging of renal cell carcinoma, should be performed.

**III-19. The answer is D.** *(Chap. 96)* Older men are the most common victims of carcinoma of the bladder. Transitional cell carcinoma, the most common histologic subtype of cancer of the bladder in this country, is associated with a more favorable prognosis than is adenocarcinoma or squamous carcinoma. Squamous carcinomas occur more frequently in Egypt, where the prevalence of *Schistosoma haematobium* is high. The prognosis in cancer of the bladder is highly linked to the stage of the disease at presentation: muscular or perivascular fat invasion offers a much bleaker outlook (45 percent 5-year survival) than does disease confined to the mucosa. Risk factors for cancer of the bladder include exposure to the aromatic amines (cigarette smoke and products of the dye, rubber, and chemical industries) but not a positive family history, as in the case of renal carcinoma. Chronic bladder irritation, such as that produced by the metabolites of cyclophosphamide as well as by recurrent stones or infections, also leads to a higher incidence of carcinoma of the bladder.

**III-20. The answer is C.** *(Chaps. 49, 278. Narins, Am J Med 72:496, 1982.)* The evaluation of patients with hypokalemia should first include a consideration of redistribution of body potassium into cells as occurs in alkalosis, beta$_2$-agonist excess with refeeding syndrome and/or insulin therapy, vitamin B$_{12}$ therapy, patients with pernicious anemia, and periodic paralysis. In periodic paralysis serum bicarbonate is normal. If the patient is hypertensive and plasma renin is elevated, renovascular hypertension or a renin-secreting tumor (including Wilms') must be considered and appropriate imaging studies must be carried out. If plasma renin levels are low, mineralocorticoid effect may be high, due either to endogenous hormone (glucocorticoid overproduction or aldosterone overproduction as in Conn's syndrome) or to exogenous agents (licorice or steroids). In a normotensive patient a high serum bicarbonate excludes renal tubular acidosis. High urine chloride excretion makes gastrointestinal losses less likely and implies primary renal potassium loss as might be seen in diuretic abuse (ruled out by the urine screen) or Bartter's syndrome. In Bartter's syndrome, hyperplasia of the granular cells of the juxtaglomerular apparatus leads to high renin levels and secondary aldosterone elevations. Such hyperplasia appears to be secondary to chronic volume depletion caused by a hereditary (autosomal recessive) defect that interferes with salt reabsorption in the thick ascending loop of Henle. Chronic potassium depletion, which frequently initially presents in childhood, leads to polyuria and weakness.

**III-21. The answer is D.** *(Chap. 274)* The syndrome described is typical of rapidly progressive glomerulonephritis with rapid onset of acute renal failure in the setting of glomerular disease (manifested by red blood cell casts and proteinuria). The patient's vomiting is consistent with the development of azotemia over a short time period. Renal biopsy is highly recommended early in the course of such a disease to define the nature and severity of the glomerular lesion for both prognostic and therapeutic purposes. The hallmark pathologic lesion associated with this clinical scenario is crescentic glomerulonephritis, the manifestation of extracapillary endothelial proliferation. Such a finding on renal biopsy carries an ominous prognosis, especially if crescents are present in more than 70 percent of glomeruli or if GFR is < 5 mL/min. Spontaneous resolution rarely occurs except in cases associated with an infectious cause, such as endocarditis and streptococcal disease. Though controlled trials are lacking, it appears that high-dose methylprednisolone given parenterally ("pulse steroids") can stave off the need for hemodialysis in some patients. Plasmapheresis may benefit some patients, especially those who have anti-glomerular basement antibodies.

**III-22.   The answer is A.**   *(Chap. 272)*   Nearly 200,000 patients in the United States require long-term dialysis. Myocardial infarction and other complications of atherosclerotic vascular disease are frequently seen among these patients because of risk factors (e.g., diabetes mellitus) as well as accelerated atherosclerosis. Carpal tunnel syndrome and other complications of dialysis-related amyloidosis, such as an accumulation of beta$_2$ microglobulin in the osteoarticular structures, may occur in patients on dialysis for more than 5 to 10 years, particularly among the elderly. Protein-calorie malnutrition is seen in up to 50 percent of these patients and contributes substantially to increased mortality and morbidity. High-output congestive heart failure resulting from anemia and/or large arteriovenous fistulas is a rare complication in the erythropoietin era but should still be considered in a dialysis patient with dyspnea. Kidney transplant recipients are at increased risk of carcinoma of the skin, non-Hodgkin's lymphoma, and EBV-associated lymphoproliferative disorders; there has been no clear-cut increase in the risk of solid tumors in patients treated with dialysis.

**III-23.   The answer is D.**   *(Chap. 275)*   Cryoglobulinemia with renal involvement is associated with hypocomplementemia in the vast majority of cases; in the past several years, it has been well recognized that hepatitis C is the culprit in most instances. Diffuse proliferative lupus nephritis (WHO class IV) is the most aggressive form of the disease and the one most often associated with hypocomplementemia and active systemic disease. Relatively early in the course of postinfectious glomerulonephritis, immune complex deposition is in full force and serum complements are low; later, these parameters normalize, usually accompanying improved renal function. Henoch-Schönlein purpura, the systemic manifestation of IgA nephropathy, is not associated with hypocomplementemia. Other causes of hypocomplementemic glomerulonephritis are GN associated with subacute bacterial endocarditis or another chronic infection (e.g., abscess), membranoproliferative GN type II (dense deposit disease), and "shunt nephritis."

**III-24.   The answer is E.**   *(Chap. 270)*   Years before dialysis was routinely available, it was well established that protein restriction (prescribed or self-imposed) could alleviate some of the symptoms of uremia; unfortunately, prolonged protein restriction led to the development of malnutrition and its associated complications. In the setting of chronic renal failure, a number of clinical studies have suggested that modest protein restriction may slow the rate of progression of renal failure, particularly in patients with glomerular disease and daily protein excretion rates >1 g/d. There are insufficient data in the setting of acute renal failure to adequately assess the importance of protein intake. However, in view of the hypercatabolism that accompanies many cases of acute renal failure, most practitioners provide adequate protein to patients (e.g., ≥1.0 to 1.2 g protein per kg per day) and provide dialysis if uremia ensues. There are no set laboratory "cutoffs" (BUN >100) that indicate the need for dialysis.

**III-25.   The answer is B.**   *(Chap. 49. Beck, N Engl J Med 301:528–530, 1979.)*   Hyponatremia can be broadly categorized as hypovolemic, euvolemic, or hypervolemic. Hepatic cirrhosis in this case is unlikely because of the absence of edema. Gastrointestinal fluid loss is unlikely because of normal blood pressure without orthostasis. Furthermore, depending on whether the fluid loss is upper (vomiting with resultant alkalosis) or lower (diarrhea with resultant acidosis), it often is accompanied by a disturbance in acid-base balance. Addison's disease is possible, although it often is associated with orthostasis, some degree of hypotension, and hyperkalemia (due to aldosterone deficiency). The uric acid can be very helpful in the differential diagnosis of hyponatremia. It is typically elevated in patients with congestive heart failure and renal failure, two other important causes of hyponatremia, and tends to be quite low in patients with SIADH.

**III-26.  The answer is D.** *(Chap. 274)*   Membranous glomerulopathy is the most common cause of nephrotic syndrome in adults. Other relatively common disorders associated with nephrosis include diabetic nephropathy (seen in conjunction with retinopathy in >90 percent of cases), focal and segmental glomerulosclerosis (primary or secondary to remote nephron loss), minimal-change disease, paraproteinemias (amyloid, light-chain deposition disease), and HIV-associated nephropathy. Other glomerular diseases, including IgA nephropathy, postinfectious glomerulonephritis (GN), and membranoproliferative GN, may manifest with heavy proteinuria (>3.5 g/d) but rarely develop into full-blown nephrotic syndrome (with edema, severe hypoalbuminemia and hyperlipidemia, etc.).

**III-27.  The answer is C.** *(Chap. 272)*   Mycobacterial peritonitis and fungal peritonitis are relatively rare but important problems, particularly in patients who receive repeated courses of antibacterial therapy for suspected or documented bacterial peritonitis. Dialysis disequilibrium is a syndrome characterized by headache, confusion, and occasionally seizures; it is seen in association with the excessively rapid correction of uremia with dialysis (usually hemodialysis). It is thought to be related to cerebral edema caused by the rapid removal of extracellular solute (urea) with resultant osmotic transfer of water into the cells. Peritoneal carcinomatosis (from ovarian or widespread gastrointestinal carcinoma) is possible in this case, although there is no history of cancer.

**III-28.  The answer is E.** *(Chap. 50. Gabuzda, Hall, Medicine 45:481–490,1966.)*   Hypokalemia impairs the renal excretion of ammonium, thereby resulting in hyperammonemia in cases of hepatic failure. The use of loop diuretics (often prescribed for the edema and ascites associated with hepatic failure) promotes kaliuresis. The alternative choices may improve hyperammonemia in selected cases.

**III-29.  The answer is E.** *(Chap. 276)*   Nephrocalcinosis is an uncommon cause of interstitial renal disease associated with a variety of metabolic disorders. The routine (with or after a meal) use of calcium-based phosphate binders rarely results in hypercalcemia, although injudicious use may lead to complications. Crohn's disease and other abnormalities of ileal fat absorption may cause nephrocalcinosis because of excessive absorption of dietary oxalate and calcium oxalate nephrolithiasis.

**III-30.  The answer is B.** *(Chap. 275)*   Undernutrition is a major problem in patients with end-stage renal disease. Overnutrition, or obesity, is also a problem in selected patient groups and is a risk factor for the development of kidney disease via its associations with diabetes, hypertension, sleep apnea, and right-sided congestive heart failure. Focal segmental glomerulosclerosis with nephrotic syndrome is seen more commonly among the obese. Peritoneal dialysis, because of continuous glucose administration, and transplantation, often resulting from glucocorticoid use, are the two renal replacement therapies commonly associated with obesity.

**III-31.  The answer is D.** *(Chap. 50)*   The key element is the anion gap, calculated as (Na + K) − Cl (normal 8 to 12). The anion gap is 32 in this case. Causes of high anion gap acidosis include diabetic or alcoholic ketoacidosis, renal failure, and the excessive ingestion of salicylates, methanol, ethanol, or ethylene glycol. The clues here are the negative Acetest (making alcoholic and/or diabetic ketoacidosis less likely) and the presence of calcium oxalate crystals (oxylate is a by-product of ethylene glycol). Hemodialysis should be provided in these cases of toxic ingestion, since the products are water-soluble and can quickly cause damage to the CNS if not promptly removed.

**III-32.** **The answer is D.** *(Chap. 270)* Cholesterol embolization (also known as atheroembolic renal disease) is characterized by pyuria, progressive renal failure (usually nonoliguric), and associated organ dysfunction (including bowel, pancreas, and CNS). Hypocomplementemia and eosinophiluria also may be seen. The urinalysis is not compatible with acute tubular necrosis because of the absence of granular casts.

**III-33.** **The answer is C.** *(Chap. 274. Joven et al., N Engl J Med, 323:579–584, 1990.)* Dyslipidemia is present in the vast majority of patients with nephrotic syndrome and typically is characterized by a relatively selective increase in LDL cholesterol. There is evidence of accelerated atherosclerosis in these patients. Although there appears to be an increased risk of myositis in patients with renal failure treated with lipid-lowering agents, the risk is relatively low (far below 20 percent). Combination therapy (e.g., an HMG-CoA reductase inhibitor and a fibric acid derivative) should be used with caution.

**III-34.** **The answer is D.** *(Chap. 271. Maschio et al., N Engl J Med 334:939–945, 1996.)* Evidence continues to accumulate that inhibition of angiotensin converting enzyme can slow the progression of chronic renal insufficiency in a variety of disease states. In general, patients with protein excretion rates in excess of 1 g per day tend to derive the greatest benefit. For reasons that are not entirely clear, patients with ADPKD tend not to benefit from this therapy (and do not appear to benefit from a low-protein diet).

**III-35.** **The answer is A-N, B-N, C-Y, D-Y, E-N.** *(Chaps. 47, 270. Kupin, Contrib Nephrol 102:1, 1993.)* Because of a beneficial effect on neuromuscular membranes, intravenous calcium infusion is the correct treatment for the cardiac disturbances caused by hyperkalemia; however, this approach does not lower serum potassium concentration. Sodium bicarbonate infusion, however, lowers serum potassium levels rapidly by causing potassium to move into cells. Intravenous infusion of glucose and insulin achieves the same result, though slightly less rapidly. Potassium-binding resins effectively remove potassium from the body but act slowly, particularly when instilled into the stomach. Persons who are in acute renal failure and have a large potassium load because of severe muscle damage may require emergency dialysis. Such persons have a profound inability to excrete magnesium, and so the administration of additional magnesium would be dangerous.

**III-36.** **The answer is A-Y, B-Y, C-Y, D-Y, E-Y.** *(Chap. 270)* Muscle cells may be sufficiently taxed during strenuous exercise (e.g., distance running) to result in cell breakdown and myoglobin release. Muscle breakdown associated with sedative overdose generally is attributed to ischemia caused by muscle compression in immobile, comatose patients. Muscle ischemia and breakdown can result from mechanical compression, vascular insufficiency, or cocaine overdose. Not only can ethanol ingestion promote muscle breakdown in a similar manner, ethanol itself has a direct toxic effect on muscle. Hypokalemia and hypophosphatemia decrease energy production by muscle cells and thus increase the risk of rhabdomyolysis in any setting. Volume depletion can contribute to decreased muscle perfusion and, more important, increase the susceptibility of the kidneys to damage from myoglobin and other muscle breakdown products.

**III-37.** **The answer is A-N, B-Y, C-N, D-Y, E-Y.** *(Chap. 47. Resnick, N Engl J Med 320:1, 1989.)* The force for bladder emptying is provided by the detrusor muscle, which is innervated by parasympathetic outflow from the sacral plexus. The involuntary control that prevents automatic bladder emptying emanates from sympathetic innervation of the bladder outlet. A sacral spinal reflex arc mediates automatic detrusor contraction when the intravesical pressure exceeds 20 cmH$_2$O (a volume of 400 mL) unless it is inhibited by cortical centers via the reticulospinal tracts. Diseases leading to damage of inhibitory neural pathways in the brain or spinal cord, such as multiple strokes, Alzheimer's disease, brain tumors, and normal-pressure hydrocephalus, create detrusor instability. In this situation the bladder will empty automatically before it is filled owing to unchecked operation of the spinal reflex arc. By contrast, conditions leading to chronic overflow incontinence caused by obstruction at the bladder neck or a hypotonic bladder caused by autonomic neuropathy can result in hydronephrosis and impaired renal function. The most common example of outflow obstruction is benign prostatic hypertrophy. Examples of conditions in which autonomic peripheral neuropathy can lead to overflow incontinence include diabetes mellitus, hypothyroidism, uremia, collagen vascular diseases, Guillain-Barré syndrome, and exposure to certain toxins (including alcohol). Cholinergic agents such as bethanechol sometimes can aid bladder emptying in those with overflow incontinence.

**III-38.** **The answer is A-Y, B-N, C-Y, D-Y, E-N.** *(Chap. 274)* Persons who have nephrotic syndrome may lose a variety of serum proteins other than albumin. Loss of thyroxine-binding globulin leads to reduced serum thyroxine levels, and loss of cholecalciferol-binding protein may combine with a decrease in albumin-bound calcium to reduce serum calcium levels. Loss of antithrombin III, protein C, or protein S and hyperfibrinogenemia have been implicated in hypercoagulability, which affects some persons who have the nephrotic syndrome. Hyperlipidemia is associated commonly with the nephrotic syndrome; the cause remains uncertain, though the lowered plasma oncotic pressure may stimulate hepatic lipoprotein synthesis. Loss of metal-binding proteins may lead to zinc or copper deficiency.

**III-38.** **The answer is A-Y, B-Y, C-N, D-N, E-Y.** *(Chap. 274)* Studies during epidemics of streptococcal disease have shown that the latent period between symptomatic pharyngitis and the appearance of poststreptococcal glomerulonephritis (PSGN) is 6 to 10 days. The latent period after cutaneous infection is more difficult to establish but appears to be longer. Persons who receive early antimicrobial therapy for streptococcal infection may develop glomerulonephritis but not mount the immune response to the streptococcal enzymes (e.g., streptolysin O) on which laboratory testing for antecedent streptococcal infection is based. Antimicrobial therapy is recommended for persons who have acute glomerulonephritis and continuing streptococcal infection. Long-term prophylaxis, however, is unwarranted because affected persons are not markedly predisposed to recurrent episodes of PSGN. For unknown reasons, PSGN leads to permanent, progressive renal insufficiency more often in adults than in children.

**III-40.** **The answer is A-Y, B-Y, C-N, D-N, E-N.** *(Reeders, Nat Genet 1:235–237, 1992.)* Most patients with adult polycystic kidney disease, an autosomal dominant disorder, are presumed to have a mutation at a locus on the short arm of chromosome 16. This particular locus is close to the gene coding for the alpha-globin chain. A highly polymorphic (genetic variability among individuals; less than 1 percent of the population is homozygous) locus is associated with the alpha-globin gene cluster. Thus, in an individual family with members manifesting the disease, a given polymorphic allele can be shown to be coinherited with the disease. Since such a polymorphism is inherited as a germ-line sequence, DNA from any tissue in the body can be extracted, cut with the proper restriction enzyme, electrophoresed, and probed with a radioactive sequence at the polymorphic region. The presence of a fragment of the size previously established to be associated with the disease suggests a predisposition to the disease. If a person lacks the relevant fragment, even if that person is homozygous at the polymorphism, the likelihood of disease is very low because of the proximity of this locus to the disease-specific gene. The biochemical defect has not been identified; patients have an increased incidence of subarachnoid hemorrhage resulting from berry aneurysms as well as pancreatic and hepatic cysts.

**III-41.** **The answer is A-Y, B-N, C-Y, D-N, E-Y.** *(Chap. 270)* The granular casts seen in the photograph are the hallmark of acute tubular necrosis (ATN) (ischemic or nephrotoxic acute renal failure). The most common cause of ATN is prerenal failure. Such an occurrence is not uncommon in major intravascular volume loss of a real or effective nature (burns, trauma, surgery with major blood loss or aortic compromise, severe pancreatitis, pregnancy-related catastrophe, severe heart failure). A second important cause of ATN is that brought on by agents directly toxic to the tubules. These agents include endogenous pigments such as hemoglobin (released in hemolytic crises) and myoglobin (released in rhabdomyolysis from any cause, including heat stroke, multiple trauma, severe exercise, and hypokalemia/hypophosphatemia). Certain antibiotics (e.g., aminoglycosides), radiographic contrast, organic solvents, and heavy metals are examples of direct tubular toxins. The renal disease caused by endocarditis would produce red blood cell casts on urinalysis. Obstructive uropathy, as exemplified by the man with prostatism, would tend to produce few abnormalities in the urinary sediment.

**III-42.** **The answer is A-N, B-Y, C-Y, D-Y, E-Y.** *(Chap. 271. Eschback, Ann Intern Med 111:992, 1989.)* Debilitating normochromic, normocytic anemia experienced by most patients with chronic renal failure (CRF) is a significant clinical problem. Fortunately, much recent evidence supports the use of recombinant human erythropoietin as a safe and effective therapy, even though bone marrow responsiveness may be somewhat decreased owing to the presence of uremic toxins. The former reliance on multiple blood transfusions was fraught with dangers, including viral infections and hemosiderosis (chronic iron overload), which can damage many organs, including the heart and gonads. Folic acid deficiency is not uncommon in these patients, since the vitamin is lost during dialysis even though the MCV is not elevated. Clotting problems in uremia are multifactorial; however, impaired platelet function can be improved safely with the administration of cryoprecipitate, desmopressin, or erythropoietin.

**III-43.** **The answer is A-Y, B-N, C-Y, D-N, E-Y.** *(Chap. 276)* Glycosuria (with a normal blood glucose concentration), proteinuria, and hyperchloremic acidosis ("normal anion gap acidosis") constitute evidence of proximal renal tubular dysfunction. Frequent nocturia, presumably resulting from an impaired ability to concentrate urine, also suggests renal insufficiency caused by a tubulointerstitial disease. Multiple myeloma may present in this manner, and similar renal abnormalities may be associated with analgesic abuse and Sjögren's syndrome. The findings presented in this case are not characteristic of primary glomerular diseases, such as diabetic nephropathy, or the membranous glomerulopathy induced by penicillamine.

**III-44.** **The answer is A-N, B-Y, C-Y, D-Y, E-Y.** *(Chaps. 278, 279)* This patient with recurrent renal calculi and nephrocalcinosis has a normal serum calcium concentration. The serum electrolyte pattern is typical of distal (type 1) renal tubular acidosis with evidence of renal potassium wasting, hyperchloremic metabolic acidosis, and an alkaline urine. The nephrocalcinosis and distal RTA could be consistent with hypervitaminosis D, medullary sponge kidney, hyperparathyroidism, sarcoidosis, or multiple myeloma. However, in all these conditions except medullary sponge kidney, an increased serum calcium concentration is responsible for the nephrocalcinosis. Intravenous pyelography would better define the defect seen in medullary sponge kidney; it shows a typical "paintbrush" pattern in the renal papillae with tiny papillary cysts containing the calcium deposits. Although medullary sponge kidney usually is not inherited, type 1 distal RTA is often hereditary, and relatives should be screened.

**III-45.** **The answer is A-N, B-Y, C-Y, D-N, E-Y.** *(Chap. 272)* Living volunteer donors should be healthy, have normal renal arteries, and have the same blood group as the recipient. The one exception to the last rule occurs in the case of a type O donor, who can donate to a recipient with any blood group, since no endothelial antigens in the ABO system are present to engender rejection. The donor and recipient should be as closely HLA-matched as possible, and the mixed lymphocyte response (MLR) should be absent. DNA typing techniques have obviated the need for MLR testing in related donors. In the case of cadaveric donor kidneys, there is a direct relationship between the degree of HLA incompatibility and graft loss. For example, there is a projected 10-year graft survival rate of 27 percent if there are five HLA mismatches but a 52 percent rate if there is only one mismatch. Chronic rejection frequently is due to nephrosclerosis, which often is initially characterized by proliferation of the intima (with eventual fibrosis) in the renal vasculature. Prophylaxis against rejection includes the use of cyclosporine, which inhibits production of the immunostimulatory molecule IL-2 by helper-inducer T lymphocytes and the mercaptopurine analogue azathioprine. Azathioprine is metabolized by the purine degradative pathway to uric acid via the action of xanthine oxidase. Thus, coadministration of the xanthine oxidase inhibitor allopurinol could interfere with drug catabolism and lead to a dangerously toxic effect of a given dose of azathioprine.

**111-46. The answer is A-Y, B-N, C-Y, D-Y, E-N.** *(Chap. 279. Coe, N Engl J Med 327: 1141–1152, 1992.)* The clinical scenario is certainly consistent with distention/irritation of the renal collecting system as a result of stone passage. Since about 75 percent of all renal stones are caused by calcium oxalate or calcium phosphate, it is likely that the scout film of the abdomen will be positive. While surgical removal (either directly or by retrograde passage of a basket) was the primary approach in the treatment of a renal stone that led to intractable pain, obstruction, bleeding, or infection, lithotripsy (stone dissolution by sound waves) is becoming the preferred alternative. Ultrasound can be applied directly via a cystoscopically placed transducer, via percutaneous flank incision, or by extracorporeal means. The composition of the kidney stone should be assessed directly, if possible. Outpatient evaluation should consist of measurements of serum electrolytes, creatinine, uric acid, serum and urine calcium, and urine oxalate and citrate. In this fashion one will screen for idiopathic hypercalciuria (the most common reason for nephrolithiasis), primary hyperparathyroidism, hyperuricosuria, distal renal tubular acidosis, and hyperoxaluria (associated with fat malabsorption, including that due to ileal resection or bypass). If the patient is found to have idiopathic hypercalciuria, thiazide diuretics are a reasonable therapeutic approach because they lower calcium excretion.

**III-47–III-49. The answers are 47-A, 48-C, 49-D.** *(Chap. 50)* All the sets of laboratory values presented in this question indicate renal insufficiency with metabolic acidosis. Calculation of unmeasured anions (anion gap) is helpful in determining the etiology of the acidosis. Ethylene glycol ingestion, for example, not only causes acute renal failure but leads to rapid accumulation of metabolic acids. Acidosis is disproportionate to the degree of renal insufficiency and is characterized by a high anion gap (choice A). Amphotericin B also causes renal insufficiency with disproportionate metabolic acidosis. Acidosis, however, is due to a distal tubular acidification defect (distal, or type 1, renal tubular acidosis) and is characterized by hyperchloremia, a normal anion gap, and inability to lower the urine pH (choice C). Urinary potassium loss also may be excessive. With moderate renal insufficiency caused by glomerulonephritis, metabolic acidosis usually is mild and the anion gap is only slightly, if at all, elevated (choice D).

The set of laboratory data in choice E illustrates moderate renal insufficiency with disproportionate hyperkalemia and hyperchloremic acidosis, so-called type IV renal tubular acidosis. A number of causes of renal insufficiency, most notably diabetic nephropathy but usually not acute glomerulonephritis, can produce these findings. The laboratory values in choice B illustrate an apparent reduction of the anion gap, which has been reported most frequently in association with multiple myeloma. The apparent reduction in unmeasured anions is due to the presence of abnormal circulating paraprotein that bears a positive charge.

# IV. DISORDERS OF THE NERVOUS SYSTEM AND MUSCLES

## *QUESTIONS*

**DIRECTIONS:** Each question below contains five suggested responses. Choose the **one best** response to each question.

**IV-1.** For the last 5 weeks a 35-year-old woman has had episodes of intense vertigo lasting several hours. Each episode is associated with tinnitus and a sense of fullness in the right ear; during the attacks, she prefers to lie on her left side. Examination during an attack shows that she has fine rotary nystagmus, which is maximal on gaze to the left. There are no ocular palsies, cranial-nerve signs, or long-tract signs. An audiogram shows high-tone hearing loss in the right ear, with recruitment but no tone decay. The most likely diagnosis in this case is

(A) labyrinthitis
(B) Ménière's disease
(C) vertebral-basilar insufficiency
(D) acoustic neuroma
(E) multiple sclerosis

**IV-2.** A 25-year-old woman presents to the emergency department with a severe, throbbing headache of the right supraorbital area for the past hour. She also complains of nausea and photophobia. She has had similar attacks in the past, often brought on by menstruation. About 45 min ago she took 400 mg of ibuprofen. Which of the following would be the best therapeutic choice at this time?

(A) Meperidine, 50 mg intramuscularly
(B) Codeine, 60 mg orally
(C) Naproxen, 750 mg orally
(D) Sumatriptan, 6 mg subcutaneously
(E) Verapamil, 300 mg orally

**IV-3.** A 29-year-old woman who uses oral contraceptives comes to the emergency room because when she looked in the mirror this morning, her face was twisted. It felt numb and swollen. While eating breakfast, she found that her food tasted different and she drooled out of the right side of her mouth when swallowing. Neurologic examination discloses only a dense right facial paresis equally involving the frontalis, orbicularis oculi, and orbicularis oris. Finger rubbing is appreciated as louder in the right ear than in the left. The physician should

(A) instruct the patient in using a patch over the right eye during sleep
(B) recommend that she discontinue the use of oral contraceptives
(C) order brainstem auditory evoked potentials to assess her hearing asymmetry
(D) inform her that her chances of substantial improvement within several weeks are only about 40 percent
(E) order an echocardiogram to rule out mitral valve prolapse as a source of emboli

**IV-4.** The distinctive tetrad of symptoms of the narcolepsy-cataplexy syndrome includes all the following EXCEPT

(A) uncontrollable daytime sleepiness
(B) sudden brief episodes of loss of muscle tone
(C) paralysis upon falling asleep
(D) confusional episodes
(E) hallucinations at the onset of sleep or wakening

**IV-5.** A 45-year-old man presents with a daily headache. He describes two attacks per day over the past 3 weeks. Each attack lasts about an hour and awakens the patient from sleep. The patient has noted associated tearing and reddening of his right eye as well as nasal stuffiness. The pain is deep, excruciating, and limited to the right side of the head. The neurologic examination is nonfocal. The most likely diagnosis of this patient's headache is

(A) migraine headache
(B) cluster headache
(C) tension headache
(D) brain tumor
(E) giant cell arteritis

**IV-6.** A 25-year-old woman who was the driver of a car struck in the rear by another car while she was stopped at a red light presents to the emergency department with neck pain as well as discomfort in the axilla, upper arm, elbow, dorsal forearm, and index and middle fingers. Coughing exacerbates the pain. Neurologic examination reveals weakness in the right second and third fingers, forearm, and wrist. The right triceps reflex is diminished. The most likely diagnosis in this case is

(A) syringomyelia
(B) cervical sprain
(C) thoracic outlet syndrome
(D) cervical disk herniation
(E) brachial plexopathy

**IV-7.** A patient with previous spells of diplopia, ataxia, dysarthria, and dizziness becomes acutely comatose. The most likely cause is

(A) basilar artery thrombosis
(B) subarachnoid hemorrhage
(C) carotid occlusion
(D) cerebellar hemorrhage
(E) pontine hemorrhage

**IV-8.** A 75-year-old woman complains of dizziness and lightheadedness while walking. The patient has had long-standing diabetes and is taking an oral hypoglycemic agent. She has no other medical problems and lives alone. Physical examination reveals visual acuity of 20/80 in both eyes and sensory neuropathy in a stocking-glove distribution. On close questioning, she denies any symptoms of "herself spinning or the world spinning." She has no apparent anxiety or depression. Orthostatic vital signs are normal. A head-tilt maneuver reveals no nystagmus. The most likely diagnosis in this case is

(A) dysequilibrium of aging
(B) benign positional vertigo
(C) Ménière's disease
(D) brainstem stroke
(E) neoplasm of the central nervous system

**IV-9.** A 35-year-old woman complaining of trouble with her "peripheral vision" is subjected to visual field examination. While one eye is tested at a time, she is asked to focus on a central target while the examiner's fingers are moved in from various directions. She is unable to distinguish objects brought laterally toward the midline, encompassing about half the visual field in each eye. Which of the following lesions would most likely account for these findings?

(A) Open-angle glaucoma
(B) Closed-angle glaucoma
(C) Multiple sclerosis
(D) Pituitary tumor
(E) Embolic occlusion of the posterior
    cerebral artery

**IV-10.** Evoked-potential testing is most useful in diagnosing

(A) brainstem involvement in stroke
(B) a clinically occult lesion in multiple sclerosis
(C) large hemispheral strokes
(D) spinal cord compression
(E) shearing of white matter tracts after
    head injury

**IV-11.** A 25-year-old weight lifter comes to the emergency department frightened by recent headaches. He recently read a newspaper article about cerebral aneurysms. He reports 5 to 10 sudden, severe headaches, all occurring during coitus, with each lasting about 1 h. The physician should

(A) recommend that the patient seek psychiatric help for his sexual dysfunction
(B) perform a CT scan with contrast and schedule four-vessel cerebral angiography to search for an aneurysm or arteriovenous malformation
(C) inform the patient that coital headache is a benign clinical syndrome that may be helped by the administration of propranolol, 20 mg three times a day
(D) tell the patient to report back to the emergency department for a cerebrospinal fluid examination and CT scan without contrast to search for subarachnoid blood
(E) determine whether other members of his family have a history of migraine

**IV-12.** A 60-year-old male diabetic patient complains of the acute onset of diplopia. He denies headache, fever, stiff neck, or other symptoms. The only abnormality on neurologic examination pertains to eye movements. The patient's right eyelid is ptotic. The pupil is deviated downward and outward. The patient cannot move the eye upward, downward, or inward. There is, however, no anisocoria, and normal pupillary responses are present bilaterally. The appropriate course of action at this time is

(A) administration of high-dose steroids
(B) administration of a topical ophthalmic beta-adrenergic blocker
(C) cerebral angiography
(D) visual field testing
(E) reexamination in 1 month

**IV-13.** Presbycusis, the hearing loss associated with aging, may affect 33 percent of people age 75 or older. The most common cause of this problem is

(A) fixation of middle ear bones
(B) tympanic membrane failure
(C) loss of neuroepithelial cells
(D) vascular lesions in central auditory pathways
(E) exposure to ototoxins such as furosemide

**IV-14.** Bradykinesia, a decreased ability to initiate volitional movements, as well as constant impedance to the examiner's efforts to extend the arm would most likely be due to lesions in which of the following structures?

(A) Anterior horn cell of the spinal cord
(B) Descending corticospinal fibers
(C) Basal ganglia
(D) Internal capsule
(E) Cerebral cortex

**IV-15.** A 70-year-old man complains of pain and stiffness in both shoulders and hips. Examination reveals atrophic shoulder girdle and gluteal musculature. Reflexes and cerebellar function are intact. There is no sensory loss. The serum creatine kinase level is normal. Temporal artery biopsy is negative. The most appropriate therapeutic strategy at this time is

(A) prednisone, 60 mg daily
(B) prednisone, 10 mg daily
(C) potassium repletion
(D) naproxen, 750 mg twice daily
(E) reassurance; no treatment is required

**IV-16.** A 65-year-old man with advanced pancreatic cancer complains of increasing abdominal pain. He is taking codeine 60 mg every 4 h. Examination reveals an alert man with a benign abdomen and normal neurologic function. The best step at this point would be to

(A) add phenytoin
(B) add indomethacin
(C) increase the dose of codeine
(D) add sustained-release morphine sulfate and use the codeine as circumstances require (prn)
(E) refer the patient for a celiac block

**IV-17.** A 55-year-old woman presents because of intermittent, brief, extreme stabbing pains in her lips and right cheek. The pain can be brought on by touching her face. The results of an examination of the structures of the face and cranial nerves are entirely normal. Appropriate initial treatment for this condition would consist of

(A) ergotamine
(B) amitriptyline
(C) propranolol
(D) carbamazepine
(E) referral to an otolaryngologist for nerve block

**IV-18.** During the evaluation of a patient with a gait disorder, it is noted that the patient is unable to identify accurately the direction of examiner-initiated movement of the great toe. Pain and temperature sense in the same distribution are intact. This abnormality reflects a lesion in which of the following structures?

(A) Posterior column on the same side as the affected toe
(B) Spinothalamic tract on the same side as the affected toe
(C) Thalamic nucleus on the same side as the affected toe
(D) Lower sensory neuron on the same side as the affected toe
(E) Frontal cortex on the opposite side from the affected toe

**IV-19.** A patient being evaluated for aphasia is unable to repeat sentences correctly or name objects properly. However, the patient's speech is effortless and melodic. There are frequent errors in word choice and obvious difficulties in comprehension. The remainder of the patient's neurologic examination is normal. Damage in which area of the brain would account for this type of aphasia?

(A) Posterior temporal and parietal lobes, dominant hemisphere
(B) Frontal and parietal lobes, dominant hemisphere
(C) Prefrontal and frontal regions, dominant hemisphere
(D) Posterior parietal and temporal lobes, nondominant hemisphere
(E) Parietal and occipital lobes, nondominant hemisphere

**IV-20.** A patient is evaluated for anisocoria. The right pupil is small and round compared with the left pupil in room light; this difference is magnified when the room is darkened. The right pupil responds briskly to light, constricts when pilocarpine is placed in the eye, and dilates when atropine is placed in the eye. Minimal dilation is produced by 4% cocaine. This patient has a lesion in the

(A) right optic nerve
(B) right iris
(C) right third nerve
(D) right sympathetic chain
(E) left occipital lobe

**IV-21.** Which of the following would help exclude the diagnosis of seizure in a patient with sudden loss of consciousness?

(A) A brief period of tonic-clonic movements at the time of falling
(B) An aura of a strange odor before falling
(C) Sudden return to normal mental function upon awakening, though with a feeling of physical weakness
(D) Urinary incontinence
(E) Laceration of the tongue

**IV-22.** A 55-year-old man who lost his job approximately 5 months ago complains of profound difficulty sleeping at night. He recently found a new job but has continued to experience difficulty sleeping. He notes that he falls asleep more easily while watching television early in the evening and feels sleepy outside the house. He is preoccupied with his inability to sleep at night. General physical examination and routine laboratory screening are unremarkable. He denies the use of alcohol, coffee, and other drugs. What is the most appropriate approach?

(A) Administration of a benzodiazepine
(B) Administration of stimulants
(C) Administration of estrogen
(D) Administration of tricyclic antidepressants
(E) No therapy

**IV-23.** A 65-year-old man presents with severe right-sided eye and facial pain, nausea, vomiting, colored halos around lights, and loss of visual acuity. His right eye is quite red, and that pupil is dilated and fixed. Which of the following diagnostic tests would confirm the diagnosis?

(A) CT of the head
(B) MRI of the head
(C) Cerebral angiography
(D) Tonometry
(E) Slit-lamp examination

**IV-24.** A 35-year-old woman presents with an apparent seizure. She was feeling well when she noted that her right thumb began suddenly to retract repetitively, followed by right hand movements. Within 1 min her right arm and the right side of her face also began to contract. About 2 min later the patient developed diffuse convulsive motor activity and loss of consciousness lasting about 5 min. After her recovery of consciousness the patient was amnestic for the event and also had about 6 h of weakness in her right arm. Which of the following is the most likely cause of this type of seizure?

(A) Herpes encephalitis
(B) Temporal lobe epilepsy
(C) Juvenile myoclonic epilepsy
(D) Abscess or tumor in the left motor strip
(E) Cerebral embolism

**IV-25.** A 19-year-old man has had an 8-year history of recurrent episodes of loss of conscious activity that last for seconds to several minutes. Sometimes he has as many as 100 of these lapses. The patient regains awareness of his environment very quickly. There is no major motor manifestation during the episodes or a period of confusion afterward. The patient's neurologic examination is totally normal. Which of the following drugs would be the most effective for this patient's problem?

(A) Phenytoin
(B) Carbamazepine
(C) Phenobarbital
(D) Ethosuximide
(E) Primidone

**IV-26.** A patient who complains of imbalance is found to walk with a wide-based gait and to sway forward and backward upon standing. Balance cannot be maintained when the patient is standing with the feet together and with the eyes open or closed. No limb ataxia or nystagmus can be elicited. These findings are most consistent with a lesion or lesions in the

(A) vestibular apparatus
(B) midline cerebellar zone
(C) intermediate cerebellar zone
(D) lateral cerebellar zone
(E) left frontal cortex

**IV-27.** Which of the following brain tumors tends to occur in immunosuppressed persons, arise in periventricular regions, and respond both clinically and radiographically to corticosteroid therapy?

(A) Glioblastoma
(B) Ependymoma
(C) Meningioma
(D) Medulloblastoma
(E) B-cell lymphoma

**IV-28.** A 59-year-old chronic alcoholic has loss of consciousness and shaking of his entire body for approximately 5 min. He is somewhat confused after this episode and is brought to the emergency department, where another episode occurs. The patient develops incontinence during the event and again is confused afterward. CT of the brain and a lumbar puncture are negative. No major metabolic abnormalities were detected on blood testing. Appropriate therapy for this condition consists of

(A) phenytoin, 1000 mg given in a slow IV push
(B) diazepam, 10 mg IV bolus
(C) phenobarbital, 400 mg given over 30 min
(D) carbamazepine, 600 mg orally daily
(E) no specific anticonvulsant therapy

**IV-29.** A patient who is being treated for temporal lobe epilepsy (complex partial seizures) and is having recurrent seizures on his chronic regimen of carbamazepine is given phenobarbital as a second drug. However, the seizures increase in frequency. What is the probable reason for the apparently deleterious effect of adding phenobarbital?

(A) Intracerebral bleeding from worsening bone marrow suppression
(B) Decreased carbamazepine level
(C) Decreased stability of CNS neuronal membranes
(D) Hypokalemia
(E) Increased intracranial pressure

**IV-30.** A person who has right hemiparesis from stroke would be LEAST likely to display

(A) left facial weakness
(B) left-gaze paresis
(C) inability to calculate
(D) left-right confusion
(E) ignoring of the deficit

**IV-31.** A 65-year-old man with a long-standing history of hypertension complains of recurrent 30-min episodes of right arm weakness occasionally associated with difficulty speaking. The results of his neurologic examination at this time are normal. Cerebral angiography reveals 80 percent stenosis of the left internal carotid artery. The most appropriate therapy at this point would be

(A) intravenous heparin with a plan to convert to oral warfarin
(B) oral warfarin
(C) aspirin
(D) ticlopidine
(E) carotid endarterectomy

**IV-32.**   A 54-year-old man with long-standing hypertension presents to the emergency department with severe occipital headache and dizziness. He has noted several hours of nausea and vomiting. Neurologic examination reveals an inability to stand. His eyes are deviated to the right side, and he has mild left-sided facial weakness. Assuming that blood is seen on CT scanning, which is the most appropriate therapeutic strategy at this time?

(A)   Intravenous high-dose dexamethasone
(B)   Intravenous mannitol
(C)   Intravenous nitroprusside
(D)   Surgical removal of a clot
(E)   Cerebral angiography

**IV-33.**   For the last 6 weeks, a 64-year-old woman has had a headache and difficulty reading. Her husband has noted a mild but progressive intellectual decline in her during this period. On examination, she has grasping reactions and myoclonic jerks when loud noises occur. CT and cerebrospinal fluid examination are normal. The most likely diagnosis is

(A)   multiple sclerosis
(B)   Alzheimer's disease
(C)   bilateral subdural hematoma
(D)   Creutzfeldt-Jakob disease
(E)   subacute sclerosing panencephalitis

**IV-34.**   The most common presenting finding or symptom of multiple sclerosis is

(A)   internuclear ophthalmoplegia
(B)   transverse myelitis
(C)   cerebellar ataxia
(D)   optic neuritis
(E)   urinary retention

**IV-35.**   A 45-year-old woman presents with a generalized tonic-clonic seizure, the first in her life. MRI evaluation reveals a midline mass along the falx cerebri. The mass enhances with gadolinium, which documents the existence of tumor vessels supplied by the external carotid artery. The optimal therapy would be

(A)   surgery
(B)   radiation
(C)   radiation plus surgery
(D)   radiation plus surgery plus chemotherapy
(E)   radiation plus chemotherapy

**IV-36.**   The most common cause of death in patients with intracerebral metastatic lesions resulting from carcinoma is

(A)   intractable seizures
(B)   infection
(C)   radiation toxicity
(D)   progressive intracerebral metastases
(E)   systemic tumor

**IV-37.**   A comatose patient is being evaluated by caloric stimulation of the vestibular apparatus. Cold-water irrigation of the right external auditory canal leads to deviation of both eyes to the right for 2 min, followed by a slow drift back to the midline. This finding is most consistent with a lesion in the

(A)   right labyrinth
(B)   midbrain
(C)   medulla
(D)   pons
(E)   cerebral hemispheres

**IV-38.**   A 68-year-old woman presents with an 18-month history of progressive loss of recent memory and inattentiveness. At this time she is having difficulty speaking, her judgment appears to be impaired, and she occasionally evidences paranoid behavior. In addition to neurofibrillary tangles, the neuropathologic findings in this condition include plaques made of

(A)   low-density lipoprotein
(B)   unesterified cholesterol
(C)   beta-amyloid protein
(D)   immunoglobulin proteins
(E)   protease inhibitor

**IV-39**   A 68-year-old man develops a rest tremor of the right hand and arm. The patient moves slowly and has a diminished range of facial expressions. He has no postural abnormalities. Which of the following drugs would be most appropriate at this time?

(A)   Deprenyl
(B)   Levodopa
(C)   Carbidopa-levodopa (Sinemet)
(D)   Bromocriptine
(E)   Benztropine

**IV-40.** A 69-year-old man is brought to the doctor by his wife because she complains that he has been "talking strangely." The patient enunciates words slowly and with difficulty. The melody of speech is abnormal. The speech is agrammatic in the sense that many prepositions and articles are omitted. When a word can be discerned, it usually is appropriate for the conversation, and the patient appears to comprehend what is said to him. The lesion accounting for this problem is most likely to be in the

(A) left frontal lobe
(B) right frontal lobe
(C) left parietal lobe
(D) right parietal lobe
(E) bilateral temporal lobes

**IV-41.** A 50-year-old woman presents to her primary care physician complaining of intermittent unprovoked attacks of severe shortness of breath, palpitations, shaking, diffuse numbness, and an intense fear of dying or going crazy. These attacks are not precipitated by any obvious anxiety-provoking situation. Moreover, the patient is particularly loath to leave her house without a companion. General physical examination and routine laboratory studies, which include normal electrolytes, thyroid function tests, electrocardiography, and continuous cardiac rhythm monitoring, have convinced the physician that there is no clear-cut organic cause of this problem. The patient is not on chronic medicine and does not abuse alcohol. The most appropriate therapy for this patient is

(A) diazepam
(B) flurazepam
(C) imipramine
(D) lithium
(E) fluphenazine

**IV-42.** A previously active 25-year-old woman presents with profound fatigue. She had an upper respiratory infection about 6 months ago from which she has never recovered. She now complains of intermittent headaches, sore throat, muscle and joint aches, and occasional feverishness. Her fatigue is so severe that she is unable to work. She now complains of excessive irritability, confusion, and inability to concentrate. Her physician has documented the presence of fever to 38.6°C (101.5°F) orally and the presence of palpable anterior cervical adenopathy both now and approximately 2 months ago. The patient has undergone an extensive workup, including complete blood count, serum chemistry analysis, HIV serology, EBV serology, CMV serology, and CT scan of the head, all of which were negative or not consistent with an acute infection. The patient has had no psychiatric or medical problems. Appropriate therapy at this time would consist of

(A) acyclovir
(B) corticosteroids
(C) vitamin $B_{12}$ injections
(D) intravenous immunoglobulin
(E) ibuprofen

**IV-43.** A 59-year-old man who has alcoholic cirrhosis but has been abstinent for 10 years has progressive dysarthria, tongue dystonia, shuffling gait, and fast tremor that worsens as his hand moves toward a target. These symptoms are most likely caused by

(A) Wilson's disease
(B) acquired hepatocerebral degeneration
(C) Wernicke's disease
(D) Marchiafava-Bignami disease
(E) paraneoplastic syndrome

**IV-44.** The most likely diagnosis for a patient with impotence and urinary incontinence who, over years, sustains tremor at rest, bradykinesia, rigidity, severe orthostatic hypotension, and anhidrosis is

(A) the autonomic form of the Landry-Guillain-Barré syndrome
(B) Shy-Drager syndrome
(C) guanethidine intoxication
(D) micturition syncope
(E) Parkinson's disease

**IV-45.** A 65-year-old man with long-standing schizo-phrenia is admitted to the general medical service because of atypical pneumonia. The patient has been on chlorpromazine for at least 10 years. In addition to find-ings related to his pneumonia and thought disorder, he repetitively smacks his lips and thrusts his tongue as well as exhibiting a bizarre stooped posture. Which of the following would be the best approach to reverse these troublesome neurologic symptoms?

(A) Administration of benztropine
(B) Administration of oxazepam
(C) Administration of propranolol
(D) Administration of levodopa-carbidopa (Sinemet)
(E) Reduction of the dose of chlorpromazine

**IV-46.** A 42-year-old man who has had difficulty con-centrating on his job lately, comes to medical attention because of irregular, jerky movements of his extremities and fingers. A sister and an uncle died in mental insti-tutions, and his mother became demented in middle age. The most likely diagnosis is

(A) alcoholic cerebral degeneration
(B) Huntington's chorea
(C) Wilson's disease
(D) Hallervorden-Spatz disease
(E) Gilles de la Tourette's disease

**IV-47.** A 72-year-old woman presents with brief, inter-mittent excruciating episodes of lancinating pain in the lips, gums, and cheek. These intense spasms of pain may be initiated by touching the lips or moving the tongue. The results of a physical examination are nor-mal. MRI of the head is also normal. The most likely cause of this patient's pain is

(A) acoustic neuroma
(B) meningioma
(C) temporal lobe epilepsy
(D) trigeminal neuralgia
(E) facial nerve palsy

**IV-48.** A 30-year-old patient presenting with a gradual decline in mental function is found to have a large lesion on CT examination of the brain. Biopsy reveals glioblas-toma multiforme. Physical examination of the skin reveals large, cream-brown cutaneous macules and numerous subcutaneous nodules. Gene mutations in which of the following account for this clinical syndrome?

(A) Rb protein
(B) Neurofibromin
(C) Hexosaminidase A
(D) KALIG-1
(E) Amyloid precursor protein

**IV-49.** Syringomyelia is characterized by all the follow-ing EXCEPT

(A) thoracic scoliosis
(B) ataxia
(C) muscle atrophy in the hands
(D) loss of pain sensation in the shoulders
(E) preservation of the sense of touch

**IV-50.** A 45-year-old man complains of severe right arm pain. He gives a history of having slipped on the ice and severely contusing his right shoulder approximately 1 month ago. At this time he has sharp, knifelike pain in the right arm and forearm. Physical examination reveals a right arm that is more moist and hairy than the left arm. There is no specific weakness or sensory change. However, the right arm is clearly more edematous than the left, and the skin appears somewhat atrophic in the affected limb. The patient's pain is most likely due to

(A) subclavian vein thrombosis
(B) brachial plexus injury
(C) reflex sympathetic dystrophy
(D) acromioclavicular separation
(E) cervical radiculopathy

**IV-51.** An 18-year-old man is brought to the emergency department because of a bicycle accident. He was riding with a group of friends who noted that the patient's bike hit a rock, the bike tumbled, and the patient's head hit the pavement. Unconsciousness lasted about 30 s. It is now approximately 1 h after the accident. At this time the patient is alert, though he has thrown up once and complains of difficulty in concentration and blurred vision. Furthermore, he is complaining of a severe frontal headache. The physical examination is notable for the absence of blood at the tympanic membranes and the mastoid processes and a completely nonfocal neurologic examination. Skull x-rays and MRI are nor-mal. The most appropriate course of action at this point is to

(A) obtain a neurosurgical consultation
(B) admit the patient to the hospital for observation
(C) administer phenytoin and admit the patient to the hospital for observation
(D) perform an electroencephalogram
(E) discharge the patient home in the care of his friends

IV-52. A 30-year-old man comes to the emergency department because he has had progressive weakness of his legs, sensory loss ascending from his toes to the level of his umbilicus, and urinary retention for the last 3 days. Examination reveals a central scotoma, absent knee and ankle jerks, and diminished pinprick sensation in the legs and abdomen up to the umbilicus. Cerebrospinal fluid contains 40 lymphocytes per cubic millimeter and a protein concentration of 0.72 g/L (72 mg/dL). This clinical picture is LEAST consistent with which of the following diagnoses?

(A) Acute idiopathic polyneuritis
(B) Acute necrotizing myelitis
(C) Postvaccinal myelitis
(D) Postinfectious myelitis
(E) Multiple sclerosis

IV-53. A 70-year-old man is brought in by his wife because of increased drowsiness and generally confused thinking over the past 2 months. Before a seemingly minor motor vehicle accident about 2 months ago, the patient had been running a small business without difficulty. There are no focal or lateralizing signs on neurologic examination. Noncontrast CT scan of the brain is normal except that there are no cortical sulci and the ventricles are small. The most likely diagnosis is

(A) Alzheimer's disease
(B) metabolic encephalopathy
(C) subdural hematoma
(D) cerebrovascular accident
(E) depression

IV-54. The bone most commonly fractured in association with an epidural hematoma is

(A) frontal
(B) parietal
(C) temporal
(D) occipital
(E) sphenoidal

IV-55. A patient presents with a rapidly progressive dementia associated with prominent myoclonic jerks that are provoked by her being startled as well as signs and symptoms of cerebellar dysfunction and emotional lability. Routine cerebrospinal fluid analysis is unremarkable. MRI shows minimal cortical loss. Electroencephalography discloses periodic sharp wave complexes on a generalized slow background. This disease is caused by

(A) a slow-virus infection
(B) deposition of fibrillary amyloid
(C) deposition of aluminum
(D) a proteinaceous infectious particle
(E) spirochetes

IV-56. A 60-year-old mildly obese woman complains of a very bothersome burning pain on the anterolateral aspect of her right thigh from the groin almost as far distally as the knee. Examination shows reduction of sensation to touch and pinprick in the affected area. There is no loss of muscle strength, and reflexes are normal. The most likely diagnosis is

(A) ruptured intervertebral disk
(B) femoral hernia
(C) nutritional neuropathy
(D) compression of the lateral femoral cutaneous nerve
(E) disruption of the lumbosacral plexus

IV-57. The major pathologic feature of idiopathic inflammatory polyneuropathy (Guillain-Barré syndrome) is

(A) loss of anterior horn cells
(B) destruction of axons
(C) inflammation of sensory ganglia
(D) wallerian degeneration
(E) segmental demyelination

IV-58. Cataracts, frontal baldness, testicular atrophy, and muscle weakness and wasting occur in association with

(A) myotonic dystrophy
(B) limb-girdle dystrophy
(C) pseudohypertrophic dystrophy
(D) facioscapulohumeral dystrophy
(E) myotonia congenita

IV-59. The form of muscular dystrophy most likely to be encountered in persons older than 50 years of age is

(A) facioscapulohumeral dystrophy
(B) oculopharyngeal dystrophy
(C) myotonic dystrophy
(D) Duchenne's dystrophy
(E) limb-girdle dystrophy

IV-60. Delayed relaxation of a muscle after voluntary contraction is characteristic of certain dystrophic diseases and periodic paralysis. This phenomenon is called

(A) myokymia
(B) myoedema
(C) myotonia
(D) contracture
(E) fibrillation

**IV-61.** A 65-year-old woman with diabetes mellitus has a 3-month history of sacral pain. In the last month a burning pain progressively developed over the lateral aspect of her left foot and was followed by loss of sensation and weakness of plantar flexion and dorsiflexion. Electromyography showed fibrillations in the left gastrocnemius, extensor hallucis, and quadriceps muscles. Nerve conduction was normal in the legs. A myelogram showed normal results. Now she complains that her knee "gives out" while she is walking; she has an absence of left knee and ankle jerks. Her physician should

(A) inform the patient that normal results on her myelogram make a diabetic neuropathy the most likely diagnosis

(B) arrange for a pelvic examination and schedule a CT scan of the pelvis to search for a malignancy compressing or infiltrating the lumbarsacral plexus

(C) arrange for a repeat myelogram because of new quadriceps weakness

(D) arrange for CT scan of the head to search for an expanding mass over the right sensorimotor strip that would affect the foot and leg

(E) reexamine her at 2-month intervals to determine the progression of her condition

**IV-62.** The weakness associated with myasthenia gravis is due to which of the following disorders in the neuromuscular junction?

(A) Reduced acetylcholine in presynaptic vesicles

(B) Presynaptic block in the release of acetylcholine

(C) Presence of antibodies against presynaptic membranes

(D) Degradation and blockage of postsynaptic receptors

(E) Damage of postsynaptic membranes by T lymphocytes

**IV-63.** A 49-year-old man with long-standing hypertension presents with right-sided weakness involving the face, arm, and leg which has evolved over the past 6 h. Neurologic examination is remarkable only for a right-sided hemiparesis without associated aphasia, papilledema, or sensory loss. CT scan done after several days most likely would reveal

(A) a small infarction in the left internal capsule

(B) a large infarction in the left cerebral cortex

(C) a left internal capsule hemorrhage

(D) a left cerebral cortical hemorrhage

(E) normal findings

**IV-64.** A 54-year-old woman with metastatic breast cancer and extensive bony involvement presents with headache and diplopia. Neurologic examination reveals no evidence of increased intracranial pressure, and the only new abnormalities are slight disorientation and the inability to abduct the right eye. Head CT without contrast is negative. Lumbar puncture reveals a mononuclear pleocytosis and elevated protein, but the results, including those of cytologic examination, are otherwise unremarkable. Among the following studies, which is the most likely to establish a diagnosis?

(A) Contrast CT of the head

(B) MRI of the head

(C) CT of the right orbit performed with bone windows

(D) Retinal angiography

(E) Repeat lumbar puncture

**IV-65.** A 27-year-old man seeks advice because he has noticed fasciculations in his calf muscles. He has no other complaints. Examination shows that muscle bulk and strength, tendon and plantar reflexes, and sensory function are all normal. He should undergo

(A) muscle biopsy

(B) sural nerve biopsy

(C) myelography

(D) electromyography

(E) none of the above

**IV-66.** Which of the following statements concerning porphyric neuropathy is true?

(A) It is rarely associated with confusion or seizures.

(B) It predominantly involves the sensory system.

(C) It is symmetric, and weakness is often more proximal than distal.

(D) It causes elevated protein concentration in cerebrospinal fluid.

(E) It is associated with inflammation of nerves.

**IV-67.** A patient has a total right hemianesthesia at the time of a cerebral infarction. One year later he complains of constant severe burning pain with occasional sharp jabs of pain in the left side of his face and left arm. The chronic pain syndrome is most likely

(A) part of a biologic depressive syndrome secondary to a right parietal lobe stroke

(B) caused by a lesion in the spinal cord affecting the right spinothalamic tract

(C) a sequela of thalamic infarction

(D) secondary to a shoulder-hand syndrome involving the side affected by the stroke

(E) tic douloureux

**IV-68.** A 55-year-old man is evaluated for weakness. Over the past few months he has noted slowly progressive weakness and cramping of his left leg. Lately he also has had some trouble swallowing food. He is awake and alert. Findings on the neurologic examination are normal except for marked atrophy with fasciculations in the muscles of both legs, hyperactive reflexes in the upper and lower extremities, a diminished gag reflex, and a positive extensor plantar response. Which of the following represents the most likely diagnosis?

(A) Cervical spondylosis
(B) Guillain-Barré syndrome
(C) Lambert-Eaton syndrome
(D) Vitamin B$_{12}$ deficiency
(E) Amyotrophic lateral sclerosis

**IV-69.** Duchenne's muscular dystrophy is characterized by

(A) autosomal dominant inheritance
(B) onset in the second decade of life
(C) normal cardiac muscle
(D) universal elevation of serum creatine kinase
(E) the requirement in prenatal diagnosis for family studies for analysis of restriction fragment length polymorphisms (RFLPs)

**IV-70.** A 68-year-old previously healthy woman develops a lilac-colored rash in a butterfly distribution about the eyes, on the bridge of the nose, and on the cheeks. She has a similar rash on her knuckles. She has had an associated muscle weakness manifested by difficulty arising from a chair and climbing stairs. She takes no medicines. Other than the rash and proximal muscle weakness, the woman's examination is unremarkable. The most appropriate subsequent procedure would be

(A) barium enema, upper GI series, intravenous pyelography, mammography, and chest x-ray
(B) hemogram, serum chemistries, Pap smear, urinalysis, mammography, and chest x-ray
(C) biopsy of an affected muscle
(D) electromyography (EMG)
(E) glucocorticoid treatment

**IV-71.** Which of the following statements correctly characterizes Wernicke's encephalopathy?

(A) The most prominently affected area is the frontal cortex, bilaterally
(B) Most patients present with the triad of encephalopathy, ophthalmoplegia, and ataxia
(C) In the absence of a response to glucose, thiamine should be administered
(D) After the patient responds to emergent treatment, profound amnesic psychosis may supervene
(E) Intake of alcohol is required to produce the full-blown syndrome

**IV-72.** Which of the following disorders is LEAST likely to produce a sensory level on neurologic examination?

(A) Myelopathy due to vitamin B$_{12}$ deficiency
(B) Neoplastic cord compression
(C) Vertebral dislocation and cord compression
(D) Acute myelitis
(E) Spinal epidural abscess

**IV-73.** A 39-year-old man presents with acute low back pain radiating into the posterior aspect of the right thigh and continuing down to the lateral aspect of the foot. On examination, the right patellar reflex is normal but the right Achilles tendon reflex is depressed compared with the left. Muscle power in the right lower extremity is full when the patient is examined in the supine position. The patient can stand on his heels and on the toes of the left foot, but the right toes are weak. Magnetic resonance imaging of the lumbosacral spine reveals a right-sided disk protrusion. The most likely site of disk pro- trusion is the

(A) L2–L3 interspace
(B) L3–L4 interspace
(C) L4–L5 interspace
(D) L5–S1 interspace
(E) S1–S2 interspace

**IV-74.** A 28-year-old woman who is 28 weeks pregnant presents with a 2-week history of burning pain in the lateral aspect of the left thigh. She has not noted back pain, weakness, or a change in bladder function. Examination reveals normal muscle strength in the legs. Deep tendon reflexes are normal. On sensory examination she notes decreased light touch in an oval-shaped area on the lateral aspect of the left thigh starting just above the knee. This most likely represents a lesion of the

(A) L3 nerve root
(B) femoral nerve
(C) lateral femoral cutaneous nerve
(D) saphenous nerve
(E) obturator nerve

**IV-75.** A 50-year-old man presents with a 2-month history of difficulty walking. He states that he trips over his toes and must lift his legs high with each step to avoid falling. He has no low back pain or sensory complaints in the legs. He is not taking medications. There is no family history of a similar problem. Thigh flexion, extension, adduction, and abduction are normal. There is mild weakness of foot dorsiflexion, inversion, and eversion. Plantar flexion of the foot is strong. Deep tendon reflexes are brisk throughout. This most likely represents

(A) bilateral L5 radiculopathy
(B) a bilateral lesion of the common peroneal nerve
(C) nutritional polyneuropathy
(D) hereditary sensorimotor polyneuropathy
(E) amyotrophic lateral sclerosis (motor neuron disease)

**IV-76.** A 4-year-old boy presents with a 3-week history of headache, ataxia, and vomiting. A head CT shows a posterior fossa mass arising from the midline cerebellum and involving the fourth ventricle. The most likely pathology of this tumor is

(A) oligodendroglioma
(B) craniopharyngioma
(C) glioblastoma multiforme
(D) medulloblastoma
(E) hemangioblastoma

**IV-77.** Which of the following is NOT a part of Parinaud syndrome?

(A) Paralysis of upward gaze
(B) Convergence nystagmus on upward gaze
(C) Skew deviation
(D) Lid retraction
(E) Normal to large pupils

**IV-78.** Correct statements regarding Gerstmann's syndrome include all the following EXCEPT

(A) affected patients have difficulty distinguishing right from left
(B) it results from a lesion of the dominant parietal lobe
(C) prosopagnosia is a prominent feature
(D) dysgraphia is a prominent feature
(E) acalculia is a prominent feature

**IV-79.** All the following are likely to be found in a patient with Wernicke's aphasia EXCEPT

(A) fluent speech output
(B) normal repetition
(C) paraphasic errors
(D) right superior quadrantanopia
(E) poor language comprehension

**IV-80.** Hypokalemic paralysis may be associated with all the following EXCEPT

(A) an autosomal dominantly inherited disorder
(B) hyperthyroidism
(C) Addison's disease
(D) diuretic abuse
(E) villous adenoma of the colon

**IV-81.** A 25-year-old woman presents with a sudden onset of diplopia. On examination she is unable to adduct the left eye past the midline. Nystagmus is noted in the right eye on abduction. Otherwise, extraocular movements are normal. The most likely location of the lesion is the

(A) right frontal lobe
(B) left labyrinth
(C) midbrain, affecting the rostral interstitial nucleus of the medial longitudinal fasciculus
(D) left occipital cortex
(E) left upper pons, affecting the medial longitudinal fasciculus

**IV-82.** A 64-year-old right-handed woman is able to produce and comprehend spoken language, repeat, write, and name objects in the left visual field. However, she is completely unable to read, including sentences she herself has recently written. Correct statements regarding this syndrome include all the following EXCEPT

(A) it may be associated with color anomia
(B) the most common location is a combination of the left occipital cortex and the left splenium of the corpus callosum
(C) the most common location is the left orbitofrontal cortex
(D) it is associated with a right homonomyous hemianopia
(E) the most common etiology is a cerebrovascular lesion

**IV-83.** A 22-year-old moderately obese woman complains of an excruciating headache over the past week. She denies other symptoms; her only medication is an oral contraceptive. On examination, the only findings are mild bilateral papilledema and a left sixth nerve palsy. MRI is normal; the ventricles are described as "slit-like." Cerebospinal fluid manometry yields a pressure of 490 mmH$_2$O. CSF chemistry and cytology are unremarkable. True statements regarding this condition include all the following EXCEPT

(A) it can be associated with venous sinus thrombosis

(B) a carbonic anhydrase inhibitor may alleviate the symptoms

(C) the patient should have close opthalmologic follow-up

(D) visual evoked potentials would be expected to be abnormal

(E) overdose of vitamin A or D and corticosteroid use or discontinuation are known precipitants

**IV-84.** True statements concerning Friedreich's ataxia include all the following EXCEPT

(A) it is the most common hereditary spinocerebellar ataxia

(B) the onset of symptoms occurs before age 25 years

(C) the molecular defect involves the expansion of a trinucleotide repeat sequence

(D) diabetes mellitus is more prevalent in Friedreich's ataxia patients than in the general population

(E) it is transmitted in an autosomal dominant manner

**IV-85.** The Prader-Willi syndrome includes all the following EXCEPT

(A) congenital hypotonia

(B) obesity and hyperphagia

(C) mental retardation

(D) deletions of the proximal long arm of chromosome 15

(E) café au lait spots

**IV-86.** A 64-year-old attorney with a 10-year history of adult-onset diabetes mellitus presents with the complaint of chronic burning dysesthesia in the feet. This symptom has been present for a year. He has been told that his pain is part of a diabetic neuropathy. He tried narcotics and antiepileptic medications in the past, but they made him too drowsy to work. The physician suggests a tricylic antidepressant. The best choice is

(A) doxepin

(B) amitryptiline

(C) imipramine

(D) nortriptyline

(E) desipramine

**IV-87.** A 35-year-old man with a history of intravenous drug abuse presents with the subacute onset of left shoulder pain. He has been evaluated by an orthopedic surgeon and a neurologist, who have found his examination normal. Plain films of the shoulder and MRI of the cervical spine, as well as electromyography, have been normal. He is undergoing physical therapy. In the office, the physician notes that he is hiccuping. Which of the following tests would be most useful?

(A) Abdominal computed tomography

(B) Barium swallow

(C) MRI of the brain

(D) Cervical myelography

(E) Gastric endoscopy

**IV-88.** A 72-year-old man with a history of hypertension and coronary artery disease is comatose in the cardiac intensive care unit after a ventricular tachycardiac arrest. Irrigation of the patient's left ear with 60 mL of cool water results in a bilateral conjugate tonic deviation of the eyes toward the left with no fast corrective movements to the midline. This finding indicates that

(A) there is a lesion between the midbrain and the pons

(B) there is danger of imminent transtentorial herniation

(C) there is an intact brainstem eye movement circuit with bilateral hemispheric dysfunction

(D) there has been an interruption in the reticular activating system

(E) the patient is in status epilepticus

**IV-89.** A 30-year-old woman presents with a complaint of visual difficulty. She bumps into objects that are beside her and has noticed that she must turn her head to either side to see things on the right and left. She also has noticed a change in her usually regular menstrual cycle. Which test is most likely to be abnormal?

(A) Visual evoked potentials
(B) Serum prolactin level
(C) Blood glucose
(D) Cerebrospinal fluid protein
(E) Neuropsychological testing

**IV-90.** A 65-year-old man with a history of hypertension and chronic obstructive pulmonary disease secondary to tobacco smoking presents to a physician after his wife notes that his left eyelid is drooping. On examination, the left pupil is 2 mm in diameter and the right is 4 mm. In dim light, the left pupil measures 2.5 mm while the right measures 5 mm. A left ptosis is seen. The skin of the face is dry bilaterally. The remainder of the neurologic examination is normal. The first step in the workup should be

(A) cerebral MRI
(B) ultrasound study of the carotid arteries
(C) chest x-ray
(D) ophthalmology consultation
(E) blood glucose determination

**IV-91.** True statements concerning Balint's syndrome include all the following EXCEPT

(A) it occurs after unilateral damage to the non-dominant occipital lobe
(B) it includes simultanagnosia
(C) the affected individual has impaired manual reaching toward visual targets
(D) movement exacerbates the symptoms
(E) it includes oculomotor apraxia

**IV-92.** A 68-year-old right-handed woman is known to have an anaplastic astrocytoma. She is able to produce grammatically correct language with no paraphasias, but her speech is uttered in a monotone that fails to convey her intended emotional meaning. There are no associated neurologic signs. The most likely location of her tumor is the

(A) right parietal lobe
(B) right frontal lobe
(C) right basal ganglia
(D) left frontal lobe
(E) left temporal lobe

**IV-93.** A 38-year-old woman complains of disturbed sleep because of an irresistible urge to move her legs. This is particularly bothersome just before she falls asleep. True statements regarding this syndrome include all the following EXCEPT

(A) the severity may wax and wane over time
(B) it can be caused by iron or folic acid deficiency anemia or renal failure
(C) it may be exacerbated by caffeine ingestion and pregnancy
(D) it is a form of narcolepsy
(E) treatment includes levodopa-carbidopa, benzodiazepines, and gabapentin

**IV-94.** A 72-year-old right-handed man with a history of atrial fibrillation and chronic alcoholism is evaluated for dementia. His son gives a history of a stepwise decline in the man's function over the past 5 years with the accumulation of mild focal neurologic deficits. On examination he is found to have a pseudobulbar affect, mildly increased muscle tone, and brisk deep tendon reflexes in the right upper extremity and an extensor plantar response on the left. This history and examination are most consistent with which of the following?

(A) Binswanger's disease
(B) Alzheimer's disease
(C) Creutzfeld-Jakob disease
(D) Vitamin $B_{12}$ deficiency
(E) Multi-infarct dementia

**IV-95.** Which of the following statements is true of Stokes-Adams attacks?

(A) Patients almost always have a family history of the disorder
(B) They are caused by high-degree atrio-ventricular block
(C) They are caused by recurrent paroxysmal tachyarrhythmias
(D) They usually are preceded by an aura
(E) Focal neurologic signs are common after these episodes

**IV-96.** All the following statements concerning anosmia and olfactory disturbances are correct EXCEPT

(A) unilateral loss of smell is an uncommon complaint
(B) cranial trauma results in unilateral or bilateral anosmia in 50 percent of cases
(C) head trauma and viral infections are the leading causes of olfactory disorders
(D) congenital anosmia and hypogonadotropic hypogonadism are the clinical hallmarks of Kallmann syndrome
(E) Cushing's syndrome can distort smell perception

**IV-97.** Routine laboratory tests used in the evaluation of dementia include all the following EXCEPT

(A) vitamin $B_{12}$
(B) Venereal Disease Research Laboratory (VDRL) test for syphilis
(C) erythrocyte sedimentation rate
(D) thyroid-stimulating hormone (TSH)
(E) serum electrolytes

**IV-98.** All of the following disorders are caused by expansion of a trinucleotide repeat sequence EXCEPT

(A) Huntington's disease
(B) Myotonic dystrophy
(C) Duchenne's muscular dystrophy
(D) Friedreich's ataxia
(E) Fragile-X syndrome

**IV-99.** All the following structures have been implicated in the generation of wakefulness EXCEPT

(A) brainstem reticular formation
(B) midbrain
(C) subthalamus
(D) emboliform nucleus
(E) basal forebrain

**IV-100.** A 12-year-old girl complains of muscle aches and difficulty climbing stairs and combing her hair. She has a rash over the malar area of her face and the extensor surfaces of her hands and fingers. True statements concerning this syndrome include all the following EXCEPT

(A) the patient probably will have an elevated erythrocyte sedimentation rate
(B) the symptoms most likely will improve with corticosteroids
(C) it may be accompanied by calcinosis cutis
(D) biopsy of an affected muscle most likely would show perifascicular atrophy
(E) biopsy of an affected muscle most likely would show fiber type grouping

**DIRECTIONS:** Each question below contains five suggested responses. For **each** of the five responses listed with each question, you are to respond either YES (Y) or NO (N). In a given item **all, some, or none** of the alternatives may be correct.

**IV-101.** Progressive gait disability in elderly persons may be due to

(A) normal-pressure hydrocephalus
(B) cervical spondylosis
(C) subdural hematoma
(D) carotid stenosis
(E) subacute combined degeneration

**IV-102.** Which of the following elements would be involved in the appreciation of pain caused by an injurious stimulus?

(A) Spinocerebellar tract
(B) Spinothalamic tract
(C) Dorsal horn of the spinal cord
(D) Red nucleus
(E) Nucleus ventralis posterolateralis

**IV-103.** A patient complains of hearing loss in the right ear. A 256-Hz tuning fork is placed in the middle of the forehead; the patient reports that he hears the tone in his right ear. He also notes better perception of a tone when the tuning fork is placed in contact with the right mastoid process than when it is placed outside his right ear. Lesions in which of the following structures could account for these findings?

(A) Eighth nerve
(B) Central auditory pathways
(C) Cochlea
(D) External auditory canal
(E) Middle ear

**IV-104.** Useful tests for myasthenia gravis would include which of the following?

(A) Repetitive motor-nerve stimulation
(B) Single-fiber electromyography
(C) Muscle biopsy
(D) Nerve conduction studies
(E) Curare challenge testing

**IV-105.** Which of the following would be consistent with a diagnosis of low back strain in a patient with low back pain?

(A) Limitation of flexion of the spine
(B) Scoliosis or straightening of the normal lordosis as noted on x-ray films
(C) Urinary retention and obstipation
(D) Sudden onset while bending over shoveling snow
(E) Absence of ankle reflex with radiating pain

**IV-106.** A lesion in the corticospinal tract rather than in an anterior horn neuron projecting to muscle cells is suggested by

(A) spasticity
(B) marked atrophy
(C) fasciculations
(D) involvement of individual muscles
(E) the presence of an extensor plantar reflex

**IV-107.** The tremor associated with Parkinson's disease is characterized by
(A) worsening with voluntary movement
(B) occurrence with flexed posture
(C) occurrence at a rate of 5 Hz
(D) association with rigidity
(E) abolition by moderate intake of alcohol

**IV-108.** Peripheral nerve damage caused by diabetes may result in

(A) relapsing weakness
(B) distal sensory neuropathy
(C) incontinence
(D) footdrop
(E) ophthalmoplegia

**IV-109.** Chronically progressive spinal cord disease with sensory and motor signs evolving over years may be due to

(A) spinocerebellar degeneration
(B) multiple sclerosis
(C) cervical spondylosis
(D) lumbar disk disease
(E) amyotrophic lateral sclerosis

**IV-110.** A person with long-standing alcoholism develops bilateral lateral-rectus (sixth-nerve) palsies. Diagnostic considerations would include

(A) brainstem hemorrhage
(B) subdural hematoma
(C) orbital fractures
(D) neurosyphilis
(E) Wernicke's encephalopathy

**IV-111.** A 60-year-old man comes to the emergency room with the sudden onset of a neurologic deficit. After examining the patient, the physician orders cerebral angiography. The results show occlusion of the left vertebral artery from its origin to the site where it joins the basilar artery. The right vertebral artery, the basilar artery, and both carotid arteries are patent. Examination in the emergency room probably disclosed

(A) left hemiparesis sparing the face
(B) deviation of the uvula to the right on phonation
(C) left appendicular ataxia
(D) left internuclear ophthalmoplegia
(E) diminished pain and temperature sensation in the right arm and leg

**IV-112.** Which of the following may occur ipsilateral to a disease process within the cavernous sinus?

(A) Ptosis
(B) Numbness of the brow
(C) Numbness of the chin
(D) Marked decrease in visual acuity
(E) Inability to elevate the eye

**IV-113.** Favorable prognostic factors for a patient's remaining seizure-free when anticonvulsants are stopped after 2 years on therapy include

(A) a normal EEG before drug withdrawal
(B) complex partial seizures with secondary generalization
(C) simple partial seizures
(D) the requirement of a single drug for seizure control
(E) few seizures before becoming seizure-free

**IV-114.** Correct statements concerning the use of lithium in psychiatry include

(A) lithium is effective for treating acute manic/ hypomanic episodes but plays no role in prophylaxis against future attacks
(B) hyperthyroidism is an important long-term complication
(C) nephrogenic diabetes insipidus is common
(D) gastrointestinal complaints and thirst are common side effects
(E) during acute mania, lithium can be administered with behavior control as the sole end-point

# IV. DISORDERS OF THE NERVOUS SYSTEM AND MUSCLES

## ANSWERS

**IV-1. The answer is B.** *(Chap. 21)* The symptoms and signs described in the question are most consistent with Ménière's disease. In this disorder, paroxysmal vertigo resulting from labyrinthine lesions is associated with nausea, vomiting, rotary nystagmus, tinnitus, high-tone hearing loss with recruitment, and, most characteristically, fullness in the ear. Labyrinthitis would be an unlikely diagnosis in this case because of the hearing loss and multiple episodes. Vertebral-basilar insufficiency and multiple sclerosis typically are associated with brainstem signs. Acoustic neuroma only rarely causes vertigo as its initial symptom, and the vertigo it does cause is mild and intermittent.

**IV-2. The answer is D.** *(Chaps. 15, 364. Welch, N Engl J Med 329:1476–1483, 1993)* While the pathophysiology of migraine remains unclear, electrical stimulation of midline dorsal raphe in the brainstem leads to characteristic pain. Pharmacologically, serotonin-mediated neurotransmission appears to be critical in the generation of migrainous pain. Sumatriptan and dihydroergotamine both work by blocking 5-hydroxytryptamine receptors (type I, especially the D subtype). While nonsteroidal anti-inflammatory agents such as ibuprofen and naproxen are helpful in patients with mild to moderate migraine, presumably by reducing inflammatory stimuli from cyclooxygenase inhibition leading to reduced prostaglandin generation, the patient in the question has too severe an attack to benefit from the additional use of this class of agents. Also, the use of narcotic analgesics as a primary therapy is no longer recommended; sumatriptan will relieve a migraine headache in approximately 75 percent of patients within 1 h of treatment. Unfortunately, because of its short half-life (with either oral or subcutaneous administration), headache recurs in up to one-third of patients. Sumatriptan-associated side effects are usually mild to moderate and highly reversible; they include reactions at the injection site, flushing sensations, and neck pain or stiffness. Although up to 5 percent of patients treated with sumatriptan experience chest tightness or pressure, myocardial ischemia is exceedingly rare. Nonetheless, this drug should not be given to those with a history of myocardial infarction, ischemic heart disease, or Prinzmetal's angina. Both beta-adrenergic antagonists and calcium channel blocking drugs are effective prophylactic agents in patients with frequent migraines.

**IV-3. The answer is A.** *(Chap. 372)* The abrupt appearance of an isolated peripheral facial palsy, which may include ipsilateral hyperacusis resulting from involvement of fibers to the stapedius and loss of taste on the anterior two-thirds of the tongue resulting from involvement of the fibers of the chorda tympani, is most often idiopathic, as in Bell's palsy. If the patient is unable to close the eye, artificial tears may be helpful during the day to prevent drying, and the eye should be patched at night to prevent corneal abrasion. Excellent recovery occurs in 80 percent of these cases. Oral contraceptives and mitral valve prolapse are not associated with the causes of this clinical picture. Evoked potentials are not helpful diagnostically.

**IV-4. The answer is D.** *(Chap. 27)* Narcolepsy is uncontrollable daytime sleepiness, and cataplexy is a sudden, brief loss of muscle tone. Sleep paralysis and hypnagogic hallucinations are common in persons with narcolepsy. A properly performed sleep electroencephalogram is useful in supporting a diagnosis of narcolepsy; in affected persons REM sleep occurs much earlier during sleep than normal. (False-positive tests can occur if the subject has recently been sleeping, awakens briefly, and then falls asleep again for the test.) Confusion and epileptic disorders are not part of the narcolepsy-cataplexy syndrome.

**IV-5. The answer is B.** *(Chap. 15)* Cluster headaches, which can cause excruciating hemicranial pain, are notable for their occurrence during characteristic episodes. Usually attacks occur during a 4- to 8-week period in which the patient experiences one to three severe brief headaches daily. There may then be a prolonged pain-free interval before the next episode. Men between ages 20 and 50 are most commonly affected. The unilateral pain usually is associated with lacrimation, eye reddening, nasal stuffiness, ptosis, and nausea. During episodes alcohol may provoke the attacks. Even though the pain caused by brain tumors may awaken a patient from sleep, the typical history and normal neurologic examination do not mandate evaluation for a neoplasm of the central nervous system. Acute therapy for a cluster headache attack consists of oxygen inhalation, although intranasal lidocaine and subcutaneous sumatriptan also may be effective. Prophylactic therapy with prednisone, lithium, methysergide, ergotamine, or verapamil can be administered during an episode to prevent further cluster headache attacks.

**IV-6. The answer is D.** *(Chap. 16)* Herniation of a lower cervical disk may be due to trauma, especially in the setting of neck hyperextension. If the disk herniates laterally, it generally will compress the nerve route exiting the lower of the two vertebrae that account for the intervertebral space. For example, if the disk between the fifth and sixth cervical vertebrae herniates, the full syndrome will be characteristic of a C6 radiculopathy: pain in the trapezius, shoulder, radial forearm, and thumb; absent biceps reflex; and preserved triceps reflex. A C7 radiculopathy caused by a disk protruding between the sixth and seventh cervical vertebrae will produce the following: pain in the shoulder blade, pectoral and medial axillary region, upper arm, elbow, dorsal forearm, and index and middle fingers; paresthesia and sensory loss in the second and third fingers or the tips of all the fingers; weakness in forearm and wrist extension as well as hand grip; and a preserved biceps reflex but a diminished triceps reflex. Coughing and sneezing often exacerbate the pain caused by a herniated cervical disk. Unlike the lateral disk syndromes mentioned above, a disk that herniates centrally may be painless but cause symptoms in the lower extremities.

**IV-7. The answer is A.** *(Chaps. 24, 366)* Patients with basilar artery stenosis frequently have spells of ischemic brainstem dysfunction before a catastrophic stroke caused by arterial thrombosis. Timely anticoagulation and allowing a higher blood pressure can arrest the progression of this potentially fatal stroke. Acute coma can occur in association with each of the cerebrovascular accidents mentioned in the question except carotid occlusion. Subarachnoid hemorrhage causes an acute increase in intracranial pressure that reduces blood flow to the brain. Unilateral cortical infarction does not cause coma, but damage to brainstem structures via infarction or compression will cause coma.

**IV-8. The answer is A.** *(Chap. 21. Froehling, JAMA 271:385–388, 1994)* The evaluation of a "dizzy" patient relies on a combination of careful history taking and neurologic examination. It is important to get a sense of whether the patient has true vertigo, which is usually manifest as the sensation that either the world or the patient is spinning. Some elderly patients complain of dizziness while ambulating or standing without true vertigo, although they may have mild lightheadedness. Typically these patients have peripheral neuropathy, myelopathy, parkinsonian rigidity, cerebellar ataxia, or poor vision. Such patients actually have multiple sensory-defect dizziness, also known as *benign dysequilibrium of aging*. Unlike patients with benign paroxysmal positional vertigo, they should not display excess nystagmus on head-tilt testing. Central lesions are unlikely given a neurologic examination that was normal except for the peripheral neuropathy and other sensory deficits.

**IV-9.** **The answer is D.** *(Chap. 28)* Knowledge of visual pathway anatomy is necessary for an understanding of visual field defects. Monocular visual field loss often results from retinal fiber loss, corresponding to lesions visible on ophthalmoscopic examination. Retinal fibers traveling in the optic nerve change direction at the optic chiasm so that the right brain appreciates left visual space and the left brain appreciates right visual space. Therefore, a discrete vertical midline characterizes all visual pathway disorders resulting from lesions at or posterior to the chiasm. Because chiasmal lesions interrupt the central fibers that mediate temporal vision (with peripheral fibers mediating more midline vision), a pituitary tumor or craniopharyngioma (which typically impinges centrally) results in loss of visual fields in the bitemporal regions. If a lesion exists well posterior to the optic chiasm, such as loss of visual cortex in the one occipital lobe as a result of an embolism in the posterior cerebral artery, a complete loss of visual perception in one field will result. For example, destruction of the right visual cortex will lead to complete left homonymous hemianopia with loss of temporal vision in the left eye and medial vision in the right eye.

**IV-10.** **The answer is B.** *(Chap. 361)* The testing of evoked potentials is of the greatest utility in detecting subclinical spinal cord and optic nerve lesions. Up to two-thirds of persons with multiple sclerosis have neurologic deficits that are evident on visual or peroneal somatic evoked potentials but *not* on physical examination. A "second lesion" of this type frequently establishes the diagnosis of multiple sclerosis. Evoked potentials may be abnormal in the other conditions listed in the question.

**IV-11.** **The answer is C.** *(Chap. 15)* Errors made in the investigation of patients with a sudden onset of severe headache can result in catastrophic subarachnoid hemorrhage from a ruptured aneurysm. Patients frequently have "warning" bleeding that causes severe headache and brings them for medical attention. Sudden headache during physical exertion is a presentation of a ruptured intracranial aneurysm. A careful cerebrospinal fluid examination is the most sensitive test, but noncontrast CT may show the subarachnoid blood and make the lumbar puncture unnecessary. A patient with a reasonable suspicion for aneurysmal bleeding should not be sent home to wait for other symptoms because the next symptom is often a catastrophic subarachnoid hemorrhage. In the patient described, however, the repeated onset of headache with coitus is characteristic of a benign coital headache syndrome. If the patient had only a single sudden coital headache, an investigation for a cerebral aneurysm would be appropriate. A family history of migraine usually is not helpful for the diagnosis of coital headache.

**IV-12.** **The answer is E.** *(Chaps. 28, 372)* Isolated lesions of the third nerve with pupillary sparing are common and usually are due to microinfarction in association with diabetes or hypertension. Thus, older patients with such a third nerve palsy can be followed expectantly in the absence of signs of subarachnoid hemorrhage or other, more diffuse processes. More detailed reinvestigation is mandated if recovery is not complete, as it usually is, within a 3-month period. The third nerve is a midline structure that contains both sympathetic motor and visceral nuclei. It innervates the ipsilateral medial rectus, inferior rectus, and inferior oblique muscles as well as the contralateral superior rectus muscle. A central nucleus innervates both levator palpebrae superioris muscles. Moreover, axons from visceral nuclei project ipsilateral parasympathetic outflow to the pupillary sphincter and ciliary ganglion, which control pupillary reflexes as well as accommodation. Therefore, a midbrain infarction (involving the nucleus of the oculomotor nerve), if complete, will produce a unilateral third nerve palsy characterized by ipsilateral ptosis and inability to turn the eye upward, downward, and inward. Bilateral ptosis and paralysis of the contralateral superior rectus muscle will result. Pupillary involvement also will be complete. More distal lesions can produce single or multiple extraocular muscle abnormalities with or without pupillary derangement. It is also important to recognize that the third nerve may be impinged along its extracranial extent. Particularly noteworthy is compression against the tentorial edge, which may occur during profound intracranial hypertension with temporal lobe herniation. In herniation the pupillary fibers are affected first, causing pupillary dilation and unresponsiveness to light. Cavernous sinus thrombosis also may affect the third nerve; this process typically affects the fourth and sixth nerves.

**IV-13.** **The answer is C.** *(Chap. 29)* The primary evaluation of a patient with hearing impairment consists of determinating of whether the loss is sensorineural (lesions in the inner ear, eighth nerve, or central auditory pathways) or conductive (lesions in the external auditory canal or middle ear). The demonstration that bone conduction is better than air conduction suggests a conductive hearing loss. About a third of persons over age 70 require a hearing aid because of presbycusis, which is manifested by a loss of discrimination for particular sounds and difficulty understanding speech in noisy environments. This is usually due to sensorineural deafness, with lesions in the neuroepithelial cells (hair cells), the neurons, or the stria vascularis of the peripheral auditory system. Though of lesser magnitude, degeneration of central auditory pathways also may be a problem in those with presbycusis. Hearing aids are the mainstay of treatment for persons with this condition; however, cochlear implants, by providing a neural prosthesis, may aid patients with profound sensorineural deafness.

**IV-14.** **The answer is C.** *(Chaps. 21, 368)* Lesions in the basal ganglia, instead of resulting in the clasp-knife spasticity and hyperreflexia of upper motor neuron lesions or the hypotonia of lower motor neuron lesions, may result in a host of movement disorders, including akinesia or bradykinesia, lead-pipe rigidity, chorea, irregular and variable continuous movements, dystonia (increased muscle tone that causes fixed abnormal postures), myoclonus (brief involuntary random muscular contractions), asterixis (quick arrhythmic movements), hemiballismus (violent flinging motion of an arm), tremor, and tics (stereotyped, purposeless, and irregularly repetitive movements). These so-called extrapyramidal syndromes do not involve the characteristic weakness of muscles or muscle groups typical of lesions of the corticospinal tracts. It is possible that these extrapyramidal syndromes can coexist with lesions in the corticospinal tract or cerebellum, and this makes precise delineation of the abnormality difficult. Other degenerative conditions, such as Shy-Drager syndrome, have many elements of Parkinson's disease (bradykinesia, bland facial expression, rest tremor, and muscular rigidity), but postural hypotension, abnormal eye movements, and Babinski's signs also may occur. In addition to dopamine, important neurotransmitters in the basal ganglia include γ-aminobutyric acid, enkephalin, and substance P.

**IV-15.** **The answer is D.** *(Chap. 22)* Polymyalgia rheumatica typically occurs in elderly patients and is characterized by complaints of weakness, stiffness, and pain in the proximal musculature. There may be an associated inflammatory arthritis, an elevated erythrocyte sedimentation rate, or an accompanying temporal arteritis. Inflammatory myositis is ruled out by the presence of normal creatine kinase levels; a muscle biopsy will show atrophy without evidence of inflammation. Unless temporal arteritis is also present, nonsteroidal anti-inflammatory agents constitute the treatment of choice; low-dose prednisone may be administered if the initial agents fail.

**IV-16.** **The answer is D.** *(Chap. 12)* The patient is already on maximal doses of a relatively weak narcotic analgesic that also has quite a few side effects. Increasing the dose of codeine or adding a nonsteroidal anti-inflammatory drug such as indomethacin is likely to be of little benefit. Neuropathic pain, unlike the somatic pain afflicting the patient, might be managed with the help of an anticonvulsant such as phenytoin. Since the patient has not failed an adequate trial of narcotics, referral for a nerve-altering intervention is premature. One should institute a sustained-release preparation of morphine, with another narcotic to be taken between doses of morphine until a sufficient level of analgesia is achieved.

**IV-17.** **The answer is D.** *(Chaps. 15, 372)* A disease of middle-aged and elderly patients, particularly women, paroxysmal facial pain (tic douloureux, trigeminal neuralgia) is usually of idiopathic origin. It may occur in association with multiple sclerosis, herpes zoster, or a tumor. Brief, intense, lancinating pains brought on by manipulation of trigger zones in the lips or face, without motor or sensory paralysis, characterize this disorder. The treatment of first choice is the anticonvulsant carbamazepine, which is effective in most patients. In cases of nonresponse or intolerance to carbamazepine, radiofrequency ablation of the gasserian ganglion of the trigeminal nerve may be beneficial.

**IV-18.** **The answer is A.** *(Chaps. 23, 369)* Peripheral nerve trunks contain fibers of various sizes. Small fibers mediate sensations of pain and temperature, and larger fibers are involved in touch, vibration, and joint position sense. Therefore, a lesion in a peripheral nerve would be expected to affect all such functions. The different fibers segregate near the dorsal roots. The smaller fibers cross and ascend in the contralateral side through the spinal cord to the brainstem and to the ventral posterior lateral nucleus of the thalamus, ultimately projecting to the parietal cortex. The larger fibers that mediate tactile and position sense project upward in the posterior columns of the spinal cord and synapse initially in the cuneate nuclei of the lower medulla; a secondary neuron crosses to ascend in the medial lemniscus and synapses in the ventral posterolateral nucleus of the thalamus with ultimate projections to the parietal cortex. Therefore, loss of joint position without loss of pain sensation would reflect a lesion in the ipsilateral posterior column, contralateral brainstem, thalamus, or parietal cortex.

**IV-19.** **The answer is A.** *(Chap. 25. Domasio, N Engl J Med 326:531–539, 1992)* Patients with Wernicke's aphasia usually have damage in an area of the posterior temporal and parietal regions, which are supplied by the lower division of the middle cerebral artery. Not only are spoken and written communication affected, auditory and visual understanding also may be deranged. At first glance, speech in a person with lesions in this area appears to be effortless and well woven together. However, because of problems in finding words, the content is often unintelligible, as there are frequent errors in word choice and substitution of incorrect phonemes (e.g., "trable" for "table"). Patients with lesions in this location rarely have associated motor defects, but problems in sensory processing are possible, depending on the degree of parietal lobe disease. As in true Broca's aphasia, these patients have difficulty repeating sentences and naming things properly. Patients with Wernicke's aphasia may experience paranoid ideation and become agitated and hostile.

**IV-20.** **The answer is D.** *(Chaps. 28, 372)* The features described in the question are consistent with sympathetic denervation of the right eye, the so-called Horner pupil. This lesion, which frequently is produced by pulmonary neoplasms of the superior sulcus, usually is associated with ipsilateral ptosis and anhidrosis. Pupillary light responses should be normal, as should the response to mydriatics [substances causing pupillary dilation (e.g., anticholinergics)] and miotics [drugs causing pupillary constriction (e.g., cholinergics, beta-adrenergic blockers)]. However, since the sympathetic nerve endings are depleted, cocaine cannot cause local release of sympathomimetic substances and is a poor mydriatic. An oculomotor palsy would also produce ipsilateral ptosis, but a dilated pupil that is poorly reactive to light on that side would be the cause of anisocoria.

**IV-21.** **The answer is C.** *(Chap. 365)* Patients with loss of consciousness resulting from a seizure usually have mental confusion, headache, and drowsiness postictally, whereas patients with a brief syncopal spell recover fully as soon as blood pressure returns to normal. Auras, urinary incontinence, and a laceration of the tongue are clues that the cause of the loss of consciousness was a seizure. Moreover, syncope rarely occurs during recumbency.

**IV-22.** **The answer is A.** *(Chap . 27)* Chronic or long-term insomnia, by definition, lasts for months or years and usually is reflective of a psychiatric or chronic medical condition, drug use (including caffeine or alcohol), or a primary sleep disorder. Psychophysiologic insomnia is characterized by preoccupation with the inability to sleep at night. The problem often is triggered by a stressful event but may persist for long periods because of the acquisition of poor sleep habits. Patients often are aroused by their own failed efforts to sleep. They more readily sleep at unusual times or places. This patient does not have narcolepsy, since excessive daytime sleep and cataplexy are not included in his syndrome. Narcolepsy may be treated with stimulants such as methylphenidate. Moreover, he has no findings suggestive of sleep apnea syndromes, which might benefit from the use of conjugated estrogens. Instead, rigorous attention to sleep hygiene, such as making sure the bedroom is used only for sleep and removing distracting stimuli at bedtime, is most appropriate. Benzodiazepine hypnotics may be helpful during the initiation of treatment by serving to allow behavioral therapy, which is probably the most specific way to treat this problem.

**IV-23.** **The answer is D.** *(Chap. 28)* The patient in question is suffering from acute angle-closure glaucoma, resulting from obstruction of the outflow of aqueous humor at the iris. The buildup of intraocular pressure can be confirmed by measurement and requires urgent treatment with hyperosmotic agents. Permanent treatment requires laser or surgical iridotomy. Angle-closure glaucoma is less common than primary open-angle glaucoma, which is asymptomatic and usually is detectable only through measurements of intraocular pressure at a routine eye examination.

**IV-24.** **The answer is D.** *(Chap. 365)* It is important to classify seizures on the basis of whether they begin in a focal area of the brain, remain localized or secondarily generalize, or are generalized from the earliest manifestation. This patient exhibited the classic "Jacksonian march," with repetitive shaking of contiguous ipsilateral body parts, caused by a demonstrable progression of epileptiform discharges in the contralateral motor cortex usually resulting from a focus from a tumor or abscess. This patient therefore had a simple partial seizure with secondary generalization. In this case the focus was obvious; in some cases the focal features can be discerned only on the basis of a postictal deficit (e.g., Todd's paralysis of an extremity). Juvenile myoclonic epilepsy begins in adolescence and is characterized by postawakening myoclonic seizures marked by sudden, brief muscle contractions involving one body part or the entire body. Complex partial seizures, also referred to as temporal lobe epilepsy (typical of herpes simplex encephalitis), involve episodic changes in behavior with loss of attachment to the environment and typically are associated with a minor automatism such as lip smacking or picking at clothes.

**IV-25.** **The answer is D.** *(Chap. 365)* Different types of seizures respond better to certain classes of anticonvulsant drugs. For example, generalized tonic-clonic seizures may be treated successfully with phenytoin, carbamazepine, phenobarbital, or valproic acid. Carbamazepine and phenytoin also are effective for the treatment of partial seizures, though persons with complex partial seizures may require more than one type of drug at a time. Partial absence seizures, such as those described in the question, are best treated with ethosuximide or valproic acid, although clonazepam (a benzodiazepine) also may be effective. The side effects of ethosuximide include ataxia, lethargy, GI irritation, skin rash, and bone marrow suppression.

**IV-26.** **The answer is B.** *(Chaps. 21, 369)* Alcoholic cerebellar degeneration is an example of a disease primarily of the midline area of the cerebellum (vermis). A characteristic cerebellar gait disorder is manifested by a wide-based walk and stance and the inability to stand with the feet together even with the eyes open. Patients complain of imbalance and frequently try to hold on to objects as they walk. However, unlike more diffuse cerebellar disease, there is no associated limb ataxia or nystagmus.

**IV-27.   The answer is E.**   *(Chap. 375. Fine, Ann Intern Med 119:1093–1104, 1993)*   Lymphoma of the brain (usually diffuse large cell) is increasingly common as a sporadic tumor and occurs frequently in immunosuppressed patients, especially those with AIDS. Its clinical sensitivity to corticosteroids can mistakenly suggest a diagnosis of multiple sclerosis, and its complete disappearance or dramatic improvement on CT after steroid therapy is baffling. Radiosensitivity is a well-known feature of most primary CNS lymphomas, which almost always are of B-cell origin.

**IV-28.   The answer is E.**   *(Chaps. 356, 365)*   When a patient presents with a generalized tonic-clonic seizure, it is important to consider alcohol as a potential etiology. Persons who heavily abuse alcohol may have seizures from a cerebral contusion or subdural hematoma caused by trauma, metabolic abnormalities, central nervous system infection, or alcohol withdrawal. Seizures taking place during alcohol withdrawal or binge drinking usually are brief tonic-clonic seizures that occur in a flurry of several over a short period of time. Once other causes for seizures in alcoholics are ruled out, it is not necessary to administer chronic antiepileptic treatment. First, such seizures tend to be self-limited and abate once withdrawal is complete or binge drinking has stopped. Second, the use of anticonvulsant medicines in this typically noncompliant group of patients with a host of other medical problems is fraught with the dangers of severe side effects.

**IV-29.   The answer is B.**   *(Chap. 365)*   Antiepileptic drugs commonly have a host of side effects. For example, phenytoin has a narrow therapeutic index and is associated with neurologic symptoms such as ataxia and nonneurologic symptoms such as gum hyperplasia, lymphadenopathy, hirsutism, and osteomalacia. Carbamazepine is notable for causing bone marrow suppression and gastrointestinal irritation as well as ataxia, dizziness, and vertigo. Phenobarbital enhances the metabolism of many other drugs via liver enzyme induction. In fact, carbamazepine levels, which are potentially increased by erythromycin, are decreased by phenobarbital. Especially if the phenobarbital is not destined to have a major therapeutic effect in this patient with complex partial seizures, the induction of a reduced carbamazepine level may actually lead to worse control. It may be necessary to increase the carbamazepine dose to achieve a therapeutic level in order to give the combination therapy an adequate trial. The bone marrow suppression of carbamazepine may produce a dose-dependent mild to moderate depression in the white blood count cell but is not notable for causing severe thrombocytopenia.

**IV-30.   The answer is E.**   *(Chap. 366)*   Before assuming that a stroke is due to hemispheral disease, clinicians should search for contralateral brainstem signs. Right hemiparesis with left facial weakness or left-gaze paresis indicates a pontine stroke, which generally is due to basilar artery branch disease. Inability to calculate (acalculia) and left-right confusion with dysgraphia are part of the Gerstmann's syndrome of left parietal stroke and may occur with right hemiparesis. Minimizing or ignoring the deficit is most typical of a right-brain lesion and is associated with a left hemiparesis.

**IV-31.   The answer is E.**   *(Chap. 366. Gilman, N Engl J Med 326:1671–1676, 1992)*   Transient ischemic attacks (TIAs) are caused by low flow in large vessels such as the internal carotid artery, embolism from an arterial or cardiac source, or lacunar (small penetrating vessel) atherosclerosis. As exemplified in this case, a low-flow TIA usually is brief and recurrent and frequently is due to a tightly stenotic atherosclerotic lesion at the internal carotid artery. Hypoperfused distal branches of the middle cerebral artery cause hip, shoulder, or arm weakness and possible aphasic symptoms, depending on the amount of territory involved. Transient recurrent monocular blindness (amaurosis fugax) also may be a manifestation of an internal carotid artery occlusion. Embolic TIAs tend to be of longer duration than the low-flow TIAs described above. Lacunar TIAs occur because of blockage of one of the intracerebral penetrating vessels arising from the middle cerebral, basilar, or vertebral arteries. On the basis of the cerebral angiography performed in this case, it is apparent that the patient in fact had a low-flow TIA caused by a tightly stenotic lesion of the internal carotid artery. Heparin may be useful for impending stroke resulting from this pathophysiology, warfarin may be appropriate after embolic phenomena, and antiplatelet agents may have prophylactic value for secondary strokes. However, the procedure of choice in this case is carotid endarterectomy. If the lesion had not been tightly stenotic (less than 70 percent stenosis), the value of such surgery would have been less clear.

**IV-32.** **The answer is D.** *(Chap. 366)* There are four major hypertensive hemorrhage syndromes. The most common site for bleeding is the internal capsule adjacent to the basal ganglia, which generally produces contralateral hemiplesia with eye deviation away from the side of the weakness. As the blood expands within the brain, stupor and coma may occur rapidly. Thalamic hemorrhage results in hemiplegia from pressure on the adjacent internal capsule as well as in a prominent sensory deficit. The eyes typically deviate downward and inward, and the pupils are unequal. Pontine hemorrhages produce a rapid onset of deep coma, quadriplegia, and pinpoint pupils that do react to light. Cerebellar hemorrhages develop over several hours and are manifested by nausea, vomiting, vertigo, dizziness, and occipital headache. The eyes tend to deviate away from the hemorrhage; there may be an ipsilateral sixth nerve palsy, blepharospasm, or ocular bobbing. Cerebellar findings tend to be limited. It is important to recognize this lesion, since it is treatable until the point of coma from brainstem compression. While osmotic therapy to reduce intracranial pressure may be helpful, the most important therapy for such infratentorial clots is surgical removal. Neurosurgical therapy for acute supratentorial clots such as those which may be caused by a thalamic or capsular hemorrhage is more controversial because of the difficulty in reaching these central areas safely.

**IV-33.** **The answer is D.** *(Chap. 367)* Very few diseases cause rapid dementia that is noticeable in a period of weeks. Among them are depression, metabolic encephalopathy, encephalitis, poisoning, Binswanger's disease (white-matter infarction), and Creutzfeldt-Jakob disease. (Alzheimer's disease has a more insidious onset.) Creutzfeldt-Jakob disease is a slow-virus infection that causes a spongiform change in the cerebral cortex; it is characterized by rapid dementia, startle myoclonus, and frequently signs of occipital and cerebellar disease. CT and cerebrospinal fluid examination are nearly always normal in affected persons; after a period of time electroencephalography shows rapid, synchronous sharp waves, a diagnostic finding.

**IV-34.** **The answer is D.** *(Chap. 376)* Optic neuritis is the initial symptom in approximately 40 percent of persons who eventually are diagnosed with multiple sclerosis. This rapidly developing ophthalmologic disorder is associated with partial or total loss of vision, pain on motion of the involved eye, scotoma affecting macular vision, and a variety of other visual-field defects. Ophthalmoscopically visible optic papillitis occurs in about half the cases.

**IV-35.** **The answer is A.** *(Chap. 375. Black, N Engl J Med 324:1555–1564, 1991)* Meningiomas are the most common type of benign brain tumor and account for 15 percent of primary CNS neoplasms. They may grow to an extremely large size before detection. Meningiomas most commonly present in women in the fifth or sixth decade. They may arise around the midline between the cerebral hemispheres, in the olfactory groove, and along the sphenoidal ridge, the foramen magnum, and the tentorium of the cerebellum. The neoplastic cells arise from pia or arachnoid tissue, though up to seven histologic subtypes have been identified. Cytogenetic analysis typically reveals abnormalities of chromosome 22. If possible, depending on the site, meningiomas should be totally removed surgically. Parasagittal tumors usually are resectable and have low recurrence rates. Chemotherapy plays no role, and radiation is reserved for postsurgical treatment for the rare malignant meningiomas and for symptomatic patients whose tumors cannot be excised completely. Meningiomas represent a stark contrast to primary high-grade malignant astrocytoma (glioblastoma), in which median survival, even with trimodality therapy, is little more than a year.

**IV-36.   The answer is E.**   *(Chap. 375)*   The most common tumors of the central nervous system by far are those derived from metastatic systemic cancer. The most common sources of intracerebral metastases are cancer of the lung in men and breast cancer in women. Melanoma, though a less common tumor, has a definite predilection for spread to the central nervous system. As patients fare better from the standpoint of their primary neoplasms compared with historical controls, as is the case for ovarian cancer or sarcoma, the incidence of intracerebral metastases rises. Headache, focal neurologic deficits, and seizures are common ways in which those with intracerebral metastases may present. Treatment usually consists of a combination of glucocorticoids and radiation therapy. However, patients with solitary lesions, particularly if they are asymptomatic in the presence of minimal systemic disease (particularly if there has been a disease-free interval longer than 1 year), should be considered for surgical resection. Though most patients with metastatic cancer to the brain improve clinically and by radiographic evaluation after treatment, their 1-year survival is less than 20 percent. The presence of intracerebral metastases is actually a marker for advanced systemic disease, since the vast majority of these patients die not from complications of therapy or from the intracerebral tumor itself but from advanced recurrent systemic malignancy.

**IV-37.   The answer is E.**   *(Chap. 372)*   Bilateral conjugate eye movement to the side of the caloric stimulation indicates integrity of the brainstem pathways from the medulla to the midbrain (where the third nerve originates), as do full conjugate oculocephalic motions (doll's-eye maneuvers). The absence of the rapid corrective phase manifested by nystagmus-like leftward gazing indicates a bilateral hemispheric lesion. Failure of an eye to adduct properly in the initial phase of the caloric response indicates a lesion in the ipsilateral third nerve (midbrain) or in the medial longitudinal fasciculus producing internuclear ophthalmoplegia. In the former case, the pupil would be dilated and the eye would be abducted at rest.

**IV-38.   The answer is C.**   *(Chap. 367. Yankner, N Engl J Med 325:1849–1857, 1991)* Alzheimer's disease is the most common cause of dementia in the elderly. It is highly prevalent, affecting up to 45 percent of those over age 85. In a relatively small percentage of cases, the disease occurs in a familial pattern; this is thought to be due to autosomal dominant inheritance with linkage to chromosome 21 or 19. The clinical beginnings of the disease tend to be subtle. The initial symptoms usually are limited to loss of recent memory. Psychiatric symptoms may then supervene and can include depression, anxiety, delusions, and paranoid behavior. An extrapyramidial component exists so that patients walk in a shuffling manner with short steps. Radiographic evaluation usually reveals neuronal atrophy. Neuropathologically, the disease is characterized by neurofibrillary tangles, which may contain an abnormally phosphorylated form of a microtubular protein known as tau, as well as spherical deposits known as senile plaques. A protein known as beta-amyloid can be found in these plaques. Certain families with inherited Alzheimer's disease have been found to harbor a point mutation in the amyloid precursor protein. From a neurotransmitter standpoint, acetylcholine, a neurotransmitter that is important in memory formation, is synthesized at abnormally low levels. The current model for the pathogenesis of Alzheimer's disease is that altered cleavage of the amyloid precursor protein generates the so-called beta-amyloid protein, which then binds to a protease inhibitor–enzyme complex, in turn preventing the normal inactivation of extracellular proteases. It is these abnormally activated extracellular proteases that may mediate the neuronal degeneration characteristic of Alzheimer's disease. Therapeutic strategies that could inhibit the generation of beta-amyloid are of potential therapeutic interest.

**IV-39.** **The answer is A.** *(Chap. 368. Standaert, Med Clin North Am 77:169, 1993)* Parkinson's disease is a chronic degenerative disease of middle-aged and elderly persons that is characterized pathologically by a decrease in dopaminergic transmission in the caudate nucleus and putamen. Early manifestations of the disease include a unilateral rest tumor with a frequency of 4 to 5 per second. The tremor may progress to involve structures on both sides of the body with eventual postural imbalance, profound restriction of movement, and eventual degeneration to a chair-bound existence. Total paralysis is highly uncharacteristic, and tendon reflexes as well as sensory examination are normal. The early stage of the disease can be treated with deprenyl, a monoamine oxidase inhibitor that slows disease progression. Treatment of more progressive Parkinson's disease requires dopamine replacement in the form of levodopa. Levodopa is given in combination with a dopa-decarboxylase inhibitor (carbidopa), which prevents bloodstream destruction of levodopa but is unable to pass through the blood-brain barrier. Carbidopa in combination with levodopa in a ratio of 1:4 or 1:10 (Sinemet) is available. Though costly, dopamine-receptor agonists such as bromocriptine may be used to lower the required dose of Sinemet. Anticholinergic drugs such as benztropine and trihexyphenidyl may constitute useful adjunctive therapy but must be used carefully because of the side effects of confusion, glaucoma, urinary retention, and progression of dementia. Amantadine, which causes the release of dopamine from presynaptic terminals, also may be useful early in the disease. Unfortunately, as the disease progresses, the therapeutic index of the levodopa-carbidopa combination decreases. If levodopa-induced hallucinations occur, clozapine may be helpful, although neutropenia may occur.

**IV-40.** **The answer is A.** *(Chap. 25)* Most lesions that lead to aphasia, a disturbance in the production or comprehension of speech and language, occur in the dominant cerebral hemisphere. Ninety percent of people are right-handed; the left hemisphere is dominant in 95 percent of right-handed people, and 50 percent of those who are left-handed. Broca's, or major motor, aphasia denotes a syndrome in which the praxis of speech is severely disturbed. This problem usually results from a large lesion in the posterior frontal lobe along the insula and sylvian fissure, not simply in Broca's area in the inferior frontal lobe. Patients have great difficulty in articulation, grammar, and writing, though comprehension and fluency are relatively well preserved. Emboli of the superior division of the left middle cerebral artery are the most common cause of this syndrome.

**IV-41.** **The answer is C.** *(Chap. 385. Shader, N Engl J Med 328:1398–1405, 1993)* Anxiety symptoms are extraordinarily common in medical patients. Such symptoms may occur as a consequence of a primary psychiatric problem or may be due to drug therapy or medical illness. There are several different subcategories of anxiety disorders, including posttraumatic stress disorder, phobic disorders (e.g., agoraphobia, social phobias, and simple phobias), obsessive-compulsive disorder, generalized anxiety disorder, and panic disorder. The most important feature of panic disorders is the sudden onset of overwhelming feelings of terror and fear associated with multiple symptoms, including dyspnea, palpitations, and faintness. Attacks usually occur away from home and tend to be recurrent. Panic disorder may well have a genetic basis insofar as it occurs to a greater degree in first-degree relatives. In addition to the elicitation of often complex medical workups for these dramatic symptoms, the morbidity of panic disorder often stems from its association with agoraphobia and the house-bound situation to which patients restrict themselves. Major depression, substance abuse, and suicide may complicate panic disorders. As in the case of a patient presenting with a generalized anxiety disorder, it is important to rule out a host of medical conditions. The list of such medical disorders is long and includes angina, carcinoid syndrome, hyperthyroidism, menopausal symptoms, mitral valve prolapse, pheochromocytoma, porphyria, pneumothorax, pulmonary embolus, and temporal lobe epilepsy. Complications also include the use or abuse of drugs such as alcohol, amphetamines, aminophylline, anticholinergics, antihistamines, caffeine, cocaine, glucocorticoids, monosodium glutamate, salicylates, and thyroid replacement drugs. The currently accepted theories concerning the etiology of panic disorder center on a genetic susceptibility to an environmental event that triggers adrenergic overload. While tricyclic antidepressants, monoamine oxidase inhibitors, and benzodiazepines are effective in the treatment of panic disorder, the drug of first choice is usually a low dose of a tricyclic such as imipramine. The newer serotonin reuptake–inhibitor antidepressants, such as fluoxetine and sertraline, also may be effective. It is important to maintain patients with panic disorder on long-term medication because the relapse rate is very high if these medicines are discontinued. The only benzodiazepine approved for use in panic disorder is alprazolam; however, clonazepam is also useful, especially in view of its longer half-life. In fact, the benzodiazepines may be used to prevent the episodes while the tricyclic dose is being increased over the 1 to 2 weeks required to achieve full therapeutic efficacy.

**IV-42.** **The answer is E.** *(Chap. 384)* Although a viral cause has been postulated, no clear-cut etiology has been demonstrated for chronic fatigue syndrome. Furthermore, while several subtle immunologic abnormalities have been documented in certain patients with this syndrome, there is no definitive diagnostic test. The diagnosis of chronic fatigue syndrome relies on the Centers for Disease Control and Prevention's working definition. A definitive diagnosis is based on the presence of both of the major criteria: persistent or relapsing fatigue that does not resolve with bed rest and is severe enough to reduce average daily activity by 50 percent and exclusion of other chronic conditions, including preexisting psychiatric diseases. The physical examination must include two of the following three physical findings by a doctor on at least two occasions 1 month apart: low-grade fever, pharyngitis, and palpable lymphadenopathy. Finally, at least six of the common symptoms must be present; these symptoms include mild fever or chills, sore throat, painful lymph nodes in the cervical chains, muscle weakness, muscle discomfort, fatigue after minimal exercise, new headaches, arthralgias, neuropsychological symptoms, and sleep disturbance. Patients who do not have the required physical findings need to fulfill eight of the symptom criteria. Since there is no specific therapy for this disease, treatment requires an understanding of the patient and the avoidance of unproven therapies such as acyclovir, vitamin $B_{12}$, intravenous gamma globulin, and steroids. Treatment should be symptom-directed. Thus, nonsteroidal anti-inflammatory agents, decongestants, and antidepressants may be helpful, depending on the symptoms. Finally, life-style modification, including a graded exercise program, minimal caffeine intake, and avoidance of complete rest, is advisable.

**IV-43.** **The answer is B.** *(Chap. 369)* Acquired hepatocerebral degeneration is a neurologic syndrome that consists mainly of extrapyramidal signs. A well-known consequence of chronic liver disease, this disorder simulates Wilson's disease in many ways, including the presence of neuropathologic lesions in the cortex, basal ganglia, and other deep nuclei. Many cases become evident after a bout of hepatic encephalopathy, but others occur insidiously in persons who never have had encephalopathy.

**IV-44.** **The answer is B.** *(Chap. 368)* The combination of autonomic insufficiency and parkinsonian symptoms is known as the Shy-Drager syndrome. The autonomic form of the Landry-Guillain-Barré syndrome causes acute autonomic paralysis but does not cause the parkinsonian symptoms of tremor at rest, bradykinesia, and rigidity. A number of antihypertensive agents cause orthostatic hypotension, but none cause parkinsonism. Micturition syncope is a condition in which syncope occurs because of vagal surge at the time of release of intravesicular pressure.

**IV-45.** **The answer is E.** *(Chap. 385. Michels, N Engl J Med 329:552–560, 628–638, 1993)* The outlook for patients with schizophrenic disorders has improved with the use of antipsychotic medications such as the phenothiazines, which include chlorpromazine, fluphenazine, and thioridazine. In particular, these medicines are useful for the treatment of the "positive" symptoms of schizophrenia, such as hallucinations and psychotic agitation. However, they are less useful against the "negative" symptoms typified by social withdrawal. In general, antipsychotic medications block dopamine neurotransmission in nigrostriatal structures. This dopamine blockade can induce extrapyramidal side effects that mimic Parkinson's disease. Although many antipsychotics have intrinsic anticholinergic action, which can result in dry mouth, hypotension, and urinary retention, the addition of benztropine, another anticholinergic medicine used in the treatment of Parkinson's disease, may be effective in treating these extrapyramidal side effects. A particularly notable side effect of antipsychotic medicines is akathisia, which is characterized by obligatory movement of the extremities and motor restlessness. Akathisia may respond to the institution of beta-blocking drugs or antiparkinsonian agents but most likely would benefit from a decrease in the dose of the neuroleptic agent. The most common serious side effect of neuroleptic medicines is tardive dyskinesia, manifest by involuntary repetitive movements of musculature such as tongue thrusting and lip smacking. Involuntary limb movements and postural dystonia also may be part of this syndrome. While newer antipsychotic medications such as clozapine may have a role to play in the treatment or amelioration of tardive dyskinesia, currently the best approach is to lower the dose of the neuroleptic agent. Of course, such reductions may not be possible without exacerbation of the underlying thought disorder.

**IV-46.    The answer is B.**    *(Chap. 367)*    Huntington's chorea, which is inherited as an autosomal dominant trait, is characterized by dementia and choreiform movements. The motor disorder may include grimacing, respiratory spasms, speech irregularity, and a dancing, jangling quality in the gait. Laboratory workup is normal except that atrophy of the caudate nucleus may be seen on a carefully evaluated CT or MRI scan. Through the use of DNA linkage analysis, patients can be tested before disease development if this is appropriate from a psychosocial standpoint. The disease-specific gene is located on the short arm of chromosome 4.

**IV-47.    The answer is D.**    *(Chap. 372)*    Brief paroxysms of severe, sharp pains in the face without demonstrable lesions in the jaw, teeth, or sinuses are called tic douloureux, or trigeminal neuralgia. The pain may be brought on by stimuli applied to the face, lips, or tongue or by certain movements of those structures. Aneurysms, neurofibromas, or meningiomas impinging on the fifth cranial nerve at any point during its course typically present with trigeminal neuropathy, which will cause sensory loss on the face, weakness of the jaw muscles, or both; neither symptom is demonstrable in this patient. The treatment for this idiopathic condition is carbamazepine or phenytoin if carbamazepine is not tolerated. When drug treatment is not successful, surgical therapy, including the commonly applied percutaneous retrogasserian rhizotomy, may be effective. A possible complication of this procedure is partial facial numbness with a risk of corneal anesthesia, which increases the potential for ulceration.

**IV-48.    The answer is B.**    *(Chaps. 363, 325)*    Neurofibromatosis type 1 is an autosomal dominant condition carried on the long arm of chromosome 17. It is characterized by tumors involving the sheaths of peripheral nerves and is associated with café au lait spots (tanned cutaneous flat lesions). The neurofibromas are rarely symptomatic, although they may occasionally entrap nerve roots. In addition to sarcomatous degeneration, central nervous system tumors, including optic glioma, glioblastoma, and meningioma, may occur in patients with neurofibromatosis. Mutations in the gene encoding the protein neurofibromin account for this disease. The structure of this protein suggests that it may have GTPase-activating properties and thus may be a tumor-suppressor gene. Neurofibromatosis type II, in which bilateral acoustic neuromas are found in addition to multiple neurofibromas, is believed to be caused by mutations in the gene that encodes the protein merlin, a 587-amino-acid cytoskeletal protein. Other neurologic disorders known to be caused by gene mutations include ocular retinoblastoma, which is caused by mutations in the Rb protein on chromosome 13; hexosaminadase A mutations, which account for Tay-Sachs disease; and KALIG-1 mutations, which give rise to Kallman's syndrome.

**IV-49.**   **The answer is B.**   *(Chap. 373)*   The most characteristic symptom of syringomyelia is loss of pain sense with preservation of touch. This phenomenon occurs most commonly over the shoulders in a capelike distribution. Tissue loss in the central gray matter of the spinal cord, where pain fibers cross to join the contralateral spinothalamic tract, is the neuropathologic process involved. Other characteristic features of syringomyelia include thoracic scoliosis and muscle atrophy of the hands. Ataxia does not occur unless the syrinx extends into the brainstem.

**IV-50.**   **The answer is C.**   *(Chap. 372)*   Pain, loss of function (without clear-cut sensory or motor deficits), and a localized autonomic impairment are called reflex sympathetic dystrophy (also known as shoulder-hand syndrome or causalgia). Precipitating events in this unusual syndrome include myocardial infarction, shoulder trauma, and limb paralysis. In addition to the neuropathic-type pain, autonomic dysfunction, possibly resulting from neuroadrenergic and cholinergic hypersensitivity, produces localized sweating, changes in blood flow, and abnormal hair and nail growth as well as edema or atrophy of the affected limb. Treatment is difficult; however, anticonvulsants such as phenytoin and carbamazepine may be effective, as they are in other conditions in which neuropathic pain is a major problem.

**IV-51.**   **The answer is E.**   *(Chap. 374. White, N Engl J Med 327:1507–1511, 1992)*   Concussion, the transient loss of consciousness consequent to blunt impact to the skull, is believed to occur because of electrophysiologic dysfunction of the upper midbrain as a result of sudden movement of the brain within the skull. About 3 percent of those with concussions also have an associated intracranial hemorrhage, but the absence of a skull fracture decreases the risk. Amnesia for events just prior to the trauma is common, as are a single episode of emesis, severe bilateral frontal headache, faintness, blurred vision, and problems with concentration. However, minor injuries are characterized by an absence of neurologic signs, normal skull x-ray, and normal CT or MRI scans. In the absence of persistent confusion, behavioral changes, decreased alertness, or focal neurologic signs, patients may be discharged to be observed by responsible individuals. Several more worrisome clinical syndromes may accompany more severe head injury. Such symptoms are characterized by (1) delirium and wishing not to be moved, (2) severe memory loss, (3) focal deficit, (4) global confusion, (5) repetitive vomiting and nystagmus, (6) drowsiness, and (7) diabetes insipidus. Positive findings on CT scan or EEG would be common with these types of postconcussive syndromes, neurosurgical evaluation would be required, and prophylactic phenytoin, glucocorticoids, and haloperidol could be considered.

**IV-52.**   **The answer is A.**   *(Chap. 373)*   Neuromyelitis optica (Devic's disease) usually occurs in association with necrotizing myelitis but also is seen in persons who have multiple sclerosis and postinfectious and postvaccinal myelitis. Neuromyelitis optica is characterized by both transverse myelitis and optic neuritis; affected persons can display signs and symptoms such as progressive sensorimotor deficits, central scotoma, and elevated protein concentration and cell count in the cerebrospinal fluid. In the case presented in the question, the presence of optic nerve involvement and the finding of a sensory level on the trunk rule out acute idiopathic polyneuritis, although the analysis of cerebrospinal fluid is not inconsistent with polyneuritis in its early stages. A diagnosis of acute spinal epidural abscess is made less likely by the presence of optic neuritis.

**IV-53.**   **The answer is C.**   *(Chap. 374)*   The cause of chronic subdural hematoma may be a trivial or inapparent injury, such as might be incurred after a sudden deceleration experienced in a motor vehicle accident. The symptoms are relatively nonspecific and usually are characterized by an intermittent headache accompanied by some degree of personality change, drowsiness, or confusion. This condition is easily confused with drug intoxication, stroke, dementia, and depression. For the patient in the question, however, the lack of focal findings argues against stroke, and the rapidity of onset would be unusual for dementia. CT scan does not define the hematomas, because they have become isodense with the passage of time (2 to 6 weeks since the injury); however, the absence of sulci and the small size of the ventricles, coupled with the clinical scenario, are highly suggestive of bilateral subdural hematomas. Surgical evacuation of the hematomas is the treatment of choice.

**IV-54.** **The answer is C.** *(Chap. 374. White, N Engl J Med 327:1507–1511, 1992)* Epidural bleeding may cause rapidly deteriorating mental status after an initial lucid interval following head trauma. Such hematomas occur in 1 to 3 percent of all head injuries. The typical profile of a patient with an acute epidural hematoma is that of an alcoholic who sustains severe trauma and fractures the squamous portion of the temporal bone, tearing the origin of dural vessels arising from the middle meningeal artery. Therefore, the most common location of an epidural hematoma is overlying the lateral temporal convexity. These hematomas expand rapidly because of the force of arterial bleeding, strip the dura from the attached inner table of the skull, and produce a characteristic bulge-type clot on CT. This dramatically evolving picture requires neurosurgical intervention, usually in the form of clot evacuation.

**IV-55.** **The answer is D.** *(Chap. 379)* Rapidly progressive dementia with myoclonus is the hallmark of Creutzfeldt-Jakob disease. While most cases are sporadic, a small percentage are familial with an autosomal dominant pattern of inheritance. In addition to dementia, myoclonus, and cerebellar signs, the electroencephalogram shows a characteristic pattern, as described in the question. CT scanning or MRI usually is not specifically helpful except that the degree of dementia is out of proportion to the degree of radiographic brain loss. Definitive diagnostic accuracy requires a brain biopsy, which would show vascular degeneration, neuronal loss, and glial hypertrophy without significant inflammation. While Creutzfeldt-Jakob disease was formerly thought to be a disease of viral etiology, it is now accepted that the cause is the deposition of a proteinaceous infectious particle (prion) devoid of nucleic acid that is encoded by a gene on the short arm of human chromosome 20. The function of this protein is at present unknown, but certain mutations in this gene have been found in families with hereditary Creutzfeldt-Jakob disease.

**IV-56.** **The answer is D.** *(Chap. 381)* Entrapment of the lateral femoral cutaneous nerve, which can occur at the site where it enters the thigh beneath the inguinal ligament near the anterior superior iliac spine, causes a sensory neuropathy known as *meralgia paresthetica*. The symptoms of this disorder, which typically occur in obese persons, include pain and decreased tactile sensation over the lateral aspect of the thigh. Treatment consists of infiltration with a local anesthetic or, if this procedure proves ineffective, surgical sectioning of the nerve.

**IV-57.** **The answer is E.** *(Chap. 381)* The inflammatory response in Guillain-Barré syndrome strips myelin between the nodes of Ranvier in peripheral nerves. This phenomenon explains both the slowing of nerve conduction and the potential for recovery. Axons are destroyed only in extensively involved areas as a secondary phenomenon. To date, no convincing evidence has emerged to support the contention that the central nervous system is involved in Guillain-Barré syndrome.

**IV-58.** **The answer is A.** *(Chap. 382)* Myotonia, muscle wasting, cataracts, testicular atrophy, and frontal baldness characterize the hereditary disorder myotonic dystrophy. The onset usually occurs in early adulthood. In affected persons, mental retardation is common, atrial arrhythmia is a frequent complication, and diabetes mellitus is more prevalent than it is in the general population. Myotonic dystrophy is the type of muscular dystrophy most commonly observed in hospitalized patients.

**IV-59.   The answer is B.**  *(Chap. 383)*   Oculopharyngeal dystrophy is a dominantly inherited disease that occurs in families of French-Canadian or middle European ancestry. Because it causes late-onset progressive ptosis and difficulty swallowing, it may be difficult to distinguish from myasthenia gravis, which is not a dystrophic muscle disease. Proximal weakness and ophthalmoplegia suggest the presence of a progressive external ophthalmoplegia.

**IV-60.   The answer is C.**  *(Chap. 383)*   Myotonia is a phenomenon in which brief, persistent contractions of a muscle occur after voluntary contraction or sometimes percussion. Myokymia refers to continuous small-muscle movement that frequently is difficult to distinguish from fasciculations. Fibrillation is the electromyographically detected spontaneous firing of muscle fibers and is not visible except in the tongue. Myoedema is a poorly defined sign, similar to myotonia, in which a ridge of percussed muscle remains contracted for 5 to 8 s. It was once thought to be related to hypoalbuminemia, but this relationship probably does not exist.

**IV-61.   The answer is B.**  *(Chap. 16)*   Malignancy in the pelvis not infrequently causes compression or infiltration of nerves exiting the spinal cord en route to the leg. This results in a stepwise progression of sensory and motor deficits in areas supplied by the involved nerve roots or trunks. Continuous pain in the distribution of a specific nerve or root is also common. In this patient the neurologic deficits began in an S1 distribution but then progressed to the L5 and finally the L4 roots, suggesting an expanding paravertebral mass. Isolated spontaneous activity of muscle fibers, called *fibrillations,* is characteristic of denervation. Nerve conduction will be normal in the leg if the lesion is proximal to the measuring electrodes, that is, in the pelvis. An expanding cortical mass also may cause progressive numbness in the foot and leg and may be missed on a CT scan that does not take cuts all the way up to the vertex. Back pain and neuropathic pain would not occur with a cortical lesion, and the reflexes under such circumstances should be hyperactive.

**IV-62.   The answer is D.**  *(Chap. 382)*   More than three-quarters of patients with myasthenia have circulating antibodies against components of the postsynaptic membrane, including acetylcholine receptors. Antibody action leads to an unfolding, or "simplification," of the membrane and consequently a reduced number of acetylcholine receptors. As a result, existing acetylcholine in the synapse is less effective in producing muscle contraction.

**IV-63.   The answer is A.**  *(Chap. 366. Fisher, Neurology 32:871, 1982)*   A pure motor hemiparesis on one side (with ipsilateral face and body involvement) and no other cortical deficits (aphasia or cortical sensory loss) suggests an internal capsular lesion. The major differential diagnosis in this setting is between a hypertensive hemorrhage and an internal capsular lacunar infarct. Both entities may present with a fluctuating course over hours; however, hemorrhages tend to produce some manifestation of increased intracranial pressure. Lacunar infarctions result from atherothrombotic and hyalinization changes in the penetrating branches of the circle of Willis, the middle cerebral artery stem, and the vertebrobasilar system. Apart from the internal capsule, common locations for lacunar infarctions include the thalamus, where they produce a pure sensory deficit, and the base of the pons, where they produce hemiparesis and dysarthria with a clumsy hand. CT scanning can document most supratentorial lacunar infarctions, whose size usually ranges from 0.5 to 2 cm.

**IV-64.   The answer is E.**  *(Chap. 375)*   The typical symptoms of neoplastic meningitis include headache, confusion, radiculopathy, and cranial nerve abnormalities in patients with a variety of tumors, including non-Hodgkin's lymphoma, leukemia, melanoma, breast cancer, lung cancer, and stomach cancer. Given these symptoms, especially with a negative CT, MRI, or both, the diagnosis of leptomeningeal metastases from breast cancer is quite likely. A single lumbar puncture is a relatively insensitive test; repeat examinations of cerebrospinal fluid often are required to establish the diagnosis of cancer that has spread to the meninges. Especially in cases where the cancer cells are "caked" onto the inferior portion of the brain, eradication by chemotherapy alone (usually methotrexate, thiotepa, or cytosine arabinoside) is difficult, and radiation therapy should be administered as well.

**IV-65.    The answer is E.**    *(Chaps. 21, 383)*    Fasciculations may occur in a variety of metabolic and toxic disorders, including amyotrophic lateral sclerosis, progressive bulbar palsy, ruptured intervertebral disk, and peripheral neuropathy. However, they should not be viewed with alarm in the absence of weakness, muscle atrophy, or loss of tendon reflexes. The best treatment a physician can offer a person who is asymptomatic except for fascicular twitches is reassurance and, if appropriate, advice to reduce coffee intake.

**IV-66.    The answer is C.**    *(Chap. 381)*    Although porphyric neuropathy may occur without involvement of the central nervous system, with acute paralysis there is frequently a history of confusion or coma. Predominantly a motor neuropathy, porphyric neuropathy can cause significant sensory loss in some persons. In this respect it may simulate inflammatory polyneuropathy, though inflammation does not occur. Curiously, protein concentration in CSF usually is normal in affected persons.

**IV-67.    The answer is C.**    *(Chap. 12)*    One of the most distressing sequelae of thalamic damage is a chronic pain syndrome (Déjerine-Roussy syndrome) that occurs months to a few years after the initial lesion. The findings of total hemianesthesia and loss of all sensory modalities in the face, arm, and leg are characteristic of thalamic infarction. Lesions of the spinothalamic tract also may cause neuropathic pain syndromes, but hemianesthesia of the face does not occur with spinal cord lesions. Parietal lobe lesions usually affect the cortical senses (i.e., two-point discrimination, graphesthesia, or stereognosia) rather than causing a total hemianesthesia. Depression is not commonly associated with burning pain. Tic douloureux is not associated with sensory loss.

**IV-68.    The answer is E.**    *(Chap. 370. Prados, Neurology 43:751, 1993)*    Amyotrophic lateral sclerosis (ALS) is an untreatable disease that results in the progressive loss of upper and lower motor neuron function. Other components of the nervous system remain intact, including the neurons required for ocular motility. Limb weakness and cramping is the first symptom, followed by muscular atrophy, fasciculations, and loss of function of the cranial nerve musculature. Early in the disease, upper-tract signs may predominate, resulting in spasticity. Pneumonia resulting from failure of clearance of secretions is usually the terminal event. Treatable causes of motor neuron diseases such as cervical spondylosis (no bulbar involvement) and lead poisoning should be excluded whenever the diagnosis of ALS is considered. Guillain-Barré syndrome produces an ascending, rapidly developing paralysis. Vitamin $B_{12}$ deficiency should lead to abnormalities in posterior column function. Lambert-Eaton syndrome is a paraneoplastic neuromuscular disorder that does not feature upper-tract signs.

**IV-69.    The answer is D.**    *(Chap. 38. Koenig, Cell 50:509, 1987)*    Duchenne's muscular dystrophy is an X-linked recessive disorder in which affected boys develop progressive weakness of limb girdle muscles beginning at age 5 or earlier. By age 12 walking is impossible, and these patients usually succumb to respiratory failure by age 25. Most muscular tissues, including cardiac tissues, are involved. An abnormally high creatine kinase level is found in all these patients before disease onset and in many female carriers. The responsible gene has been identified. This 2000-kb gene codes for a product termed dystrophin, a 400-kDa protein localized to the muscle plasma membrane. Since about 60 percent of these patients have an exon deletion or duplication in the dystrophin gene, it is possible to test directly for these genetic abnormalities in utero, obviating the need for more cumbersome family studies to determine RFLPs for linkage.

**IV-70.   The answer is D.**   *(Chap. 383. Dalakas, N Engl J Med 325:1487, 1991)*   This patient displays the characteristic heliotropic rash, with knuckle involvement and proximal muscle weakness, typical of dermatomyositis. Although a biopsy could be done, the disease is patchy and the absence of lymphocytic infiltration would not rule out the diagnosis. EMG is diagnostic in about 40 percent of affected persons. Since the diagnosis is straightforward and dermatomyositis frequently is associated with malignancy in those over age 60, it is reasonable to screen for cancer. In addition to the common epithelial malignancies, myeloproliferative disorders can be heralded by dermatomyositis. However, an unfocused radiologic diagnostic attack definitely should be suspended in favor of the simple and cost-effective tests outlined in choice B. Although steroids probably will be symptomatically beneficial even in those with malignancies, their use probably should be delayed until the screening is completed. If an early neoplasm can be found and treated, the dermatomyositis may respond without the need to resort to the dangers of high-dose glucocorticoid therapy.

**IV-71.   The answer is D.**   *(Chap. 386. Charness, N Engl J Med 321:442, 1989)*   Wernicke's encephalopathy is a consequence of thiamine (vitamin $B_1$) deficiency. Although it is most commonly observed in chronic alcoholics in this country, well-documented cases have occurred in prisoners of war in whom alcohol played no role. Certain areas in the thalamus, hypothalamus, midbrain, floor of the fourth ventricle, and cerebellar vermis are prone to destruction as a consequence of thiamine deficiency. While most patients present with some form of abnormal mental functioning, the classic triad of ophthalmoplegia, confusion, and ataxia is rarely encountered. As can be seen in autopsy series, many patients frequently go undiagnosed. When the diagnosis is suspected, thiamine should be administered before glucose, since glucose can precipitate worsening of the disease. Thiamine will relieve the ocular palsies within hours, although improvement in ataxia and in apathy and confusion takes longer. Many of those who recover from the acute encephalopathy will be left with a profound defect in memory and learning known as *Korsakoff's psychosis.*

**IV-72.   The answer is A.**   *(Chap. 373)*   The finding of a clear sensory level above which pinprick is felt but below which sensation is absent is the *sine qua non* of spinal cord disease. The segmental level at which sensory loss begins also indicates the corresponding cord level of the lesion. Other typical signs of spinal cord disease, such as hypertonicity and hyperreflexia, may be absent in acute lesions; bladder function, however, is invariably affected if the lesion is severe. Myelopathy caused by a deficiency of vitamin $B_{12}$ only rarely gives a vague sensory level on the trunk.

**IV-73.   The answer is E.**   *(Chap. 16)*   A disk at the L2-L3 interspace would compress the L2 root. There may be weakness of hip flexion and sensory loss along the upper border of the thigh below the inguinal ligament. No tendon reflex is mediated by this root. A lesion of the L3 root would cause weakness of hip flexion and knee extension and sensory loss over the midportion of the anterior thigh. No tendon reflex is mediated by this root. A lesion of the L4 root would result in a depressed or absent patellar reflex, weakness of knee extension and foot dorsiflexion, and sensory loss over the anterior knee and the medial portion of the foreleg. A lesion of the L5 root would result in weakness of knee flexion, dorsiflexion of the ankle and great toe, and weakness of inversion and eversion of the foot. Sensory loss would be noted over the lateral aspect of the foreleg and the dorsal surface of the foot. A lateral disk protrusion at the S1-S2 interspace would compress the S1 nerve root. The S1 root mediates the Achilles tendon reflex, innervates part of the gastrocnemius, and provides sensation to the lateral aspect and sole of the foot.

**IV-74.   The answer is C.**   *(Chap. 16)*   A lesion of the L3 root would produce symptoms that include the anterior portion of the thigh. There also may be weakness of hip flexion and knee extension. The same is true for the femoral nerve. The saphenous nerve is the cutaneous sensory continuation of the femoral nerve and supplies the medial aspect of the foreleg. The obturator nerve primarily supplies motor innervation to the thigh adductors but has a small sensory component at the medial thigh. The area described in the question corresponds to the lateral femoral cutaneous nerve. A lesion of this nerve is referred to as meralgia paresthetica. This nerve, which is made up of fibers from the L2 and L3 roots, travels over the bony rim of the pelvis and under the inguinal ligament to enter the thigh. It is a thin nerve that is easily compressed in patients with weight gain, those who wear a heavy work belt, and pregnant subjects. An intrapelvic mass also may cause compression of this nerve.

**IV-75.    The answer is E.** *(Chaps. 16, 370)* Choices A through D would involve depressed or absent reflexes and include sensory symptoms and signs on examination. A lesion of the common peroneal nerve would not cause weakness of foot inversion. The combination of subacute, painless distal muscle weakness with brisk tendon reflexes is most consistent with amyotrophic lateral sclerosis, a disease of unknown etiology in which there is loss of both upper and lower motor neurons.

**IV-76.    The answer is D.** *(Chap. 375)* An oligodendroglioma is a tumor that arises from oligodendrocytes in the white matter of the cerebral hemispheres. It is most common in early to middle adulthood. Although craniopharyngioma is more common in children than in adults, it commonly arises in a suprasellar location. Glioblastoma multiforme, the most aggressive glial tumor, is most commonly located within the cerebral hemispheres of older adults. Cerebellar hemangioblastoma, a tumor associated with von Hippel-Lindau syndrome, usually is cystic and rarely occurs in childhood. Medulloblastomas are commonly seen in childhood, are more common in males than in females, and arise from the cerebellar vermis. In contrast, when seen in adults, medulloblastomas frequently occupy the cerebellar hemispheres.

**IV-77.    The answer is C.** *(Chap. 372)* Parinaud syndrome is associated with a lesion of the rostral dorsal midbrain. It is most often seen with tumors of the pineal gland, hydrocephalus, and multiple sclerosis. The structures involved include the superior colliculus and the pretectum. Choices A, B, D, and E may be seen in this syndrome. Skew deviation most commonly results from a lesion of the cerebellum or cerebellar outflow tracts in the brainstem.

**IV-78.    The answer is C.** *(Chap. 25)* Gerstmann's syndrome results from a lesion of the dominant parietal lobe and consists of dysgraphia, acalculia, finger agnosia, and loss of or difficulty with left-right discrimination. Prosopagnosia, or the inability to recognize faces, results from bilateral damage to the visual association areas of the occipital lobe.

**IV-79.    The answer is B.** *(Chap. 25)* Wernicke's aphasia is caused by a lesion in the posterior superior temporal gyrus of the dominant hemisphere. It is characterized by impaired language comprehension, inability to repeat, and fluent speech output with paraphasic errors. The only associated neurologic sign may be a right superior quadrantanopia secondary to the proximity of the inferior optic radiation to Wernicke's area in the left temporal lobe.

**IV-80.    The answer is C.** *(Chap. 383)* Hypokalemic paralysis occurs most commonly in the setting of medical conditions that cause low serum potassium. Inherited hypokalemic paralysis usually is an autosomal dominant disorder and may be associated with hyperthyroidism. Hyperadrenalism may cause a hyperkalemic paralysis.

**IV-81.    The answer is E.** *(Chap. 372)* A lesion of the right frontal lobe involving the cortical gaze center would result in a gaze preference to the right. A left labyrinthine lesion would cause bilateral nystagmus and vertigo. The rostral interstitial nucleus of the medial longitudinal fasciculus (MLF) controls vertical gaze, which is not affected in this case. A lesion of the left occipital cortex would result in a right homonymous hemianopia. The MLF connects the horizontal gaze center in the pons with the oculomotor nuclei. Lesions of the MLF, which are common in multiple sclerosis, result in an internuclear ophthalmoplegia, or failure of adduction of the eye on the side of the lesion, accompanied by contralateral nystagmus.

**IV-82.** **The answer is C.** *(Chap. 25)* The syndrome described in the question is alexia without agraphia. This clinical syndrome is caused by isolation of the intact language network in the left hemisphere from visual input secondary to damage to the left occipital lobe and a posterior portion of the splenium of the corpus callosum. Damage to the left occipital lobe results in a right homonymous hemianopia and occasionally color anomia. The patient is unable to read because visual input to the intact right occipital lobe cannot reach the language network in the left hemisphere as a result of the interruption of crossing fibers in the splenium. There is most frequently a cerebrovascular etiology.

**IV-83.** **The answer is D.** *(Chaps. 15, 28)* Headache associated with papilledema and a sixth nerve palsy points to increased intracranial pressure. A normal cranial MRI, with the exception of "slit-like" ventricles, and increased CSF pressure along with normal CSF parameters are consistent with a diagnosis of pseudotumor cerebri, or benign intracranial hypertension. Those affected are usually young obese females. Although cases are idiopathic, an underlying venous thrombosis may be present; this may be associated with an inherited coagulopathy with or without the use of oral contraceptives. Other precipitants include vitamin A and vitamin D intoxication, the use of tetracycline antibiotics and lithium, and the use or tapering of corticosteroids. After treatment of the underlying disorder, if any, treatment may include serial lumbar punctures, a carbonic anhydrase inhibitor, optic nerve sheath fenestration, or a lumboperitoneal shunt. Treatment is undertaken to relieve the symptoms and preserve vision, which may be compromised by chronic papilledema. For this reason, these patients should have full visual field testing at presentation and ophthalmologic follow-up.

**IV-84.** **The answer is E.** *(Chap. 369)* Friedreich's ataxia (FA) is the most common of the inherited spinocerebellar ataxias, displaying autosomal recessive inheritance. The molecular defect recently was shown to involve a GAA trinucleotide repeat expansion on chromosome 9. Affected persons usually present with progressive ataxia before age 25. Other symptoms include progressive dysarthria, pyramidal-type weakness with bilateral extensor plantar responses, posterior column sensory loss, and an axonal sensory polyneuropathy with absent deep tendon reflexes in the lower extremities. Scoliosis and pes cavus (skeletal deformities) also may be seen in these patients. Nearly all FA patients have abnormal ECGs and many experience supraventricular tachyarrhythmias secondary to cardiac involvement. Diabetes mellitus and glucose intolerance are more common in FA patients than in the general population.

**IV-85.** **The answer is E.** *(Chap. 43)* Prader-Willi syndrome is caused by the inheritance of a paternally derived deletion in the proximal long arm of chromosome 15. This region contains several "imprinted" genes, the function of which depends on the sex in which they are located. In this particular situation, the gene, the absence of which is necessary for the development of the Prader-Willi syndrome, normally is expressed on the paternal chromosome but not on the maternal chromosome. In Prader-Willi syndrome, the patient inherits the nonexpressed gene from the mother and the deleted gene from the father. The clinical hallmarks of the syndrome include congenital hypotonia, obesity, hyperphagia, hypogonadism, and mental retardation. The inverse situation occurs in Angelman syndrome ("happy puppet" syndrome). This syndrome is caused by the inheritance of the same deletion in the proximal long arm of the mother's chromosome 15.

**IV-86.** **The answer is E.** *(Chap. 12)* All the tricyclic antidepressants listed in the question are moderately effective in relieving neuropathic pain. Desipramine is the least sedating among these choices.

**IV-87.** **The answer is A.** *(Chap. 12)* Abdominal CT might demonstrate an abscess just beneath the diaphragm on the left. This process irritates the diaphragm, causing hiccups and referred pain to the left shoulder. The convergence of the visceral and cutaneous sensory inputs onto a single spinal pain transmission neuron is the anatomic basis of the referred pain. Spinal pain transmission neurons at the C3, C4, and C5 levels receive cutaneous input from the shoulder and visceral input from the diaphragm. Because pain sensation usually comes from the skin, activity evoked in spinal pain neurons from visceral structures is mislocalized by the patient to the dermatome innervated by the same spinal segment (so-called referred pain). The other tests listed in the question would not reveal the visceral irritant that produces his symptoms.

**IV-88.** **The answer is C.** *(Chap. 24)* In the evaluation of a comatose patient, eye movements provide invaluable information about the function of the central nervous system and can help localize the cause of coma to hemispheric versus brainstem. The evaluation described in the question is the oculovestibular reflex, which gives the examiner information about the eye movement circuit from the external auditory canal to the pons and midbrain. In an awake patient with normally functioning hemispheres and brainstem, irrigation of one external auditory canal with cool water results in a tonic conjugate gaze of both eyes toward the side of the irrigation, followed by a fast corrective saccade in the reverse direction. If the patient has suffered bihemispheric damage (e.g., anoxic, metabolic), as in this case, the tonic deviation occurs without the quick corrective saccade.

**IV-89.** **The answer is B.** *(Chap. 28)* This scenario is most consistent with a pituitary tumor compressing the optic chiasm and causing a bitemporal hemianopia. This midline tumor would initially compress the center of the chiasm, damaging the retinal fibers arising from the nasal portion of the retina, which cross in the chiasm. These nasal retinal fibers carry information from the temporal visual fields.

**IV-90.** **The answer is C.** *(Chap. 28)* The classic triad of Horner's syndrome consists of ipsilateral miosis, ptosis, and anhidrosis. However, the anhidrosis is often absent or difficult to appreciate. The majority of cases are idiopathic, but Horner's syndrome may be caused by a neoplasm impinging on the sympathetic chain or sympathetic cervical ganglia. Damage to the sympathetic contribution to the third cranial nerve results in paresis of the iris dilator muscle. Given this patient's history of smoking and lack of any other abnormalities on examination that would raise a suspicion of intracerebral pathology, a chest x-ray to look for an apical tumor (Pancoast's tumor) compressing the sympathetic chain or superior cervical ganglion would be the next best step in the workup.

**IV-91.** **The answer is A.** *(Chap. 25)* Balint's syndrome occurs after bilateral involvement of the network required for spatial orientation in the parietal lobes. This syndrome includes difficulty with orderly visuomotor scanning of the environment (oculomotor apraxia), diminished ability to reach toward visual targets (optic ataxia), and inability to integrate visual information from the center of gaze with more peripheral vision (simultanagnosia). Movement exaggerates the deficits.

**IV-92.** **The answer is B.** *(Chap. 25)* A tumor located in the left posterior frontal lobe (Broca's area) might be expected to result in nonfluent aphasia and a right hemiparesis involving the face and arm to a greater degree than the leg. Damage to the posterior superior left temporal gyrus (Wernicke's area) would result in fluent aphasia and possibly a right superior quadrantanopia. A tumor located in the right parietal lobe may cause a syndrome of left hemineglect and denial of the deficit (anosagnosia). A lesion of the right basal ganglia would result in a contralateral movement disorder. The syndrome described in the question is motor aprosodia, or the inability to convey emotional meaning through melodic stress and intonation, while the ability to produce grammatically correct language remains intact. This situation results from involvement of the right frontal lobe.

**IV-93.  The answer is D.**  *(Chap. 27)*  The symptoms described in the question correspond to the restless leg syndrome (RLS), a chronic disorder characterized by an irresistible urge to move the legs, especially while one is lying in bed before sleeping. It may be primary or secondary. This disorder, which may be inherited, is more common in women than in men. Secondary restless leg syndrome may be caused by iron or folic acid deficiency, anemia, or renal failure. The symptoms may wax and wane over time and may be exacerbated by caffeine and pregnancy. Virtually all affected persons exhibit periodic limb movements during sleep. It is not a form of narcolepsy, which is characterized by excessive daytime sleepiness, cataplexy, hypnagogic and hypnopompic hallucinations, and sleep paralysis. All of the treatments listed may be used to alleviate symptoms.

**IV-94.  The answer is E.**  *(Chaps. 26, 367)*  All the choices given in the question are causes of or may be associated with dementia. Binswanger's disease, the cause of which is unknown, often occurs in patients with long-standing hypertension and/or atherosclerosis; it is associated with diffuse subcortical white matter damage and has a subacute insidious course. Alzheimer's disease, the most common cause of dementia, is also slowly progressive and can be confirmed at autopsy by the presence of amyloid plaques and neurofibrillary tangles. Creutzfeld-Jakob disease, a prion disease, is associated with a rapidly progressive dementia, myoclonus, rigidity, a characteristic EEG pattern, and death within 1 to 2 years of onset. Vitamin $B_{12}$ deficiency, which often is seen in the setting of chronic alcoholism, most commonly produces a myelopathy that results in loss of vibration and joint position sense and brisk deep tendon reflexes (dorsal column and lateral corticospinal tract dysfunction). This combination of pathologic abnormalities in the setting of vitamin $B_{12}$ deficiency is also called *subacute combined degeneration*. Vitamin $B_{12}$ deficiency also may lead to a subcortical type of dementia. Multi-infarct dementia, as in this case, presents with a history of sudden stepwise declines in function associated with the accumulation of bilateral focal neurologic deficits. Brain imaging demonstrates multiple areas of stroke.

**IV-95.  The answer is B.**  *(Chaps. 20, 230)*  Stokes-Adams attacks are a form of cardiac syncope resulting from a high degree of atrioventricular block, which may be persistent or intermittent. Usually there are no premonitory symptoms with these attacks, which occur when cardiac asystole lasts longer than approximately 8 s. Prompt and complete recovery after the attacks is the rule, with focal neurologic signs being rare. These episodes may occur several times per day, and an ECG taken between attacks may be normal as a result of the transitory nature of the atrioventricular block. This disorder is not familial. Recurrent paroxysmal tachyarrhythmias are another cause of cardiac syncope, which results from a sudden drop in cardiac output.

**IV-96.  The answer is B.**  *(Chap. 29)*  Olfactory disorders are most frequently caused by head trauma and viral infections; the former is more common in children and teenagers, and the latter is more common in adults. Cranial trauma is followed by unilateral or bilateral anosmia in 5 to 10 percent of cases. Unilateral anosmia is an uncommon complaint, whereas bilateral olfactory disturbance often brings a patient to medical attention because of a perceived loss of taste sensation. Endocrine disorders such as diabetes mellitus, hypothyroidism, and Cushing's syndrome may distort smell perception. Congenital anosmias are rare. Kallmann syndrome is a disorder of neuronal migration with hypothalamic and olfactory bulb abnormalities; congenital anosmia and hypogonadotropic hypogonadism are the clinical features.

**IV-97.** **The answer is C.** *(Chaps. 26, 367)* The laboratory workup of dementia is somewhat controversial, as most of the screening tests employed have a low yield. However, some relatively inexpensive tests can rule out treatable causes of dementia and are certainly worth ordering. Serum vitamin $B_{12}$, VDRL, TSH, and electrolytes are among the tests that can identify correctable metabolic, endocrinologic, and infectious causes of dementia.

**IV-98.** **The answer is C.** *(Chap. 363)* All the choices listed in the question are known to be caused by an expansion of a trinucleotide repeat sequence, with the exception of Duchenne's muscular dystrophy, which results from a recessively inherited or spontaneous mutation in the dystrophin gene. In trinucleotide repeat disorders, affected patients have a greater number of repeats (e.g., of a CAG or CCG sequence) than is present in the general population. These repeat sequences tend to be "unstable" and achieve greater lengths with each succeeding generation. This accounts for the phenomenon of "genetic anticipation," in which the clinical disorder is more severe and has an earlier age at onset with succeeding generations. However, this phenomenon is not common to all trinucleotide repeat disorders; Friedreich's ataxia, an autosomal recessively inherited spinocerebellar degeneration which does not display this phenomenon, was recently shown to be caused by a GAA repeat on chromosome 9.

**IV-99.** **The answer is D.** *(Chap. 27)* Structures A through C and E have all been implicated in the generation of wakefulness or EEG arousal. The generation of sleep, by contrast, has been localized to the thalamus, the medullary reticular formation, or the basal forebrain. The emboliform nucleus is one of the "roof nuclei" of the cerebellum and has not been implicated in the generation of circadian rhythms.

**IV-100.** **The answer is E.** *(Chaps. 21, 383)* The syndrome described in the question is pediatric dermatomyositis, an inflammatory myopathy. It is characterized by myalgias, proximal weakness, a "heliotrope" rash over the malar aspect of the face and extensor surfaces, elevated ESR, and response to corticosteroids. The pathologic hallmark on muscle biopsy is perifascicular atrophy, which is thought to be due to preferential inflammation of the perifascicular capillaries. Fiber type grouping, on the other hand, is the pathologic signature of neurogenic muscle disease. In adults, dermatomyositis is associated with an underlying malignancy at a rate of approximately 20 to 30 percent. This is not true of childhood dermatomyositis.

**IV-101.** The answer is A-Y, B-Y, C-N, D-N, E-Y. (Chap. 21) Normal-pressure hydrocephalus and cervical spondylosis typically present with gait difficulty: short steps (sometimes mistaken for parkinsonism) and leg stiffness with slowness of step, respectively. Subacute combined degeneration may produce spasticity of gait as part of its lateral column (corticospinal) damage. Subdural hematoma generally does not cause isolated gait difficulty, and carotid stenosis causes either transient ischemic attacks or strokes but not a progressive syndrome of any sort.

**IV-102.** **The answer is A-N, B-Y, C-Y, D-N, E-Y.** *(Chap. 12)* Owing to the release of substances from damaged tissue (e.g., histamines, prostaglandins) or from the circulation (e.g., bradykinin), sensory stimuli activate free nerve endings in the skin. Such nerves terminate in the segmental dorsal horn of the spinal cord. Substance P and other neurotransmitters released from terminals stimulate transmission via the long axons composing the spinothalamic tract that terminate in the thalamic nucleus ventralis posterolateralis (VPL). VPL fibers project to the cerebral somatosensory cortex. Descending pathways that mediate analgesia project from the periaqueductal gray region in the midbrain to the medullary midline raphe nuclei. Raphe nuclei neurons in turn project to dorsal horn nuclei, where painful afferent impulses may be modified. This system contains many opiate receptors. Another descending pain inhibitory pathway, which projects from the pontine locus coeruleus to the dorsal horn of the spinal cord, mediates its effects by alpha-adrenergic signals.

**IV-103.    The answer is A-N, B-N, C-N, D-Y, E-Y.**    *(Chap. 29)*    Localization of the tone in the affected ear when the tuning fork is placed in the midline position (Weber's test) suggests unilateral conductive loss (external or middle ear), while perception in the unaffected ear suggests sensorineural hearing loss. A tone heard louder by bone conduction than by air conduction (Rinne's test) also suggests conductive rather than sensorineural hearing loss. Assuming that the patient's bone conduction is normal (since he perceived the tone when the fork was at the mastoid process) and that only his air conduction is diminished, one can presume that the lesion is in the external auditory canal or the middle ear. A common cause of conductive hearing loss in the elderly is otosclerosis (stapes footplate fusion), which is potentially treatable by surgical reconstructive procedures involving the middle ear.

**IV-104.    The answer is A-Y, B-Y, C-N, D-N, E-N.**    *(Chaps. 361, 382)*    Conventional electromyography (EMG) and nerve conduction studies as well as muscle biopsy procedures are not useful in an evaluation of myasthenia gravis, because myasthenia is not a disease of muscle or nerve. (Electron microscopy of muscle can show unfolding of the postsynaptic muscle membrane, but this procedure is not commonly done.) Curare testing to precipitate myasthenic weakness is dangerous, undependable, and mainly of historical interest. Single-fiber EMG measures the timing of firing of two fibers in the same motor unit. The timing between pairs is inconsistent in myasthenia, giving rise to "jitter" in the oscilloscope tracing; this finding is virtually diagnostic of myasthenia. Repetitive stimulation of motor nerves to observe a decremental response also is a useful procedure in testing for myasthenia gravis.

**IV-105.    The answer is A-Y, B-Y, C-N, D-Y, E-N.**    *(Chap. 16)*    Low back pain without a ruptured disk or other nerve damage is common. It requires bed rest, the administration of muscle relaxants, and time for recovery. It often is precipitated by lifting while the spine is flexed or laterally rotated. X-rays may show the nonspecific signs of paravertebral muscle spasm: straightening of the normal lumbar lordosis or scoliosis. Because of pain and spasm, the patient cannot flex the spine normally. Signs of damage to the nervous system distinguish patients with a more serious disorder. Bowel and bladder difficulty accompanies damage to sacral roots or the spinal cord. Perineal sensation and rectal tone should be tested along with individual muscle strength, stretch reflexes, Babinski's reflexes, and dermatomal sensation. Abnormal results on any of these tests suggest that there is nerve injury in addition to muscular strain.

**IV-106.    The answer is A-Y, B-N, C-N, D-N, E-Y.**    *(Chap. 21)*    The distinction between upper motor neuron and lower motor neuron lesions is critical in clinical medicine. Lesions proximal to the anterior horn cells (in general, the cerebral motor cortex or the corticospinal tract) produce the characteristic upper motor neuron syndrome of spasticity, increased reflexes, and an extensor plantar response (Babinski's sign). By contrast, atrophy of the muscles in a paretic limb suggests lower motor neuron disease. Such disorders, which may affect individual muscles, are accompanied by fascicular twitches, which are manifestations of the hyperactivity of the diseased motor unit(s).

**IV-107.    The answer is A-N, B-Y, C-Y, D-Y, E-N.**    *(Chaps. 21, 368)*    Rest tremor, which frequently is associated with Parkinson's disease, occurs at a rate of four to five beats per second. The rest tremor of Parkinson's disease is associated with flexed posture, slowness of movement, rigidity, postural instability, and suppression by willful activity. Many tremors that worsen during movement are exaggerations of the normal physiologic tremor. The essential-familial tremor is a faster action tremor (about 8 Hz) that is responsive to moderate doses of alcohol or beta-adrenergic blockade.

**IV-108.** **The answer is A-N, B-Y, C-Y, D-Y, E-Y.** *(Chap. 381)* Acute mononeuropathy involving the oculomotor or peroneal nerves should prompt an investigation for diabetes. A neuropathy that is progressive, distal, and primarily sensory is most characteristic of diabetes but also may occur with an occult neoplasm. The autonomic neuropathy of diabetes usually coexists with the sensory type, but the sensory neuropathy may be mild. Relapsing neuropathy is more typical of idiopathic polyneuritis.

**IV-109.** **The answer is A-Y, B-Y, C-Y, D-N, E-N.** *(Chap. 370)* Several disorders produce chronic progressive spinal cord disease with sensory and motor involvement. Syndromes of spinocerebellar degeneration may involve the motor and sensory spinal cord systems in addition to causing ataxia. Multiple sclerosis usually causes a relapsing illness but can cause a progressive, usually cervical myelopathy in elderly women. Cervical spondylosis, or bony compression of the cervical cord by osteophytic bars, is another common cause of myelopathy in the elderly. Lumbar disk compression of the cauda equina, which is made up of peripheral nerves, does not cause spinal cord signs. Amyotrophic lateral sclerosis is a disease of spinal cord motor neurons and corticospinal tracts but has no sensory signs.

**IV-110.** **The answer is A-N, B-Y, C-N, D-N, E-Y.** *(Chaps. 372, 368)* Bilateral lateral-rectus palsies that develop acutely in alcoholic persons should suggest Wernicke's encephalopathy, which requires prompt treatment with thiamine. Bilateral sixth-nerve malfunction may be a falsely localizing sign resulting from increased intracranial pressure, as in subdural hematoma, but does not occur as an isolated disturbance caused by intrinsic brainstem diseases (e.g., hemorrhage). Orbital fractures usually entrap the fourth nerve, less commonly the sixth; only rarely is the palsy bilateral. Although neurosyphilis can cause cranial nerve palsies from adhesive meningitis, palsy of oculomotor-related nerves is a rarity.

**IV-111.** **The answer is A-N, B-Y, C-Y, D-N, E-Y.** *(Chap. 366)* Unilateral occlusion of a vertebral artery typically results in Wallenberg's lateral medullary syndrome. With an infarct on the left, this is likely to include damage to the left ninth and tenth cranial nerves, the left inferior cerebellar peduncle, and the spinothalamic fibers subserving pain and temperature on the right side. Vertigo and nystagmus are common since the lower vestibular complex may be affected. Horner's syndrome also is common with a smaller pupil and ptosis *ipsilateral* to the lesion. Only rarely is the medullary pyramid involved (Babinski-Nageotte syndrome), which results in a *contralateral* hemiparesis that spares the face; hypoglossal weakness may then be present ipsilateral to the lesion. Lesions of the median longitudinal fasciculus that produce internuclear ophthalmoplegia occur in the pons and midbrain in the territory of branches of the basilar artery.

**IV-112.** **The answer is A-Y, B-Y, C-N, D-N, E-Y.** *(Chap. 372)* Cranial nerves III, IV, and VI all pass through the cavernous sinus, so that complete ophthalmoplegia, including ptosis, may result from a disease process there. Since the supraorbital and maxillary divisions of the fifth nerve, but not the mandibular branch, pass through the cavernous sinus, the brow and cheek may be numb, but not the chin. The optic nerve will be involved only if the process extends superiorly.

**IV-113.** **The answer is A-Y, B-N, C-Y, D-Y, E-Y.** *(Chap. 365. Callahan, N Engl J Med 318: 942, 1988)* Although many patients with epilepsy require anticonvulsants throughout life, about half remain seizure-free long enough to warrant a trial without medications, many of which have imposing side effects. Favorable prognostic factors for remaining seizure-free include few seizures before control is attained, control on single first-choice drug therapy, a history of simple partial seizures or primary generalized seizures, the absence of a structural lesion, and a normal EEG before drug withdrawal. Even if a patient has had a long seizure-free interval (GT 2 years) and has a good chance of remaining seizure-free without anticonvulsants, the drug should be tapered over 3 to 6 months. Moreover, the patient and the physician should be aware of the consequences of a relapse and should be willing to accept the risk.

IV-114.   **The answer is A-N, B-N, C-Y, D-Y, E-N.** *(Chap. 385)* Lithium has revolutionized the treatment of bipolar affective disorders. It is effective both during acute mania and in the prevention of recurrent attacks. Although side effects—particularly gastrointestinal upset, mild tremor, and thirst—are common, the drug is safe if used carefully. The lithium dose should be titrated to serum levels: control of mania should be achieved at a level between 0.8 and 1.4 mmol/L, and maintenance levels should be between 0.6 and 1.0 mmol/L. Lithium intoxication is manifested by depression of mental status; treatment is mainly supportive. Other important long-term side effects include hypothyroidism (by inhibiting the secretion of thyroid hormone) and renal complications. Effects on the renal tubules produce nephrogenic diabetes insipidus with polyuria, polydipsia, and impaired urinary concentrating ability in about 25 percent of patients on the drug.

# V. DISORDERS OF THE RESPIRATORY SYSTEM

## QUESTIONS

**DIRECTIONS:** Each question below contains five suggested responses. Choose the **one best** response to each question.

**V-1.** A young male is brought to the emergency department after having been submerged for a prolonged period in a nearby pond. Cardiopulmonary resuscitation was performed at the scene. The patient is being ventilated by mask and bag upon arrival in the emergency department. A brief examination reveals that the patient has no obvious sites of trauma and is conscious but not communicative. His blood pressure is 90/60, pulse is 120, temperature is 36°C (96.8°F), and respiratory rate is 30. Cardiac rhythm reveals sinus tachycardia. Pulse oximetry reveals oxygen saturation of 83 percent. Which of the following is the best method to reverse the patient's apparent hypoxemia?

(A) Administration of sodium bicarbonate
(B) Administration of acetazolamide
(C) Administration of supplemental oxygen
(D) Application of continuous positive airway pressure and administration of supplemental oxygen
(E) Administration of supplemental oxygen and endotracheal suction to remove aspirated fluid

**V-2.** A patient who is being evaluated for shortness of breath is found to have an arterial $P_{O_2}$ of 7.9 kPa (59 mmHg) while breathing room air at sea level and an arterial $P_{O_2}$ of 8.1 kPa (61 mmHg) while breathing 40% inspired $O_2$. The arterial $P_{CO_2}$ is normal. Which of the following conditions would be LEAST likely to account for these findings? *RF type 1*

(A) Idiopathic pulmonary fibrosis
(B) Atelectasis
(C) *Klebsiella* pneumonia
(D) Cardiogenic pulmonary edema
(E) Osler-Rendu-Weber syndrome

**V-3.** A 63-year-old man has pneumococcal pneumonia with extensive air-space consolidation in the left upper and left lower lobes. He complains of extreme shortness of breath when positioned with his left side down. An arterial blood sample drawn in this position shows a $P_{O_2}$ of 6.2 kPa (46 mmHg); 10 min earlier, an arterial blood sample drawn while his right side was dependent had revealed a $P_{O_2}$ of 8.2 kPa (66 mmHg). The most likely explanation for the drop in $P_{O_2}$ when the man was lying on his left side is *→ diseased*

(A) increased blood flow to the dependent lung
(B) reduced ventilation to the dependent lung
(C) increased airway resistance in the dependent lung
(D) accumulation of interstitial edema in the dependent lung
(E) increased stiffness of the chest wall on the dependent side

**V-4.** A 65-year-old man presents with progressive shortness of breath. Other than a history of heavy tobacco abuse, the patient has a benign past medical history. Breath sounds are absent two-thirds of the way up on the left side of the chest. Percussion of the left chest reveals less resonance than normal. While you place your hand on the left side of the chest and have the patient say "ninety-nine," no tingling is appreciated in the hand. The trachea appears to be deviated toward the left. Which of the following diagnoses is most likely?

(A) Bacterial pneumonia
(B) Viral pneumonia
(C) Bronchial obstruction
(D) Pleural effusion *Stony dull*
(E) Pneumothorax *- Hyperresonant*

*R      L*
*BS Absent ↓ percussion ↓ trans.*

**157**

**V-5.** The best way to make a diagnosis of cystic fibrosis in a patient suspected of having this disorder is

(A) sweat chloride test
(B) sputum culture
(C) pulmonary function testing
(D) stool for fetal fat content
(E) DNA analysis

**V-6.** A 21-year-old college student with no prior medical problems begins working as a laboratory technician. He subsequently presents because of several recent episodes of shortness of breath, cough, fever, chills, and malaise. Each episode has lasted several days. The patient is seen during the recovery phase of an episode of this type; findings at physical examination are normal. Chest x-ray reveals several ill-defined, diffuse, patchy infiltrates. The laboratory evaluation is positive only for an increased erythrocyte sedimentation rate. Pulmonary function studies display reduced lung volumes.

On further questioning, it is learned that these episodes begin on days when the patient is required to tend to experiments involving laboratory rats at the animal facility. What is the best treatment for this condition?

(A) Inhaled cromolyn sodium
(B) Prednisone
(C) Inhaled beclomethasone
(D) Discontinuation of visits to the animal facility
(E) No treatment

**V-7.** The primary pathophysiologic problem in idiopathic pulmonary fibrosis is believed to be

(A) microorganism-mediated activation of pulmonary neutrophils
(B) immune complex–mediated activation of alveolar macrophages
(C) direct immune complex–mediated pulmonary interstitial damage
(D) primary fibroblast proliferation
(E) viral-mediated pulmonary epithelial damage

**V-8.** A 59-year-old man with a long-standing smoking history presents with persistent dyspnea. His $FEV_1$ is 1.0 L/min, arterial blood gas reveals $P_{O_2}$ of 60 mmHg, $P_{CO_2}$ of 40 mmHg, pH 7.45, and $O_2$ saturation of 90 percent. He has hyperlucent lungs on chest x-ray and decreased breath sounds on physical examination. The patient's current medical regimen consists of theophylline (300 mg twice daily) and inhaled isoproterenol. The most important addition to the patient's therapy would be

(A) trimethoprim-sulfamethoxazole
(B) substitution of albuterol for isoproterenol
(C) oxygen therapy
(D) prednisone
(E) addition of inhaled beclomethasone

**V-9.** Although asthma is a heterogeneous disease, a given individual with asthma would be most likely to

(A) relate a personal or family history of allergic diseases
(B) conform to a characteristic personality type
(C) display a skin-test reaction to extracts of airborne allergens
(D) demonstrate nonspecific airway hyperirritability
(E) have supranormal serum immunoglobulin E

**V-10.** A diagnosis of allergic bronchopulmonary aspergillosis in a person who has asthma, recurrent pulmonary infiltrates, and eosinophilia would be supported by all the following findings EXCEPT

(A) delayed, tuberculin-type skin-test reaction to *Aspergillus fumigatus*
(B) sputum culture positive for *A. fumigatus*
(C) immediate skin test reaction to *A. fumigatus*
(D) marked elevation of the serum immunoglobulin E level
(E) radiographic evidence of bronchiectasis

**V-11.** A 22-year-old woman with a history of intermittent wheezing in response to exercise presents to the emergency room with shortness of breath. Her attack occurred during an aerobics class. At this point she is having obvious difficulty breathing and has diffuse wheezes on pulmonary examination. $O_2$ saturation is 95 percent by pulse oximetry. The most effective treatment at this point would be

(A) intravenous aminophylline
(B) inhaled cromolyn sodium
(C) inhaled albuterol
(D) intravenous hydrocortisone
(E) inhaled beclomethasone

**V-12.** The dyskinetic ciliary syndromes, including Kartagener's syndrome, can produce all the following manifestations EXCEPT

(A) bronchiectasis
(B) sinusitis
(C) recurrent bronchitis
(D) interstitial pulmonary fibrosis
(E) infertility

**V-13.** A patient with advanced adult respiratory distress syndrome (ARDS) has suffered a pneumothorax after being exposed to 10 cmH$_2$O positive end-expiratory pressure (PEEP). Which of the following modes of mechanical ventilation would be best?

(A) Assist/control mode of ventilation
(B) Synchronized intermittent mandatory ventilation
(C) Pressure-control ventilation
(D) Pressure-support ventilation
(E) Continuous positive airway pressure

**V-14.** A 48-year-old Haitian man presents with shortness of breath. Chest x-ray reveals a right pleural effusion extending about halfway up the chest. The patient has no other known medical problems and is on no medicines. The rest of the general physical examination is unremarkable. Diagnostic thoracentesis reveals the following: lactate dehydrogenase 1.7 μkat/L (100 U/L), glucose 6.4 mmol/L (150 mg/dL), and amylase 1.6 μkat/L (90 U/L). Cell count reveals 1000 red cells per microliter and 1000 white cells per microliter (differential: 50 percent neutrophils, 25 percent lymphocytes, and 25 percent monocytes). A ventilation-perfusion lung scan is indeterminate on the right side because of the large effusion, but there are no ventilation-perfusion mismatches elsewhere. The next most appropriate step would be

(A) pulmonary arteriogram
(B) abdominal CT
(C) chest CT
(D) needle biopsy of pleura
(E) administration of isoniazid with ethambutol

**V-15.** A 45-year-old woman presents with fever and cough. She has had no past medical problems and was well until about 3 days ago. Physical examination is remarkable for a temperature of 39°C (102.2°F) and the presence of diffuse rales on chest examination. Except for an elevated white count with a left-shifted differential, her blood tests are normal. Chest radiography reveals patchy bilateral infiltrates. She is unable to produce sputum. She has resting hypoxemia and requires hospital admission. Which is the most reasonable choice of antibiotics at this time?

(A) Penicillin G
(B) Cefotaxime
(C) Erythromycin
(D) Ampicillin plus sulbactam
(E) Ampicillin plus sulbactam plus erythromycin

**V-16.** A 60-year-old man with emphysema and bronchitis is brought to an emergency room by an ambulance crew that has been giving him oxygen by mask. Three days ago, he noted that his sputum had changed color and increased in amount. His wife called the ambulance when he became suddenly short of breath and confused. On arrival at the hospital, he is somnolent. Midinspiratory crackles and diffuse expiratory wheezes are audible on examination of the chest, and he has marked peripheral edema and ascites. Hemoglobin is 180 g/L (18 g/dL). Arterial blood gases are pH 7.08, P$_{O_2}$ is 19.8 kPa (148 mmHg), and P$_{CO_2}$ is 14.2 kPa (106 mmHg). The most appropriate immediate therapy for this man would be

(A) intravenous infusion of sodium bicarbonate
(B) endotracheal intubation and assisted ventilation
(C) administration of isoetharine by air-compressor nebulizer
(D) discontinuation of supplemental oxygen
(E) subcutaneous injection of epinephrine

**V-17.** A 34-year-old man complains of shortness of breath after minimal exertion. He has no systemic symptoms. He developed a nonproductive cough 10 months ago. A chest x-ray, which was reportedly normal, was done at that time. Examination now reveals a respiratory rate of 28 breaths per minute, and diffuse end-inspiratory crackles are heard over his lower lung fields. His chest x-rays are shown below. An arterial $P_{O_2}$ measured while the patient is breathing room air is 55 mmHg, and arterial $P_{CO_2}$ is 26 mmHg. Routine blood counts are normal. The next step in his evaluation should be

(A) angiotensin converting enzyme level
(B) transbronchial biopsy
(C) bronchoalveolar lavage
(D) salivary gland biopsy
(E) serology for rheumatoid factor

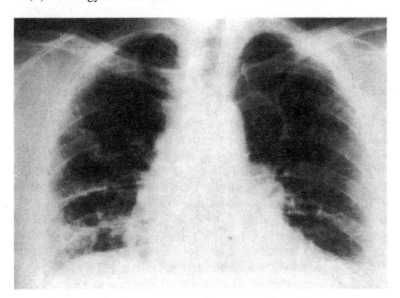
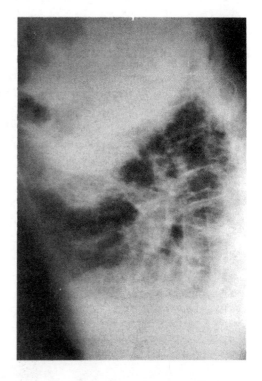

**V-18.** A 23-year-old woman complains of dyspnea and substernal chest pain on exertion. Evaluation for this complaint 6 months ago included arterial blood-gas testing, which revealed pH 7.48, $P_{O_2}$ 79 mmHg, and $P_{CO_2}$ 31 mmHg. Electrocardiography then showed a right axis deviation. Chest x-ray now shows enlarged pulmonary arteries but no parenchymal infiltrates, and a lung perfusion scan reveals subsegmental defects that are thought to have a "low probability for pulmonary thromboembolism." Echocardiography demonstrates right heart strain but no evidence of primary cardiac disease. The most appropriate diagnostic test now would be

(A) open lung biopsy
(B) Holter monitoring
(C) right-heart catheterization
(D) transbronchial biopsy
(E) serum $\alpha_1$-antitrypsin level

**V-19.** A 53-year-old man is noted to be tachypneic and confused 48 h after suffering multiple orthopedic and internal injuries in an automobile accident. Chest x-ray is interpreted as normal, but arterial blood-gas values are as follows: pH 7.49, $P_{O_2}$ 52 mmHg, and $P_{CO_2}$ 30 mmHg. The course of action most likely to confirm the diagnosis of this man's condition would be to

(A) order a ventilation-perfusion scan
(B) order pulmonary angiography
(C) order impedance plethysmography
(D) order blood testing for fibrin split products
(E) repeat the physical examination

**V-20.** All the following statements about obstructive sleep apnea syndrome are true EXCEPT

(A) men are affected more often than women
(B) systemic hypertension is a common finding
(C) alcohol can be a contributing factor
(D) estrogens are frequently useful
(E) personality changes may be the presenting complaint

**V-21.** A 54-year-old man has a nonproductive cough and exertional breathlessness. He also notes low-grade fever, malaise, and a weight loss of 7 kg (15 lb) over 6 weeks. His white blood cell count is 13,500/$\mu$L. He has a history of mild asthma. A chest x-ray discloses peripheral lung infiltrates. The most likely diagnosis is

(A) idiopathic pulmonary fibrosis
(B) alveolar proteinosis
(C) polymyositis
(D) chronic eosinophilic pneumonia
(E) lymphangiomyomatosis

**V-22.** Owing to profound hypoxemia, tracheal intubation is performed on a drowning victim, and mechanical ventilation is begun. Inspired oxygen concentration is 80%. Initially, the man is agitated and fights the respirator. Arterial blood gases are obtained and show pH 7.21, $P_{O_2}$ 70 mmHg, and $P_{CO_2}$ 56 mmHg. The most appropriate management step at this time would be to

(A) add positive end-expiratory pressure (5 cmH$_2$O)
(B) sedate the man and control his ventilation
(C) infuse sodium bicarbonate intravenously
(D) raise the inspired oxygen concentration
(E) initiate extracorporeal membrane oxygenation

**V-23.** One week after a right total hip replacement a 65-year-old woman develops the sudden onset of shortness of breath. A workup reveals normotension, a prominent second heart sound, hypoxemia, sinus tachycardia with new right axis deviation on the electrocardiogram, and a normal chest x-ray. Oxygen is administered. Impedance plethysmography is consistent with a large proximal clot in the left leg. Which of the following would be the most reasonable next step?

(A) Performance of a pulmonary angiogram
(B) Performance of perfusion scintigraphy
(C) Administration of tissue plasminogen activator
(D) Administration of heparin
(E) Administration of warfarin

**V-24.** Which of the following is LEAST likely to be associated with cystic fibrosis?

(A) Intestinal obstruction
(B) Sinusitis
(C) Steatorrhea
(D) Dextrocardia
(E) Clubbing

*Questions V-25–V-26.*

A 35-year-old man seeks medical attention for breathlessness on exertion. He has never smoked cigarettes and has not been coughing. One sibling died of respiratory failure at 40 years of age. His three children are healthy. Physical examination reveals him to be tachypneic as he exhales through pursed lips. His chest is tympanitic to percussion, and breath sounds are poorly heard on auscultation. Chest x-ray shows flattened diaphragms with peripheral attenuation of bronchovascular markings that is most noticeable at the lung bases.

**V-25.** Expected results of the pulmonary function testing of the man described above would include

(A) increased lung elastic recoil
(B) increased total lung capacity
(C) reduced functional residual capacity
(D) increased vital capacity
(E) increased diffusing capacity

**V-26.** Initial laboratory assessment of the man described above should include all the following EXCEPT

(A) acid starch gel
(B) measurement of sweat chloride concentration
(C) immunoelectrophoresis
(D) complete spirometry
(E) arterial blood-gas determination

**V-27.** Correct statements concerning the pathogenesis of $\alpha_1$-antitrypsin deficiency include all the following EXCEPT

(A) emphysema results from an inability to inhibit alveolar destruction by neutrophils
(B) clinical deficiency of $\alpha_1$-antitrypsin usually results from one of several missense mutations that cause a truncated mRNA
(C) the disease is inherited in a dominant fashion
(D) mutations of the $\alpha_1$-antitrypsin gene of the S type produce less severe emphysema than do mutations of the Z type
(E) treatment with purified $\alpha_1$-antitrypsin can raise the serum level to that associated with lung protection

**V-28.** To decrease the likelihood of drug toxicity, the theophylline dose should be reduced in a patient with asthma in each of the following circumstances EXCEPT

(A) age greater than 70
(B) azithromycin use for *Mycoplasma* pneumonia
(C) congestive heart failure
(D) marijuana abuse
(E) allopurinol use for gout

**V-29.** Known consequences of asbestos exposure include all of the following EXCEPT

(A) pulmonary fibrosis
(B) pleural effusion
(C) small cell carcinoma
(D) peritoneal mesothelioma
(E) pleural plaques

**V-30.** In which of the following clinical circumstances would it be appropriate to use a rigid bronchoscope instead of a flexible fiberoptic bronchoscope?

(A) A 22-year-old male with known HIV infection who complains of shortness of breath and has diffuse interstitial infiltrates on chest x-ray
(B) A 65-year-old male with a long history of smoking who has shortness of breath and right upper lobe collapse
(C) A 33-year-old female with a history of acute myeloid leukemia complaining of severe dyspnea who is currently 4 months after an allogeneic bone marrow transplant and has a reticulonodular pulmonary infiltrate
(D) A 50-year-old female with a heavy smoking history who currently complains of intermittent hemoptysis
(E) A 28-year-old male with a history of acute myeloid leukemia who is currently 30 days after an allogeneic bone marrow transplant with a significant pulmonary hemorrhage and bilateral alveolar infiltrates on chest x-ray

**V-31.** The most common initial symptom of byssinosis is

(A) wheezing
(B) dyspnea on exertion
(C) cough
(D) hemoptysis
(E) chest tightness

**V-32.** A 27-year-old female with a history of common variable immunodeficiency has had many upper and lower respiratory tract infections. She now presents with a third episode of recurrent cough and copious purulent sputum production, which is sometimes blood-tinged. She is afebrile, and her pulmonary exam is normal. Chest radiography reveals the presence of several parallel linear opacities and a few ringlike shadows. The diagnosis that most likely accounts for this patient's symptoms is

(A) bronchiectasis
(B) non-small-cell lung cancer
(C) *Mycoplasma* infection
(D) viral pneumonia
(E) pulmonary thromboembolism

**V-33.** In which of the following situations would single-lung transplantation be contraindicated?

(A) A 48-year-old male with chronic obstructive pulmonary disease and an $FEV_1$ of 20 percent of the predicted value
(B) A 50-year-old male with idiopathic pulmonary fibrosis, resting hypoxia, and a total lung capacity of 50 percent of the predicted value
(C) A 23-year-old female with primary pulmonary hypertension with a mean pulmonary artery pressure of 70 mmHg
(D) A 23-year-old female with cystic fibrosis and an $FEV_1$ of 20 percent of the predicted value
(E) A 25-year-old male with an $\alpha_1$-antitrypsin deficiency and resting hypoxia

**V-34.** A 50-year-old male chronic alcoholic presents with a 2-week history of fever, night sweats, cough, productive sputum, and pleuritic chest pain. The patient has had a recent negative HIV test and has no other medical problems. Chest x-ray reveals a 3-cm cavitary lesion in the posterior segment of the left lower lobe. This cavity contains an air-fluid level. Which of the following is the most likely etiologic agent?

(A) *S. pneumoniae*
(B) *H. influenzae*
(C) *Mycobacterium tuberculosis*
(D) *Mycoplasma pneumoniae*
(E) *Actinomyces*

**V-35.** A 55-year-old male presents with several months of dyspnea and a nonproductive cough. Physical examination reveals dry crackles at both lung bases. Chest radiography and high-resolution computed tomography reveal a bibasilar reticular nodular pattern in the lung fields. Spirometry reveals reductions in total lung capacity, vital capacity, and residual volume. The carbon monoxide diffusion capacity is reduced to 35 percent of normal. Resting arterial hypoxemia is demonstrated on arterial blood-gas testing. Transbronchial biopsy results reveal an increase in inflammatory cells on the alveolar surface, predominantly macrophages, as well as diffuse intraalveolar fibrosis. The mainstay of therapy at this point would be

(A) oral prednisone
(B) oral cyclophosphamide
(C) 4-week course of oral azithromycin
(D) lung transplantation
(E) bronchodialator therapy

**V-36.** A 19-year-old normal nonsmoking female has a moderately severe pulmonary embolism while on oral contraceptive pills. Which of the following is the most likely predisposing factor?

(A) Abnormal factor V
(B) Abnormal protein C
(C) Diminished protein C level
(D) Diminished protein S level
(E) Diminished antithromin III level

**V-37.** A 65-year-old male presents for an evaluation because he is "feeling poorly." Symptoms include morning headache and poor sleep quality. He is quite tired during the day and frequently falls asleep while he reads or watches television. Physical examination reveals a ruddy complexion but is otherwise unremarkable. Laboratory examination is normal except for elevations in hematocrit and plasma $HCO_3^-$ concentration. Polysomnography demonstrates a decreased ventilatory response to hypercapnia and many episodes of central apnea (no diaphragmatic activity is noted). The maximum respiratory pressure that he generates against an occluded airway is normal. Spirometry and blood gases are normal. Of the following, which is the most likely cause of the patient's problem?

(A) Obstructive sleep apnea
(B) Ankylosing spondylitis
(C) Amyotrophic lateral sclerosis
(D) Myasthenia gravis
(E) Carotid body dysfunction

**V-38.** All the following are typical manifestations of chronic hyperventilation EXCEPT

(A) dyspnea
(B) seizures
(C) tetany
(D) muscle weakness
(E) clubbing

**V-39.** Which of the following circumstances leading to the acute respiratory distress syndrome and the necessity for mechanical ventilation would have the best prognosis?

(A) A 33-year-old male with a heroin overdose
(B) A 68-year-old male with an acute myocardial infarction and 2 h of hypotension
(C) A 25-year-old male poststatus a gunshot wound, major volume loss, hypotension, and acute renal failure
(D) A 21-year-old female with acute myeloid leukemia with gram-negative sepsis during induction therapy
(E) A 45-year-old fireman with severe smoke inhalation injury and arterial $Pa_{O_2}$ of 60 mmHg despite 100 percent $F_{I_{O_2}}$

**V-40.** All the following represent strategies to deal with the complications of mechanical ventilation EXCEPT

(A) thoracostomy placement for barotrauma-induced pneumothorax
(B) prophylactic antibiotics
(C) reduce inspired oxygen tension
(D) hemodynamic monitoring
(E) sucralfate

**V-41.** A 65-year-old man with chronic bronchitis presented to the emergency room 2 weeks ago with acute respiratory failure. He was intubated and treated with diuretics and antibiotics. However, after apparent improvement during a 1-week stay in the intensive care unit on mechanical ventilation, he has failed three attempts at being weaned from the ventilator. All the following factors could account for the difficulty in removing this patient from the ventilator EXCEPT

(A) overdiuresis
(B) benzodiazepines
(C) a $P_{CO_2}$ too high before extubation
(D) hypokalemia
(E) hypothyroidism

**DIRECTIONS:** Each question below contains five suggested responses. For **each of the** five responses listed with each item, you are to respond either YES (Y) or NO (N). In a given item **all, some,** or **none** of the alternatives may be correct.

**V-42.**  Hypoxemia occurring after pulmonary thrombo-embolism can result from

(A)  lowered mixed venous $P_{O_2}$ resulting from heart failure

(B)  perfusion of atelectatic areas

(C)  increased dead-space ventilation in the area of vascular occlusion

(D)  perfusion of areas poorly ventilated because of airway constriction

(E)  inadequate time for oxygen diffusion secondary to a reduction in the capillary bed

**V-43.**   Which of the following conditions would be likely to result in an increased residual volume on plethysmographic pulmonary function testing?

(A)  Emphysema

(B)  Sarcoidosis

(C)  Cystic fibrosis

(D)  Fracture of the cervical spine

(E)  Kyphoscoliosis

**V-44.**   A 51-year-old man develops pancreatitis associated with the passage of a gallstone. His treatment includes meperidine and intravenous normal saline. Two days later he becomes anxious, tachypneic, and short of breath. An emergency chest x-ray demonstrates diffuse, bilateral interstitial and alveolar infiltrates. A year ago he suffered a myocardial infarction, but since then he has had no evidence of congestive heart failure. In this case, adult respiratory distress syndrome can be distinguished from cardiogenic pulmonary edema by

(A)  measurement of lung water

(B)  measurement of protein concentration in edema fluid

(C)  measurement of pulmonary artery wedge pressure

(D)  measurement of lung compliance

(E)  calculation of the alveolar-arterial $P_{O_2}$ difference

# V. DISORDERS OF THE RESPIRATORY SYSTEM

## ANSWERS

**V-1. The answer is D.** (*Chap. 394. Modell, N Engl J Med 328:253–256, 1993.*) Ninety percent of drowning patients aspirate fluid; however, the vast majority aspirate less than 22 mL/kg. Although aspiration of fresh water can produce acute hypervolemia with dilutional hyponatremia and possibly even hemolysis, these are rare occurrences. Aspiration of seawater can cause hypovolemia with ensuing hypernatremia. In the absence of documentation of such an electrolyte problem, no specific therapy is required. Aspiration of water of any type leads to considerable venous admixture (i.e., ventilation-perfusion abnormalities), which can produce hypoxemia. The most important therapeutic maneuvers, after resuscitation on the scene, are to provide supplemental oxygen, intravenous access, and transportation to a hospital where the patient can be evaluated for adequacy of ventilation, cardiac function, and blood volume. The best way to reverse drowning-associated hypoxemia consists of the application of continuous positive airway pressure (CPAP). CPAP may be combined with mechanical inflation of the lung as needed; mechanical inflation may be particularly effective in those who have aspirated fresh water, which leads to a change in the surface-tension characteristics of pulmonary surfactant. Correction of severe metabolic acidosis with bicarbonate is controversial. Finally, the universal need for corticosteroid therapy and antibiotics is no longer accepted.

**V-2. The answer is A.** (*Chap. 250*) The general mechanisms responsible for hypoxemia include alveolar hypoventilation, impaired diffusion, ventilation-perfusion inequality, and shunting (blood bypassing ventilated areas of the lung). In each of these cases, except for shunting, the arterial $P_{O_2}$ increases significantly when the inspired $P_{O_2}$ is raised. Examples of shunts (which could account for the lack of response to oxygen therapy described in the question) include congenital heart disease that produces direct right-to-left intracardiac flow (usually associated with pulmonary hypertension), intrapulmonary vascular shunting (i.e., congenital telangiectatic disorders such as Osler-Rendu-Weber syndrome), and, most commonly, perfused alveoli that are not ventilated because of atelectasis or fluid buildup (pneumonia or pulmonary edema). Since impaired diffusion usually is not severe enough to lead to disordered gas exchange except during exercise, most cases of normocapnic hypoxemia are due to ventilation-perfusion mismatch. Many processes that affect the lungs (alveolar disease, interstitial lung disease, pulmonary vascular disease, airway disease) do so unevenly, leading to some areas with adequate perfusion and poor ventilation and some with good ventilation and poor perfusion.

**V-3. The answer is A.** (*Chap. 250*) In a person standing erect, blood flow per unit volume increases from the apex of the lung to the base. Ventilation also increases from the apex to the base, but the gradient is less than that for blood flow, making the ventilation-perfusion ratio lower at the bottom of the lung than it is at the top. Both ventilation and perfusion are affected by posture; as a general rule, the dependent regions are better perfused than ventilated and have the lowest ratio of ventilation to perfusion. Thus, a person with unilateral air-space disease may have an increase in venous admixture when the diseased lung is dependent. In that situation, blood flow increases to the diseased lung, perfusing atelectatic and poorly ventilated alveoli, and hypoxemia ensues.

**V-4.    The answer is C.**   (*Chap. 249*)   In evaluating a patient with shortness of breath, examination of the thorax is crucial. Tracheal deviation to the left indicates either a pleural effusion on the right or loss of volume on the left. Volume loss typically is due to an obstructed bronchus that produces atelectasis in the affected segment or lobe. Loss of aerated lung will be reflected in dullness to percussion, absent breath sounds on auscultation, and a decrease in tactile fremitus. A consolidative process such as bacterial pneumonia may well produce increased fremitus as well as bronchial breath sounds and whispered pectoriloquy, since sounds are well transmitted through a consolidated area. In a pneumothorax, a percussion of the chest would reveal hyperresonance, although breath sounds and fremitus would be absent. A possible cause of obstruction and atelectasis of a large amount of left lung tissue could be obstruction of a major bronchus by carcinoma of the lung, especially in an older patient who is a heavy smoker.

**V-5.    The answer is A.**   (*Chap. 257. Stutts, Science 269:847, 1995.*)   Cystic fibrosis, an autosomal recessive disease, results from a mutation in a gene on chromosome 7. Because of the multiple potential mutations that have been described in this gene, it is currently not feasible to use DNA-based diagnosis to identify patients with this disorder or heterozygous carriers. The gene codes for a protein called the cystic fibrosis transmembrane regulator (CFTR), which is a single-chain 1480 amino acid–containing protein that functions as a cyclic AMP–regulated chloride channel. All affected tissues, including airway and intestinal epithelium, sweat ducts, and exocrine pancreatic ducts, express an abnormal CFTR protein. The most common mutation in this protein is an absence of phenylalanine in amino acid position 508, resulting from a 3-basepair DNA deletion. A consequence of this and the other mutations in the CFTR protein is failure of normal calcium chloride transport. Therefore, secretions are dehydrated and poorly cleared. The diagnosis of cystic fibrosis now depends on a combination of clinical criteria and a demonstration that sweat chloride values are abnormally low. About half of the 1 to 2 percent of patients with cystic fibrosis who have normal sweat chloride values have a specific single G to T mutation in the CFTR gene.

**V-6.    The answer is D.**   (*Chap. 253*)   Given the temporal relationship of the symptoms to the work with rats, serologic evidence for inflammation, the nonspecific radiographic findings, and the restrictive pulmonary physiology suggested by spirographic examination, the most likely diagnosis is acute hypersensitivity pneumonitis, with male rat urine probably being the offending antigen. Without treatment, the patient could develop the subacute or chronic form of the disease with potentially serious physiologic impairment. While steroids can be helpful in severe or chronic cases, the best therapy is to remove the offending antigen or remove the patient from an environment where exposure is inevitable. This approach is difficult when the patient's life-style or livelihood requires a radical change; in the case presented, however, simply restricting the student's laboratory efforts to those not involving direct animal care seems relatively nondisruptive.

**V-7.    The answer is B.**   (*Chap. 259*)   Bronchoalveolar lavage in patients with idiopathic pulmonary fibrosis, a chronic inflammatory disorder of the lower respiratory tract characterized by dyspnea and reticulonodular infiltrates on chest radiography, discloses an abundance of alveolar macrophages. Probably related to locally generated immune complexes, alveolar macrophages become activated and then produce several mediators that recruit and induce fibroblast proliferation, which causes secondary damage. Macrophage-derived mediators believed to be important in this process include fibronectin, a 200-kDa dimeric glycoprotein that interacts with connective tissue matrix as well as specific receptors on fibroblasts, and platelet-derived growth factor, whose beta chain is encoded by the c-*sis* proto-oncogene. Platelet-derived growth factor is believed to play an important role in recruiting fibroblasts to the site of inflammation. Macrophages also produce chemotaxins such as leukotriene $B_4$ and interleukin 8, which attract neutrophils and eosinophils into the region.

**V-8.    The answer is C.**  (*Chap. 258. Oswald-Mammosser, Chest 107:1193, 1995.*)  The patient has evidence of obstructive lung disease on the basis of hyperinflation, decreased breath sounds, decreased $FEV_1$, and a heavy smoking history. He has chronic hypoxemia and a moderate degree of $CO_2$ retention. He may have an intermediate syndrome between emphysema and chronic bronchitis. Smoking cessation, yearly vaccination against influenza, and a one-time vaccination against *S. pneumoniae* infection are indicated. There are no definitive data to support the use of chronic antibacterial prophylaxis or systemic glucocorticoids, though occasional patients will benefit from steroid therapy given either systemically or by inhalation. The major issue is hypoxemia, which should be treated with continuous (at least nocturnal) oxygen therapy. Several trials have documented the benefit of oxygen therapy for lowering mortality, improving neuropsychological status, and decreasing the incidence of heart failure. Albuterol, a selective beta$_2$ agonist, induces bronchodilation with few cardiac side effects; however, the benefit of oxygen therapy is likely to be much greater than that of changing the inhaled sympathomimetic.

**V-9.    The answer is D.**  (*Chap. 252*)  The importance of immune mechanisms in the pathogenesis of asthma is suggested by the common association between the disease and the presence of allergic diseases, skin-test sensitivity, and increased serum IgE levels. In addition, many susceptible persons develop bronchospasm after inhalation challenge with airborne allergens. A large proportion of asthmatic subjects, however, have none of these markers of immunologic activity and are classified as having idiosyncratic asthma. When tested for bronchial hyperirritability with various nonantigenic bronchoprovocational agents (e.g., histamine and cold air), asthmatic subjects are found to be more sensitive than normal, and the bronchoconstriction is generally reversible after exposure to a beta-adrenergic agonist; the reason for this airway hyperirritability, which is a common feature of all asthmatic persons, is unknown. Although psychologic factors certainly influence the expression of asthma, no single personality type is considered "asthmatic."

**V-10.    The answer is A.**  (*Chap. 253*)  Allergic bronchopulmonary aspergillosis is a hypersensitivity pneumonitis that involves an allergic reaction to antigens from *Aspergillus* spp., most commonly *A. fumigatus*. The diagnosis should be suspected in asthmatic persons who have recurrent pulmonary infiltrates associated with peripheral blood or sputum eosinophilia. Suggestive laboratory findings include serum immunoglobulin E levels elevated to many times normal and the presence of aspergilli in the sputum. Antigenic skin testing is positive both in immediate (type I, wheal and flare) reaction and reaction evident after 4 to 6 h (type III, erythema and induration). Delayed, tuberculin-type (type IV, cell-mediated) reactions, however, do not occur. Serum precipitins to aspergilli are found in the majority of affected persons. The inflammatory response leads to dilatation of central airways and often is evident radiographically as mucoid impaction.

**V-11.    The answer is C.**  (*Chap. 252. McFadden, Am J Med 99:651, 1995.*)  Asthmatic patients who present with an acute attack and lack signs of impending ventilatory collapse should be treated with an inhaled aerosolized beta$_2$ agonist such as albuterol or isoproterenol. Such medicines can be given up to every 20 min by inhaled nebulizer for three doses, with the frequency reduced thereafter. Such drugs are five times more effective than intravenous aminophylline. Intravenous or inhaled steroids will have a delayed onset of action, if they are destined to be beneficial at all. Patients should be reassured that mortality from asthma is unlikely; however, it is nonetheless advisable to respect an acute asthmatic attack, especially one accompanied by $CO_2$ retention.

**V-12.    The answer is D.**  (*Chap. 256*)  Cilia, which are responsible for the motility and mucous clearance functions of many cell types, are composed of a double tubular structure. Abnormalities in one of the anatomic components of cilia can lead to a lack of coordinated ciliary action. Kartagener's syndrome, the best known of the dyskinetic ciliary syndromes, is caused by an absence of the inner or outer dynein arms normally present in functional cilia. Impaired ciliary motion is most prominently reflected in the lack of sperm motility and the impaired epithelial function of the fallopian tubes and respiratory tract. Infertility results from impaired motility of sperm and epithelial function of fallopian tubes, while chronic sinopulmonary infections result from impaired function of the respiratory tract. Recurrent bronchitis and pneumonia caused by impaired removal of airway secretions can lead to diffuse bronchiectasis with abnormally dilated airways and copious sputum production but not to interstitial pulmonary fibrosis.

**V-13.  The answer is C.**  (*Chap. 266*)   A patient with the stiff lungs characteristic of the adult respiratory distress syndrome often requires the institution of 0 to 5 cmH$_2$O of positive end-expiratory pressure to maintain adequate oxygenation. However, such high pressures may disrupt lung tissue, causing subcutaneous emphysema or pneumothorax. Patients with such complications probably are best served by the use of pressure-control ventilation, in which a given pressure is imposed at the airway opening during the inspiratory phase and delivers whatever tidal volumes and inspiratory flow rates are possible on the basis of set pressure. In addition to its use in situations where barotrauma has occurred, pressure-control ventilation may be helpful in postoperative thoracic surgical patients who have newly created suture lines. Because of the asynchronous nature of pressure-control ventilation relative to the patient's own ventilatory efforts, such ventilation usually requires heavy sedation. However, newer modifications of pressure-control ventilation allow the patient to initiate breaths to be given at a set pressure, allowing its use without such sedation.

**V-14.  The answer is D.**  (*Chap. 262. Berkmann, Postgrad Med J 69:12, 1993.*)   The initial step in the evaluation of a pleural effusion is the determination of the presence of either a transudative effusion, usually caused by congestive heart failure, cirrhosis, or nephrotic syndrome, or an exudative pleural effusion, which may be due to a host of causes. The working definition of an exudative effusion is one that meets any of the following criteria: (1) pleural fluid to serum protein concentration ratio greater than 0.5, (2) pleural fluid to serum lactic dehydrogenase (LDH) concentration ratio greater than 0.6, (3) pleural fluid LDH concentration greater than two-thirds of the upper limit of normal serum LDH. This patient's effusion is an exudate. Additional studies to be done include measurement of pleural glucose and cultures for bacterial mycobacteria and fungi. If the glucose is less than 60 mg/dL, malignancy, empyema, or rheumatoid pleuritis should be considered. Esophageal rupture, pancreatitis, and malignancy can cause an elevated pleural fluid amylase. If no diagnosis is apparent after the above studies, occult pulmonary embolism should be considered. If there is still no diagnosis based on these studies, it is then appropriate to perform a needle biopsy of the pleura with particular attention to histologic analysis for tuberculosis or cancer.

**V-15.  The answer is E.**  (*Chap. 255. Fang, Medicine 69:307–316, 1992.*)   Patients who require hospitalization for pneumonia acquired in the community optimally receive prompt microbiologic diagnosis. Recent studies have shown that about one-third of patients with such community-acquired pneumonias are alcohol abusers or have COPD. The potential microbiologic etiology for this spectrum of disease is *S. pneumoniae*, *H. influenzae*, *Legionella* spp., *Chlamydia*, anaerobes, *S. aureus*, and *Mycoplasma*. If the likelihood of pneumococcal pneumonia is high on the basis of the sputum Gram stain, penicillin and ampicillin still remain the drugs of choice, given a relatively low rate of penicillin-resistant organisms. However, if the likelihood of aerobic bacterial infection is high, second-generation cephalosporins such as cefotaxime are appropriate. If anaerobic infection is considered likely, metronidazole or ampicillin plus sulbactam should be used. In the current case, given the lack of clear-cut microbiologic evidence for a specific infection, the absence of sputum, and the equivocal findings on the chest x-ray, *Chlamydia* or *Legionella* should be strongly considered. The best empiric regimen in this situation would be ampicillin plus sulbactam in addition to erythromycin. A microbiologic diagnosis should be made in the next few days to allow narrowing of the antibiotic regimen.

**V-16. The answer is B.** (*Chap. 258*)  Certain persons with severe obstructive lung disease appear to respond to uncontrolled oxygen therapy by dangerously reducing their minute ventilation. Because they are relatively insensitive to changes in arterial $P_{CO_2}$, hypoxemia is the major ventilatory stimulus in these persons. When hypoxemia is suddenly treated with supplemental oxygen therapy given in an uncontrolled fashion, ventilation drops and worsening ventilation-perfusion relationships occur, arterial $P_{CO_2}$ rises, acidosis results, and coma may develop. However, abrupt removal of supplemental oxygen may precipitate life-threatening hypoxemia. Because acidosis must nevertheless be reversed rapidly by increasing ventilation, endotracheal intubation should be performed, followed by mechanical ventilation of a sufficient amount to return arterial pH to the physiologic range. Inhaled bronchodilators cannot be given to comatose, unintubated persons. Epinephrine is relatively ineffective in persons with acute or chronic respiratory failure and is dangerous in elderly, acidemic patients.

**V-17. The answer is B.** *(Chap. 259)*  The chest x-rays presented show diffuse, severe interstitial infiltrates without hilar adenopathy. Although sarcoidosis may produce this radiographic picture, it is also compatible with idiopathic interstitial pneumonitis, hypersensitivity pneumonitis, collagen vascular disease, inhalation of inorganic dusts, and many other processes. The degree of respiratory system dysfunction demonstrated by this patient necessitates rapid evaluation and a definitive histologic diagnosis so that appropriate therapy can be initiated. Angiotensin converting enzyme levels, although elevated in many patients with sarcoidosis, are not sufficiently sensitive or specific to replace tissue biopsy in the workup of persons with interstitial infiltrates. Although biopsy of extrapulmonary tissue may demonstrate noncaseating granulomas in patients with sarcoidosis, such biopsies may be negative in patients with active disease. A pathologic diagnosis is absolutely required in patients presenting with interstitial lung disease of uncertain etiology. Fiberoptic bronchoscopy should be performed to rule out infection or malignancy; an accompanying transbronchial biopsy may yield a diagnosis about 25 percent of the time. Bronchoalveolar lavage to assess the degree of inflammation may be helpful in monitoring disease activity, but its precise role in interstitial lung disease has not been defined. Despite its relatively low yield, the relatively low risk makes an attempt at transbronchial biopsy reasonable before definitely obtaining tissue at open lung biopsy.

**V-18. The answer is C.**  [*Chap. 260. Rich, Primary Pulmonary Hypertension, in Braunwald E (ed), Heart Disease, 1996.*]  Primary pulmonary hypertension is an uncommon disease that usually affects young women. Early in the illness affected persons often are diagnosed as psychoneurotic because of the vague nature of presenting complaints, for example, dyspnea, chest pain, and evidence of hyperventilation without hypoxemia on arterial blood-gas testing. However, progression of the disease leads to syncope in approximately one-half of cases and signs of right heart failure on physical examination. Chest x-ray typically shows enlarged central pulmonary arteries with or without attenuation of peripheral markings. The diagnosis of primary pulmonary hypertension is made by documentation of elevated pressures by right heart catheterization and exclusion of other pathologic processes. Lung disease of sufficient severity to cause pulmonary hypertension would be evident by history and on examination. Major differential diagnoses include thromboemboli and heart disease; outside the United States, schistosomiasis and filariasis are common causes of pulmonary hypertension, and a careful travel history should be taken.

**V-19. The answer is E.**  (*Chap. 261*)  The clinical triad of dyspnea, confusion, and petechiae in a person who has had recent long-bone fractures establishes the diagnosis of fat embolism syndrome. This disorder, which usually occurs within 48 h of injury, may lead to respiratory failure and death. Petechiae most often are found across the neck, in the axillae, and in the conjunctivae; however, their appearance is often evanescent. No laboratory test is specific for fat embolism.

**V-20.   The answer is D.**   (*Chap. 264. Fujita, Ear Nose Throat J 72:67, 1993.*)   Obstructive sleep apnea syndrome is a complex entity that involves intermittent upper-airway obstruction during sleep. Most of the manifestations, such as hypertension, cor pulmonale, chronic fatigue, personality changes, and disordered sleep behavior, resolve when obstruction is bypassed by a tracheostomy or endotracheal tube. Although the syndrome is more common in men, the prevalence increases in women after menopause. Alcohol and sedatives can exacerbate ventilatory obstruction by decreasing upper-airway muscle tone. Treatment of severe obstructive sleep apnea includes tricyclics to improve upper-airway muscle tone, uvulopalatopharyngoplasty to create a more spacious airway, continuous nasal positive airway pressure to prevent muscular collapse, and tracheostomy to bypass the obstruction completely. Estrogens, which once were thought to be beneficial in improving respiratory drive, are not now considered a mainstay of treatment.

**V-21.   The answer is D.**   (*Chap. 253. Hayakawa, Chest 105:1462, 1992.*)   Chronic eosinophilic pneumonia is an interstitial lung disorder of unknown cause that produces a systemic illness characterized by fever, weight loss, and malaise. Although lung biopsy shows an eosinophilic infiltrate involving both the interstitium and the alveolar space, there may not be an associated eosinophilia in the peripheral blood. The diagnosis should be suggested by the "photonegative pulmonary edema" pattern, with central sparing and nonsegmental, patchy infiltrates in the lung periphery. This disorder often responds dramatically to corticosteroid therapy. Idiopathic pulmonary fibrosis and polymyositis produce diffuse reticular, nodular, or reticulonodular infiltrates on chest x-ray. Alveolar proteinosis is a rare disorder that most often produces a diffuse air-space filling pattern radiating from hilar regions on chest x-ray, often with air bronchograms. Alveolar proteinosis does not cause fever unless it is complicated by an infection such as nocardiosis. Lymphangiomyomatosis is also rare. It occurs exclusively in women of childbearing age. The chest x-ray shows reticulonodular infiltration, but the lungs often appear hyperinflated. Lymphangiomyomatosis is complicated by pleural effusion and pneumothorax but not by fever.

**V-22.   The answer is B.**   (*Chap. 266. Hinson, Annu Rev Med 43:341, 1992.*)   Some persons who become agitated or anxious on a mechanical ventilator receive inadequate ventilation because they are breathing out of phase with the machine. The man described in the question has adequate oxygenation; a $P_{O_2}$ of 70 mmHg means that his hemoglobin is more than 90 percent saturated. However, he is hypoventilating and has developed an acute respiratory acidosis. Positive end-expiratory pressure (PEEP) improves oxygenation by raising the lung volume and reducing shunting, but it does not have a large effect on carbon dioxide clearance. Therefore, the appropriate first step in management would be to administer a sedative and control the man's ventilation to reduce arterial $P_{CO_2}$ and raise pH.

**V-23.   The answer is D.**   (*Chap. 261*)   Patients at high risk for thromboembolic disease include those who have had recent anesthesia, recent childbirth, heart failure, leg fracture, prolonged bed rest, obesity, estrogen use, or cancer. The clinical scenario presented is highly consistent with a pulmonary embolism arising from venous thrombosis of a proximal lower extremity in a postoperative patient. While the electrocardiogram is usually normal except for sinus tachycardia, the finding of new right-sided heart strain is compatible with a significant pulmonary embolus. The positive impedance plethysmogram for an above-the-knee venous thrombosis obviates the need for additional diagnostic testing. The patient must receive antithrombotic therapy (heparin) in an attempt to inhibit clot growth, promote resolution, and prevent recurrence. Warfarin requires several days to achieve anticoagulation and is therefore not appropriate in the acute setting. While thrombolytic therapy can clearly hasten the resolution of thrombi and may be appropriate for large, deep venous thromboses and pulmonary embolisms large enough to cause hypotension, its role in altering the natural history of this disorder has not been defined. Furthermore, recent surgery is a contraindication to the use of thrombolytic agents, which, even in the case of more specific newer agents such as tissue plasminogen activator, carry significant hemorrhagic risk. Lower-molecular-weight heparins (e.g., enoxaporin) have several potential advantages, including a longer half-life and a more predictable dose response, compared with unfractioned heparin; however, this newer agent has not received FDA approval for the treatment of pulmonary embolism or deep venous thrombosis.

**V-24.    The answer is D.**    (*Chap. 257*)    Although the majority of patients with cystic fibrosis are diagnosed in childhood, a significant number of patients are not identified until their late teens, twenties, or even thirties. Accurate diagnosis requires that the sweat chloride test be given to all patients with clinical features of cystic fibrosis. Airway obstruction resulting from bronchiectasis is associated with sinusitis and infertility in males with both cystic fibrosis and the immotile cilia syndrome, but only males with immotile cilia have Kartagener's syndrome (bronchiectasis, sinusitis, and dextrocardia). Patients with cystic fibrosis may have any of several gastrointestinal manifestations including obstruction, intussusception, fecal impaction, volvulus, portal hypertension, and steatorrhea. Steatorrhea is a manifestation of pancreatic insufficiency. Nearly all patients with cystic fibrosis display clubbing.

**V-25.    The answer is B.**    (*Chap. 258*)    The man described in the question presents with physical signs (pursed lip breathing, chest hyperexpansion) and radiographic evidence (flattened diaphragms, attenuated markings) suggestive of obstructive lung disease with loss of lung tissue. Reduced expiratory air-flow rates are produced by narrowing of airways (e.g., in asthma), loss of airways (e.g., in bronchiolitis obliterans), or loss of elastic tissue (e.g., in emphysema). Pathophysiologically, these conditions cause increased resistance as airways are narrowed or collapse as well as decreased driving pressure that represents loss of elastic recoil. Air trapping and reduced lung recoil lead to an increase in both total lung capacity (TLC) and functional residual capacity (FRC), which is the volume at which the tendency of the lung to recoil inward is just balanced by the tendency of the chest to recoil outward. Although TLC is increased, vital capacity, the maximum amount of gas that can be exhaled from the lungs with a single breath, is reduced owing to the great increase in residual volume produced by gas trapping. Not only is vital capacity reduced, it takes longer to empty the lungs; thus, forced expiratory volume in 1 s ($FEV_1$) is reduced as a percentage of vital capacity. When alveolar capillaries are destroyed by emphysema, the diffusing capacity, which reflects in part the surface area of alveolar membrane available for gas exchange, is reduced.

**V-26.    The answer is B.**    (*Chap. 258*)    To establish baseline information in persons who have emphysema, spirometry should be performed, and for persons with significant complaints or physical findings, arterial blood gases also should be checked. Although cigarette smoking accounts for the vast majority of cases of emphysema, a small percentage of persons who develop this illness have had no exposure to tobacco products. A subset of this nonsmoking, emphysematous population is deficient in $\alpha_1$-antitrypsin, which is a protease inhibitor that normally is found in the serum. It is currently believed that release of proteolytic enzymes from inflammatory cells accounts for the lung destruction that typifies emphysema, and $\alpha_1$-antitrypsin deficiency, a familial disorder, the genotype of which is acid starch gel and immunoelectrophoresis, permits this destruction to occur unimpeded. Exercise testing is not necessary as an initial screening test for emphysema but should be considered before oxygen therapy is prescribed. A male who has emphysematous respiratory failure, gives no history of respiratory infections, and has children would not have cystic fibrosis (affected men are sterile); therefore, a sweat chloride test would not be a useful procedure.

**V-27.    The answer is C.**    (*Chap. 258*)    Reduced serum levels of the antiprotease $\alpha_1$-antitrypsin, which is synthesized primarily in the liver, are associated with an inability to control the alveolar-damaging effects of neutrophil elastase and clinical emphysema. $\alpha_1$-Antitrypsin is encoded by a 7-exon gene spanning 12.2 kilobases on chromosome 14. Common disease-producing mutations of the normal M gene are the Z type, in which a single amino-acid substitution results in a hyperaggregative, improperly processed protein, and the S type, which results in a product with a shortened half-life and also is due to a single amino-acid change. Heterozygotes (either M2 or M5) appear to have sufficient, albeit reduced, levels of $\alpha_1$-antitrypsin to prevent severe lung damage. Since the S type produces less clinical antiprotease "deficiency," the pulmonary disease produced in SS homozygotes is much less severe than that seen in patients whose genotype is ZZ. Intravenous administration of normal human purified $\alpha_1$-antitrypsin can increase serum levels to a point at which sufficient antiprotease activity is provided to protect alveoli from elastase-induced damage.

**V-28.   The answer is D.**   (*Chap. 252*)   Although inhaled sympathomimetics are now considered the first-choice treatment for acute asthmatic attacks, methylxanthines such as theophylline are effective bronchodilators and continue to be used extensively in this disorder. The therapeutic plasma concentration is 10 to 20 μg/mL, but the dose required to achieve these levels varies widely, depending on the clinical situation. The theophylline dose should be reduced in any condition in which the clearance of this drug is significantly impaired, such as in the very young, the elderly, and those with liver or cardiac dysfunction. Many drugs interfere with the metabolism of theophylline. Some commonly used agents, including allopurinol, propranolol, cimetidine, and erythromycin, interfere with theophylline clearance and thus lead to increased levels of this methylxanthine. Drugs that activate hepatic microsomal enzymes, such as cigarettes, marijuana, phenobarbital, and phenytoin, may lower theophylline levels.

**V-29.   The answer is C.**   (*Chap. 254*)   Inhalation of asbestos fibers for 10 years or more may lead to interstitial fibrosis that typically begins in the lower lobes and later spreads to the middle and upper lung fields. This fibrosis is associated with a restrictive pattern on pulmonary function testing. The chest x-ray shows linear densities, thickening or calcification of the pleura (pleural plaques), and, in severe cases, honeycombing. Exposure to asbestos also may cause exudative pleural effusions. These effusions are often bloodstained and may be painful. The diagnosis may be elusive if a careful occupational exposure is not obtained. These effusions are benign, but affected persons may later sustain malignant mesotheliomas of the pleura or peritoneum. Unlike pulmonary fibrosis, pleural effusions and mesotheliomas may develop after brief exposures to asbestos, often exposures of 1 to 2 years. Mesotheliomas are not associated with cigarette smoking, but the combination of exposure to asbestos and cigarette smoking has a multiplicative effect on the risk of development of lung cancer. Exposure to asbestos increases the risk for both adenocarcinoma and squamous cell (but not small cell) carcinoma of the lung; this suggests that lung cancer screening may be useful in selected individuals.

**V-30.   The answer is E.**   (*Chap. 251*)   The flexible fiberoptic bronchoscope is ideal for many clinical situations, including those designed to determine many endobronchial pathologic states, including tumors, granulomas, bronchitis, foreign bodies, and sites of bleeding. Washing or infiltration of a higher volume of sterile saline (bronchoalveolar lavage) can be used to detect abnormal cells or recover pathogens such as *P. carinii* in patients with HIV infection. Brushing or biopsy at the surface of an endobronchial lesion can enhance the recovery of cellular material or tissue that can be very helpful in detecting neoplasms or infection. Pulmonary hemorrhage can complicate a transbronchial biopsy if the patient is at risk for a bleeding diathesis. Pneumothorax can occur if the forceps are too close to the pleural surface. Because a rigid bronchoscope has a larger suction channel and allows ventilation, this instrument is still useful for the retrieval of foreign bodies and the suctioning of massive hemorrhages.

**V-31.** **The answer is E.** (*Chap. 254*)  Pulmonary disease secondary to cotton dust exposure is one of the most common occupational lung diseases. During the production of yarn for cotton, linen, and rope making, exposure to cotton, flax, or hemp produces a host of respiratory symptoms. Exposure to cotton dust (byssinosis) is characterized as chest tightness toward the end of the first day of the workweek. Such symptoms are associated with a significant drop in the forced expiratory volume during the workday. Although most workers have no recurrence after the workweek, up to 25 percent may have a progressive symptom complex consisting of recurrent chest tightness, eventually leading to an obstructive pattern on pulmonary function testing. The chest tightness appears to be due to bronchospasm, which may be reversible with bronchodilators. The best treatment is a reduction of dust exposure.

**V-32.** **The answer is A.** (*Chap. 256*)  Bronchiectasis represents an abnormal permanent dilation of the bronchi, typically on the basis of chronic destruction and inflammation caused by repetitive infection or other chronic insults. Many infectious agents, including adenovirus, influenza virus, *Staphyloccoccus aureus*, tuberculosis, and anaerobic infection, can each predispose a patient to the bronchiectatic state. Problems of primary immune defenses such as immunoglobulin deficiency, primary cilliary disorders, and cystic fibrosis also can produce dilated bronchi. This anatomic problem leads to recurring cough and purulent sputum production, frequently associated with hemoptysis resulting from friable, inflamed airway mucosa. Repetitive bronchiectatic episodes tend to produce increased problems. Physical examination is nonspecific; however, the chest radiograph is frequently abnormal, and the findings may include cystic spaces caused by saccular bronchiectasis or the so-called tram track (parallel linear shadows) or rings (produced if the inflamed thickened airways are seen in cross section). Treatment requires elimination of the underlying problem (e.g., by immunoglobulin infusions), improved clearance of tracheobronchial secretions, control of infection, and the use of bronchodilators to reverse airflow obstruction.

**V-33.** **The answer is D.** (*Chap. 267*)  Emphysema, either smoking-induced or resulting from $\alpha_1$-antitrypsin deficiency, is the indication for almost 50 percent of all single-lung transplants. It is important to determine the optimal lung transplant window in which the patient has severe limitations secondary to his or her disease but has not passed the point at which lung transplant surgery would be dangerously complicated. Life expectancy of less than 2 years and severe obstructive lung disease ($FEV_1$ of less than 30 percent of the predicted value) are required. Patients with pulmonary fibrosis must have profound impairment of total lung capacity and resting hypoxia; those with pulmonary hypertension need to be severely functionally limited and have pulmonary artery pressures greater than 50 mmHg. Patients with cystic fibrosis must also have severe limitations in expiratory capacity as well as abnormalities in arterial blood gases. They are not candidates for single-lung transplantation because of the risk of disseminated infection. Instead, they require a bilateral lung transplant or a related donor bilobe transplant to reduce the likelihood of disseminated infection. In each of the other situations, single-lung transplantation can be performed with acceptable risk and tangible benefit for the patient.

**V-34.** **The answer is E.** (*Chap. 255*)  Microbial pathogens may enter the lung by several routes, including aspiration of organisms that colonize the oropharynx, inhalation of infectious aerosols, direct inoculation (e.g., from tracheal intubation or stab wounds), and hematogenous dissemination from an extrapulmonary site. In a chronic alcoholic, presumably with a higher likelihood of aspiration of oral contents, one must seriously consider the presentation of an aspiration pneumonia caused by anaerobic oral flora. Moreover, certain oral anaerobes, such as *S. aureus*, *S. pneumoniae* serotype III, aerobic gram-negative bacilli, oral anaerobes, *M. tuberculosis*, and fungi, produce tissue necrosis and pulmonary cavities. *H. influenzae*, *M. pneumoniae*, and other type serotypes of *S. pneumoniae* are less likely to cause cavities. Cavities associated with *M. tuberculosis* do have air-fluid levels but are typically in the upper lobe as a result of the fact that they require high oxygen tension for optimal growth. By contrast, a cavity containing an air-fluid level in a dependent, fully ventilated, fully draining bronchopulmonary segment suggests that the culprit is an oral anaerobe. One particular oral anaerobe, *Actinomyces* spp., can produce a chronic fibrotic necrotizing process that can cross tissue planes to involve the pleural space, ribs, vertebrae, and subcutaneous tissue with the eventual discharge of sulfur granules.

**V-35.** **The answer is A.** (*Chap. 259. Hunninghack, Am J Respir Crit Care Med 151:915, 1995.*)  This patient presents with the classic history, physical findings, and pathologic findings consistent with idiopathic pulmonary fibrosis. This is an unrelenting interstitial lung disease which produces scarring and ablation of alveoli with a concomitant restrictive lung pattern. If progressive and/or unresponsive to therapy, the disease will lead to progressive loss of pulmonary function and ultimately to right-sided heart failure. The primary cause is unknown, although the pathophysiology clearly involves the activation of alveolar macrophages, with secondary cytokine release causing alveolar damage with associated fibrosis. Once the diagnosis is made, even at an advanced stage, a trial of glucocorticoids is indicated. High-dose steroid therapy for 8 weeks usually is initiated with gradual tapering if objective improvement is noted. Cyclophosphamide may be useful in patients who are unresponsive to glucocorticoids. The dose of cyclophosphamide should be titrated to ensure that the total neutrophil count does not drop below $1000/\mu L$. Drugs such as penicillamine, cyclosporine, and colchicine, each of which could potentially play a role in inhibiting macrophage-produced growth factors, remain investigative. Although measures to prevent progressive restrictive physiology include diuretics and oxygen for congestive heart failure, rapid treatment of infection, and the routine use of prophylactic pneumococcal influenza vaccine, in the situation of a patient who is in otherwise good medical condition but has profoundly deranged pulmonary physiology secondary to fibrosis, lung transplantation should be considered.

**V-36.** **The answer is A.** (*Chap. 261. Ridker, N Engl J Med 332:912, 1995.*)  Many patients who develop pulmonary thromboembolism have an underlying inherited predisposition that remains clinically silent until they are subjected to an additional stress, such as the use of oral contraceptive pills, surgery, or pregnancy. The most frequently inherited predisposition to thrombosis is so-called activated protein C resistance. The inability of a normal protein C to carry out its anticoagulant function is due to a missense mutation in the gene coding for factor V in the coagulation cascade. This mutation, which results in the substitution of a glutamine for an arginine residue in position 506 of the factor V molecule, is designated the factor V Leiden gene. Based on the Physicians Health Study, about 3 percent of healthy male physicians carry this particular missense mutation. Carriers are clearly at an increased risk for deep venous thrombosis and also for recurrence after the discontinuation of coumadin. The allelic frequency of factor V Leiden is more common than are all other identified inherited hypercoagulable states combined, including deficiencies of protein C, protein S, and antithrombin III and disorders of plasminogen.

**V-37.** **The answer is E.** (*Chap. 263*)  The hypoventilation syndromes are defined as disorders which yield to hypercapnia (usually a $Pa_{CO_2}$ in the range of 50 to 80 mmHg). The clinical manifestations of such a syndrome include respiratory acidosis with a compensatory rise in the plasma bicarbonate concentration and a decrease in chloride concentration. The hypercapnia leads to an obligatory decrease in the arterial oxygen tension with subsequent cyanosis and secondary polycythemia. Moreover, chronic hypercapnia can induce pulmonary vasoconstriction which can eventually lead to right ventricular failure. Problems of hypoventilation normally are exacerbated at night, leading to worsened hypercapnia during sleep with subsequent morning headache and daytime somnolence with eventual intellectual impairment. A polysomnogram can distinguish whether the defect is in the metabolic control system (chemoreceptors or brainstem initiating neurons) versus the neuromuscular system (brainstem neurons, spinal cord, respiratory nerves) or in the ventilatory apparatus (e.g., chest wall, lungs, airways) itself. Those with a central problem such as higher CNS malfunction or chemoreceptor insufficiency have normal spirometry, blood gases, and tests of voluntary hyperventilation. However, they would have a markedly blunted response to hypoxia or hypercapnia. Respiratory neuromuscular dysfunction that produces a decrease in the ability to exhale would lead to an abnormal spirometric evaluation and also would make it impossible for the patient to generate normal inspiratory and expiratory muscle pressures against a closed airway. Those with problems with the venilatory apparatus, such as those which typically occur in obstructive sleep apnea, would be able to generate adequate expiratory and inspiratory muscle pressures and generally would have markedly abnormal blood gases (e.g., a widened arterial alveolar oxygen tension gradient).

**V-38.   The answer is E.**   (*Chap. 263*)   In all cases of chronic hyperventilation the mechanism involves an increase in respiratory drive that may well be physiologic (e.g., chronic hypoxemia) but can be detrimental because of the ensuing alkalemia. This disturbance in blood pH can produce neurologic symptoms such as dizziness, syncope, and seizure activity caused by cerebral vasoconstriction. The neuromuscular side effects of chronic alkalemia can include paresthesia, muscle weakness (from hypophosphatemia), and hypocalcemia-induced carpopedal spasm tetany. The primary respiratory alkalosis can lead to central sleep apnea. The disorders that most frequently lead to unexplained hyperventilation are pulmonary vascular diseases such as chronic thromboembolism and anxiety. In patients who have symptoms clearly secondary to hyperventilation, inhalation of a low concentration of carbon dioxide can be helpful.

**V-39.   The answer is A.**   (*Chap. 265. Milberg, JAMA 273:306, 1995.*)   The acute respiratory distress syndrome is a condition characterized by hypoxemic respiratory failure resulting from noncardiogenic pulmonary edema. Whatever the initial insult, the final common pathway of diffuse lung injury represents a cascade of cellular events that are associated with cytokine production by inflammatory cell activation and the production of inflammatory mediators which damage alveolar and pulmonary endothelial cells, leading to increased vascular permeability and loss of surfactant production by type II pneumocytes. When the injury is severe, mechanical ventilation is required. Despite the critical involvement of the inflammatory response in the generation of acute respiratory distress syndrome, glucocorticoids have shown no benefit in the treatment of this condition, except in childhood meningococcemia and *P. carinii* pneumonia. Although mortality rates for acute respiratory distress syndrome range from 50 to 70 percent, it is likely that improvements in therapy are reducing this dire outcome. Age greater than 65 years, multiorgan system failure, sepsis, and severe gas exchange disturbances are all negative prognostic factors. However, those with uncomplicated overdoses tend to have a relatively improved outcome. Those who survive are likely to return to the preexisting level of function.

**V-40.   The answer is B.**   (*Chap. 266*)   Enterotracheal intubation with positive-pressure mechanical ventilation may save lives in multiple settings associated with respiratory failure. This highly invasive technique has both direct and indirect effects on many organ systems. Lung complications include barotrauma (especially in the setting of the use of high levels of positive end-expiratory pressure), nosocomial pneumonia, oxygen toxicity, tracheal stenosis, and deconditioning of respiratory muscles. If a clinically significant pneumothorax occurs (e.g., associated with hypoxemia, decreased lung compliance, and hypotension), placement of a thoracostomy tube is required. While nosocomial pneumonia is common in patients intubated for more than 72 h because of aspiration of oral pharyngeal contents caused by leaks around the endotracheal tube cuff, the use of prophylactic antibiotics is not indicated. Moreover, it can be difficult to distinguish between colonization and true infection, since virtually all ventilated patients can be shown to have potentially pathogenic bacteria in the lower respiratory tract. Oxygen toxicity, which may result from the effect of oxygen free radicals on lung tissues, needs to be managed with the conservative use of inspired oxygen tensions. Right-sided heart hemodynamic monitoring often is required to provide optimal levels of intravascular volume replacement in these patients. It is important to maintain adequate venous return, but increased lung water also must be avoided. Mild to moderate cholestasis and stress ulceration are two important gastrointestinal effects of mechanical ventilation. If the total bilirubin values are greater than 4.0 mg/dL, it is likely that a cause of liver damage other than intubation is operative. Prophylactic therapy with sucralfate or an $H_2$-receptor antagonist is helpful in preventing stress-related ulcers in intubated patients.

**V-41.  The answer is C.**  (*Chap. 266*)  There are many reasons why patients fail removal from assisted ventilation. Sedatives, which are commonly prescribed earlier in the hospital stay for agitation or sleep, may not have been discontinued or metabolized and could contribute to impairment of respiratory drive. Persistent secretions that could be removed by suctioning also might contribute to the problem. A very important issue is maintenance of a continued drive to breathe. The central respiratory centers are sensitive to blood pH and will promote ventilation when sufficient acidosis (greater than that normally noted in a bronchitic patient with chronic $CO_2$ retention) ensues. Thus, creation of metabolic alkalosis with diuretic therapy or running the assisted minute ventilation too high (i.e., lower $P_{CO_2}$ and higher pH than normal for the patient) could account for failed extubation. Neuromuscular weakness caused by diuretic-induced hypokalemia, malnutrition, and occult hypothyroidism are potential factors leading to difficulty in independent ventilation and trouble in weaning.

**V-42.  The answer is A-Y, B-Y, C-N, D-Y, E-N.**  (*Chap. 261*)  Hypoxemia occurs commonly after massive pulmonary thromboembolism, although normal arterial oxygen tension does not exclude the diagnosis. The most important mechanism producing hypoxemia in this setting is an increase in venous admixture caused by continued perfusion of poorly ventilated areas. Ventilation may be decreased by atelectasis or by airway constriction in response to the release of bronchoactive mediators. A fall in cardiac output that produces a low mixed venous $P_{O_2}$ can increase the effect of venous admixture. Increased dead-space ventilation would not be a cause of hypoxemia.

**V-43.  The answer is A-Y, B-N, C-Y, D-Y, E-N.**  (*Chap. 250*)  The volume remaining in the lungs at the conclusion of a complete forced expiration is termed the *residual volume* and can be determined either by the body plethysmography or by helium dilution methods. At the residual volume there is a balance between the intrinsic outward recoil of the chest wall and the force maintained by the respiratory muscles to decrease lung volumes further. Therefore, increases in the residual volume can result from the functionally weak musculature of the chest wall that might be observed in neuromuscular disorders that affect the ability to expire forcefully (Guillain-Barré syndrome, muscular dystrophies, cervical spine injury). Furthermore, diseased airways will collapse at low lung volumes, preventing further emptying and also producing an abnormally high residual volume. Thus, any condition in which airway obstruction plays a major role (chronic bronchitis, emphysema, asthma, cystic fibrosis) may be associated with increased residual volume. By contrast, pulmonary parenchymal disease (e.g., sarcoidosis) produces normal expiration and reduced lung volumes. If inspiratory dysfunction is the primary chest wall problem (as in kyphoscoliosis and obesity), residual volume will be relatively unaffected or slightly decreased.

**V-44.  The answer is A-N, B-Y, C-Y, D-N, E-N.**  (*Chap. 265. Kolleff, N Engl J Med 332:27, 1995.*)  The adult respiratory distress syndrome (ARDS) is a clinical triad of hypoxemia, diffuse lung infiltrates, and reduced lung compliance not attributable to congestive cardiac failure. This syndrome's many causes suggest its complex pathogenesis. However, the pathologic outcome is the same: an increase in lung water caused by an increase in alveolar capillary permeability. This noncardiogenic pulmonary edema is identical to congestive cardiac pulmonary edema in its effect on the mechanical properties of the lung and on gas exchange. Just as in cardiac pulmonary edema, the increase in lung water associated with ARDS produces interstitial edema and alveolar collapse, and so the affected lung becomes stiff and the alveolar-arterial oxygen tension difference widens. Unlike cardiac edema, however, the increase in lung water in ARDS occurs as a result of an increase in alveolar capillary permeability and is not due to an increase in hydrostatic forces. Edema fluid in ARDS therefore often contains macromolecules (such as serum proteins), and measurement of pulmonary artery wedge pressure is normal or low. In clinical practice, determination of pulmonary artery wedge pressure is the most helpful discriminant between ARDS and cardiac failure.

# VI. ENDOCRINE, METABOLIC, AND GENETIC DISORDERS

## QUESTIONS

**DIRECTIONS:** Each question below contains five suggested responses. Choose the **one best** response to each question.

**VI-1.** The use of repeated phlebotomy in the treatment of persons with symptomatic hemochromatosis may be expected to result in

(A) increased skin pigmentation
(B) improved cardiac function
(C) return of secondary sex characteristics
(D) decreased joint pain
(E) an unchanged 5-year survival rate

**VI-2.** A 19-year-old man has had a 5-year history of hyperglycemic episodes and glycosuria. However, he has never been hospitalized for diabetic ketoacidosis. Which of the following statements regarding the mode of inheritance of his disease is correct?

(A) This disease is inherited in an autosomal recessive fashion
(B) If the patient has children, they will have approximately a 50-percent chance of developing diabetes
(C) The diabetic susceptibility gene in this patient resides on human chromosome 6
(D) The patient is likely to carry one of a limited number of HLA-D locus alleles
(E) The patient has an unusual susceptibility to a viral infection

**VI-3.** Which of the following studies is most sensitive for detecting diabetic nephropathy?

(A) Serum creatinine level
(B) Creatinine clearance
(C) Urine albumin
(D) Glucose tolerance test
(E) Ultrasonography

**VI-4.** Which of the following statements concerning intensive insulin therapy for diabetes (the use of an external insulin pump or three or more daily insulin injections guided by frequent blood glucose monitoring) is correct?

(A) All patients with diabetes mellitus should receive such therapy
(B) It has been definitively shown that compared with standard therapy, such intensive therapy reduces the likelihood of retinopathy in patients with insulin-dependent diabetes mellitus
(C) Such therapy will consistently return blood glucose to normal levels, but a reduction of long-term complications has not been demonstrated
(D) With careful monitoring, an increase in the number of hypoglycemic episodes is avoided
(E) Intensive insulin therapy failed to reduce the level of glycosylated hemoglobin

**VI-5.** Evidence of continuing ovarian estrogen production in a 29-year-old woman who is being evaluated for secondary amenorrhea is provided by

(A) normal plasma estrone and luteinizing hormone (LH) levels
(B) a normal plasma prolactin level
(C) an increase in plasma estradiol level after the administration of human chorionic gonadotropin (hCG)
(D) the appearance of menses after a short course of progesterone therapy
(E) a lack of hot flashes

**VI-6.** Which of the following inhibits growth hormone secretion from the anterior pituitary gland?

(A) Somatostatin
(B) Growth hormone–releasing hormone
(C) Hypoglycemia
(D) Arginine
(E) Serotonin

**VI-7.** A 7-year-old girl is referred for evaluation of vaginal bleeding for 2 months. The mother says that she has not been exposed to exogenous estrogens. Physical examination reveals height at the 98th percentile, Tanner stage III breast development, and no axillary or pubic hair. No abdominal or pelvic masses are palpated. Neurologic examination is normal. Radiographic and laboratory evaluations reveal the following:

Brain MRI: normal pituitary and hypothalamus
Bone age: 10 years
Urinary 17-ketosteroids: 1.7 μmol
    (0.5 mg)/g creatinine/24 h
Urinary gonadotropins: undetectable

The appropriate next step in the management of this girl would be

(A) exploratory laparotomy
(B) treatment with medroxyprogesterone acetate
(C) measurement of plasma androstenedione level
(D) abdominal CT scanning and/or pelvic sonography
(E) karyotype analysis

**VI-8.** A 40-year-old man presents with an insidious onset of fatigue, headaches, muscle weakness, and paresthesias. Physical examination reveals hypertension, an enlarged tongue, wide spacing of the teeth, and a doughy appearance to the skin. Which of the following laboratory results would be INCONSISTENT with the expected diagnosis?

(A) Serum prolactin = 35 μg/L (35 ng/mL)
(B) Serum glucose = 8.6 mmol/L (155 mg/dL)
(C) Elevated insulin-like growth factor (IGF-I)
(D) Growth hormone concentration = 0.2 μg/L (0.2 ng/mL) 1 h after oral administration of 100 g glucose
(E) Elevated 16F bending protein 3 (1 GF BP3)

**VI-9.** Which of the following statements concerning the diagnosis of pheochromocytoma is correct?

(A) Measurement of plasma catecholamines is the preferred initial screening test
(B) Random urine samples are equivalent in diagnostic accuracy to the measurement of catecholamines or catecholamine metabolites in a 24-h urine collection
(C) After collection, the urine should be treated with dilute sodium hydroxide and refrigerated
(D) The ideal time to collect urine is during a period of clinical stability
(E) Strenuous exertion may falsely elevate the level of free urinary catecholamines

**VI-10.** A 42-year-old man (indicated by the star in the family history below) has renal failure as a result of Alport's syndrome, which consists of nephritis associated with sensorineural deafness and is inherited as an autosomal dominant defect. He is being evaluated for a renal transplant from a living related donor. The best candidate for evaluation as a potential kidney donor for this man would be his

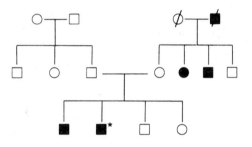

■ Renal failure
／ Deceased

(A) mother
(B) father
(C) unaffected brother
(D) sister

**VI-11.** Peripheral blood cells are obtained from the members of a family; the DNA is extracted, treated with restriction endonuclease E run on an agarose gel, transferred to nitrocellulose paper, probed with a 4-kilobase (kb) radiolabeled segment of DNA, and exposed to x-ray film. In the following pattern, solid blocks indicate segments of DNA hybridizing to the probe and numbers indicate DNA length in kilobases. What most likely accounts for the fact that only one band appears in the son and only one (different) band appears in the daughter?

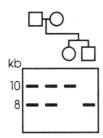

(A) A gene deletion in each child
(B) Chromosome segregation in the offspring
(C) Linkage disequilibrium in the offspring
(D) Parents who are heterozygotes for restriction fragment length polymorphism
(E) Loss of the restriction site for endonuclease E in both the children

**VI-12.** A 42-year-old alcoholic man has eaten poorly for the last 10 days but has continued to drink. His family brings him to the emergency room. On neurologic examination he is confused but otherwise normal. Blood glucose concentration is 2.8 mmol/L (50 mg/dL). Intravenous infusion of a bolus of 50% glucose solution is given. His confusion worsens, and he develops horizontal nystagmus, ataxia, and a heart rate of 130 beats per minute. At this point, the man's physician should

(A) order an immediate CT scan of the head
(B) perform a lumbar puncture
(C) administer another bolus of 50% glucose solution
(D) administer intravenous folic acid, 5 mg
(E) administer intramuscular thiamine, 50 mg

**VI-13.** A 24-year-old woman with a several-year history of chronic, debilitating, cramping abdominal pain has been evaluated several times for this problem. In each case the possibility of psychogenic causes has been raised because of the absence of abdominal tenderness, fever, and leukocytosis during the episodes. The patient has had intermittent vomiting, constipation, arm and chest pain, and difficulty in urination. She also complains of increasing leg weakness. The attacks of abdominal pain often are associated with anxiety, insomnia, and disorientation. A prior workup has also included abdominal angiography, abdominal CT, and endoscopy. The results of all the diagnostic studies were normal. The patient's current physical examination and routine laboratory examination, including complete blood count and serum chemistries, are unremarkable. The urinary pyrrole porphobilinogen excretion is elevated. Which of the following is the most appropriate advice for this patient?

(A) The patient's offspring may be at risk only if the father is also a carrier of this disease
(B) Intravenous administration of heme may ameliorate the attacks
(C) Narcotic analgesics should not be used during acute attacks
(D) The patient should avoid aspirin
(E) The patient should avoid prolonged exposure to the sun

**VI-14.** After apical scars are found on chest x-ray in a 48-year-old postmenopausal woman, chemoprophylaxis with isoniazid is begun. Two months later the woman complains of weakness, nausea, and tingling in the feet. Physical examination is unremarkable, and routine blood and urine test results are normal. Four weeks later she has a grand mal seizure and is admitted to the hospital. Findings on the admission physical include seborrheic dermatitis, glossitis, and absent ankle and knee tendon reflexes; hematologic testing reveals microcytic anemia. At this point, the woman's physician should

(A) order immediate electroencephalography
(B) order CT of the brain
(C) discontinue isoniazid and begin treatment with rifampin
(D) administer intramuscular pyridoxine, 100 mg, and then give 50 mg orally daily
(E) administer intramuscular cyanocobalamin, 100 μg, and then give 100 μg daily for 1 week

**VI-15.** A 78-year-old man who lives alone and prepares his own food is found to have numerous ecchymotic areas on the posterior aspect of his lower extremities. On closer examination of the skin, he has hemorrhagic areas around hair follicles; the hairs are fragmented. Splinter hemorrhages are present in the nail beds, and several hematomas are present in the muscles of the arms and legs. Except for the absence of teeth, the rest of the physical examination is unremarkable. Laboratory examination reveals a normal PT, PTT, and CBC, except for a hematocrit of 28 percent (red blood cell indices are normal). This clinical syndrome is most likely due to a deficiency of

(A) vitamin A
(B) vitamin C
(C) folate
(D) vitamin K
(E) pyridoxine

**VI-16.** A 20-year-old woman has a history of multiple fractures since childhood, kyphoscoliosis, bluish-gray teeth, and conductive hearing loss. Examination of the face reveals blue sclerae. Several relatives on her mother's side have been similarly affected. She has no history of physical abuse or abnormal serum chemistries. The most likely mechanism of the patient's abnormalities is

(A) excessive deposition of normal collagen fibrils in bone
(B) inability to convert procollagen to collagen
(C) mutation in the gene for type I procollagen
(D) mutation in the gene for type II procollagen
(E) mutation in the gene for type III procollagen

**VI-17.** A clinical presentation that includes long thin extremities, dislocation of the ocular lens, and aortic aneurysms is most likely due to a derangement in which of the following molecules?

(A) Procollagen type I
(B) Procollagen type II
(C) Proteoglycan
(D) Elastin
(E) Fibrillin

**VI-18.** A 25-year-old man with a renal allograft and a history of an intracerebral abscess is evaluated for profound polyuria. He is admitted to the hospital for a water deprivation test. No fluids are given after 12 midnight. By 11 A.M. he has lost 1 kg, and urine osmolality has been 120 mosm/kg for the last 3 h. Plasma osmolality is 320 mosm/kg (serum sodium is 155 mmol/L). At 11 A.M. 1 μg desmopressin is given by subcutaneous injection; 45 min later the urine osmolality is measured at 121 mosm/kg. The patient is then allowed to drink. Treatment of this patient should include

(A) vasopressin tannate in oil
(B) hydrochlorothiazide
(C) desmopressin
(D) chlorpropamide
(E) demeclocycline

**VI-19.** A person with hypercalcemia caused by sarcoidosis probably would have all but which one of the following?

(A) An abnormal chest x-ray
(B) Increased absorption of calcium from the gastrointestinal tract
(C) Hypercalciuria
(D) Increased serum parathyroid hormone level
(E) Hypergammaglobulinemia

**VI-20.** The most likely etiology for the eating disorder anorexia nervosa is

(A) decreased levels of luteinizing hormone–releasing hormone (LHRH)
(B) decreased levels of growth hormone
(C) decreased levels of insulin-like growth factor I (somatomedin C)
(D) low levels of serum thyroxine
(E) psychiatric disorder

**VI-21.** A 45-year-old obese man without known medical problems complains of feeling very sleepy during the day and often falling asleep while listening to friends. The most likely cause of this patient's problem is

(A) narcolepsy
(B) upper airway obstruction at night
(C) glucocorticoid excess
(D) growth hormone excess
(E) estrogen excess

**VI-22.** A 67-year-old man with chronic arthritis is found to have passed a uric acid stone after an episode of renal colic. On workup he is found to have multiple radiolucent stones in the left renal pelvis, uric acid excretion of 5.4 mmol/d (900 mg/d), a serum uric acid concentration of 580 μmol/L (9.8 mg/dL), a serum creatinine concentration of 160 μmol/L (1.8 mg/dL), and monosodium urate crystals in an effusion in the left knee. The drug of choice for long-term therapy in this patient is

(A) probenecid alone
(B) probenecid and sodium bicarbonate
(C) allopurinol
(D) colchicine
(E) sulfinpyrazone

**VI-23.** An obese woman has hypertriglyceridemia without hypercholesterolemia. The most appropriate first step in the treatment of this woman would be

(A) weight reduction
(B) nicotinic acid
(C) gemfibrozil
(D) clofibrate therapy
(E) bile acid–binding resin therapy

**VI-24.** An X-linked recessive disease characterized by nephrolithiasis, arthritis, self-mutilative behavior, and mental retardation is associated with

(A) failure to excrete uric acid because of inherited defective renal tubular function
(B) failure to excrete uric acid because of xanthine oxidase mutation
(C) uric acid overproduction caused by inherited acceleration of purine degradation
(D) increased urate production caused by an inability to convert purine bases to ribonucleotides
(E) increased urate production caused by increased levels of phosphoribosylpyrophosphate

**VI-25.** In designing a hormone replacement program for patients with coexistent thyroid and adrenal failure,

(A) the dose of glucocorticoid must be increased slowly once thyroid replacement has been initiated
(B) the dose of thyroid hormone must be increased slowly once glucocorticoid replacement has been initiated
(C) mineralocorticoid replacement also must be included if combined therapy is required
(D) thyroid replacement must not be initiated until treatment with glucocorticoid has been instituted
(E) growth hormone replacement also must be included if combined therapy is required

**VI-26** A 20-year-old man presents with weakness. Physical examination reveals mild jaundice and a liver two fingers beneath the right costal margin. Laboratory evaluation is remarkable for the presence of elevated hepatic transaminases (four times normal). Other laboratory results are negative, including serology for hepatitis A, B, and C; ANA; rheumatoid factor; iron; and iron binding. Serum ceruloplasmin is 50 mg/L (5 mg/dL). The patient denies intake of alcohol and exposure to known hepatotoxins. The most appropriate treatment is

(A) liver transplantation
(B) interferon-α
(C) penicillamine
(D) glucocorticoids
(E) desferrioxamine

**VI-27.** A 45-year-old man who works in the metal smelting industry was involved in an accident in which he was exposed to a great deal of dust and manufacturing by-products. Several days after this episode he developed jaundice, nausea, vomiting, diarrhea, and shortness of breath. Physical examination demonstrated icteric sclerae and tachycardia. Laboratory evaluation revealed hematocrit 32 percent, WBC count 14,000/μL, and platelet count 350,000/μL. Urinalysis disclosed no red cells or white cells per high-power field, but there were several granular casts. The urine dipstick was positive for blood and protein. Liver function tests included aspartate aminotransferase (SGOT) level 1.3 μkat/L (80 U/L), alanine aminotransferase (SGPT) level 2 μkat/L (120 U/L), total bilirubin 85.5 μmol/L (5 mg/dL), and direct bilirubin 17.1 μmol/L (1 mg/dL). ECG revealed T-wave inversion in all leads. Plain x-ray of the abdomen revealed patchy densities. The most appropriate diagnostic measurement would be of

(A) urinary arsenic
(B) serum lead
(C) erythrocyte protoporphyrin
(D) serum cadmium
(E) serum thallium

**VI-28.** Cholestyramine and colestipol are binding resins that are used to treat patients with hypercholesterolemia. Their serum-cholesterol-lowering effects are thought to be mediated by

(A) causing mild diarrhea and a mild degree of fat malabsorption
(B) binding of intestinal cholesterol, thus decreasing its net absorption from dietary sources
(C) decreasing the intestinal synthesis of very-low-density lipoproteins
(D) interrupting the enterohepatic circulation of cholesterol by sequestering bile acids in the intestine
(E) none of the above

**VI-29.** A 35-year-old woman ingests a hundred 325-mg acetaminophen tablets in a suicide attempt. She is immediately brought to the emergency room by friends. The appropriate therapeutic strategy is

(A) administration of activated charcoal
(B) administration of activated charcoal plus acetylcysteine therapy
(C) chelation therapy
(D) administration of phenytoin (Dilantin)
(E) acetylcysteine therapy

**VI-30.** The reason for acute renal failure after the ingestion of antifreeze is

(A) direct ethanol toxicity on renal tubules
(B) direct ethylene glycol toxicity on renal tubules
(C) toxicity of ethylene glycol metabolites to renal tubules
(D) insufficient renal perfusion as a result of circulatory collapse induced by ethylene glycol
(E) urinary obstruction caused by oxalic acid stones

**VI-31.** Obese persons are at an increased risk for all the following disorders EXCEPT

(A) hypothyroidism
(B) cholelithiasis
(C) diabetes mellitus
(D) hypertension
(E) hypertriglyceridemia

**VI-32.** Which of the following would be the most likely finding in a patient who has taken an overdose of a tricyclic antidepressant?

(A) Elevated hepatic transaminases
(B) Prolongation of the QRS complex on the electrocardiogram
(C) Urinary incontinence
(D) Metabolic alkalosis
(E) Anemia

**VI-33.** A 25-year-old man complains of diffuse bone pain. Physical examination is remarkable for the presence of an enlarged spleen (9 cm below the left costal margin). CBC discloses pancytopenia. A bone marrow examination reveals normal hematopoiesis; however, large multinucleated, macrophagelike cells engorged with cytoplasmic fibrils are present. The relevant family history includes Eastern European Jewish origins. An appropriate therapeutic intervention in this patient is administration of

(A) penicillamine
(B) desferrioxamine
(C) aglucerase
(D) leuprolide
(E) none of the above

**VI-34.** Which of the following regimens is best for the preoperative management of a patient with a known pheochromocytoma?

(A) Propranolol alone
(B) Propranolol followed by phenoxybenzamine
(C) Phenoxybenzamine followed by propranolol
(D) Prazosin alone
(E) Propranolol followed by prazosin

**VI-35.** Match the following statement with the disease it most aptly describes: A disease in which an affected person will bear, on average, both normal and affected offspring in equal proportion, with children of either sex equally likely to be affected, characterized by a delayed age of onset, and in which patients are more than 90 percent likely to have inherited an abnormal gene from a parent.

(A) Manic-depressive psychosis
(B) Myasthenia gravis
(C) Hemophilia A
(D) Neurofibromatosis
(E) Huntington's chorea

**VI-36.** Each of the following may be a direct consequence of severe magnesium deficiency EXCEPT

(A) digitalis-induced arrhythmias
(B) hypocalcemia
(C) hypokalemia
(D) hyponatremia
(E) confusion

**VI-37.** A 55-year-old woman presents to her physician with mild fatigue. Her past medical history is unremarkable. She is taking no medication. No abnormalities are detected on physical examination. The only abnormality detected on routine blood testing is an elevated calcium [2.96 mmol/L (11.9 mg/dL)] and a serum inorganic phosphorus of 0.65 mmol/L (2 mg/dL). An immunoreactive parathyroid hormone level is undetectable. The most likely etiology for this patient's high serum calcium is

(A) primary hyperparathyroidism
(B) malignancy
(C) hypervitaminosis
(D) hyperthyroidism
(E) familial hypocalciuric hypercalcemia

**VI-38.** A 64-year-old man seeks medical attention because of an annoying cough. Physical examination is remarkable only for supraclavicular lymphadenopathy. Chest x-ray shows a parahilar mass and paratracheal lymph node enlargement. Serum and urine chemistries are as follows:

Sodium: 120 mmol/L
Potassium: 4 mmol/L
Bicarbonate: 23 mmol/L
Serum osmolality: 250 mosmol/kg $H_2O$
Urine osmolality: 600 mosmol/kg $H_2O$
Urine sodium: 80 mmol/L

The most likely pathophysiologic basis for this man's hyponatremia is

(A) production of a vasopressin-like molecule by tumor tissue
(B) production of authentic vasopressin by tumor tissue
(C) potentiation of vasopressin action on the renal tubule by a tumor product
(D) stimulation of neurohypophyseal vasopressin secretion by a tumor product
(E) central nervous system metastases resulting in loss of vasopressin regulation

**VI-39.** Patients who are heterozygous for defective copies of the genes coding for either lipoprotein lipase or apoprotein CII will exhibit which of the following abnormalities?

(A) Excessive chylomicronemia
(B) Excessive amounts of low-density lipoprotein in serum
(C) Excessive amounts of very-low-density lipoprotein in serum
(D) Excessive amounts of chylomicron remnant
(E) Excessive amounts of intermediate-density lipoproteins

**VI-40.** A 32-year-old man sustains a myocardial infarction. He relates a history of early myocardial infarctions in several aunts and uncles. Moreover, it is noted that he has nodular swellings in the Achilles tendon and other tendons in the dorsum of the hand. A serum cholesterol is 10 mmol/L (400 mg/dL). A defect in which of the following proteins is the most likely etiology of this patient's clinical problem?

(A) Apoprotein E
(B) Apoprotein CII
(C) Lipoprotein lipase
(D) Lipoprotein B
(E) LDL receptor

**VI-41.** In persons with congenital adrenal hyperplasia resulting from inherited defects of adrenal steroid C-21 hydroxylase, excessive androgen production is the result of

(A) autonomous adrenal production of steroids
(B) autonomous pituitary production of ACTH
(C) extraglandular formation from large amounts of nonandrogenic adrenal steroids
(D) failure of production of an adrenal product necessary for negative feedback on pituitary ACTH secretion
(E) positive feedback on pituitary ACTH secretion by abnormal adrenal products

**VI-42.** A 38-year-old woman with obesity, dermal striae, and hypertension is referred for endocrinologic evaluation of possible cortisol excess. The woman receives a midnight dose of 1 mg of dexamethasone; a plasma cortisol level drawn at 8 A.M. the next day is 386 nmol/L (14 $\mu$g/dL). At this point in the evaluation the most appropriate diagnostic maneuver would be

(A) CT scanning of the pituitary gland
(B) abdominal CT scanning
(C) measurement of 24-h 17-hydroxycorticosteroid excretion in urine
(D) measurement of a 24-h urine free cortisol
(E) a 2-day high-dose dexamethasone suppression test (2.0 mg every 6 h for 48 h)

**VI-43.** In a 36-year-old woman who has had insulin-dependent diabetes mellitus since age 14, hyperkalemia is being evaluated. On physical examination her blood pressure is 146/96 mmHg. Laboratory evaluation discloses the following:

Fasting plasma glucose: 6 mmol/L (110 mg/dL)
Serum creatinine: 194 $\mu$mol/L (2.2 mg/dL)
Serum sodium: 135 mmol/L
Serum potassium: 6.2 mmol/L
Serum chloride: 116 mmol/L
Serum bicarbonate: 14 mmol/L

After a short ACTH infusion test, the plasma cortisol concentration increases from 386 to 717 nmol/L (14 to 26 $\mu$g/dL). After the administration of 80 mg of furosemide and 3 h of upright posture, the plasma renin activity and aldosterone concentration are unchanged from baseline values. The most appropriate therapeutic regimen to correct the electrolyte imbalance would be

(A) administration of fludrocortisone
(B) administration of furosemide
(C) administration of hydrocortisone and furosemide
(D) hemodialysis
(E) administration of potassium-binding anion-exchange resins

**VI-44.** A 22-year-old woman who has had diabetes mellitus for 6 years now wishes to become pregnant. She takes 32 units of NPH insulin each morning, and her urine glucose values (done twice daily) are "usually trace or 1+." Her hemoglobin $A_{1c}$ level is 9.8 percent (normal, 5 to 8 percent). She takes oral contraceptive pills. Her physician should advise her that

(A) home glucose monitoring and a daily regimen of multiple subcutaneous injections of regular insulin are necessary now
(B) oral contraceptive agents can falsely elevate $HbA_{1c}$ levels
(C) attempts to achieve better diabetic control can wait until she has become pregnant
(D) the current insulin regimen probably will be adequate until the last trimester of pregnancy
(E) hospitalization probably will be necessary for most of her pregnancy to ensure normal delivery and perinatal survival

**VI-45.** A 24-year-old man with diabetes since age 9 years sees his physician for a routine checkup. He has no complaints and is taking 40 units NPH and 5 units regular insulin each morning as prescribed. Ophthalmoscopic examination reveals the findings in Plate E. On the basis of these findings, his physician should recommend

(A) vitrectomy
(B) photocoagulation
(C) hypophysectomy
(D) follow-up examination in 3 months
(E) more vigorous control of the blood sugar level

**VI-46.** In a 40-year-old man with long-standing hypogonadism resulting from total surgical castration for bilateral seminomas at age 17, the effectiveness of testosterone cypionate therapy can best be monitored by the assessment of

(A) plasma testosterone level
(B) plasma luteinizing hormone (LH) level
(C) plasma testosterone cypionate level
(D) change in muscle mass
(E) frequency of nocturnal erections

**VI-47.** During a routine checkup, a 67-year-old man is found to have a level of serum alkaline phosphatase three times the upper limit of normal. Serum calcium and phosphorus concentrations and liver function test results are normal. He is asymptomatic. The most likely diagnosis is

(A) metastatic bone disease
(B) primary hyperparathyroidism
(C) occult plasmacytoma
(D) Paget's disease of bone
(E) osteomalacia

**VI-48.** The most important regulator of serum $1,25(OH)_2$ vitamin D concentration is

(A) serum calcium
(B) serum magnesium
(C) serum 25(OH) vitamin D
(D) parathyroid hormone
(E) prolactin

**VI-49.** Diseases inherited in a multifactorial genetic fashion (i.e., not autosomal dominant, autosomal recessive, or X-linked) and seen more frequently in persons bearing certain histocompatibility antigens include

(A) gluten-sensitive enteropathy
(B) neurofibromatosis
(C) adult polycystic kidney disease
(D) Wilson's disease
(E) cystic fibrosis

**VI-50.** A 20-year-old competitive swimmer is examined because of primary amenorrhea. Her height is 170 cm (67 in.), and she weighs 50 kg (110 lb). Her breasts are well developed. Findings on pelvic examination are normal, and the pubic hair appears to be normal. Cervical mucus is abundant and demonstrates ferning on drying. Urine spot and blood tests for pregnancy are negative. She is given 10 mg of medroxyprogesterone acetate twice a day for 5 days, and 3 days later she experiences menstrual bleeding for the first time. The most likely cause of the amenorrhea is

(A) functional hypothalamic amenorrhea
(B) 45,X gonadal dysgenesis
(C) polycystic ovarian disease
(D) chromaphobe adenoma of the pituitary
(E) prolactinoma of the pituitary

**VI-51.** A 21-year-old woman is examined because of secondary amenorrhea. Cyclic menses had commenced at age 14 years. When she was 19 years old she became pregnant and was hospitalized during the sixth month of that pregnancy because of bleeding and hypotension that proved to be the result of a spontaneous abortion with retained placental fragments; she received 10 units of blood, and a dilation and curettage was performed. No menses have occurred during the 2 years since the hospitalization. She now wishes to become pregnant.

Findings on physical examination, including a rectopelvic examination, are normal. Results on complete blood counts, SMA-12, and chest x-ray are within normal limits. Serum thyroid-stimulating hormone concentration is 1.5 mU/L and an 8 A.M. plasma cortisol measurement is 470 nmol/L (17 μg/dL). No menstrual bleeding occurs after the administration of 10 mg medroxyprogesterone acetate per day for 10 days or cyclic estrogen and progestogen (1.25 mg conjugated estrogens by mouth each day for 3 weeks with 10 mg medroxyprogesterone acetate per day for the last 7 days). At this point the most appropriate diagnostic study would be

(A) CT scan of the pituitary with contrast
(B) CT scan of the abdomen followed by wedge resection of the ovaries
(C) hysterosalpingography
(D) metyrapone test
(E) chromosomal analysis

**VI-52.** A 36-year-old woman has noticed the absence of menses for the last 4 months. A pregnancy test is negative. Serum levels of luteinizing hormone and follicle-stimulating hormone are elevated, and the serum estradiol level is low. These findings suggest

(A) bilateral tubal obstruction
(B) panhypopituitarism
(C) polycystic ovarian disease
(D) premature menopause
(E) exogenous estrogen administration

**VI-53.** A newborn infant with ambiguous genitalia develops vomiting and profound volume depletion. A diagnosis of congenital adrenal hyperplasia resulting from C-21 hydroxylase deficiency would be supported by all the following findings EXCEPT

(A) elevated urinary 17-ketosteroid concentration
(B) elevated plasma 11-deoxycortisol concentration
(C) elevated plasma 17-hydroxyprogesterone concentration
(D) elevated plasma androstenedione concentration
(E) elevated urinary pregnanediol and pregnanetriol concentrations

**VI-54.** In women with gonadal dysgenesis, development of malignancy in the streak gonads is most likely to occur when the karyotype is

(A) 46XX$_i$ (isochrome X)
(B) 46,XX
(C) 45,X
(D) 45,X/46,XY mosaicism
(E) 45X,46XX mosaicism

**VI-55.** The most common presentation of primary hyperparathyroidism is

(A) bone fracture
(B) increased serum creatinine
(C) osteitis fibrosa cystica
(D) calcium kidney stones
(E) asymptomatic hypercalcemia

**VI-56.** A 34-year-old woman has had three hospital admissions during the last year because of nephrolithiasis. The rate of 24-h urinary calcium excretion has been above the normal range on all three occasions, and serum calcium concentrations were between 2.5 and 2.8 mmol/L (10.2 and 11.5 mg/dL). The serum phosphorus concentration was 0.77 mmol/L (2.4 mg/dL), and the parathyroid hormone level was 229 nL eq/mL (normal, less than 150 nL eq/mL). The most appropriate management at this time would be

(A) to begin administration of prednisone, 40 mg daily, and taper the dose over a period of 4 weeks
(B) to administer thiazide diuretics to decrease calcium excretion
(C) symptomatic treatment of renal lithiasis only
(D) calcium supplementation to prevent progressive bone loss
(E) surgical exploration of the neck

**VI-57.** Which of the following conditions is LEAST likely to cause hyperthyroidism associated with low thyroidal radioactive iodine uptake (RAIU)?

(A) Subacute thyroiditis
(B) Struma ovarii
(C) Choriocarcinoma
(D) Ingestion of exogenous levothyroxine
(E) Recent intravenous pyelography

**VI-58.** Each of the following conditions is characteristic of the presentation of osteomalacia in adults EXCEPT

(A) bowing of the tibia
(B) pseudofractures
(C) long-bone pain
(D) proximal muscle weakness
(E) hypophosphatemia

**VI-59.** A 61-year-old woman noticed severe sharp pain in her back after lifting a suitcase. A compression fracture of the T11 vertebral body is identified on x-ray examination. Routine laboratory evaluation discloses a serum calcium concentration of 2 mmol/L (8.0 mg/dL), a serum phosphorus concentration of 0.77 mmol/L (2.4 mg/dL), and increased serum alkaline phosphatase activity. The serum parathyroid hormone level was subsequently found to be elevated as well. The most likely diagnosis is

(A) Paget's disease of bone
(B) ectopic parathyroid hormone secretion
(C) primary hyperparathyroidism
(D) postmenopausal osteoporosis
(E) vitamin D deficiency

**VI-60.** A 60-year-old woman has lower-back pain. Radiographic examination reveals diffuse demineralization and a compression fracture of the fourth lumbar vertebra. The serum calcium concentration is 2.8 mmol/L (11.5 mg/dL). The blood count is normal. This clinical picture is most compatible with the presence of which of the following conditions?

(A) Postmenopausal osteoporosis
(B) Paget's disease
(C) Primary hyperparathyroidism
(D) Multiple myeloma
(E) Osteomalacia

**VI-61.** Which of the following conditions is LEAST likely to be associated with a low serum 25(OH) vitamin D level?

(A) Dietary deficiency of vitamin D
(B) Chronic severe cholestatic liver disease
(C) Chronic renal failure
(D) Anticonvulsant therapy with phenobarbital or phenytoin
(E) High-dose glucocorticoid therapy

**VI-62.** In a person with severe protein starvation, which of the following conditions would be LEAST likely to increase the amount of protein needed to achieve positive nitrogen balance?

(A) Renal failure
(B) Gastrointestinal fistula
(C) Sepsis
(D) Simultaneous caloric malnutrition
(E) Thyrotoxicosis

**VI-63.** A 25-year-old previously healthy woman develops Sheehan's syndrome (infarction of the pituitary) after an intrapartum hemorrhage. Which of the following tests will be abnormal the day after her pituitary ceases to function?

(A) Total $T_3$
(B) ACTH stimulation test
(C) Total $T_4$
(D) IGF-I
(E) Insulin tolerance test

**VI-64.** Four weeks postpartum, a 32-year-old woman develops palpitations, heat intolerance, and nervousness. She is diagnosed with hyperthyroidism. Her thyroid is not enlarged or tender. The 24-h uptake of radioactive iodine is 1 percent. The most appropriate treatment for this woman is

(A) radioactive iodine ablation of her thyroid gland
(B) methimazole
(C) prednisone 60 mg a day followed by a rapid taper
(D) a beta blocker
(E) iodine drops (SSKI)

**VI-65.** A 23-year-old woman is diagnosed with Graves' disease shortly after discovering she is pregnant. Appropriate therapy includes

(A) radioactive iodine to ablate her thyroid gland
(B) propylthiouracil therapy with the goal of maintaining her thyroid function tests in the high-normal or slightly high range
(C) methimazole therapy
(D) a beta blocker
(E) propylthiouracil therapy with care taken to maintain her thyroid function tests in the mid-normal range

**VI-66.** A 33-year-old healthy woman who is taking no medications develops amenorrhea and galactorrhea. Her prolactin level is 45 ng/mL. IGF-I and 24-h free cortisol measurements are normal. MRI reveals a 2.5-cm by 2.0-cm sellar mass which nearly abuts the optic chiasm. Formal visual fields are normal. Probable diagnosis and appropriate treatment are

(A) prolactinoma requiring immediate surgery
(B) prolactinoma requiring treatment with a dopamine agonist
(C) nonfunctioning pituitary adenoma requiring surgery
(D) prolactinoma requiring serial MRIs plus oral contraceptives
(E) nonfunctioning pituitary adenoma requiring serial MRIs plus oral contraceptives

**VI-67.** An 81-year-old man is found by his family to be disoriented and confused. In the emergency room, he is found to be hypoglycemic. He is afebrile, but his physical exam is otherwise normal. A bolus of intravenous dextrose is administered, and the patient quickly recovers. His glucose is 122 mg/dL, and his neurologic exam has returned to baseline. Further history reveals that the patient has type 2 diabetes mellitus, for which he takes a sulfonylurea. He also has a history of congestive heart failure, for which he was hospitalized three times last year. Which of the following statements reflects appropriate management?

(A) He should be hospitalized
(B) The sulfonylurea should be discontinued and replaced with metformin, a medication which does not cause hypoglycemia
(C) The patient may be discharged from the emergency room without further intervention
(D) The patient may be discharged from the emergency room on a reduced dose of sulfonylurea
(E) He should undergo a workup for a possible insulinoma

**VI-68.** Causes of hypertriglyceridemia include all the following EXCEPT

(A) alcohol
(B) diabetes mellitus
(C) obesity
(D) cigarette smoking
(E) pregnancy

**VI-69.** A 70-year-old woman has a quantitative digital radiography (QDR) bone density test. She is found to have a bone density more than two standard deviations below the average peak bone mass (*t*-score) and below the average age-matched bone density (*z*-score). All the following could be part of an appropriate therapeutic plan EXCEPT

(A) alendronate
(B) estrogen
(C) weight-bearing exercise
(D) pamidronate
(E) nasal calcitonin

**VI-70.** A 41-year-old previously healthy woman presents to an emergency room complaining of nausea and vomiting. Her calcium is found to be 11.7 mg/dL with an albumin of 4.0 g/dL. Hyperparathyroidism is diagnosed, and an exploration of her four parathyroid glands reveals one large parathyroid tumor, which is removed. One day after the operation the patient complains of paresthesias in her hands and around her mouth. Her calcium is 7.3 mg/dL. Her phosphorus is 1.8 mg/dL. Four months later she still requires aggressive calcium and vitamin D supplementation. The most likely etiology of her hypocalcemia is

(A) hypoparathyroidism secondary to inadvertent surgical removal of all four parathyroid glands
(B) hypoparathyroidism secondary to atrophy of the three remaining parathyroid glands
(C) hungry bone syndrome
(D) parathyroid cancer
(E) magnesium deficiency

**VI-71.** Six hours after a transsphenoidal resection of his growth hormone–secreting tumor, a 33-year-old man complains of increased thirst. His urine output has been 350 mL/h for the last 2 h. Urine specific gravity is 1.001, and urine osmolality is 210 mmol/kg. A serum sodium is 147 mg/dL. Appropriate management at this time includes

(A) administering 2 μg DDAVP subcutaneously once and encouraging the patient to drink water when thirsty
(B) performing a water deprivation test
(C) placing the patient on 500mL/d fluid restriction
(D) administering 2μg DDAVP subcutaneously BID and encouraging the patient to drink water when thirsty
(E) obtaining an MRI of the brain

**VI-72.** A 73-year-old man in the intensive care unit is suspected of having panhypopituitarism. He is hypotensive and is not responding to antibiotics or pressors. He reports lack of libido, fatigue, cold intolerance, and recent weight gain. His cortisol is 135 nmol/L (4.8 $\mu$g/dL), TSH 0.3 $\mu$U/mL, $T_4$ 289 nmol/L (4.5 $\mu$g/dL), total $T_3$ 0.63 nmol/L (40 ng/mL), $T_3$RU 26 percent, LH 0.2 IU/L, FSH 0.5 IU/L, GH 2 $\mu$g/L. Testosterone is below normal. What conclusions can you make about this patient's pituitary function?

(A) He has panhypopituitarism. He should be started immediately on 100 mg hydrocortisone intravenously q 6 h, levothyroxine, and testosterone.

(B) He has normal pituitary function, and other reasons for his symptoms should be investigated.

(C) The status of his pituitary-adrenal axis is unclear. He should be given dexamethasone, and a cosyntropin stimulation test should be performed. Thyroid hormone and testosterone replacement are unnecessary.

(D) The status of his pituitary-adrenal axis is unclear. He should be given dexamethasone, and a cosyntropin stimulation test should be performed. Thyroid hormone and testosterone replacement should be started.

(E) He has panhypopituitarism. He should be started immediately on 100 mg hydrocortisone intravenously q 6 h and levothyroxine. The testosterone replacement can wait until he is out of the intensive care unit.

**VI-73.** A 73-year-old woman is admitted to the hospital with chest pain. An astute intern sends her for thyroid function tests after learning that the patient has gained 50 lb over the last year and suffers from cold intolerance. Cardiac catheterization reveals three-vessel disease, and coronary artery bypass is recommended. While preparing the patient for surgery the next day, the intern checks the thyroid function tests. The TSH is 81 mU/mL. What course of action is most appropriate?

(A) Postpone the surgery, start levothyroxine replacement at 0.025 mg/d, and increase the dose slowly. When the patient is euthyroid, recommend surgery.

(B) Give $T_3$ to make the patient euthyroid quickly so that surgery need be postponed no more than a week.

(C) Proceed to surgery as scheduled. Start levothyroxine postoperatively.

(D) Check a cosyntropin stimulation test, because she may have hypopituitarism and surgery may be dangerous without glucocorticoid replacement.

(E) Start propylthiouracil therapy before surgery.

**VI-74.** A 32-year-old woman is diagnosed as having Cushing's disease. A transsphenoidal procedure is performed. Two days after the surgery a 24-h urine free cortisol is 5.5 nmol/d (2 $\mu$g/d). Six weeks later, a repeat 24-h urine free cortisol is 8.3 nmol/d (3 $\mu$g/d). Her thyroid function tests are normal. What is the most likely explanation for these results, and what therapy should be initiated?

(A) The patient's Cushing's disease is cured, and she needs no further therapy.

(B) The patient's Cushing's disease is cured, and she should be treated with corticosteroids.

(C) The patient still has Cushing's disease.

(D) The patient never had Cushing's disease.

(E) The surgeon has inadvertently induced permanent adrenal insufficiency by removing normal pituitary tissue. She requires treatment with corticosteroids.

**VI-75.** A 45-year-old woman presents with weakness, central obesity, wide purple striae, and facial plethora. She is not taking exogenous corticosteroids. She does not drink alcohol. She is not depressed, though she complains of insomnia. A 1-mg dexamethasone suppression test is performed. The patient's 8 A.M. cortisol after receiving the dexamethasone at midnight the night before is 303.5 nmol/L (11 $\mu$g/dL). A 24-h urine free cortisol is 580 nmol/d (210 $\mu$g/d). A high-dose dexamethasone suppression test (2 mg q 6 hours $\times$ 2 days) is performed. The 24-h urine free cortisol on the second day is 50 nmol/d (18 $\mu$g/d). Where is the tumor which is causing the Cushing's syndrome?

(A) Pituitary
(B) Adrenal gland
(C) Ectopic
(D) It is unclear from the information given. The tumor could be in the pituitary or could be ectopic.
(E) It is unclear from the information given. The tumor could be in the adrenal gland or could be ectopic.

**VI-76.** A 64-year-old man is admitted with angina and found to be hyperthyroid. He is scheduled for a cardiac catheterization. What effect is the procedure likely to have on his thyroid function?

(A) None
(B) Exacerbate the hyperthyroidism
(C) Improve the hyperthyroidism
(D) If the hyperthyroidism is secondary to Graves' disease, it may improve; if it is secondary to toxic multinodular goiter, the hyperthyroidism may worsen
(E) If the patient has Graves' disease, the hyperthyroidism may worsen; if he has toxic multinodular goiter, it may improve

**VI-77.** A 25-year-old female nurse presents with palpitations and heat intolerance. Her thyroid is not painful. TSH is less than 0.01 mU/L, free $T_4$ is 243 nmol/L (19 μg/dL), $T_3$ resin uptake is 38 percent, and total $T_3$ is 3.6 nmol/L (230 ng/dL). The 24-h radioactive iodine uptake is 0 percent. Thyroglobulin is low. What is the most likely diagnosis?

(A) Graves' disease
(B) Silent thyroiditis
(C) Subacute thyroiditis
(D) Toxic multinodular goiter
(E) Thyrotoxicosis factitia

**VI-78.** All the following are indications for parathyroidectomy in patients with hyperparathyroidism EXCEPT

(A) kidney stones
(B) advanced age
(C) osteoporosis
(D) calcium level >2.85 mmol/L (11.5 mg/dL)
(E) decreased creatinine clearance

**VI-79.** All the following are true statements concerning multiple endocrine neoplasia type I (MEN I) EXCEPT

(A) its mode of inheritance is autosomal dominant
(B) hyperparathyroidism is its most common manifestation
(C) it is caused by a mutation in the c-RET proto-oncogene
(D) the hyperparathyroidism usually is caused by four-gland hyperplasia, not by an adenoma
(E) pituitary tumors occur in more than half of MEN I patients

**VI-80.** A 19-year-old man with type I diabetes mellitus presents to the emergency room with nausea and vomiting. His arterial pH is 7.16 with potassium of 5.4 mmol/L, bicarbonate of 7 mmol/L, sodium of 132 mmol/L, and glucose of 26 mmol/L (475 mg/dL). Appropriate management of this case probably would include the administration of all the following EXCEPT

(A) bicarbonate
(B) potassium
(C) insulin
(D) intravenous dextrose
(E) intravenous fluids

**VI-81.** Patients with polyglandular autoimmune syndrome type II (Schmidt's syndrome) often manifest all the following EXCEPT

(A) diabetes mellitus
(B) mucocutaneous candidiasis
(C) adrenal insufficiency
(D) gonadal failure
(E) hypothyroidism

**VI-82.** Common causes of hypoglycemia in hospitalized patients include all the following EXCEPT

(A) insulin
(B) sulfonylureas
(C) alcohol
(D) adrenal insufficiency
(E) renal failure

**VI-83.** All the following are characteristics of generalized lipodystrophy (also called lipoatrophic diabetes) EXCEPT

(A) the acquired form often develops after an infectious illness
(B) the congenital form is autosomal recessive
(C) loss of body fat is the central feature
(D) metabolic abnormalities such as insulin resistance, hyperglycemia, and hypertriglyceridemia are characteristic
(E) linear growth is retarded during childhood

**VI-84.** A 24-year-old woman with type I diabetes mellitus presents with 6 h of vomiting. She is diagnosed with diabetic ketoacidosis (DKA). On presentation to the hospital, her arterial pH is 7.20, her glucose is 24 mmol/L (430 mg/dL), her potassium is 5.7 mmol/L, and her serum inorganic phosphorus is 1.2 mmol/L (3.6 mg/dL). However, after the initiation of treatment for DKA, the serum inorganic phosphorus quickly falls to 0.43 mmol/L. Which of the following statements is true?

(A) She probably has severe phosphorus deficiency
(B) Phosphorus therapy should be administered
(C) Most patients with DKA are severely depleted of phosphorus
(D) The fact that her serum inorganic phosphorus concentration was high on presentation is reassuring
(E) Patients with DKA and severe phosphorus deficiency usually have been vomiting for several days before presentation

**VI-85.** Causes of hypomagnesemia include all the following EXCEPT

(A) beta blockers
(B) chronic pancreatic insufficiency
(C) poorly controlled diabetes mellitus
(D) alcoholism
(E) aminoglycosides

**VI-86.** Causes of hypercholesterolemia include all the following EXCEPT

(A) nephrotic syndrome
(B) anorexia nervosa
(C) thiazides
(D) progestogens
(E) hyperthyroidism

**VI-87.** All the following are forms or complications of simple (background) diabetic retinopathy EXCEPT

(A) increased capillary permeability
(B) retinal detachment
(C) microaneurysms
(D) cotton-wool spots
(E) dot and blot hemorrhages

**VI-88.** A 75-year-old man with type II diabetes mellitus presents with severe ear pain, drainage, fever, and leukocytosis. In addition, he has facial nerve paralysis and there is soft tissue swelling around the ear. All the following are true statements about his condition EXCEPT

(A) it usually is caused by *Pseudomonas aeruginosa*
(B) the mortality rate is 50 percent
(C) a 4-week course of ticarcillin or carbenicillin plus tobramycin is the treatment of choice
(D) surgical debridement may be necessary
(E) a mound of granulation tissue usually is present at the junction of the osseous and cartilaginous portions of the ear

**VI-89.** All the following are characteristic of an infection with rhinocerebral mucormycosis EXCEPT

(A) it usually develops during or after an episode of diabetic ketoacidosis (DKA)
(B) it is a rare fungal infection
(C) if it is not treated, death usually occurs in a week to 10 days
(D) it often presents with pain, periorbital and perinasal swelling, and decreased lacrimation
(E) it usually is treated with aggressive debridement and amphotericin B

**VI-90.** All the following interact with seven-transmembrane-domain receptors EXCEPT

(A) insulin
(B) LH
(C) TSH
(D) parathyroid hormone
(E) epinephrine

**VI-91.** All the following medications are known to cause hyperprolactinemia EXCEPT

(A) metoclopramide
(B) levothyroxine
(C) haloperidol
(D) reserpine
(E) cocaine

**VI-92.** All the following medications are known to cause hypoglycemia EXCEPT

(A) sulfonamides
(B) pentamidine
(C) propranolol
(D) salicylates
(E) thiazides

**DIRECTIONS:** Each question below contains five suggested responses. For **each** of the five responses listed with each item, you are to respond either YES (Y) or NO (N). In a given item **all, some, or none** of the alternatives may be correct.

**VI-93.**  Anovulatory cycles are characterized by

(A)  elevated levels of plasma progesterone
(B)  dysmenorrhea
(C)  an absent luteal phase
(D)  lack of a normal LH and FSH surge
(E)  irregular uterine bleeding

**VI-94.**  A 15-year-old boy has had hypothyroidism since early childhood. For several years he has noticed frequent episodes of numbness and tingling of his hands, occasionally accompanied by muscle spasms. Physical examination reveals a positive Chvostek sign, short stature, and short left fourth metacarpals (absent knuckles). The boy's mother is also short and has absent knuckles. Serum calcium concentration is 1.9 mmol/L (7.5 mg/dL). Further investigation of the boy's disorder would be expected to reveal

(A)  antibodies to parathyroid and thyroid tissue
(B)  elevated parathyroid hormone concentration
(C)  a diminished increase in urinary cyclic AMP in response to the administration of parathyroid hormone
(D)  calcification of the basal ganglia
(E)  moniliasis

**VI-95.**  Protein malnutrition commonly occurs in association with energy-deficient diets because

(A)  diets low in carbohydrate and fat cause acute protein malabsorption
(B)  amino acids are diverted from protein synthesis into oxidative metabolism
(C)  normal protein synthesis requires an adequate energy supply
(D)  normal protein metabolism occurs only if fat in the diet is adequate
(E)  it is common for diets to be deficient in both protein and energy

**VI-96.**  Appropriate dietary restrictions have been successful in treating patients who have which of the following inherited metabolic disorders?

(A)  Phenylketonuria
(B)  Familial lipoprotein lipase deficiency
(C)  Hyperprolinemia
(D)  Tay-Sachs disease
(E)  Galactosemia

**VI-97.**  A 34-year-old man with alcoholic cirrhosis is admitted to the hospital for evaluation of abdominal swelling, which has become progressively worse over the last 2 weeks. On physical examination he is noted to be cachectic; the liver is enlarged, ascites and edema are present, and stool is heme-positive. Measurement of which of the following parameters would be useful in determining the extent of this man's protein malnutrition?

(A)  Blood ammonia concentration
(B)  Serum albumin and transferrin levels
(C)  Present body weight as a percentage of ideal body weight
(D)  Midarm circumference and triceps skin-fold thickness
(E)  Ratio of 24-h creatinine excretion to height

**VI-98.**  In which of the following situations is total parenteral nutrition (TPN) indicated as the first choice to provide partial or complete nourishment?

(A)  A 34-year-old man has an acute exacerbation of Crohn's disease and develops an ileocolic fistula
(B)  A 70-year-old woman has chest and limb injuries and extensive burns after an airplane crash
(C)  A 26-year-old woman has extensive small-bowel resection for life-threatening regional enteritis
(D)  A 53-year-old man scheduled to undergo elective surgery for gallstones will be unable to eat or drink for 5 days
(E)  A 26-year-old woman is unable to swallow because of a relapse of myasthenia gravis

**VI-99.**  In a patient with hypercholesterolemia, which of the following may be an appropriate treatment to lower the serum cholesterol concentration?

(A)  Cholestyramine
(B)  Nicotinic acid
(C)  Lovastatin
(D)  Gemfibrozil
(E)  A low-cholesterol diet

**VI-100.** Hypertriglyceridemia is frequently encountered in patients with diabetes mellitus. True statements regarding this association include which of the following?

(A) The predisposition to both diseases may be independently inherited

(B) Insulin deficiency is a major factor contributing to the hypertriglyceridemia

(C) Some patients eventually need specific pharmacologic treatment for the hypertriglyceridemia

(D) Acute pancreatitis may occur with uncontrolled diabetes mellitus and elevation of triglyceride levels

(E) Hypertriglyceridemia may resolve with adequate control of the diabetes

**VI-101.** Characteristic manifestations of Nelson's syndrome (a pituitary tumor arising after bilateral adrenalectomy) include

(A) hyperpigmentation

(B) erosion of the sella turcica

(C) increased urinary 17-ketosteroid excretion

(D) failure of high doses of dexamethasone to suppress plasma cortisol levels

(E) elevated plasma ACTH levels

**VI-102.** In a person who has Cushing's syndrome, the diagnosis of functioning adrenal carcinoma would be suggested by

(A) a palpable abdominal mass

(B) markedly increased urinary excretion of 17-ketosteroids

(C) high plasma levels of ACTH

(D) failure to suppress 17-hydroxycorticosteroid secretion with high-dose dexamethasone

(E) failure to suppress urine free cortisol with low-dose dexamethasone

**VI-103.** A 30-year-old man, the father of three children, has had progressive breast enlargement during the last 6 months. He does not use any drugs. Physical examination is remarkable only for bilateral gynecomastia; testicular size is normal. Evaluation at this time might include

(A) blood sampling for SGOT and serum alkaline phosphatase and bilirubin levels

(B) blood sampling for plasma estradiol, testosterone, and human chorionic gonadotropin levels

(C) a 24-h urine collection for the measurement of 17-ketosteroids

(D) chromosomal karyotype

(E) breast biopsy

**VI-104.** True statements concerning type 1 diabetes mellitus include which of the following?

(A) Direct vertical transmission has been shown by pedigree analysis to occur with a high prevalence

(B) The concordance rate for monozygotic twins less than 40 years of age is over 80 percent

(C) The risk of type 1 diabetes is increased in persons carrying HLA antigens B8, B15, DR3, or DR4

(D) Circulating islet cell antibodies usually are present in patients with juvenile-onset type 1 diabetes studied soon before or soon after the onset of symptoms

(E) Mumps virus and coxsackievirus have been identified as possible causative agents in juvenile-onset type 1 diabetes

**VI-105.** The diagnosis of diabetes mellitus is certain in which of the following situations?

(A) Abnormal oral glucose tolerance in a 24-year-old woman who has been dieting

(B) Successive fasting plasma glucose concentrations of 8, 9, and 8.5 mmol/L (147, 165, and 152 mg/dL) in an asymptomatic, otherwise healthy businesswoman

(C) Hyperglycemic ketoacidosis that developed in an 18-year-old man after surgical reduction of a fractured leg

(D) Persistent asymptomatic glycosuria in a 30-year-old woman

(E) Hyperglycemic hyperosmolar coma that developed in a 73-year-old man after a stroke

**VI-106.** Characteristics of hyperosmolar coma include

(A) blood glucose concentration greater than 33 mmol/L (600 mg/dL)

(B) marked elevation of serum free fatty acids

(C) association with thrombosis and bleeding from disseminated intravascular coagulation

(D) occurrence in elderly persons with maturity-onset diabetes

(E) best initial therapeutic response with large volumes of free water and large doses of insulin

**VI-107.** A 45-year-old woman has had diabetes for the last 8 years and has been treated with either oral hypoglycemic agents or insulin. She has been doing well on human NPH insulin for the last several months. However, in the last week she has developed symptoms of hyperglycemia. Doubling her insulin dose does not help, and she is admitted to the hospital. Physical examination of this nonobese woman shows no sign of infection, ketoacidosis, or Cushing's syndrome. After admission, the insulin dose is increased progressively to 240 units daily, but blood glucose concentration never falls below 19 mmol/L (350 mg/dL). True statements regarding this woman's condition include which of the following?

(A) IgG anti-insulin antibodies are likely to be present in high titer
(B) Cell-surface insulin receptors are likely to be decreased in number
(C) Anti-insulin-receptor antibodies, increased erythrocyte sedimentation rate, and other signs of autoimmune disease are likely to be present
(D) Insulin desensitization procedures should be instituted
(E) Treatment should include high-dose prednisone

**VI-108.** Which of the following would be associated with a poor prognosis for the development of (or progression of) symptomatic renal failure in a 29-year-old woman who has had type 1 diabetes mellitus since the age of 14 years?

(A) Urine albumin excretion of 0.12 to 0.17 g/d on three separate occasions
(B) Urine protein excretion of 0.55 to 0.62 g/d on three separate occasions
(C) Diastolic blood pressure of 110 to 123 mmHg
(D) Nocturia, three times per night
(E) Insulin requirement greater than 120 units per day

**VI-109.** A 40-year-old physician's assistant has had episodic confusion, diaphoresis, and palpitations for the past 4 weeks. She has had several nightmares and three syncopal episodes. Fasting hypoglycemia with inappropriately elevated plasma insulin concentration is documented in the hospital. Plasma C-peptide concentration also is increased. Her physician should

(A) measure plasma insulin antibody levels
(B) measure plasma proinsulin levels
(C) measure plasma or urine sulfonylurea levels
(D) perform an abdominal CT scan
(E) consult a surgeon for pancreatic surgery

**VI-110.** Causes of fasting hypoglycemia that are due primarily to overutilization of glucose include

(A) carnitine deficiency
(B) hepatoma
(C) insulinoma
(D) congestive heart failure from cor pulmonale
(E) hypopituitarism

**VI-111.** Testosterone replacement in a patient with Klinefelter syndrome (47,XXY) would be indicated in order to

(A) maintain spermatogenesis
(B) prevent antisocial behavior
(C) maintain sexual potency
(D) cause the disappearance of gynecomastia
(E) promote virilization

**VI-112.** Correctly matched deficiencies of specific trace elements and their recognized features include

(A) zinc deficiency: hyperkeratosis and alopecia
(B) zinc deficiency: gonadal atrophy
(C) copper deficiency: fever
(D) cobalt deficiency: anemia
(E) selenium deficiency: heart failure

**VI-113.** Increased gonadal production of estrogen is characteristic of

(A) testicular feminization
(B) polycystic ovarian disease
(C) persistent follicle cyst
(D) third trimester of pregnancy
(E) arrhenoblastoma

**VI-114.** Known causes of ambiguous genitalia include

(A) the sex-chromosome pattern XYY
(B) the mosaic sex-chromosome pattern 45,X/46,XY
(C) single-gene mutations that impair androgen action
(D) hypogonadotropic hypogonadism
(E) maternal ingestion of a virilizing drug during pregnancy

**VI-115.** True statements describing persons who have Klinefelter syndrome include which of the following?

(A) They are 20 times as likely as normal men to develop breast cancer
(B) They may have a normal peripheral-blood karyotype and testes of average size
(C) They have an increased incidence of hypospadias
(D) They almost always are mentally deficient and socially maladjusted
(E) Diagnosis usually is not made until after puberty

**VI-116.** A 40-year-old woman with known alcoholism is hospitalized because of dizziness and muscle aches. Serum phosphorus concentration is 0.3 mmol/L (0.9 mg/dL) several days after admission. Clinical signs and symptoms associated with hypophosphatemia include

(A) waddling gait
(B) irritability and apprehension
(C) elevated concentration of serum creatine phosphokinase
(D) bacterial infection
(E) congestive cardiomyopathy

**VI-117.** Correct statements concerning hypervitaminosis D include which of the following?

(A) It may result from prolonged sun exposure.
(B) It usually results from a single excessive dose of vitamin $D_2$ or $D_3$.
(C) The consequences include hypercalcemia, hypercalciuria, and renal impairment.
(D) Anephric patients can develop vitamin D toxicity.
(E) Serum 1,25(OH) vitamin D levels are elevated.

**VI-118.** A 25-year-old woman presents to her internist complaining of fatigue. Although she does not seem to be depressed, she admits to a diminished appetite and loss of interest in sex. She is also intolerant of the cold and notes that her hair is falling out. She has trouble caring for her 1½-year-old child and recounts a very difficult parturition with a great deal of blood loss. She is on no medicines, has been amenorrheic since the birth of the child, and did not nurse the infant. Which of the following tests would help diagnose her problem?

(A) Measurement of growth hormone 1 h after insulin administration
(B) Measurement of plasma cortisol 1 h after insulin administration
(C) Measurement of urinary free cortisol
(D) Thyroid function tests and TSH
(E) ACTH stimulation test

**VI-119.** Manifestations of hypothyroidism include

(A) diminished QRS voltage on ECG
(B) depressed serum cholesterol
(C) microcytic anemia
(D) increased serum creatine phosphokinase
(E) increased serum lactic dehydrogenase

**VI-120.** A 25-year-old man presents with a several-month history of fatigue, weakness, anorexia, and nausea. Physical examination reveals a slightly emaciated, thin, tanned man whose baseline blood pressure is 90/60. He complains of extreme light-headedness during the assessment of orthostatic vital signs. Laboratory evaluation reveals hyponatremia and hyperkalemia. The plasma cortisol level fails to rise significantly 60 min after intramuscular administration of 250 μg cosyntropin. Which of the following conditions could have caused this clinical picture?

(A) Withdrawal from prolonged (> 1 year) administration of steroids for asthma
(B) Disseminated tuberculosis
(C) Craniopharyngioma
(D) Disseminated cytomegalovirus infection
(E) Esophageal candidiasis requiring long-term high-dose ketoconazole therapy

**VI-121.** Established complications of oral contraceptive use include

(A) deep venous thrombosis
(B) thromboembolic stroke
(C) hypertension
(D) endometrial cancer
(E) breast cancer

**VI-122.** In which of the following porphyria syndromes may the diagnosis be made on the basis of a positive Watson-Schwartz reaction in the urine (detection of porphobilinogen)?

(A) Intermittent acute porphyria
(B) Congenital erythropoietic porphyria
(C) Protoporphyria
(D) Porphyria cutanea tarda
(E) Variegate porphyria

**VI-123.** Correct statements concerning inherited defects of metabolism include which of the following?

(A) Niemann-Pick disease is caused by a deficiency of glucosylceramidase and is associated with a characteristic bone marrow storage cell
(B) The incidence of disease resulting from hexosaminidase deficiency has been reduced in North America by heterozygote detection programs
(C) Errors in glycogen elongation or branching are incompatible with a normal life expectancy
(D) Early diagnosis of phenylketonuria is possible but is of little therapeutic benefit
(E) Cystinuria, the most common inborn error of amino acid transport, is associated with increased urinary excretion of all dibasic amino acids

# VI. ENDOCRINE, METABOLIC, AND GENETIC DISORDERS

## ANSWERS

**VI-1. The answer is B.** *(Chap. 342)* In persons with symptomatic hemochromatosis, repeated phlebotomy, by removing excessive iron stores, results in marked clinical improvement. Specifically, the liver and spleen decrease in size, liver function improves, cardiac failure is reversed, and skin pigmentation ("bronzing") diminishes. Carbohydrate intolerance may abate in up to half of all affected persons. For unknown reasons, there is no improvement in the arthropathy or hypogonadism (resulting from pituitary deposition of iron) associated with hemochromatosis. The 5-year survival rate increases from 33 to 90 percent with treatment; prolonged survival may actually increase the risk of hepatocellular carcinoma, which affects one-third of persons treated for hemochromatosis. However, if phlebotomy is begun in the precirrhotic stage, which is possible with effective genetic screening, liver cancer will not develop.

**VI-2. The answer is B.** *(Chap. 334)* Although non-insulin-dependent diabetes mellitus disease (nonketogenic) is familial, the exact mode of inheritance is not known except for the specific variant known as maturity-onset diabetes of the young (MODY), which is manifested by mild hyperglycemia without ketosis. On the basis of family studies, this disease is inherited in an autosomal dominant fashion with almost complete penetrance. Therefore, 50 percent of the children of a diabetic parent with MODY will develop the disease. There is linkage between MODY and mutations in the glucokinase gene on the short arm of chromosome 7. This abnormality is not present in ordinary nonketotic diabetics. Unlike the case in insulin-dependent diabetes, no HLA relationships have been identified. Moreover, an autoimmune etiology for the disease is not felt to be important; this is also a distinctive feature compared with typical juvenile-onset insulin-dependent diabetes.

**VI-3. The answer is C.** *(Chap. 334. Nathan, N Engl J Med 328:1676–1685, 1993.)* Nephropathy is a leading cause of death in diabetic patients. Diabetic nephropathy may be functionally silent for 10 to 15 years. Clinically detectable diabetic nephropathy begins with the development of microalbuminuria (30 to 300 mg of albumin per 24 h). The glomerular filtration rate actually may be elevated at this stage. Only after the passage of additional time will the proteinuria be overt enough (0.5 g/L) to be detectable on standard urine dipsticks. Microalbuminuria precedes nephropathy in patients with both non-insulin-dependent and insulin-dependent diabetes. An increase in kidney size also may accompany the initial hyperfiltration stage. Once the proteinuria becomes significant enough to be detected by dipstick, a steady decline in renal function occurs, with the glomerular filtration rate falling an average of 1 mL per minute per month. Therefore, azotemia begins about 12 years after the diagnosis of diabetes. Hypertension clearly is an exacerbating factor for diabetic nephropathy.

**VI-4. The answer is B.** *(Chap. 334. The Diabetes Control and Complications Trial Research Group, N Engl J Med 329:977–986, 1993.)* After many years of uncertainty, the NIH-sponsored multicenter Diabetes Control and Complications Trial established the fact that intensive therapy was more effective than standard therapy in reducing the development of retinopathy, the progression of retinopathy in patients who already had mild disease, and the occurrence of microalbuminuria and clinical neuropathy. There was, however, an increased likelihood of severe hypoglycemia despite the intensive monitoring practiced in the treated group. Enrollment required the presence of insulin-dependent diabetes mellitus for 1 to 5 years; therefore, these results cannot be definitively generalized to all patients with diabetes, although it is possible that patients with non-insulin-dependent diabetes mellitus also may benefit from strict glucose control. Patients in the intensively treated arm of this trial exhibited better control of blood glucose levels and lower levels of glycosylated hemoglobin. However, return of blood glucose to normal was not achieved. Moreover, patients who undertake such intensive therapy must be highly motivated and capable of withstanding its physical and emotional rigors.

**VI-5.**    **The answer is D.**    *(Chaps. 52, 337)*   Progesterone therapy results in secretory differentiation of an estrogen-primed proliferative endometrium, and the endometrium is sloughed after progesterone withdrawal only if it has been stimulated first by estrogen. Thus, in a woman being evaluated for secondary amenorrhea, the appearance of menses after a short course of progesterone is indicative of an estrogen-primed endometrium and provides good evidence of ovarian estrogen secretion. Estrone levels do not reflect direct ovarian estrogen secretion because estrone is derived principally from the peripheral conversion of androstenedione, which is secreted from the adrenal glands as well as from the ovaries. A woman with amenorrhea caused by hypogonadotropic hypogonadism, also called hypothalamic amenorrhea, has deficient ovarian estrogen secretion but may demonstrate an increase in plasma estradiol after human chorionic gonadotropin (hCG) administration. Prolactin secretion is increased by estrogen stimulation, accounting for a slightly higher mean prolactin level in women compared with that in men. However, a normal prolactin level is not evidence of persistent estrogen secretion. Although hot flashes are common in menopause, a low-estrogen state, they are not seen in hypothalamic amenorrhea, a common cause of secondary amenorrhea and a low-estrogen state.

**VI-6.**    **The answer is A.**    *(Chap. 328)*   Growth hormone, also known as somatotropin, is secreted by somatotroph cells, which account for 50 percent of the anterior pituitary glands. The release of growth hormone from the anterior pituitary is pulsatile in nature, increasing after meals, with exercise, and during slow-wave sleep. Growth hormone, which is necessary for normal growth, exerts its effects through mediators such as somatomedins and insulin-like growth factors. In addition to its involvement in growth, somatotropin is involved in stimulating the incorporation of amino acids into protein and inhibiting glucose uptake by tissues. By the latter effect, growth hormone helps restore low blood sugars to normal and is therefore a counterregulatory hormone to insulin. Both hypoglycemia and insulin stimulate growth hormone release, as does the presence of free amino acids such as arginine. Hypothalamic secretagogues also control growth hormone release. These molecules include the stimulatory hormone growth hormone–releasing hormone and the inhibitory hormone somatostatin (somatotropin release–inhibitory factor). The former is probably more important, since sectioning of the pathways between the hypothalamus and the anterior pituitary results in inhibition of growth hormone release. Other neurotransmitters influence growth hormone release, including hypothalamus-derived dopamine, which stimulates growth hormone–releasing hormone. Alpha-adrenergic agonists stimulate growth hormone release, and alpha-adrenergic blockers inhibit growth hormone increases. Serotonin agonists stimulate growth hormone release; this perhaps accounts for the nocturnal surge in growth hormone secretion.

**VI-7.**    **The answer is D.** *(Chaps. 52, 337)*   In a 7-year-old girl, isosexual precocity that is associated with undetectable levels of gonadotropins and urinary 17-ketosteroid levels appropriate for her chronologic age is most likely due to an estrogen-secreting tumor. Tumor localization procedures, such as abdominal CT and pelvic sonography, should be performed before laparotomy. Plasma androstenedione measurement is unlikely to be helpful if urinary 17-ketosteroid excretion is low or normal. In idiopathic precocious puberty, a diagnosis of exclusion, urinary gonadotropins are normal for chronologic age or are elevated; in addition, if plasma gonadotropins are measured frequently during a 24-h period, the characteristic pubertal nocturnal surge should be seen in patients with idiopathic precocious puberty.

**VI-8.    The answer is D.**    *(Chap. 328)*    Growth hormone excess in adults results in a clinical syndrome known as acromegaly, an insidious disease characterized by bony and soft tissue overgrowth, enlargement of the jaw and tongue, wide spacing of the teeth, and coarsened facial features. Hypertension may occur as a result of expansion of plasma volume and total body sodium. Laryngeal hypertrophy leads to a hollow-sounding voice. A moist, oily, doughy handshake is also characteristic. Because of the slow onset, relatives and friends who see the patient daily may not notice these changes. The diagnosis is more likely to be made by those who have not seen the patient before or for many years.

Laboratory abnormalities include abnormal glucose tolerance and mild hyperprolactinemia. The reason for growth hormone excess in virtually all patients with acromegaly is a pituitary adenoma. Useful screening tests for the diagnosis of acromegaly include measurements of glucose-suppressed growth hormone concentrations (60 min after the oral administration of 100 g glucose, growth hormone normally should be suppressed to a value less than 1 μg/L) and IGF binding protein 3. IGF-I concentrations are elevated secondary to the high levels of growth hormone. Once a laboratory test has confirmed the clinical suspicion of acromegaly, MRI or CT should be undertaken to define the presumptive pituitary adenoma.

**VI-9.    The answer is E.**    *(Chap. 333)*    Since provocative testing plays a very small role in the diagnosis of pheochromocytoma, the most frequently employed assays include measurement of catecholamines or catecholamine metabolites in a single 24-h urine sample. The three assays used include measurement of vanillylmandelic acid, metanephrines, and unconjugated ("free") catecholamines. Accuracy of diagnosis depends on the collection of a full 24-h urine sample that is treated with acid and refrigerated during and after the collection. The diagnostic yield would be increased if the 24-h urine collection included a time period during which the patient experienced a hypertensive paroxysm. False-positive increases in urinary free catecholamine excretion may occur if the patient is taking methyldopa, levodopa, or sympathomimetic amines. Endogenous plasma and urinary catecholamines also may be increased during hypoglycemia, strenuous exercise, and significant central nervous system disease. Urinary metanephrines and vanillylmandelic acid are also falsely positive in situations in which endogenous catecholamines may be increased or if the patient is receiving a monoamine oxidase inhibitor. Since plasma catecholamines are highly subject to endogenous variation in catecholamine secretion, they have not been particularly useful as an initial screening test for the diagnosis of pheochromocytoma.

**VI-10.    The answer is B.**    *(Chaps. 274, 348)*    Many autosomal dominant disorders vary in the time of onset and the severity of expression. Therefore, persons such as the two apparently unaffected siblings who are at risk for the development of hereditary nephritis, even in the absence of overt evidence of renal impairment, are poor renal donor candidates. In addition, the mother is clearly a carrier and a poor candidate. The father is the best close relative to evaluate as a potential donor.

**VI-11.    The answer is D.**    *(Chap. 65)*    One of the most important techniques for identifying the genomic sites responsible for inherited diseases and for prenatal diagnosis is the identification of restriction fragment length polymorphisms (RFLPs). Such RFLP sites are the consequences of variable sequences that may or may not allow a specific restriction endonuclease (an enzyme recognizing a specific, usually four- to seven-base DNA sequence) to cut at that site. In the Southern blots of the depicted family, the parents are heterozygous for a restriction site that is 2 kb away from one nonpolymorphic site and 8 kb away from another nonpolymorphic site in the other direction (which is the section the probe recognizes). In one of each of the parents' chromosomes the polymorphic site is present; in the other chromosome it is not. Thus, upon digestion of the parents' DNA, both a 10-kb fragment, representing the chromosome that lacks the polymorphic site, and an 8-kb fragment, representing the chromosome that has this site, exist. The son has inherited the chromosome with the site present from both his father and his mother, while the daughter has inherited the chromosome without the sequence that does not allow the extra cut from both parents. If the polymorphic sequence that allows cutting were associated with an autosomal recessive disease (by virtue of its being proximate on the genome), then such a marker could be used to predict the presence of the disease in the son or a fetus with a similar pattern on Southern blotting of DNA.

**VI-12.   The answer is E.** *(Chap. 79)*   The causes of thiamine deficiency in alcoholic persons include poor dietary intake, impaired absorption and storage, and accelerated destruction of thiamine diphosphate. Both the cardiovascular and the neurologic signs of thiamine deficiency (beriberi) can become abruptly evident after the administration of glucose to thiamine-depleted asymptomatic persons. Nystagmus, ataxia, and confusion, often accompanied by ophthalmoplegia, are strongly suggestive of Wernicke's encephalopathy; cardiovascular involvement may be signaled by tachycardia as an early manifestation of peripheral vasodilation. Thiamine should be administered promptly—preferably before glucose is given—to any person in whom subclinical thiamine deficiency is suspected.

**VI-13.   The answer is B.** *(Chap. 343)*   Acute attacks of abdominal pain that are often precipitated by diet or drugs such as barbiturates, sulfonamides, anticonvulsants, and alcohol and that have no clear-cut etiology despite an aggressive diagnostic workup may be due to acute intermittent porphyria. The porphyrias are inherited or acquired disorders of heme biosynthesis. Acute intermittent porphyria, which is caused by an autosomal dominant mutation, is characterized by a half-normal level of HMB synthase (the enzyme that catalyzes the condensation of four pyrrole porphobilinogen molecules to form the linear tetrapyrrole hydroxymethylbilane, which ultimately undergoes cyclization). Heterozygotes are prone to a host of sympathomimetic symptoms and psychological problems in addition to recurrent abdominal pain. Peripheral neuropathy, which is due to axonal degeneration of motor neurons, also may occur. The diagnostic test of choice is demonstration of increased urinary pyrrole porphobilinogen excretion as well as increased levels of urinary δ-aminolevulinic acid. Usually there is no skin disease, even after sun exposure. During acute attacks, narcotics may be given without fear of exacerbation of the attack; phenothiazines also may be administered safely. Heme therapy, presumably by including feedback inhibition of early heme biosynthesis, can abrogate attacks. However, recovery from the severe motor neuropathy may take years.

**VI-14.   The answer is D.** *(Chap. 79)*   The combination of peripheral neuritis, dermatitis, glossitis, microcytic anemia, and convulsions suggests the presence of pyridoxine deficiency. Naturally occurring pyridoxine deficiency is rare owing to the widespread distribution of the vitamin in food. Clinical deficiency is frequent, however, because many commonly used drugs act as pyridoxine antagonists. Pyridoxal phosphate is the active cofactor for numerous enzymatic reactions in amino acid metabolism and in heme synthesis; it is also important for normal neuronal excitability. Estrogens inhibit the role of pyridoxine in tryptophan metabolism, and hydrazines such as isoniazid can inhibit various enzymes that use pyridoxine as a cofactor and thus induce convulsions. Cycloserine and penicillamine act similarly. The appropriate management for persons receiving drugs capable of causing pyridoxine deficiency is dietary supplementation (at least 30 mg of pyridoxine daily); overt deficiency, when present, requires immediate parenteral therapy.

**VI-15.   The answer is B.** *(Chap. 79. Revler, JAMA 253:805, 1985.)*   Humans, unlike many animals, are incapable of synthesizing ascorbic acid from D-glucose and require exogenous vitamin C. Ascorbic acid functions as a redox agent, and its most important role is in the synthesis of appropriately hydroxylated collagen. Features of scurvy result from defective collagen synthesis and include capillary fragility resulting in ecchymoses (caused by impaired collagen formation in blood vessels), poor wound healing, and abnormal hair development. This syndrome is common in edentulous, elderly men who reside alone and ingest a diet deficient in milk, fruits, and vegetables. Resolution of bleeding occurs rapidly after the administration of oral ascorbic acid. Vitamin A deficiency tends to produce night blindness and xerophthalmia. Bleeding is seen in vitamin K deficiency but should be accompanied by an elevated prothrombin time caused by impaired synthesis of clotting factors. The anemia of folate deficiency, which is often seen in concert with scurvy, is macrocytic. Patients with insufficient quantities of available pyridoxine can develop seizures.

**VI-16.   The answer is C.**   *(Chap. 348)*   Osteogenesis imperfecta, which usually is transmitted in an autosomal dominant fashion, results in brittle bones because of a generalized decrease in bone mass. Although the clinical course is variable, some patients have multiple fractures in childhood, undergo some remission during puberty, and begin to suffer fractures again later in life. Associated abnormalities include blue sclerae, brown or translucent bluish-gray discoloration of the teeth, and progressive hearing loss. The family history is usually positive. The most common molecular defect is a mutation in one of the two genes coding for type I procollagen. Some mutations result in a decreased synthesis of pro-α I collagen genes, whereas other mutations result in the synthesis of structurally abnormal procollagen alpha chains. Most patients with Ehlers-Danlos syndrome have a defect in the synthesis of type III procollagen, and those with chondrodysplasia have a defect in the gene for type II procollagen.

Type I collagen is the most abundant of the 18 different collagens identified thus far. It is composed of two identical chains: alpha I and alpha II. After procollagen chains are translated from messenger RNA in ribosomes, they pass into the rough endoplasmic reticulum, where hydrophobic signal peptides at the *N* terminus are cleaved (resulting in up to a 50 percent reduction of protein mass). Additional posttranslational modification includes conversion of proline residues to hydroxyproline and hydroxylation of lysine residues. After the requisite number of posttranslational conversions, the protein can fold into its native triple-helical conformation.

**VI-17.   The answer is E.**   *(Chap. 348)*   Marfan syndrome, which is inherited in an autosomal recessive fashion, is characterized by long thin extremities, reduced vision from dislocation of the lens (ectopia lentis), and proximal aortic aneurysms. This disease must be distinguished from homocysteinuria, which also may cause ectopia lentis, congenital arachnodactyly, and familial aortic aneurysms. Patients with Marfan syndrome are usually tall and have severe chest deformities, including pectus excavatum and pectus carinatum. Mitral valve prolapse and dilation of the aortic root are not uncommon and may be detected by echocardiography early in life. Most patients with Marfan syndrome have mutations in the gene for fibrillin, a glycoprotein of 350 kDa. Fibrillin is a major component of elastin-associated microfibrils, which are abundant in large blood vessels and the lens suspensory ligaments.

**VI-18.   The answer is B.**   *(Chap. 350)*   The evaluation of polyuric syndromes should include simultaneous measurements of urine and plasma osmolality. Ideally, the plasma osmolality should be elevated so that the determination of an inappropriately dilute urine is possible. Such an effort may require an overnight water deprivation test. This test must be carried out carefully to ensure that a dangerous level of dehydration does not occur. Once 1 kg of body weight is lost and the plasma osmolality is elevated, the finding of a urine osmolality stable for 3 h at a low level confirms the diagnosis of diabetes insipidus. At that point vasopressin is administered, and the urine osmolality is checked between 30 and 60 min thereafter. In cases of central diabetes insipidus, the rise in urine osmolality exceeds 9 percent, whereas in nephrogenic diabetes insipidus, which frequently is due to renal dysfunction, as in the case presented, there is little, if any, increment. The treatment for nephrogenic diabetes insipidus can include the administration of diuretics to cause a fall in glomerular filtration rate and a concomitant increase in proximal tubular fluid resorption, decreased distal fluid delivery, and diminished production of dilute urine. This therapeutic strategy should be accompanied by sodium restriction.

**VI-19.**   **The answer is D.**   *(Chaps. 353, 354)*   The hypercalcemia of sarcoidosis usually is associated with disseminated disease. Therefore, almost all persons with sarcoidosis who have hypercalcemia also have an abnormal chest x-ray (diffuse fibronodular infiltration, marked enlargement of hilar nodes, or both). This is an important point in the differential diagnosis of hypercalcemia—sarcoidosis is unlikely as a cause of hypercalcemia if the chest x-ray is normal. Hypergammaglobulinemia is another helpful clue to the presence of sarcoidosis. The hypercalcemia of sarcoidosis is thought to be the consequence of increased synthesis of $1,25(OH)_2$ vitamin $D_3$ and the subsequent increased intestinal absorption of calcium. The elevated serum calcium concentration in sarcoidosis causes a decreased level of serum parathyroid hormone, resulting in marked hypercalciuria.

**VI-20.**   **The answer is E.**   *(Chap. 76)*   A host of endocrinologic abnormalities may occur as a consequence of the loss of muscle mass and fat in patients with severe anorexia nervosa. The disease usually begins shortly after puberty and is characterized by profound weight loss caused by a lack of caloric intake and a high level of physical activity. Other features include cold intolerance caused by a secondary defect in regulatory thermogenesis, hypothalamic amenorrhea, hypokalemia, low serum immunoglobulins, normal or elevated growth hormone levels, decreased levels of somatomedin C, and low serum triiodothyronine concentrations. Again, all these abnormalities seem to result from, rather than cause, the eating disorder. Most authorities favor a psychiatric etiology. Unfortunately, the benefits of psychiatric intervention and behavior modification have been somewhat marginal. Hospitalization may be required to save the patient's life if the anorexia nervosa is quite severe.

**VI-21.**   **The answer is B.**   *(Chap. 75)*   Grossly obese patients are more likely than are the nonobese to have high blood pressure, peripheral vascular disease, cerebrovascular disease, diabetes, and hyperlipidemia. The so-called Pickwickian syndrome, which is characterized by hypersomnolence during the day, is thought to be due to nocturnal upper airway obstruction that leads to hypoxemia and hypercapnia and causes arousal with each episode. This chronic arousal pattern at night causes sleep deprivation and daytime somnolence. The obese habitus, in addition to sleep-induced relaxation of the throat muscles, is believed to cause the aforementioned upper airway obstruction. These patients tend to develop blunted respiratory responses to hypercapnia and hypoxemia as well as ventilation-perfusion mismatches. Progestational agents stimulate the ventilatory response in such patients. Hyperinsulinemia, insulin resistance, diabetes, and hyperlipidemia may all be more common in obese persons but are not believed to play a role in the obesity-hypoventilation syndrome or in daytime somnolence.

**VI-22.**   **The answer is C.**   *(Chaps. 279, 344)*   Colchicine is useful in the treatment of acute gouty arthritis but not in that of chronic tophaceous gout. However, it can be a useful ancillary drug in the treatment of chronic gout at the start of allopurinol therapy to prevent the precipitation of acute gouty arthritis. Chronic gout can be treated either with uricosuric agents (probenecid and sulfinpyrazone) or with an inhibitor of uric acid synthesis (allopurinol). The ideal candidate for uricosuric agents is a patient under age 60 years who has normal renal function, a uric acid excretion of less than 700 mg/day, and no history of renal stones. Specific indications for choosing allopurinol over a uricosuric agent include the presence of uric acid nephrolithiasis, high uric acid excretion, and impairment of renal function; hence, allopurinol is the appropriate initial drug in this patient. Combinations of allopurinol and uricosuric agents may be employed when uric acid levels cannot be controlled with either drug alone.

**VI-23.**   **The answer is A.**   *(Chap. 341)*   Whether hypertriglyceridemia in an overweight person is due to familial hypertriglyceridemia, multiple lipoprotein-type hyperlipidemia, or sporadic hypertriglyceridemia, the primary mode of therapy should be weight reduction. Dietary saturated fats should be restricted as part of the weight reduction regimen. Hypothyroidism and diabetes mellitus, if present, should be treated, and the use of alcohol and oral contraceptives should be avoided. If these measures are inadequate, drug therapy with nicotinic acid or gemfibrozil should be tried. Bile acid–binding resins such as cholestyramine and colestipol are used in the treatment of hypercholesterolemia but are not useful for treating hypertriglyceridemia.

**VI-24.** **The answer is D.** *(Chap. 344)* Uric acid is the end product of purine metabolism. The serum urate level depends on dietary ingestion of purines as well as endogenous sources of purine production. Such sources include de novo purine biosynthesis and "salvage" of purine bases by hypoxanthine phosphoribosyltransferase (HPRT). HPRT catalyzes the addition of phosphated sugars to purine bases to form the ribonucleotides inosine monophosphate and guanosine monophosphate. Increased salvage activity prevents de novo synthesis by reducing phosphoribosylpyrophosphate (PRPP) levels and thus increasing the concentrations of the inhibitory ribonucleotides. A salvage pathway deficiency resulting from an increase in PRPP synthetase or a decrease in HPRT function will cause the overproduction of purines from the 11-step de novo pathway. Therefore, persons deficient in HPRT develop hyperuricemia and nephrolithiasis as well as gouty arthritis. Complete deficiency of HPRT, which is known as the Lesch-Nyhan syndrome, also is typified by self-mutilation and choreoathetosis.

**VI-25.** **The answer is D.** *(Chap. 331)* When coexistent adrenal insufficiency is suspected, it is important that thyroid replacement not be initiated until treatment with a glucocorticoid has begun. Adrenocortical insufficiency can be precipitated by an increase in the clearance rate of glucocorticoids engendered by correction of the hypothyroid state.

**VI-26.** **The answer is C.** *(Chap. 345)* The hallmark of Wilson's disease is the accumulation of excess copper deposits. The precise reason for this increased deposition of copper is not known, but serum ceruloplasmin levels are low because of secondary inhibition of formation of this protein as a result of the excess of copper. Whatever the reason, the ability of hepatocytes to store copper is exceeded, and this mineral ultimately is released in the blood with subsequent uptake in extrahepatic sites, including the brain and Descemet's membrane of the cornea (which produces the characteristic Kayser-Fleischer rings). Liver disease may take the form of acute hepatitis, fulminant hepatitis, cirrhosis, or chronic active hepatitis, as in this patient. Neurologic manifestations such as tremors, spasticity, chorea, drooling, and unusual psychiatric behavior may be primary. The diagnosis can be made because of a depressed serum concentration of ceruloplasmin in the presence of Kayser-Fleischer rings or a low serum ceruloplasmin in the presence of an elevated hepatic concentration of copper determined on a liver biopsy specimen. The mainstay of therapy for Wilson's disease is orally administered penicillamine, which removes and detoxifies the excess copper deposits. Problems associated with penicillamine treatment include sensitivity and the need for lifelong therapy. The one contraindication to the use of penicillamine therapy is fulminant hepatitis (usually accompanied by Coombs-negative hemolytic anemia). This syndrome is almost always fatal if a liver transplant cannot be performed.

**VI-27.** **The answer is A.** *(Chap. 397)* Arsenic toxicity may occur after exposure to inorganic arsenic compounds, which are used in insecticides, wood preservatives, and the glass manufacturing industry. Arsine gas is produced by metal smelting and refining, lead plating, and the manufacture of silicon microchips. Both acute and chronic toxicity resulting from ingestions may be noted. Arsine gas combines with globin to produce severe hemolysis with anemia, hemoglobinuria, and hematuria some 3 to 4 h after ingestion. Additional findings may include gastrointestinal complaints such as nausea, vomiting, and diarrhea as well as malaise, tachycardia, and dyspnea. Massive acute ingestions can lead to cardiovascular collapse, renal failure, delirium, coma, and seizures. Arsenic deposits may be seen on plain radiographs of the abdomen and in hair and nails for long periods after the initial exposure. Other laboratory abnormalities may include abnormal results of liver function tests, electrocardiac abnormalities (QT prolongation and T-wave inversion), anemia, leukocytosis, leukopenia, hemoglobinemia, proteinuria, and cellular casts in the urine. Once the acute toxic ingestion is dealt with by induction of vomiting, arsenic chelation must be considered with agents such as dimercaprol. The best way to assess the results of treatment is by ensuring that 24-h urine arsenic levels fall to less than 67 nmol.

**VI-28. The answer is D.** *(Chap. 341)* Cholestyramine and colestipol are bile acid–binding resins that decrease the reabsorption of bile acids from the intestine, thus secondarily decreasing the enterohepatic circulation of cholesterol. The liver responds to the acid depletion by increasing the synthesis of bile acids. The additional cholesterol required for bile acid synthesis is obtained by the liver by increasing the number of receptors for low-density lipoproteins (LDL), which in turn lowers the plasma level of LDL. The most common side effects of these resins are constipation and bloating, although mild steatorrhea may occur when they are used in high doses.

**VI-29. The answer is B.** *(Chap. 391. Snilkstein, N Engl J Med 319:1557–1562, 1988.)* Once a significant dose of acetaminophen is ingested, the normal detoxifying pathways—sulfation and glucuronidation—become saturated. This process, however, depletes hepatic glutathione, an important protector against oxidative injury. Oxidants cause hepatic necrosis and, if the ingested dose is great enough, fatal hepatic failure. However, one cannot wait for evidence of abnormal transaminases to begin therapy. As is almost certainly the case with this patient, given the high number of tablets ingested, a serum acetaminophen level is going to be high and will indicate the need for antidote therapy. For patients who arrive within 4 h after the ingestion, the initial treatment should include activated charcoal. This strategy does not interfere with the primary therapy: *N*-acetylcysteine. The earlier the treatment starts, the better off the patient will be. Therapy with *N*-acetylcysteine, if given orally, should be continued for 72 h.

**VI-30. The answer is C.** *(Chap. 391)* Ethylene glycol is an important component of antifreeze as well as hydraulic fluids and windshield cleaners. It is metabolized by alcohol dehydrogenase to glycoaldehyde and then is successively oxidized to glycolic acid, glyoxylic acid, and oxalic acid. Ethanol, which is preferentially metabolized by alcohol dehydrogenase compared with ethylene glycol, may be used to prevent buildup of end-stage oxidative metabolites of ethylene glycol. Ethylene glycol is directly responsible for the CNS depression seen in an overdose with this agent. However, its metabolite, glycolic acid, is responsible for the metabolic acidosis, increased anion gap, and renal damage, which frequently is manifested as acute tubular necrosis. Oxalic acid may precipitate as calcium oxalate crystals in various locations, including the brain, heart, and kidney. If patients do not suffer from the cardiopulmonary collapse that may acutely accompany a massive overdose, acute tubular necrosis, which occurs 12 to 24 h after ingestion, usually is reversible. In addition to supportive measures and ethanol infusions in cases of severe ingestions, hemodialysis will treat the complications of renal failure and remove ethylene glycol from the circulation.

**VI-31. The answer is A.** *(Chap. 75)* Although only a minority of obese persons have diabetes mellitus, more than 80 percent of type 2 diabetics are obese. Obesity appears to be a major contributory factor to the development of diabetes, largely through its effects on insulin sensitivity. A clear relationship also exists between hypertension and obesity in adults, though the mechanism is unclear. Hypertriglyceridemia is associated commonly with obesity and correlates with the degree of obesity; increased hepatic production of very-low-density lipoproteins (VLDL) from free fatty acids is felt to be the major cause of increased triglyceride levels in obese persons, although peripheral defects in VLDL clearance may be present in some. Weight loss can reduce or reverse all these complications. The prevalence of cholelithiasis is increased with increasing adiposity, but the same cannot be said of hypothyroidism—only a small percentage of hypothyroid persons are obese, and an even smaller fraction of obese persons are hypothyroid.

**VI-32.  The answer is B.**  *(Chap. 391)*  Tricyclic compounds are commonly used in depressed patients and thus are frequently employed during suicide attempts. Their primary mode of action may be to block the uptake of synaptic transmitters in the central nervous system, but the side effects are due primarily to their central and peripheral anticholinergic activity, peripheral alpha-blocking activity, and quinidine-like effects on the heart. In mild overdoses, anticholinergic effects such as mydriasis, urinary retention, confusion, and tachycardia may be seen. In more significant overdoses, cardiac toxicity, seizures, and hypotension may occur. Arrhythmias, including ventricular tachyarrhythmias and bradycardias, are typical. Prolongation of the QRS complex to more than 100 ms correlates with an increased risk of cardiac arrhythmias and seizures. Treatment includes gastric lavage, supportive care, anticonvulsants if seizures have occurred, and sodium bicarbonate, lidocaine, and phenytoin to treat ventricular tachyarrhythmia. Physostigmine, an acetylcholinesterase inhibitor, may reverse the anticholinergic effects of mild poisoning, but this drug should not be administered during severe poisoning because of the possibility of cardiac toxicity.

**VI-33.  The answer is C.**  *(Chap. 346. Beutler, N Engl J Med 325:1354, 1991.)*  Gaucher disease, an autosomal recessive syndrome, is caused by a deficiency of the enzyme glucocerebrosidase. The absence of this enzyme results in the accumulation of extremely insoluble glucocerebroside as a result of failure of lysosome-mediated glycolipid degradation. The gene encoding this enzyme is on the long arm of chromosome 1. In North America, this disease is most commonly due to a point mutation of cDNA nucleotide 1226, typically found in Jewish persons of Eastern European origin. Though some types of Gaucher disease can present with dramatic neurologic manifestations or cause death early in life, the most common type is the adult-onset, or type I, variety. The disease is manifested by hepatomegaly and splenomegaly, which may contribute to thrombocytopenia. Hepatic involvement can result in fibrosis and abnormal liver function. Bone involvement—particularly flaring of the distal femur, aseptic necrosis of the femoral heads, and bone infarcts—is a common complication. Laboratory abnormalities include pancytopenia, abnormal results of liver function tests, and elevation of serum acid phosphatase. While the diagnosis should be made on the basis of the clinical presentation, bone marrow examinations are frequently performed to evaluate the associated hematologic abnormalities. Such an examination will invariably reveal the presence of so-called Gaucher cells, which are storage macrophages that contain excessive amounts of glucocerebroside, identified as engorgement with a fine, scroll-like pattern. The diagnosis can be confirmed by determination of leukocyte β-glucosidase activity. While splenectomy is effective in correcting the thrombocytopenia and anemia, the bone disease is of course not affected by this procedure. A major recent change in therapy for Gaucher disease has been the availability of aglucerase, the commercially produced modified glucocerebrosidase (mannose-terminated). Therapy with this agent appears to be effective and safe; however, the cost can range to several hundred thousand dollars per year. Other potential therapeutic strategies include allogeneic transplantation or autologous transplantation of stem cells into which a normal glucocerebrosidase gene has been inserted. This gene transfer approach has not been clinically applied.

**VI-34.  The answer is C.**  *(Chap. 333. Bravo, N Engl J Med 311:1298, 1984.)*  Pheochromocytomas produce and secrete catecholamines, which may lead to paroxysmally high blood pressure. Approximately 80 percent of these tumors are solitary adrenal lesions, but 10 percent are bilateral and 10 percent are extraadrenal. Pheochromocytoma also is associated with familial multiple endocrine neoplasia types IIa and IIb (hyperparathyroidism and medullary carcinoma are the other endocrinologic manifestations). Once the diagnosis is confirmed, usually by documenting excess urinary catecholamine metabolites over a 24-h period plus localization by CT scanning, it is important to prepare the patient for surgery by preventing the effects of catecholamine release through treatment with phenoxybenzamine, a long-acting alpha-adrenergic blocker. Liberal salt intake also should be instituted to help restore the contracted plasma volume to normal before surgery. Beta blockers should not be given before alpha blockade has been established because of the potential for hypertension as a result of the antagonism of beta-mediated vasodilation in skeletal muscle beds. However, propranolol is useful in treating the reflex tachycardia induced by phenoxybenzamine. While prazosin is an effective agent for the treatment of hypertensive crises associated with pheochromocytoma, its use as a primary agent in the management of this disorder has not been established.

**VI-35.** **The answer is E.** *(Chap. 65)* Autosomal dominant diseases are manifest in the heterozygous state, when only one abnormal gene is present, with the corresponding allele being normal. Consequently, there is a 50 percent chance that the offspring of an affected heterozygote will inherit the mutant allele. Furthermore, affected individuals will bear an equal number of normal and affected offspring. There is no sex predilection for such a disease. In many autosomal dominant disorders, the affected person may not have an affected parent. This occurs because the mutations leading to such disorders are often spontaneous. The parent in whose germ cell the mutation arose will be clinically normal, as will the parent's other children. However, since the mutation is now present in the reproductive cells of an affected individual, such a patient will transmit the disease to half of his or her children. Some autosomal dominant diseases, such as tuberous sclerosis and achondroplasia, arise in spontaneous mutations in about 80 percent of cases; Marfan syndrome and neurofibromatosis do so in about 30 to 40 percent of cases. By contrast, Huntington's chorea, adult polycystic kidney disease, and familial hypercholesterolemia have a much lower incidence of occurrence resulting from spontaneous mutations. Other characteristics of many autosomal dominant disorders that are not seen in recessive syndromes are delayed age of onset and variability of clinical expression. For example, the neurologic abnormalities associated with Huntington's chorea frequently do not present until the fourth or fifth decade. Second, the multiple endocrine neoplasia syndromes manifest themselves with abnormalities in various organs within the same kindred. Hemophilia A is an X-linked recessive disorder, and hemochromatosis is autosomal recessive. Myasthenia gravis is inherited in a polygenic fashion but is more common in patients who harbor an HLA-B8 histocompatibility antigen locus.

**VI-36.** **The answer is D.** *(Chap. 357)* Magnesium deficiency may occur as a result of generalized nutritional insufficiency or lack of supplementation in programs of total parenteral nutrition. Other causes include gastrointestinal malabsorption of any cause, chronic diarrhea, chronic alcoholism, increased renal excretion (from cisplatin, amphotericin B, aminoglycosides, or loop diuretics), and various endocrine disorders (e.g., hyperparathyroidism, hypoparathyroidism, diabetic ketoacidosis, Conn's syndrome, and syndrome of inappropriate secretion of vasopressin). The clinical sequelae of severe magnesium deficiency [<0.5 mmol/L (1.0 meq/L)] include anorexia, vomiting, lethargy, paresthesias, muscle cramps, irritability, decreased attention span, and confusion. Hypocalcemia, as a result of diminished responsiveness and the release of parathyroid hormone, may be severe enough to produce tetany. About half of patients with hypomagnesemia may become hypokalemic (the mechanism is unclear, but secondary hyperaldosteronism may play a role). Low levels of serum calcium, potassium, and magnesium all serve to promote dangerous cardiac arrhythmias, especially in a patient receiving digitalis. Hyponatremia is not a known consequence of hypomagnesemia, although the syndrome of inappropriate secretion of vasopressin may cause a low serum magnesium.

**VI-37.** **The answer is B.** *(Chap. 354. Burtis, N Engl J Med 322:1106–1112, 1990.)* Patients who present with hypercalcemia and hypophosphatemia should be thought of as having an excess of parathyroid hormone activity. Patients with nonparathyroid hormone–like mediated hypercalcemia, such as those with excessive levels of vitamin D caused by intoxication or sarcoidosis or by increased bone turnover as in hyperthyroidism, would not be expected to have a low serum phosphate. Second, patients with familial hypocalciuric hypercalcemia, an autosomal dominant trait, often have normal or slightly low levels of immunoreactive parathyroid hormone. Thus, those with hypercalcemia and hypophosphatemia without elevated levels of parathyroid hormone are likely to have the hypercalcemia of malignancy. The clinical setting usually but not invariably makes this diagnosis obvious. It is now clearly recognized that many solid tumors, including carcinomas of the lung and kidney, may produce a parathyroid hormone–related protein that will not be identified by the currently available assays that detect true parathyroid hormone elaborated from the parathyroid gland. This parathyroid-related protein synthesized by tumors bears striking amino acid homology to that of native parathyroid hormone with regard to amino acids 1 through 13 but is thereafter unique. In fact, it is now recognized that the majority of patients with cancer and hypercalcemia have humoral hypercalcemia, as determined by elevated urinary cyclic AMP excretion.

**VI-38.   The answer is B.**   *(Chap. 330)*   Patients with lung cancer, particularly small cell carcinoma, frequently present with the syndrome of inappropriate vasopressin (AVP, antidiuretic hormone) secretion. Indeed, more than half of patients with such tumors show evidence of inappropriate secretion of AVP, even when serum sodium concentration remains normal. AVP is produced by the tumor tissue itself and is chemically identical to arginine vasopressin secreted by the neurohypophysis. Central nervous system lesions of infectious, inflammatory, and vascular etiologies also can result in inappropriate AVP secretion, but intracerebral metastases from lung carcinomas usually are not responsible for inappropriate AVP secretion.

**VI-39.   The answer is A.**   *(Chap. 341)*   Dietary triglycerides in cholesterol are packaged by gastrointestinal epithelial cells into large lipoprotein particles called chylomicrons. After secretion into the intestinal lymph and passage into the general circulation, chylomicrons bind to the enzyme lipoprotein lipase, which is located on endothelial surfaces. This enzyme is activated by a protein contained in the chylomicron, apoprotein CII, liberating free fatty acids and monoglycerides, which then pass through the endothelial cells and enter adipocytes or muscle cells. Therefore, complete inactivation of either lipoprotein lipase or apoprotein CII as a result of the inheritance of two defective copies of the relevant gene results in an accumulation of chylomicrons (type I lipoprotein elevation) that is due to failure of conversion to the chylomicron remnant particle. Patients with familial lipoprotein lipase deficiency usually present in infancy with recurrent attacks of abdominal pain caused by pancreatitis. They also have eruptive xanthomas resulting from triglyceride deposition. Treatment should consist of a low-fat diet that may be supplemented by medium-chain triglycerides, which are not incorporated into chylomicrons. The absence of functional apoprotein CII, with consequent failure to activate lipoprotein lipase, presents with a similar phenotype, although the affected patients are typically detected at a somewhat later age than are patients with familial lipoprotein lipase deficiency.

**VI-40.   The answer is E.**   *(Chap. 341. Brown, Science 232:34, 1986.)*   The most common hyperlipidemic syndrome known to be caused by a single gene defect is familial hypercholesterolemia, an autosomal dominant disorder caused by a mutant LDL receptor. Heterozygotes have a two- to threefold elevation in serum cholesterol because of a reduction in the ability of the liver and other tissues to take up cholesterol-rich LDL lipoprotein particles from the plasma. The clinical features of this syndrome usually are manifest by premature and accelerated coronary atherosclerosis as well as by tendon xanthomas, particularly in the Achilles tendon and tendons near the knee, the elbow, and the dorsum of the hand. These nodules are caused by deposits of lipid-swollen macrophages. The extremely high LDL levels lead to an enhanced infiltration of cholesterol into the artery wall after episodes of endothelial damage, thus leading to enhanced atherosclerosis. The presence of very elevated plasma cholesterol levels, the occurrence of tendon xan-thomas, and a family history of atherosclerosis or hyperlipidemia are highly suggestive of familial hypercholesterolemia.

**VI-41.   The answer is D.**   *(Chap. 332)*   In the various forms of congenital adrenal hyperplasia, including steroid C-21 hydroxylase deficiency, both pituitary and adrenal regulatory mechanisms function appropriately. The enzymatic defect in cortisol production results in an absence of the product (cortisol) necessary for feedback inhibition of ACTH secretion by the pituitary gland. ACTH in turn causes the production of increased amounts of cortisol precursors such as 17-hydroxyprogesterone, which is converted to androgens by the adrenal gland. Therapy with appropriate doses of glucocorticoid causes suppression of pituitary ACTH and adrenal androgen secretion, indicating that inhibiting and stimulating control mechanisms of the hypothalamic-pituitary-adrenal axis can function normally.

**VI-42.   The answer is D.**   *(Chaps. 328, 332)*   In a single-dose overnight dexamethasone suppression test, which is a screening procedure in the workup of possible cortisol excess, suppression of plasma cortisol concentration to less than 140 nmol/L (5 μg/dL) implies normal hypothalamic-pituitary-adrenal feedback and excludes a diagnosis of Cushing's syndrome. However, failure to suppress plasma cortisol after this procedure is not necessarily diagnostic and must be investigated further. Several factors can affect the validity of screening dexamethasone testing. For example, in 10 to 15 percent of cases obesity interferes with normal suppression of cortisol after an overnight dexamethasone test. However, obese persons uniformly show normal excretion of free cortisol in urine [<275 nmol/d (<100 μg/d)]. A 24-h urine free cortisol or 2-day low-dose dexamethasone test is necessary to exclude or establish the diagnosis of Cushing's syndrome in all persons with an abnormal or equivocal 1-mg overnight dekamethanone suppression test. The high-dose test, which is reserved for patients with established Cushing's syndrome, serves to delineate the specific cause. Imaging procedures should be performed only after a diagnosis of cortisol excess has been established.

**VI-43.   The answer is B.**   *(Chap. 332)*   Hyporeninemic hypoaldosteronism occurs most commonly in adults with diabetes mellitus in association with mild renal failure, metabolic acidosis, and hyperkalemia. The defect in aldosterone synthesis is almost certainly caused by hyporeninism, since in these patients aldosterone secretion increases promptly after the administration of ACTH but not after salt restriction or postural changes. Most patients respond to the administration of potent mineralocorticoids (fludrocortisone), diuretics such as furosemide, or both, but in general mineralocorticoids should not be the sole therapeutic agents in patients with hypertension. Furosemide will treat both the hyperkalemia and the acidosis; this diuretic will be more effective if sodium intake is reduced. Hemodialysis may be useful in emergency situations to correct hyperkalemia. Potassium restriction and enhancement of potassium excretion with anion-exchange resins are both likely to predispose to total-body potassium deficits.

**VI-44.   The answer is A.**   *(Chap. 334. Coustan, N Engl J Med 319:1663, 1988.)*   The prognosis for pregnancies complicated by diabetes mellitus has improved markedly, and perinatal mortality has decreased to the point where infant survival is similar to that in the population at large. This improved outcome is a result of aggressive treatment of maternal hyperglycemia and advances in the techniques of fetal surveillance and neonatal care. When mean maternal blood glucose levels exceed 8.3 mmol/L (150 mg/dL) in the third trimester, perinatal mortality is almost six times that associated with mean maternal glucose levels below 5.6 mmol/L (100 mg/dL). Congenital malformations, the leading cause of perinatal mortality in infants of diabetic pregnancies, remain a problem; such abnormalities are thought to be related to poor glucose control early in the first trimester (during early embryogenesis), a time when many women do not yet know they are pregnant. Optimal care of a diabetic woman who wishes to become pregnant requires that a major attempt be made to achieve as normal a mean blood glucose concentration as possible before conception and throughout the duration of the pregnancy. Hospitalization may be required for education or treatment of complications but should not be necessary for extended periods of time. Multiple subcutaneous injections of insulin or continuous subcutaneous injection of insulin should be considered to provide "tight" control in all diabetic women who wish to become pregnant.

**VI-45.   The answer is B.**   *(Chap. 334)*   Dot hemorrhages and several larger lesions near the disk (caused by superficial retinal bleeding) are characteristic changes of background diabetic retinopathy. However, the presence of innumerable fine frondlike vessels extending around and partly covering the disk is indicative of the neovascularization of proliferative retinopathy, which requires urgent treatment. The therapy of choice is photocoagulation by xenon arc or ruby or argon laser, which significantly improves the visual prognosis in patients with proliferative retinopathy. Hypophysectomy is no longer used to treat proliferative retinopathy because of the morbidity and lack of effectiveness of the procedure. Vitrectomy should be reserved for more advanced cases, such as nonresolving vitreal hemorrhage and retinal detachment.

**VI-46.   The answer is A.**   *(Chap. 336)*   Testosterone esters are hydrolyzed by esterases in the blood as they are absorbed from the oily depots in which they are administered, and as a consequence, the esters themselves rarely can be detected in blood. Therefore, the effectiveness of therapy with agents such as testosterone cypionate can be monitored by measuring the plasma levels of testosterone itself. In men with recent onset of hypogonadism, plasma LH levels should be suppressed into the normal range by testosterone, but when LH levels have been high for many years, LH secretion becomes semiautonomous and may not return to the normal range for many months or years after the restoration of blood testosterone levels to normal. The frequency of nocturnal erections may or may not reflect plasma testosterone levels on a day-to-day or week-to-week basis, and muscle mass depends on factors in addition to plasma testosterone levels, including exercise level.

**VI-47.   The answer is D.**   *(Chap. 358)*   Paget's disease of bone is relatively common, and the incidence increases with age. An estimated prevalence of 3 percent in persons over age 40 years is a generally accepted figure. Most frequently, the disease is asymptomatic and is diagnosed only when the typical sclerotic bones are incidentally detected on x-ray examinations done for other reasons or when increased alkaline phosphatase activity is recognized on routine laboratory measurements. The etiology is unknown, but increased bone resorption followed by intensive bone repair is thought to be the mechanism that causes increased bone density and increased serum alkaline phosphatase activity as a marker of osteoblast activity. Since increased mineralization of bone takes place (although in an abnormal pattern), hypercalcemia is not present unless a severely affected patient becomes immobilized. Hypercalcemia in fact would be an expected finding in a patient with primary hyperparathyroidism, bone metastases, or plasmacytoma, with plasmacytoma typically producing no increase in alkaline phosphatase activity. Osteomalacia resulting from vitamin D deficiency is associated with bone pain and hypophosphatemia; normal or decreased serum calcium concentration produces secondary hyperparathyroidism, further aggravating the defective bone mineralization.

**VI-48.   The answer is D.**   *(Chap. 354)*   A major function of parathyroid hormone is to act as a trophic hormone to regulate the rate of formation of $1,25(OH)_2$ vitamin D. The mechanism by which parathyroid hormone exerts this effect may be secondary to its effects on phosphorus metabolism. Other hormones, including prolactin and estrogen, also may play a role in stimulating the production of $1,25(OH)_2$ vitamin D.

**VI-49.   The answer is A.**   *(Chap. 65)*   Many common diseases are known to "run in families" yet are not inherited in a simple Mendelian fashion. It is likely that the expression of these disorders depends on a family of genes that can impart a certain degree of risk and then be modified by subsequent environmental factors. The risk of the development of disease in a relative of an affected person varies with the degree of relationship; first-degree relatives (parents, siblings, and offspring) have the highest risk, which in itself varies with the specific disease. Many of these multifactorial genetic diseases are inherited in a greater frequency in persons with certain HLA (major histocompatibility system) types. For example, there is a tenfold increased risk of celiac sprue (gluten-sensitive enteropathy) in persons who harbor HLA-B8. This genotype also imparts increased risk for chronic active hepatitis, myasthenia gravis, and Addison's disease. The incidence of diabetes mellitus is much higher in those expressing HLA-D3 and HLA-D4. Spondyloarthropathies, psoriatic arthritis (HLA-B27), hyperthyroidism (HLA-DR3), and multiple sclerosis (HLA-DR2) are other examples of diseases with histocompatibility predispositions. By contrast, Wilson's disease and cystic fibrosis are inherited in an autosomal recessive fashion and adult polycystic kidney disease and neurofibromatosis are among the disorders inherited in an autosomal dominant manner.

**VI-50.   The answer is C.**   *(Chaps. 52, 337)*   The fact that withdrawal bleeding occurred after the administration of progestogen indicates that estrogen was being produced. Women with chronic anovulation who react in this way are said to be in the state of "estrus" because of acyclic production of estrogen. This diagnostic response clearly excludes causes of amenorrhea associated with suppression of ovarian function, including pituitary disease, either functional or organic, and conditions associated with streak gonads. The most likely cause of amenorrhea in such a situation is polycystic ovarian disease (PCOD), in which the ovaries produce androgens that can be converted to estrogens (largely estrone) in extraglandular tissues. In most women with PCOD, menarche occurs at the expected time and amenorrhea supervenes after a variable time. However, in some women this disorder has an early onset and may cause primary amenorrhea. Other causes of anovulation in the presence of estrogen include estrogen-secreting tumors of the ovary and adrenal tumors.

**VI-51.   The answer is C.**   *(Chaps. 52, 337)*   Asherman's syndrome, or destruction of the endometrium, occurs after vigorous curettage, usually in association with postpartum hemorrhage or therapeutic abortion. The diagnosis is confirmed by hysterosalpingography or by direct visualization of the scarred endometrium using a hysteroscope. Treatment consists of dilation and curettage, followed by the insertion of an intrauterine device for 8 weeks.

**VI-52.   The answer is D.**   *(Chaps. 52, 337)*   Low circulating levels of estrogens coupled with elevated gonadotropin levels exclude the presence of pituitary disease and indicate primary ovarian failure, which is premature at this patient's age. Bilateral tubal obstruction would cause infertility but not amenorrhea. Polycystic ovarian disease is associated with typical physical findings of weight gain and hirsutism, an earlier age of onset, and elevated circulating levels of estrogens.

**VI-53.   The answer is B.**   *(Chaps. 332, 339)*   The clinical situation described in the question is characteristic of congenital adrenal hyperplasia caused by a deficiency of either C-21 hydroxylase or 3β-ol-dehydrogenase. Urinary 17-ketosteroids are elevated in both disorders, whereas urinary pregnanediol and pregnanetriol and plasma 17-hydroxyprogesterone and androstenedione levels are elevated in association with C-21 hydroxylase deficiency. Plasma 11-deoxycortisol is elevated in patients with C-11 hydroxylase deficiency, a disorder producing hypertension because of overproduction of mineralocorticoids and consequently not associated with vomiting and volume depletion. Congenital adrenal hyperplasia caused by C-21 hydroxylase deficiency, the most common cause of ambiguous genitalia in newborns, results in virilization of females at birth and premature androgenation of males.

**VI-54.   The answer is D.**   *(Chap. 339)*   Tumors of the streak gonads are unusual in the common forms of gonadal dysgenesis, including those associated with normal karyotypes

(46,XX), X-chromosome deletion (45,X), structurally abnormal X chromosomes (46,XX$_i$), and X chromosome mosaicism (45,X/46,XX). However, malignant tumors of the streaks (so-called gonadoblastomas) are common when gonadal dysgenesis is associated with cell lines containing Y chromosomes or fragments of Y chromosomes. Consequently, the gonadal streaks should be resected whenever a Y chromosome is present in a woman with gonadal dysgenesis.

**VI-55.  The answer is E.**  *(Chap. 354)*  Persons who have hyperparathyroidism can present with manifestations of hypercalcemia, such as kidney stones or osteitis fibrosa cystica, a form of bone involvement characteristic of the disease. However, with the widespread application of biochemical screening as a routine tool in patient evaluation, more and more patients are diagnosed early in the course of the disease, when it is manifested only by asymptomatic hypercalcemia. At present, this is the most common source of diagnoses of hyperparathyroidism. A solitary parathyroid adenoma is the most common cause of this entity.

**VI-56.  The answer is E.**  *(Chaps. 279, 354)*  Patients with primary hyperparathyroidism are usually asymptomatic, and mild degrees of hypercalcemia in such patients usually can be managed with adequate hydration. Whether observation alone is appropriate in these patients is controversial, especially when the diagnosis is made at a young age, since surveillance of renal function and bone status is lifelong and cumbersome. However, definitive treatment is clearly indicated when complications arise. In this patient, hypercalcemia and nephrolithiasis constitute a clear-cut indication for surgical treatment of the hyperparathyroidism. An additional reason would be to prevent bone loss in this young woman that would place her at increased risk for the development of skeletal complications at a later time. Glucocorticoids are usually ineffective in the management of primary hyperparathyroidism and would affect bone metabolism negatively, besides producing other serious side effects when administered on a long-term basis. Thiazide diuretics and calcium supplementation are contraindicated in this patient because of the risk of inducing hypercalcemia.

**VI-57.  The answer is C.**  *(Chap. 331)*  Radioactive iodine uptake (RAIU) is often a useful test in distinguishing among the various causes of hyperthyroidism. Elevation of RAIU above the normal range usually indicates thyroid hyperfunction (some persons with hyperthyroidism have a normal or low RAIU). Painless thyroiditis is a variant of chronic lymphocytic thyroiditis associated with transient thyrotoxicosis from the release of pre-formed hormone. Radiographic contrast studies such as intravenous pyelography and oral cholecystography use organic media that release iodide and thus serve as sources for the dilution of administered radioactive iodine; as a result, RAIU may be falsely low for as long as 6 months. *Thyrotoxicosis factitia* is the term used to designate thyrotoxicosis resulting from the ingestion of thyroid hormones. Ingestion of liothyronine (T$_3$) results in a low serum thyroxine (T$_4$) concentration, while the ingestion of levothyroxine leads to elevations of both T$_4$ and T$_3$. In either case, feedback of exogenous thyroid hormone decreases TSH secretion and lowers RAIU. Struma ovarii, which is an ovarian tumor with thyroidlike tissue that releases thyroid hormone, is a rare cause of thyrotoxicosis. Measurement of RAIU over the thyroid gland would not, of course, detect the abdominal source of increased RAIU in women affected with struma ovarii. Choriocarcinoma releases factors with TSH-like activity that enhance the uptake of radioactive iodine.

**VI-58.  The answer is A.**  *(Chap. 355)*  Osteomalacia and rickets both are characterized by defective mineralization of bone; osteomalacia affects the adult skeleton, and rickets impairs the developing skeleton. Muscle weakness, hypocalcemia, hypophosphatemia, skeletal pain, and pseudofractures are cardinal features of both forms of osteomalacia. Bowing of the tibia, although common in children who have rickets, is not prominent in affected adults.

**VI-59.  The answer is E.**  *(Chap. 355)*  The combination of hypocalcemia, hypophosphatemia, elevated serum parathyroid hormone levels, and bone fractures is consistent with a diagnosis of osteomalacia in this patient. In the absence of other gastrointestinal or renal abnormalities leading to malabsorption or increased renal loss of calcium or phosphorus, vitamin D deficiency is likely to be present. Inadequate intake of vitamin D and calcium together and limited exposure to the sun are common in this age group. Postmenopausal osteoporosis is associated with vertebral and hip fractures as well, but laboratory abnormalities are not present. Primary hyperparathyroidism is associated with increased serum calcium concentration, as is ectopic parathyroid hormone secretion (although the existence of the latter has been questioned). Paget's disease of bone does not produce hypocalcemia, and it causes typical sclerotic changes on x-ray examination.

**VI-60.** **The answer is C.** *(Chap. 355)* The presenting findings in both primary hyperparathyroidism and multiple myeloma can include hypercalcemia and vertebral compression fractures. The absence of several key features—anemia, elevated erythrocyte sedimentation rate, abnormal serum protein electrophoresis, and Bence Jones proteinuria—is helpful in eliminating the possibility of multiple myeloma. If doubt remains about the diagnosis of myeloma, a marrow aspiration should be performed. The presence of hypercalcemia makes unlikely the diagnoses of osteomalacia, which is associated with hypocalcemia, and osteoporosis and Paget's disease, which are associated with normal blood calcium values.

**VI-61.** **The answer is C.** *(Chaps. 353, 354)* Measurement of the serum concentration of 25(OH) vitamin D, the major circulating form of vitamin D, can be used to assess the adequacy of dietary intake and absorption of the vitamin. (Vitamin D also is made in the skin in the presence of sunlight.) Once ingested or synthesized, vitamin D is metabolized to 25(OH) vitamin D in the liver. This reaction is not tightly regulated, and an increase in dietary intake or endogenous production of vitamin D is reflected by linear elevations of serum 25(OH) vitamin D levels. Levels are reduced in patients with severe chronic parenchymal and cholestatic liver disease but usually are normal in patients with renal failure. Anticonvulsant drugs and glucocorticoids induce hepatic microsomal enzymes, which metabolize vitamin D and 25(OH) vitamin D into inactive products; this phenomenon, along with other complex effects on calcium metabolism, helps explain why these drugs cause osteopenia.

**VI-62.** **The answer is A.** *(Chaps. 74, 78)* In most malnourished persons, positive nitrogen balance can be achieved by providing 1 g of amino acids per kilogram of ideal body weight. However, in the presence of abnormal protein losses (e.g., from burn exudates, pancreatic secretions, or gastrointestinal fistula) or hypermetabolic states (sepsis, trauma, hyperthyroidism), additional protein intake must be provided. Similarly, daily protein requirements are increased in the presence of caloric deficiency because amino acids are used for oxidative metabolism and gluconeogenesis. Renal insufficiency and hepatic insufficiency are examples of "nitrogen accumulation diseases." When the kidneys are unable to excrete urea, ammonia may be used for the net synthesis of nonessential amino acids; thus, the need for nonessential nitrogen is reduced. In hepatic failure, amino acid catabolism is decreased, and so even normal protein intake may be deleterious.

**VI-63.** **The answer is E.** *(Chap. 328)* Because the half-life of $T_4$ is approximately 1 week, the total $T_4$ will still be normal the day after the pituitary ceases to function. $T_3$ is derived primarily from $T_4$, and so it will still also be normal. IGF-I is a useful test for detecting growth hormone excess as occurs in acromegaly, but it is not a sensitive test of growth hormone deficiency. In addition, IGF-I would not fall rapidly to a new steady level. Likewise, an ACTH stimulation test would be normal even though the patient had adrenal insufficiency. The adrenal glands would have not yet atrophied and could still respond to exogenous ACTH. A test more likely to detect adrenal insufficiency in this case would be an insulin tolerance test, in which a small dose of regular insulin is administered in a monitored setting to induce hypoglycemia therapy stimulation and the release of counterregulatory hormones, including cortisol. Increased cortisol secretion in this case relies on the pituitary's ability to release ACTH, not just on the adrenal's ability to respond to ACTH. The insulin tolerance test should never be performed in elderly patients and patients with heart disease.

**VI-64.**  **The answer is D.**  *(Chap. 331)*   This patient has postpartum thyroiditis, which occurs in 5 to 9 percent of all postpartum women. Appropriate treatment is symptomatic because the hyperthyroidism is caused by the release of preformed thyroid hormone from a damaged thyroid gland. Therefore, therapies aimed at decreasing the formation of thyroid hormone, such as methimazole, or at inhibiting its release, such as SSKI, will be ineffective. Radioactive iodine also will be ineffective, since it will not be taken up by the damaged thyroid gland (reflected in the 1 percent 24-h iodine uptake). In addition, the hyperthyroidism will resolve spontaneously. Steroids are effective in subacute thyroiditis, which is characterized by a tender thyroid and often is preceded by a viral illness, but are not used in postpartum thyroiditis. Therapies, such as beta blockers, aimed at treating symptoms are the most effective treatment.

Postpartum thyroiditis is a form of lymphocytic thyroiditis, a painless inflammation of the thyroid that is thought to be autoimmune in etiology. About one-third of patients enter a hypothyroid phase after experiencing hyperthyroidism. Eighty percent of these women recover normal thyroid function, but 20 percent remain hypothyroid and require indefinite replacement therapy. Therefore, serial thyroid function testing is indicated.

**VI-65.**  **The answer is B.**  *(Chaps. 7, 331. Daniels, Endocrine Pract 1:287, 1995.)*   Radioactive iodine should never be given to a pregnant woman. In addition, both methimazole and beta blockers should be avoided in pregnant women. Methimazole may lead to an increased incidence of aplasia cutis, a fetal scalp defect. Beta blockers may lead to neonatal hypoglycemia. Antithyroid drugs, including propylthiouracil, cross the placenta and affect fetal thyroid function. Studies have shown that when a treated pregnant woman's thyroid function is in the mid-normal range, the fetus is hypothyroid. When the mother's thyroid tests are maintained in the high-normal or slightly hyperthyroid range, the fetus is likely to have normal thyroid function. Severe maternal hyperthyroidism is potentially dangerous for the fetus, but mild maternal hyperthyroidism poses a much smaller risk.

**VI-66.**  **The answer is C.**  *(Chap. 328)*   Although the most common pituitary tumor is a prolactinoma, this tumor is more likely a nonfunctioning pituitary adenoma. Though the prolactin level is elevated, one would expect it to be much higher with a prolactinoma this large. The mildly elevated prolactin most likely results from compression of the infundibular stalk. This tumor should be removed, as it is macroscopic and near the optic chiasm. Further growth could result in impairment of the patient's vision. The surgery usually is performed using a transsphenoidal approach, a technique which avoids the morbidity of a craniotomy and carries minimal risk in the hands of an experienced surgeon.

**VI-67.**  **The answer is A.**  *(Chap. 334. DeFronzo, N Engl J Med 333:541, 1995. Groop, Diabetes Care 15:737, 1992.)*   Sulfonylureas have long half-lives. One such agent, chlorpropamide, has a half-life of 24 h. Though the patient's glucose is normal after an intravenous dextrose infusion, he may become hypoglycemic again hours later. He therefore should be hospitalized with careful monitoring of glucose and mental status until the effects of the sulfonylurea have resolved. Though metformin does not cause prolonged hypoglycemia, it is contraindicated in patients with organ failure, as the combination may predispose to lactic acidosis. Sulfonylurea administration is by far the most likely cause of this man's first episode of hypoglycemia, and a workup for insulinoma is unlikely to be revealing.

**VI-68.**  **The answer is D.**  *(Chap. 341)*   Cigarette smoking has been shown to be associated with low HDL but not with hypertriglyceridemia. Alcohol, diabetes mellitus, obesity, and pregnancy are all causes of hypertriglyceridemia. In addition, many medications may cause hypertriglyceridemia, including estrogen, isotretinoin, beta blockers, glucocorticoids, and thiazides.

**VI-69.** **The answer is D.** *(Chap. 353. Liberman, N Engl J Med 333:1437, 1995.)* Alendronate, a bisphosphonate in the same class as etidronate, was recently approved for the treatment of osteoporosis. It has been shown to increase bone density and decrease fracture rates. It is taken in the morning, a half hour before eating, to maximize its absorption. Its most common complication is esophagitis, and so it is recommended that it be taken with a full glass of water and that the patient remain upright for at least half an hour after taking the pill. Pamidronate, another bisphosphonate, can be given only intravenously and is not used for osteoporosis. Estrogen replacement therapy, weight-bearing exercise, and nasal calcitonin have all demonstrated efficacy in the treatment of osteoporosis. Nasal calcitonin may not be as effective as estrogen or alendronate and usually is not chosen as a first-line treatment.

**VI-70.** **The answer is C.** *(Chap. 354)* Hypoparathyroidism would cause a high, not low, phosphate. Transient hypoparathyroidism caused by atrophy of the remaining parathyroid glands may occur after parathyroid adenoma removal. However, this condition would be expected to resolve over 24 to 48 h. Magnesium deficiency may cause hypocalcemia, but this process is mediated through impairment of parathyroid hormone (PTH) secretion and end-organ resistance to PTH. Therefore, magnesium deficiency also would be expected to result in a high serum phosphate. Parathyroid cancer would be expected to cause hypercalcemia if it was not completely removed at surgery. However, complete excision could result in hypoparathyroidism because of atrophy of the other parathyroid glands. Again, one would expect this to resolve rapidly. Hungry bone syndrome occurs when calcium-starved bones that have been under the influence of high PTH take up calcium avidly after the removal of a parathyroid adenoma. Aggressive calcium supplementation may be necessary for months after surgery. Risk factors for the development of this syndrome include a high preoperative alkaline phosphatase level and a large tumor.

**VI-71.** **The answer is A.** *(Chap. 328)* This patient has postoperative diabetes insipidus, a common complication of surgery in the area of the hypothalamus. A water deprivation test is not necessary for the diagnosis because the patient already manifests the elements necessary to make the diagnosis: a serum sodium greater than normal, accompanied by inappropriately dilute urine. Fluid restriction could be dangerous in this patient, who could develop life-threatening hypernatremia. Instead, the patient should be encouraged to drink when thirsty and should be given one dose of DDAVP. If the patient's thirst mechanism is intact, he will be thirsty until his serum sodium level corrects. He should not be placed on a standing dose of DDAVP BID, as the effects of the first dose may not have resolved 12 h later. In addition, postoperative diabetes insipidus can be followed by SIADH, leading to iatrogenic hyponatremia caused by this regimen. Instead, the patient should be given one dose of DDAVP, be encouraged to drink when thirsty, and have his serum sodium monitored twice a day. The urine osmolality or specific gravity and urine output also should be monitored. A brain MRI is not necessary unless there is no other evidence of a central nervous system complication, since this is a common, expected, and usually transient complication of this type of neurosurgery. Classically, these patients experience a short period of diabetes insipidus, followed by an episode of SIADH, followed by diabetes insipidus. In practice, many patients do not experience all three stages.

**VI-72.** **The answer is C.** *(Chap. 328)* This patient may have hypopituitarism, but it is unclear from his laboratory results. A random cortisol of 4.8 μg/dL in the middle of the stress of hypotension and an illness severe enough to warrant an intensive care unit are quite suggestive of adrenal insufficiency (though one cannot differentiate between primary and secondary causes with a cortisol alone). However, the patient's cortisol level is not diagnostic, and dexamethasone should be given to this critically ill patient to provide him with adequate glucocorticoid coverage while a cosyntropin stimulation test is performed. Dexamethasone will not interfere with the performance of the cosyntropin stimulation test. This will ensure that an accurate diagnosis is made before the patient is committed to lifelong glucocorticoid therapy. Hydrocortisone, prednisone, and methylprednisolone all cross-react with the cortisol assays and produce falsely elevated values. The thyroid function tests could reflect secondary hypothyroidism, but it is more likely that they represent the sick euthyroid state, since the TSH is only mildly low and the total $T_3$ is proportionally lower than the free $T_4$ index. Thyroid hormone replacement in patients with the sick euthyroid syndrome has not been shown to improve the outcome. The low testosterone, accompanied by the low LH and FSH, provides evidence of secondary hypogonadism. Of note, severe illness can produce temporary hypogonadism. In these cases, testosterone recovers when the patient recovers. This patient could have hypogonadism, but one must wait until he recovers from his illness to determine this definitively. Further, though testosterone is important for his long-term health, it will not contribute to recovery from his acute illness.

**VI-73.** **The answer is C.** *(Chap. 331. Laderson, Am J Med 77:261, 1984.)* A TSH of 81 mU/mL is evidence of primary hypothyroidism. Studies have shown that hypothyroidism does not significantly increase cardiac surgery mortality, and giving thyroid hormone before surgery could exacerbate cardiac ischemia angina. Therefore, cardiac surgery should not be delayed while one waits for thyroid hormone levels to be restored. In patients with primary hypothyroidism and heart disease, thyroid hormone should be replaced gradually, starting with a low dose of 0.025 mg a day and increasing the dose slowly. Rapid replacement with the shorter-acting $T_3$ (Cytomel) may exacerbate the patient's angina, as might the fluctuations in thyroid hormone levels. There is no evidence that this patient has hypopituitarism, since the high TSH provides evidence of primary, not secondary, hypothyroidism. Propylthiouracil is a medication that may be given to a person with hyperthyroidism, not one with hypothyroidism.

**VI-74.** **The answer is B.** *(Chaps. 330, 332)* After an ACTH-producing tumor is removed from the pituitary, the patient will have adrenal insufficiency and require corticosteroids for a year. Normal ACTH-producing pituitary cells have atrophied but do eventually recover to function normally. The patient should have been started on corticosteroids at the time of surgery with a slow taper over a period of months. The choice of dexamethasone as the corticosteroid would allow accurate assessment of the hypothalamic-pituitary-adrenal axis in the immediate postoperative setting. Prednisone could be initiated in place of dexamethasone after testing is completed. It would be very unusual to remove enough normal ACTH-producing pituitary cells to cause adrenal insufficiency while leaving enough TSH-producing cells to maintain normal thyroid function.

**VI-75.** **The answer is D.** *(Chaps. 330, 332. Oldfield, N Engl J Med 325:897, 1991.)* Pituitary tumors suppress with high-dose dexamethasone and are more common than adrenal and ectopic tumors. Suppression is defined as a greater than 90 percent decrease in the 24-h urine free cortisol on the second day. However, some ectopic ACTH-producing tumors, particularly carcinoids, also are suppressed with high-dose dexamethasone. The next step in localizing the tumor is the performance of a petrosal sinus catheterization. Concomitant administration of CRH during this procedure will increase its accuracy. If peripheral ACTH levels are more than double central levels, the tumor is most likely ectopic. If, however, the central ACTH levels are more than double the peripheral levels, the tumor is more likely to be pituitary in origin. If testing suggests a pituitary origin, an MRI with and without gadolinium is warranted. If testing suggests an ectopic source, locating the tumor can be difficult. One might start with a fine-cut CT scan of the lungs. Octreotide scans sometimes may be helpful in locating ectopic tumors. If the 24-h urine free cortisol had not suppressed, one would expect the tumor to be either adrenal or ectopic in origin.

**VI-76.** **The answer is D.** *(Chap. 331)* The contrast used in catheterization procedures contains iodine. Iodine tends to worsen hyperthyroidism caused by autonomous nodules, whereas it inhibits the release of thyroid hormone in patients with autoimmune thyroid disease such as Graves' disease and Hashimoto's thyroiditis. Iodine-containing medications sometimes are used in the treatment of Graves' disease. If a patient is known to have an autonomous nodule, he or she should receive an antithyroid drug such as methimazole or propylthiouracil before undergoing catheterization. Further, the antithyroid medication should be continued for at least 2 weeks after the procedure.

**VI-77.  The answer is E.**  *(Chap. 331)*  This entity of self-induced thyrotoxicosis is most commonly seen in medical and paramedical personnel and in those with easy access to thyroid hormone. Weight loss induction is one motivation for taking the unprescribed thyroid hormone in supraphysiologic doses. The patient's thyroid is suppressed because of negative feedback. Therefore, the 24-h radioactive iodine uptake is low, as in thyroiditis. This entity can be distinguished from thyroiditis by the presence of a low thyroglobulin. Graves' disease and toxic multinodular goiters cause an elevated 24-h radioactive iodine uptake.

**VI-78.  The answer is B.**  *[Chap. 354. Consensus Development Panel, Ann Intern Med 114(7): 593, 1991].*  Kidney stones, osteoporosis, a markedly elevated calcium level, and a decreased creatinine clearance are all considered indications for surgical removal of a parathyroid adenoma. Another indication for surgery is elevated 24-h urine calcium, but this sometimes can be treated with a thiazide diuretic. Poor follow-up and young, not old, age are other indications for surgery. It is increasingly recognized that avoidance of surgery is desirable in some patients. Close follow-up rather than surgery is particularly appealing for patients who have no complications attributable to hyperparathyroidism, who are unlikely to live long enough to develop complications, and in whom surgery poses a particularly great risk, such as the elderly.

**VI-79.  The answer is C.**  *(Chap. 340. Chandrasekharappa, Science 276:404, 1997.)*  MEN I is characterized by hyperparathyroidism, pancreatic islet cell tumors, and pituitary tumors. The hyperparathyroidism can be particularly difficult to manage, as it usually is caused by four-gland hyperplasia and recurs after surgery. Hyperparathyroidism is the most common manifestation of the syndrome. Most individuals are affected by age 40. Islet cell tumors are the second most common manifestation of MEN I. Pituitary tumors occur in more than half of MEN I patients. The most common type of pituitary tumor found in this population is a prolactinoma. The gene implicated in the pathogenesis of MEN I has been cloned. It is located on chromosome 11 and has been named MENIN. MEN I is inherited in an autosomal dominant fashion. A c-RET proto-oncogene mutation has been identified in 93 to 95 percent of patients with MEN II, not in those with MEN I.

**VI-80.  The answer is A.**  *(Chap. 334)*  The mainstay of therapy for diabetic ketoacidosis (DKA) is insulin and intravenous fluids. DKA cannot be reversed without insulin. The usual fluid deficit is 3 to 5 L, and both salt solutions and free water are needed. Because glucose levels drop more quickly than ketones disappear from the plasma, it is usually necessary to give intravenous dextrose when the blood glucose level drops below about 14 to 16.7 mmol/L (250 to 300 mg/dL). This allows continued administration of insulin to clear the ketones from the blood. Although the serum potassium concentration is high, there is a total body potassium deficit of several hundred millimoles. The potassium concentration will drop quickly as the pH rises, causing potassium to enter cells. Bicarbonate therapy is not recommended unless the arterial pH falls below 7.10 or 7.00 because the rapid alkalinization may impair oxygen delivery to tissues and impair left ventricular function. In addition, insulin therapy is effective in reversing the acidemia without the assistance of bicarbonate therapy.

**VI-81.  The answer is B.**  *(Chap. 340).*  Polyglandular autoimmune syndrome type II (Schmidt's syndrome) is characterized by lymphocytic infiltration of the adrenal and thyroid glands along with type I diabetes mellitus in about half of affected families. Hypogonadism is also common. A few patients develop transient hypoparathyroidism caused by antibodies that compete with parathyroid hormone for binding to the parathyroid receptor. Mucocutaneous candidiasis does not occur as part of this syndrome. Instead, it occurs in most patients with polyglandular autoimmune syndrome type I.

**VI-82.** **The answer is D.** *(Chap. 335)* Insulin, sulfonylureas, and alcohol are estimated to cause 60 percent of episodes of hypoglycemia in hospitalized patients. Most of the other 40 percent of cases can be accounted for by renal failure, liver disease, malnutrition, and sepsis. Insulinomas, solid tumors, enzymatic defects, and hormonal deficiencies, including adrenal insufficiency, can cause hypoglycemia. However, they are rare, not common, causes of hypoglycemia in hospitalized patients.

**VI-83.** **The answer is E.** *(Chap. 352)* Generalized lipodystrophy is characterized by loss of body fat and metabolic abnormalities, including insulin resistance, hyperglycemia, hypertriglyceridemia, and a high metabolic rate despite normal thyroid function. The congenital form is autosomal recessive, while the acquired form often develops after an illness such as measles, chickenpox, whooping cough, or infectious mononucleosis. Other abnormalities associated with this disorder include paradoxical fatty engorgement of the liver and enlarged kidneys and genitalia. Mental retardation is seen in about half the congenital cases. Linear growth is accelerated in the first few years of life, but epiphyses close early so that the final height is usually normal.

**VI-84.** **The answer is D.** *(Chap. 356)* Less than 5 percent of cases of DKA are accompanied by severe phosphorus deficiency, though serum inorganic phosphorus often falls after therapy for DKA is initiated as phosphorus is shifted into cells. Patients who present in DKA with hypokalemia and hypophosphatemia are more likely to be severely potassium- and phosphorus-depleted and probably will require treatment with phosphorus. Such a patient usually has been sick for many days, has maintained a good fluid intake, and has not had significant vomiting. The insulin deficiency and metabolic acidosis mobilize intracellular phosphate stores, and the patient excretes the phosphorus briskly for days before presentation.

**VI-85.** **The answer is A.** *(Chap. 357)* The most common cause of magnesium deficiency in adults is intestinal malabsorption and steatorrhea. This can result from chronic pancreatic insufficiency, short bowel syndromes, or nontropical sprue, for example. Other causes of hypomagnesemia include poorly controlled diabetes mellitus, hyperaldosteronism, the syndrome of inappropriate vasopressin secretion (SIADH), alcoholism, and medications such as diuretics, cisplatin, cyclosporine, and aminoglycosides, all of which cause magnesium wasting in the urine. Beta agonists, not beta blockers, can cause transient hypomagnesemia because magnesium is taken up into adipose tissue as fatty acids are released.

**VI-86.** **The answer is E.** *(Chap. 341)* Hypothyroidism, not hyperthyroidism, is a secondary cause of hypercholesterolemia and accounts for 2 percent of all cases of hyperlipidemia. The nephrotic syndrome can cause increases in LDL, VLDL, or both. Obstructive liver disease, anorexia nervosa, acute intermittent porphyria, and drugs such as progestogens, cyclosporine, and thiazides can all cause hypercholesterolemia.

**VI-87.** **The answer is B.** *(Chap. 334)* Diabetic retinopathy is divided into two categories: simple (background) and proliferative. Background retinopathy precedes proliferative retinopathy. The first retinal abnormality seen is increased capillary permeability (which can be demonstrated by injecting florescein and observing leakage of dye into the vitreous humor). This is followed by occlusion of retinal capillaries with subsequent microaneurysm formation. Arteriovenous shunts, dot and blot hemorrhages, and dilated veins are all manifestations of background retinopathy. Cotton-wool spots represent microinfarcts, and hard exudates probably represent leakage of proteins and lipids from damaged capillaries. Proliferative retinopathy is characterized by new vessel formation and scarring. The neovascularization probably is stimulated by hypoxia secondary to vascular occlusion. The complications of proliferative retinopathy include vitreal hemorrhage and retinal detachment.

**VI-88.** **The answer is C.** *(Chap. 334)* This patient has malignant external otitis, which usually is caused by *Pseudomonas aeruginosa*. It tends to occur in older patients with diabetes mellitus who present with severe ear pain, drainage, fever, leukocytosis, and soft tissue swelling around the ear. The facial nerve is paralyzed in about 50 percent of cases, and this subset carries a poor prognosis with a 50 percent mortality rate. A mound of granulation tissue usually is present at the junction of the osseous and cartilaginous portions of the ear. The treatment of choice is a 6-week course of ticarcillin or carbenicillin plus tobramycin. In addition, surgical debridement is often necessary.

**VI-89.** **The answer is D.** *(Chap. 334)* Rhinocerebral mucormycosis is a rare and devastating fungal infection associated with diabetes mellitus. It usually develops during or after diabetic ketoacidosis (DKA). Patients usually present with the sudden onset of periorbital and perinasal swelling, pain, bloody discharge, and increased, not decreased, lacrimation. Tissue necrosis, cranial nerve palsies, and thrombosis of the internal jugular vein or cavernous sinus may occur. The treatment of choice is amphotericin B plus aggressive debridement. If untreated, mucormycosis is uniformly fatal, usually within 7 to 10 days.

**VI-90.** **The answer is A.** *(Chap. 327)* Insulin interacts with a protein tyrosine kinase receptor, not a seven-transmembrane-domain receptor. Seven-transmembrane-domain receptors include the alpha- and beta-adrenergic receptors and receptors for parathyroid hormone, vasopressin, angiotensin II, glucagon, serotonin, dopamine, LH, FSH, TSH, and prostaglandins. The action of the hormone-receptor complex is mediated by guanine nucleotide-binding proteins (G proteins).

**VI-91.** **The answer is B.** *(Chap. 328)* Medications are important causes of hyperprolactinemia. Drugs implicated in hyperprolactinemia include dopamine-blocking drugs (e.g., phenothiazines, butyrophenones, metoclopramide, resperidone) and dopamine-depleting drugs (e.g., methyldopa and reserpine). In addition, chronic cocaine use can cause hyperprolactinemia. Severe primary hypothyroidism can cause hyperprolactinemia either through the increase in the thyroid-releasing hormone (TRH) level or through a decrease in dopaminergic tone. Therefore, levothyroxine would not be expected to cause hyperprolactinemia.

**VI-92.** **The answer is E.** *(Chap. 335)* Drugs are important causes of hypoglycemia. Insulin, sulfonylureas, disopyramide, and pentamidine all cause hypoglycemia through hyperinsulinemia. Sulfonamides and salicylates may interact with the sulfonylurea receptor. Thiazides can cause an exacerbation of glucose intolerance and worsen hyperglycemia.

**VI-93.** **The answer is A-N, B-N, C-Y, D-Y, E-Y.** *(Chaps. 52, 337)* The luteal phase of the menstrual cycle follows ovulation and is characterized by an increase in progesterone secretion by the corpus luteum. With anovulatory cycles, the corpus luteum does not form and progesterone levels remain low. Furthermore, with anovulatory cycles, the characteristic surge of LH and FSH at midcycle is absent and menses are usually painless. Irregular estrogen breakthrough bleeding that occurs with anovulatory cycles is the consequence of persistent ovarian estradiol secretion and an absence of luteal-phase progesterone secretion.

**VI-94.** **The answer is A-N, B-Y, C-Y, D-Y, E-N.** *(Chap. 354)* Familial hypocalcemia, short stature, and abnormalities of the metacarpal and metatarsal bones are characteristic features of congenital pseudohypoparathyrophy (Albright's hereditary osteodystrophy). The underlying defect is renal resistance to the action of parathyroid hormone, caused in many patients by a mutation in a guanyl-nucleotide-binding protein. Although plasma levels of parathyroid hormone are elevated, urinary cyclic AMP is low, and there is a diminished response of urinary cyclic AMP to the exogenous administration of the hormone. The basal ganglia are frequently calcified. No antibodies to parathyroid tissue can be demonstrated, and unlike the situation in idiopathic hypoparathyroidism, the frequency of monilial infection is not increased. Hypothyroidism is common in persons with pseudohypoparathyroidism; it is usually a result of resistance to TSH resulting from the same defect in membrane adenylate cyclase activity that causes resistance to parathyroid hormone.

**VI-95.**    **The answer is A-N, B-Y, C-Y, D-N, E-Y.** *(Chap. 74)*    Whenever caloric intake is deficient, amino acids are utilized as energy substrates and for gluconeogenesis to maintain an adequate blood level of glucose, which is especially important for metabolism in the brain. Thus, protein synthesis is compromised when energy requirements are not met by nonprotein calories. Stated in another way, energy undernutrition predisposes to protein starvation even when the protein supply is otherwise adequate. Nevertheless, it should be kept in mind that diets deficient in energy frequently are deficient in protein as well. Carbohydrates have a protein-sparing effect if given in sufficient quantities, but this effect does not hold true for fat. Low-carbohydrate and low-fat diets do not produce a selective protein malabsorption, although generalized malabsorption occurs in patients with severe chronic malnutrition.

**VI-96.**    **The answer is A-Y, B-Y, C-N, D-N, E-Y.** *(Chap. 67)*    Several inborn errors of metabolism can be treated successfully by the appropriate dietary restriction of a substrate or its precursors. Mental retardation and other problems associated with galactosemia and phenylketonuria can be prevented by a reduced intake of galactose or phenylalanine, respectively, during childhood. Restriction of neutral fats can prevent pancreatitis in persons with lipoprotein lipase deficiency. Neither hyperprolinemia nor Tay-Sachs disease is treatable by dietary management.

**VI-97.**    **The answer is A-N, B-Y, C-N, D-Y, E-Y.** *(Chap. 74)*    Several methods are useful in assessing protein undernutrition. Clinically, the ratio of 24-h urinary creatinine excretion to height is a sensitive and practical measure of muscle mass; it is decreased in the presence of protein malnutrition. Reduced blood levels of proteins synthesized by the liver, such as albumin and transferrin, are also characteristic findings with protein starvation. Anthropometric assessment of midarm circumference and triceps skin-fold thickness are measures of the mass of muscle and adipose tissue, respectively. While in many instances calculation of body weight as a percentage of ideal body weight is a good measure of lean body mass plus adipose tissue, the presence of ascites and edema makes this assessment unreliable. Blood ammonia levels may indicate protein overload from intestinal causes (e.g., gastrointestinal bleeding) but are not helpful in assessing protein nutrition. The combination of a careful clinical history and a thorough examination is also a reproducible and valid technique to evaluate nutritional status; however, many cachectic patients are unable to provide a detailed history.

**VI-98.**    **The answer is A-Y, B-Y, C-Y, D-N, E-N.** *(Chap. 78)*    As a general rule, when patients cannot eat a normal diet, cannot absorb an oral diet efficiently, or deteriorate in health with oral feeding, total parenteral nutrition (TPN) is needed to provide partial or complete nourishment. Bowel rest, a frequent indication for TPN, is important in treating exacerbations of inflammatory bowel disease, intestinal fistulas, and pancreatitis. While medium-chain triglycerides can be helpful, TPN is the best form of management for short bowel syndrome (over 70 percent resected). Persons who are markedly hypermetabolic from severe trauma, burns, or sepsis, for example, also may be helped by supplemental parenteral nutrition even when some oral intake is possible. Well-nourished patients who are not expected to be able to eat for 10 to 14 days should receive TPN to avoid excess wasting and malnutrition. It is unclear whether the decrease in negative nitrogen balance that results from the administration of TPN for a week or less to otherwise healthy people is of clinical significance. Patients who are unable to swallow for long periods (e.g., because of stroke, neuromuscular disorders, or coma) are best treated with enteral feedings.

**VI-99.**    **The answer is A-Y, B-Y, C-Y, D-N, E-Y.** *(Chap. 341. Havel, J Clin Invest 81:1653, 1988.)*    Appropriate therapy for patients who have familial hypercholesterolemia begins with a diet that is low in cholesterol and saturated fats and high in polyunsaturated fats. The administration of nicotinic acid (which blocks hepatic cholesterol synthesis) and bile acid–binding resins such as cholestyramine and colestipol may be required if diet alone constitutes insufficient therapy. Drugs, such as lovastatin, that inhibit 3-hydroxy-3 methylglutaryl coenzyme A, the rate-limiting step in cholesterol biosynthesis, are an effective treatment for patients with hypercholesterolemia. Gemfibrozil and clofibrate are used mainly in the treatment of hypertriglyceridemia.

**VI-100.** **The answer is A-Y, B-Y, C-Y, D-Y, E-Y.** *(Chaps. 334, 341)* Diabetic patients with insulin deficiency may show massive elevation of the serum level of triglycerides, with the concomitant risk of developing acute pancreatitis, as well as eruptive xanthomas, lipemia retinalis, and hepatomegaly. Adequate insulin replacement restores lipoprotein lipase activity and decreases hepatic production of very-low-density lipoproteins by impairing fatty acid mobilization from the adipose tissue. However, hypertriglyceridemia also occurs in well-controlled diabetic patients (generally obese), in whom it may be present as an independently inherited trait, as shown by family studies. Specific drug therapy may be required in this group of patients when diet and adequate control of the diabetic state fail to return triglyceride levels to normal.

**VI-101.** **The answer is A-Y, B-Y, C-N, D-N, E-Y.** *(Chap. 328)* The development of a pituitary adenoma in a patient who has undergone bilateral adrenalectomy for the treatment of Cushing's disease is termed Nelson's syndrome. This disorder is characterized by hyperpigmentation, erosion of the sella turcica, and high plasma ACTH levels. Because of adrenalectomy, urinary 17-ketosteroid excretion usually is low; plasma cortisol levels are determined by the regimen of replacement therapy.

**VI-102.** **The answer is A-Y, B-Y, C-N, D-Y, E-Y.** *(Chap. 332)* Adrenal carcinomas are likely to present as abdominal masses and secrete large amounts of adrenal androgens, resulting in markedly elevated urinary 17-ketosteroid excretion. Neoplastic secretion of adrenal steroids characteristically is not suppressed with low doses (0.5 mg every 6 h for 2 days) or high doses (2 mg every 6 h) of dexamethasone because it is not regulated by ACTH. Indeed, ACTH levels are usually immeasurably low in persons with adrenal carcinoma.

**VI-103.** **The answer is A-Y, B-Y, C-Y, D-N, E-N.** *(Chap. 338)* Pathologic gynecomastia develops when the effective testosterone-to-estrogen ratio is decreased owing to diminished testosterone production (as in primary testicular failure) or increased estrogen production. The latter may arise from direct estradiol secretion by a testis stimulated by luteinizing hormone or human chorionic gonadotropin or from an increase in peripheral aromatization of precursor steroids, most notably androstenedione. Elevated androstenedione levels may result from increased secretion by an adrenal tumor (leading to an elevated level of urinary 17-ketosteroids) or decreased hepatic clearance in patients with chronic liver disease. A variety of drugs, including diethylstilbestrol, heroin, digitalis, spironolactone, cimetidine, isoniazid, and tricyclic antidepressants, also can cause gynecomastia. In the case presented in the question, the history of paternity and the otherwise normal physical examination indicate that a karyotype is unnecessary, and the bilateral breast enlargement essentially excludes the presence of carcinoma and thus the need for biopsy.

**VI-104.** **The answer is A-N, B-N, C-Y, D-Y, E-Y.** *(Chap. 334. Harrison, Diabetes 38:815, 1989.)* There is considerable disagreement regarding the genetics of diabetes mellitus, but certain aspects appear to be clear-cut. Genetic factors are probably permissive for the development of type 1 (immune-mediated) and are related more directly to the development of type 2 (non-immune-mediated) diabetes. The genetic locus for diabetes appears to be located near the HLA genes on the sixth chromosome. The presence of HLA antigen B8 or B15 increases the risk for developing type 1 diabetes nearly threefold, antigens DR3 and DR4 fourfold to fivefold, and antigen combinations (e.g., B8/B15) up to tenfold. However, homozygosity for a high-risk allele (e.g., DR3/DR3) does not increase the risk further. Evidence implicates positions 45 and 57 of the $DQ_\beta$ chain as having importance in determining genetic susceptibility to type 1 diabetes. The concordance rate for monozygotic twins under 40 years of age is less than 50 percent. Pedigree analysis has shown a very low prevalence of vertical transmission for type 1 diabetes. The onset of juvenile diabetes has a seasonal variation and may follow mumps, hepatitis, or coxsackievirus infections, among others. These infections in genetically predisposed persons are theorized to produce an immune response with the development of cytotoxic islet cell antibodies, which complete the destruction of the beta cells. This theory would explain why circulating islet cell antibodies usually are detectable soon after the onset of type 1 diabetes. In some cases anti-islet-cell antibodies have been demonstrated in twins of diabetics destined to develop the disease even before glucose tolerance became abnormal.

**VI-105.** **The answer is A-N, B-Y, C-Y, D-N, E-Y.** *(Chap. 334)* The occurrence of hyperglycemic ketoacidosis or hyperglycemic hyperosmolar coma is diagnostic of diabetes mellitus. Similarly, persistent fasting hyperglycemia [glucose concentration greater than 7.8 mmol/L (140 mg/dL)], even if it is asymptomatic, has been recommended by the National Diabetes Data Group as a criterion for the diagnosis of diabetes. However, abnormal glucose tolerance—whether after eating or after a standard "glucose tolerance test"—can be caused by many factors (e.g., anxiety, infection or other illness, lack of exercise, or inadequate diet). Similarly, glycosuria may have renal as well as endocrinologic causes. Therefore, these two conditions cannot be considered diagnostic of diabetes.

**VI-106.** **The answer is A-Y, B-N, C-Y, D-Y, E-N.** *(Chap. 334)* Diabetic, hyperosmolar, nonketotic coma is a medical emergency that usually occurs as a complication of maturity-onset diabetes. Typically, affected persons are elderly (often living alone or in a nursing home), have a history of recent stroke or infection, and are unable to drink sufficient water to balance urinary fluid losses. These factors combine to cause sustained hyperglycemic diuresis with profound volume depletion and decreased urine output. Presenting features often include signs of circulatory compromise as well as central nervous system manifestations ranging from confusion or seizures to coma. Ketoacidosis is absent, perhaps because the concentration of portal-vein insulin is high enough to prevent full activation of hepatic ketogenesis. Serum levels of free fatty acids are generally lower than in diabetic ketoacidosis, and although hypertonicity is marked, measured serum sodium concentration is kept from being significantly elevated by the profound hyperglycemia. Infections are common, and disseminated intravascular coagulation can occur as a result of elevated plasma viscosity (both bleeding and in situ thrombosis have been reported). Although the administration of free water eventually becomes necessary, the treatment of salt deficits has the highest initial therapeutic priority. Several liters of isotonic saline should be given over the first 2 h, followed by half-normal saline and then a 5% glucose solution when blood glucose levels approach normal. Hypotonic fluids should not be used initially because most of the water enters the intracellular compartment, possibly leading to cerebral edema, rather than remaining in the plasma and interstitial spaces, where it is needed to support the circulation. Insulin also is required, but usually in lower doses than in patients with diabetic ketoacidosis.

**VI-107.** **The answer is A-Y, B-N, C-N, D-N, E-Y.** *(Chap. 334. Flier, Diabetes 41:1207, 1992.)* Chronic insulin resistance is defined as a need for more than 200 units of insulin per day for several days in the absence of infection or ketoacidosis. This definition was based on the assumption that the normal human pancreas produces this much insulin daily; in fact, normal daily insulin production is probably 30 to 40 units, so that relative resistance is present when more than this amount is required to control blood sugar levels. The most common causes of insulin resistance are obesity and anti-insulin antibodies of the IgG type. Antibodies develop within 60 days of the initiation of insulin therapy in nearly all diabetic persons. It is assumed that the binding of insulin by these antibodies is the major cause of severe insulin resistance, but the correlation between antibody titer and resistance is not always close. Uncontrolled hyperglycemia is the major consequence of insulin resistance, although ketoacidosis also may result. A history of discontinuous insulin use is common, and concomitant insulin allergy occurs in a minority of affected persons. Most patients require high doses of steroids, which frequently begin to take effect in a few days.

Acanthosis nigricans is a cutaneous disorder that is associated with two types of insulin resistance: type A, in which young women show accelerated growth, evidence of virilization, and decreased numbers of insulin receptors, and type B, in which older women have anti-insulin-receptor antibodies and other symptoms and signs of autoimmune disease (arthralgias, positive assay for antinuclear antibody, and others). The absence of acanthosis nigricans in the woman described in the question makes it unlikely that decreased numbers of insulin receptors or the presence of anti-insulin-receptor antibodies is playing a role in her insulin resistance.

**VI-108.** **The answer is A-Y, B-Y, C-Y, D-N, E-N.** *(Chap. 334)*    Approximately 40 percent of patients with type 1 diabetes mellitus sustain diabetic nephropathy. The progression of renal disease is markedly accelerated by hypertension, and even mild degrees of hypertension in diabetic patients should be treated aggressively. A hallmark of diabetic nephropathy is the presence of so-called macroproteinuria (excretion of more than 0.55 g/d), and once this phase is reached, there is a steady decline in renal function. So-called microalbuminuria, the excretion of 0.03 to 0.3 g/d of albumin, is also statistically predictive of the progression of renal disease. In contrast, nocturia is usually a manifestation of undertreatment of diabetes and is an indication not of renal failure but of an osmotic diuresis. There is no clear-cut relation between insulin requirement and the development of any of the long-term complications of diabetes, including nephropathy; the development of these complications correlates better with the duration than with the severity of diabetes mellitus.

**VI-109.** **The answer is A-N, B-Y, C-Y, D-N, E-N.** *(Chap 335. Grunberger, Ann Intern Med 108:252, 1988.s)*    Because factitious hypoglycemia resulting from insulin injection or sulfonylurea ingestion is common, the finding of hyperinsulinemia associated with a low blood sugar concentration can no longer be considered diagnostic of an islet cell tumor (insulinoma). Suspicion of factitious disease should be especially high in medical personnel and in the relatives of diabetics. The alpha and beta subunits of insulin are cleaved from proinsulin in the beta cell and are released in equimolar amounts with the connecting (C) peptide; elevation of plasma C-peptide levels signifies endogenous hyperinsulinemia, because exogenous insulin administration suppresses beta-cell function. Therefore, the triad of fasting hypoglycemia, hyperinsulinemia, and elevated plasma C-peptide levels is consistent with either endogenous hyperinsulinemia or the ingestion of a sulfonylurea; documentation of the latter in urine or plasma would be diagnostic. Proinsulin usually is released into the circulation in small quantities. However, in patients with insulinoma, proinsulin concentration frequently exceeds 20 percent of total insulin; ingestion of a sulfonylurea, by contrast, does not cause a disproportionate elevation of plasma proinsulin levels. Insulin antibody measurements in this case would not be expected to be helpful; antibodies may not develop for several months after the start of insulin injections, and the high C-peptide levels essentially rule out an exogenous source of insulin. However, in some circumstances antibodies to specific species of insulin can be identified and hence establish that exogenous insulin has been taken. Attempts to localize an islet cell tumor by radiologic means should be done only after factitious types of hypoglycemia have been excluded.

**VI-110.** **The answer is A-Y, B-Y, C-Y, D-N, E-N.** *(Chap. 335)*    Hypoglycemia caused by over-utilization of glucose can be associated with either high or low insulin levels. Hypoglycemia associated with hyperinsulinism can occur in persons who have a pancreatic insulinoma or who take exogenous insulin or ingest sulfonylurea drugs. Low plasma insulin levels can be associated with overutilization of glucose; examples include large, solid extrapancreatic tumors (e.g., hepatoma and sarcoma), in which high levels of insulin-like growth factors may play a role, and systemic carnitine deficiency, in which peripheral tissues are unable to use free fatty acids for energy production and the liver cannot synthesize ketone bodies. Underproduction of glucose may occur with acquired liver disease, such as hepatic congestion resulting from right-sided heart failure or viral hepatitis, or with hormone deficiencies, such as adrenal insufficiency and hypopituitarism.

**VI-111.   The answer is A-N, B-N, C-Y, D-N, E-Y.**   *(Chap. 336)*   Klinefelter syndrome frequently is not diagnosed in patients until the time of expected puberty or during adult life when incomplete virilization or another manifestation of androgen deficiency first becomes apparent. Testosterone replacement is likely to promote virilization and restore potency in these patients. However, if gynecomastia is already present, testosterone replacement therapy does not produce regression of the breast tissue and may even aggravate the gynecomastia. Surgical resection of the breast is usually necessary in this situation. Since the basic testicular lesion consists of progressive hyalinization of the seminiferous tubules, spermatogenic function is irreversibly impaired, and no form of hormonal therapy is effective in maintaining spermatogenesis. Even in normal persons, testosterone treatment produces hypospermia because of the inhibition of gonadotropin production. Although antisocial behavior may be a part of Klinefelter syndrome, it is unlikely to be a manifestation of androgen deficiency and is not correctable by testosterone replacement.

**VI-112.   The answer is A-Y, B-Y, C-N, D-Y, E-Y.**   *(Chap. 80)*   Deficiencies of trace elements (metals present at concentrations less than 1 $\mu$g per gram of tissue) can be due to dietary deficiency, malabsorption (as in chronic diarrhea), or the administration of total parenteral nutrition. Iron, copper, selenium, and zinc form stable complexes with enzymes. Selenium, for example, is a component of glutathione peroxidase and therefore functions as an antioxidant. Selenium deficiency results in myocardial necrosis. Zinc is required in tissues with a high cellular turnover, such as the gonads, and pregnant women and developing fetuses are at particular risk for zinc deficiency. Zinc deficiency dermatitis includes hyperkeratotic lesions and alopecia. Since cobalt is a component of vitamin $B_{12}$, deficiencies of this metal result in megaloblastic anemia. Copper deficiency may result in anemia, pigmentation abnormalities, hypothermia, and scurvylike skeletal changes.

**VI-113.   The answer is A-Y, B-N, C-Y, D-N, E-N.**   *(Chaps. 337, 339)*   In persons with testicular feminization, estradiol secretion by the testes is markedly increased (but not to the level produced by normal ovaries); the mechanism is lack of suppression of luteinizing hormone by testosterone and consequently increased stimulation of gonadal testosterone and estradiol secretion. Ovaries containing follicle cysts may be a source of increased estrogen production, particularly during the postmenopausal years, when gonadotropin levels are very high. The increase in estrogen production that is characteristic of polycystic ovarian disease is the consequence of peripheral conversion of androstenedione to estrogen, not of direct gonadal production. During the third trimester of pregnancy estrogen production is increased because of the formation of estrogen by the placenta rather than by the ovary. Arrhenoblastoma is a virilizing ovarian tumor and does not secrete estrogen.

**VI-114.   The answer is A-N, B-Y, C-Y, D-N, E-Y.**   *(Chap. 339)*   Ambiguous genitalia result when androgen production (or action) is defective in a male fetus or when androgen production is enhanced in a female fetus. Such aberrations can arise from a variety of causes. The most common cause is congenital adrenal hyperplasia, followed by mixed gonadal dysgenesis, which is a nonfamilial aberration of the sex chromosomes that interferes with normal sexual development, including 45,X/46,XY mosaicism. Examples of single-gene mutations leading to abnormal sexual differentiation include the Reifenstein syndrome, in which genetic males have incompletely developed male genitalia because of androgen resistance, and 5$\alpha$-reductase deficiency, in which testosterone cannot be converted to dihydrotestosterone. The historical use of progestational agents to treat pregnant women presenting with threatened abortion was associated with variable degrees of hypospadias in male offspring. Hypogonadotropic hypogonadism is associated with microphallus in male infants but not with hypospadias or abnormal sexual differentiation. Men whose chromosome pattern is 47,XYY are anatomically normal.

**VI-115.   The answer is A-Y, B-Y, C-N, D-N, E-Y.**   *(Chap. 339)*   Phenotypic men who have two or more X chromosomes have Klinefelter syndrome. Although the diagnosis of Klinefelter syndrome may be suspected prepubertally owing to the increased length of the lower body segment, most affected persons first present postpubertally with signs of decreased testosterone production and small testes. The risk of breast cancer is 20 times that of normal men (and one-fifth that of women), presumably as a consequence of long-term estrogen stimulation of the breast. Mosaic chromosome patterns (46,XY/47,XXY) are found in 10 percent of affected persons, 70 percent of whom display the mosaicism only in the testes, which may be normal in size. Hypospadias is not increased in incidence in affected persons. Although mental deficiency and social maladjustment occur with increased frequency in persons with Klinefelter syndrome, most patients with the disorder have normal mental and social competence.

**VI-116.** **The answer is A-Y, B-Y, C-Y, D-Y, E-Y.** *(Chap. 356)* Persistent hypophosphatemia is characterized by varying degrees of anorexia, dizziness, bone pain, proximal muscle weakness, cardiomyopathy, and waddling gait. Severe hypophosphatemia may result in rhabdomyolysis, which is heralded by a sharp elevation in the serum creatine phosphokinase concentration. A consequence of reduced levels of 2,3-diphosphoglycerate and ATP in erythrocytes is reduced tissue oxygenation. Leukocyte dysfunction resulting in defective phagocytosis makes a hypophosphatemic patient more susceptible to bacterial and fungal infection. Nervous system dysfunction, manifested by irritability and apprehension progressing to obtundation, may occur upon refeeding. Persons with alcoholism may develop severe hypophosphatemia shortly after hospitalization, probably related to the combined effects of glucose administration and phosphorus deficiency resulting from diminished intake. Correction of phosphorus deficits leads to a prompt reversal of the abnormalities.

**VI-117.** **The answer is A-N, B-N, C-Y, D-Y, E-N.** *(Chaps. 353, 354)* Vitamin D toxicity generally occurs after chronic ingestion of large doses of vitamin $D_2$ or $D_3$ (usually in excess of 50,000 to 100,000 IU daily for months). Ingestion of a single large dose of vitamin $D_2$ or $D_3$ does not cause acute toxicity because excessive quantities are stored in body fat and released slowly into the bloodstream. Some vitamin D metabolites, such as $1,25(OH)_2$ vitamin D, could conceivably cause toxicity after a single overdose. Hypervitaminosis D has not been reported after prolonged sun exposure, partly because the vitamin is released slowly from the skin after its conversion from previtamin D. Hypervitaminosis D causes hypercalcemia, hypercalciuria, and soft tissue calcification, particularly in the kidneys. It is believed that high circulating levels of 25(OH) vitamin D directly stimulate intestinal calcium absorption and bone resorption, since toxicity can occur in anephric persons.

**VI-118.** **The answer is A-Y, B-Y, C-N, D-Y, E-Y.** *(Chap. 328)* The enlarged pituitary gland of pregnancy is particularly vulnerable to ischemic necrosis (Sheehan's syndrome) if hypotension occurs in the postpartum period. Symptoms and signs of panhypopituitarism even several years after a difficult childbirth are consistent with this condition. Continued amenorrhea, decreased libido, cold intolerance typical of hypothyroidism, and loss of hair should therefore prompt an evaluation for anterior pituitary hypofunction. Lowering the blood sugar by giving a small amount of IV insulin normally triggers the release of counterregulatory hormones, including growth hormone and cortisol. The urinary free cortisol itself is not helpful, since a normal or low value is compatible with a stressless period, not just with panhypopituitarism. Since the patient probably has central hypothyroidism, the TSH will be inappropriately low in the face of low peripheral hormone. The response to ACTH stimulation should be blunted because the adrenal glands are not "primed" to respond to the pituitary release. Treatment of panhypopituitarism consists of hydrocortisone and thyroid hormone. Growth hormone injections are rarely required.

**VI-119.** **The answer is A-Y, B-N, C-N, D-Y, E-Y.** *(Chap. 331)* Hypothyroidism should be suspected in the setting of certain laboratory findings that are not clearly associated with an obvious explanation. In addition to an increased ratio of preejection period to left ventricular ejection time on cardiac systolic time intervals, decreased QRS amplitude on electrocardiographic examination is common. Elevated creatine phosphokinase and lactic dehydrogenase serum values may mimic a myocardial infarction. Hypothyroidism also is typically associated with macrocytic red blood cell indices caused by coexistent pernicious anemia or unknown factors. Serum cholesterol is elevated in many patients with primary hypothyroidism.

**VI-120.** **The answer is A-N, B-Y, C-N, D-Y, E-Y.** *(Chap. 332)* Weakness, hypotension, weight loss, nausea, and vomiting are all present in over 80 percent of patients with adrenal insufficiency, as documented by the failure of exogenously administered ACTH to effect a rise in the serum cortisol level. Hyperpigmentation, resulting from the melanocyte-stimulating hormone released in excess along with ACTH in cases of primary adrenal failure, is not seen in cases of secondary failure that occur because of suppressed ACTH. The best example of the latter condition is long-term steroid administration, which depresses ACTH release. Any cause of panhypopituitarism, such as a brain tumor's invasion of the sellar region, also can lead to adrenal failure on a secondary basis. Measurement of serum ACTH will distinguish between primary and secondary adrenal insufficiency. Destruction of the adrenal glands may occur as a consequence of infection with mycobacteria, cytomegalovirus, histoplasmosis, coccidioidomycosis, or cryptococcosis. Noninfectious causes of adrenal gland failure include bilateral tumor metastasis, bilateral hemorrhage, amyloidosis, sarcoidosis, autoimmune disease, and the administration of certain medications (e.g., rifampin, ketoconazole, and phenytoin).

**VI-121.** **The answer is A-Y, B-Y, C-Y, D-N, E-N.** *(Chap. 337)* Death rates associated with oral contraceptive use in women under age 40 are lower than those in women who use no contraception. The increased death rate in those not taking oral contraceptives probably is due to their higher pregnancy rate and the consequent risks associated with pregnancy. However, even with the low estrogen dose in current contraceptive pills, there are risks. The most serious are due to the tendency toward hypercoagulability induced by these agents and the increased relative risk for deep venous thrombosis, pulmonary embolism, and thromboembolic stroke. Smoking and advanced age both increase the incidence of these complications. Five percent of women taking oral contraceptives develop significant hypertension, which possibly is due to an estrogen-induced rise in angiotensinogen synthesis. Rare complications involving the liver include peliosis hepatitis (blood-filled venous lakes) and cholestatic jaundice. There is no convincing evidence to implicate oral contraceptives as a cause of increased risk of breast cancer (though such agents should not be used in the known or suspected presence of an estrogen-responsive neoplasm); their use is associated with a decreased risk of endometrial and ovarian cancer in women taking them for more than 10 years.

**VI-122.** **The answer is A-Y, B-N, C-N, D-N, E-Y.** *(Chap. 343)* The porphyrias represent disorders of heme biosynthesis. The biochemical abnormalities and clinical manifestations depend on the step that is blocked and the accumulation of precursor metabolites. Congenital erythropoietic porphyria is a rare autosomal recessive disorder that results from a defect in the enzyme uroporphyrinogen II cosynthase, which is expressed solely in maturing erythroid cells. Porphobilinogen is preferentially converted to uroporphyrinogen I and then to coproporphyrinogen I. These metabolites account for the red urine observed in children with this disorder, but excretion of porpholbilinogen is normal. Intermittent acute porphyria, characterized by attacks of recurrent neurologic and psychiatric dysfunction, is an autosomal dominant deficiency of porphobilinogen deaminase, the enzyme that converts porphobilinogen to uroporphyrinogen I. Thus, urinary levels of porphobilinogen are high during attacks. Hereditary coproporphyria is a similar disease caused by partial deficiency of coproporphyrinogen oxidase. A deficiency of protoporphyrinogen oxidase, the next to last enzyme involved in heme synthesis, leads to variegate porphyria manifested by attacks of neuropsychiatric dysfunction and photosensitivity and overexcretion of the proximal metabolite, porphobilinogen. Porphyria cutanea tarda, which is an inherited or acquired deficiency of hepatic uroporphyrinogen decarboxylase, is not associated with excess porphobilinogen production, probably because aminolevulinic acid synthase activity is not enhanced. Mild skin photosensitivity is the major manifestation of protoporphyria, and is due to a deficiency of ferrochelatase, the final enzyme in heme biosynthesis. Protoporphyrins may accumulate in erythrocytes, but urinary porphobilinogen is normal.

**VI-123.**   **The answer is A-N, B-Y, C-N, D-N, E-Y.**   *(Chaps. 346, 347, 349, 350)*   In Niemann-Pick disease, accumulation of sphingomyelins occurs usually because of a sphingomyelinase deficiency. Organomegaly and neurologic involvement are clinical features, but there is highly variable expression that depends on the subtype. The most common lysosomal storage disease, adult Gaucher disease, is characterized by splenomegaly, pancytopenia, hepatic dysfunction, and bone pain. Accumulation of glucosylceramides presumably accounts for the clinical manifestations and for the distinctive Gaucher cell observed on bone marrow examinations. Tay-Sachs disease, which is caused by a deficiency of hexosaminidase A with concomitant accumulation of sphingolipids, presents as rapidly progressive neurologic deterioration during infancy and with a characteristic macular cherry-red spot. Heterozygote detection programs (enzyme assays in Ashkenazi Jews) have reduced the incidence of this disease in North America.

Diseases of glycogen metabolism can result in disorders whose pathophysiology is based either on hepatic hypoglycemia, as in von Gierke's disease (glucose-6-phosphatase deficiency), or on muscle-energy deficiency, as in McArdle disease (muscle phosphorylase deficiency). Muscle-energy diseases generally result in painful cramping or myoglobinemia after exercise, and so strenuous exercise should be avoided. These diseases are otherwise compatible with a normal life.

A defect in the phenylalanine hydroxylase enzyme complex leads to accumulation of phenylalanine in blood and urine with associated brain damage. The plasma phenylalanine concentration usually does not rise until the institution of protein feedings but is abnormal by the fourth day of life. A diet low in phenylalanine, if instituted during the first month of life, can avert mental retardation. Screening all newborns for blood phenylalanine concentration has been beneficial in this regard.

Excessive urinary excretion of the dibasic amino acids cysteine, lysine, arginine, and ornithine as a result of impaired tubular reabsorption is the pathophysiologic hallmark of cystinuria, the most common inborn error of amino acid transport. Because of the insolubility of cysteine, the primary clinical manifestation of this disorder is cysteine nephrolithiasis.

# VII. IMMUNOLOGIC, ALLERGIC, AND RHEUMATIC DISORDERS

## QUESTIONS

**DIRECTIONS:** Each question below contains five suggested responses. Choose the **one best** response to each question.

**VII-1.** Of the following, which is expressed earliest in B-cell development?

(A) Surface immunoglobulin D
(B) Surface immunoglobulin G
(C) Surface immunoglobulin M
(D) Cytoplasmic μ chains
(E) Fc receptors

**VII-2.** A 29-year-old man with episodic abdominal pain and stress-induced edema of the lips, tongue, and occasionally larynx is likely to have low functional or absolute levels of which of the following proteins?

(A) C5A (complement cascade)
(B) IgE
(C) T-cell receptor, alpha chain
(D) Cyclooxygenase
(E) C1 esterase inhibitor

**VII-3.** A 35-year-old woman comes to the local health clinic because for the last 6 months she has had recurrent urticarial lesions, which occasionally leave a residual discoloration. She also has had arthralgias. Sedimentation rate obtained now is 85 mm/h. The procedure most likely to yield the correct diagnosis in the case would be

(A) a battery of wheal-and-flare allergy skin tests
(B) measurement of total serum immunoglobulin E (IgE) concentration
(C) measurement of C1 esterase inhibitor activity
(D) skin biopsy
(E) patch testing

**VII-4.** A 23-year-old man seeks medical attention for perennial nasal congestion and postnasal discharge. He states he does not have asthma, eczema, conjunctivitis, or a family history of allergic disease. His nasal secretions are rich in eosinophils. The test most likely to yield a specific diagnosis in this setting is

(A) serum IgE level (competitive radioimmunosorbent technique)
(B) serum IgE level (radiodiffusion technique)
(C) elimination diet test
(D) skin testing
(E) sinus x-rays

**VII-5.** A patient undergoing evaluation for possible infection with *M. tuberculosis* develops a skin wheal 48 h after intradermal placement of TB purified-protein derivative (PPD). Which of the following cellular events accounts for these findings?

(A) IL-7-induced B-cell activation and secretion of antibodies
(B) IL-3-mediated B-cell activation and induction of help for T-cell activation
(C) Monocyte-derived IL-6 activation of T cells
(D) Complement-mediated endothelial cell damage
(E) CD44-mediated monocyte adhesion to endothelial cells

**VII-6.** The hyperviscosity syndrome is most characteristic of which of the following plasma cell disorders?

(A) Multiple myeloma
(B) Heavy chain disease
(C) Indolent myeloma
(D) Waldenstrom's macroglobulinemia
(E) Primary amyloidosis

**VII-7.** A 47-year-old man has had fever, weight loss, arthralgias, pleuritic chest pain, and midabdominal pain for the last 2 months. One week ago he noticed difficulty dorsiflexing his right great toe. Blood pressure is 150/95 mmHg (he has always been normotensive), and laboratory studies reveal anemia of chronic disease, high erythrocyte sedimentation rate, and polymorphonuclear leukocytosis. The chest x-ray is clear. The most likely diagnosis is

(A) giant cell arteritis
(B) allergic granulomatosis
(C) Wegener's granulomatosis
(D) polyarteritis nodosa
(E) hypersensitivity vasculitis

**VII-8.** Which of the following statements regarding the renal involvement associated with systemic lupus erythematosus is true?

(A) Clinically apparent renal disease occurs in 90 percent of affected persons
(B) Interstitial nephritis is a rare finding on renal biopsy
(C) Renal biopsy is not initially necessary in patients with deteriorating renal function and active urine sediment
(D) Renal disease is uncommon in patients with high-titer anti-double-stranded DNA antibodies
(E) Urinalysis in affected persons usually reveals proteinuria but little sediment and no red blood cells

**VII-9.** A 25-year-old woman presents with a history of recurrent expectoration of foul-smelling sputum and intermittent fevers. Chest x-ray discloses characteristic "tram-tracking" bronchial thickening. Physical examination reveals coarse rhonchi in the right chest and splenomegaly. Blood test results are normal except for low levels of serum IgG and IgA. Her past medical history is remarkable for frequent upper respiratory infections and for a history of diarrhea 3 years ago due to Giardia lamblia infection. The most appropriate therapy would be

(A) corticosteroids
(B) corticosteroids and an alkylating agent
(C) monthly intravenous immunoglobulin
(D) splenectomy
(E) bone marrow transplantation

**VII-10.** All of the following statements regarding the epidemiology of HIV infection are correct EXCEPT

(A) the risk of transmission following skin puncture from a needle contaminated with blood from an HIV-infected patient is less than 0.5 percent
(B) most cases of AIDS are now among IV drug users
(C) the risk of transmission from a single donor unit of blood is approximately 1/500,000
(D) most pediatric cases of AIDS arise because of vertical transmission from an infected mother
(E) there is no convincing evidence that saliva can transmit HIV

**VII-11.** Each of the following would be an acceptable initial therapeutic regimen for an HIV-infected patient EXCEPT

(A) zidovudine/didanosine
(B) zidovudine monotherapy
(C) didanosine monotherapy
(D) zidovudine/zalcitabine
(E) zidovudine/lamivudine

**VII-12.** All the following statements concerning the HLA-D region on the sixth human chromosome are correct EXCEPT

(A) it is located outside the major histocompatibility gene complex
(B) it encodes proteins involved in the mixed lymphocyte response
(C) it encodes proteins expressed only on certain immune effector or closely related cells
(D) siblings matched for HLA-A, -B, and -C antigens will usually be matched at the D region
(E) it is located close to genes encoding for complement components

**VII-13.** Which of the following statements best describes the role of polymerase chain reaction (PCR) in the diagnosis of HIV infection?

(A) It should be used if the western blot is indeterminate
(B) It is a useful screening test
(C) It should be used if two consecutive serologic tests (ELISA) are positive
(D) It should be used if the initial serologic test is positive, but the second is negative
(E) It has no real role

**VII-14.** All of the following statements about the protease inhibitors are true EXCEPT

(A) patients taking indinavir should be encouraged to drink large quantities of fluids to prevent nephrolithiasis

(B) ritonavir is a powerful inhibitor of cytochrome P450 which complicates the use of other drugs metabolized by this pathway

(C) saquinavir is well tolerated, but has poor bioavailability

(D) even a mild increase in bilirubin warrants stopping indinavir use to prevent fatal hepatotoxicity

(E) maintaining continuous drug administration at the optimal dosage levels is important in preventing the development of resistance

**VII-15.** All the following statements concerning the ataxia-telangiectasia syndrome are correct EXCEPT

(A) it is inherited in an autosomal recessive manner

(B) the cause is adenosine deaminase deficiency

(C) malignancy is a common cause of death

(D) bronchiectasis may occur

(E) both humoral and cellular limbs of the immune system are affected

**VII-16.** All the following statements regarding the treatment of patients with HIV infection are true EXCEPT

(A) use of zidovudine (ZDV) therapy during pregnancy reduces the risk of vertical transmission to less than 10 percent

(B) HIV RNA assays should not be relied upon in making decisions about changing a patient's antiviral regimen

(C) though a useful agent in antiviral therapy, zidovudine monotherapy is a suboptimal regimen

(D) primary prophylaxis of *Mycobacterium avium* complex has clearly demonstrated efficacy in preventing bacteremia and improving survival

(E) breast feeding is a potential mode of HIV transmission and should be discouraged in women who are HIV-infected

**VII-17.** Which of the following statements regarding central nervous system disease in patients with HIV infection is correct?

(A) The most common cause of central nervous system disease is the AIDS dementia complex

(B) The most common cause of seizures is cryptococcal meningoencephalitis

(C) Antiretroviral agents have no role

(D) The most common finding on MRI is multiple white matter lesions

(E) Actual histologic evidence of direct HIV involvement is rare

**VII-18.** Which of the following statements concerning Kaposi's sarcoma in patients with HIV infection is INCORRECT?

(A) The decreasing incidence of Kaposi's sarcoma is likely a result of safer sexual practices

(B) Lymph node involvement implies metastatic spread and portends more aggressive disease and a poor prognosis

(C) The chest x-ray in pulmonary Kaposi's characteristically shows bilateral lower-lobe infiltrates and pleural effusions

(D) The most important determinant of response to interferon is the CD4+ count, not tumor burden

(E) In general, the tumor tends to respect issue planes and is rarely invasive

**VII-19.** A 32-year-old HIV-infected homosexual man complains of increasing dyspnea, fever, and a nonproductive cough. His peripheral CD4+ T-lymphocyte count is 100/μL. Each of the following pathogens is associated with this patient's illness EXCEPT

(A) *Pneumocystis carinii*

(B) cytomegalovirus

(C) *Mycoplasma pneumoniae*

(D) *Cryptococcus neoformans*

(E) *Mycobacterium tuberculosis*

**VII-20.** All the following are compatible with illness induced by therapeutic administration of antithymocyte globulin EXCEPT

(A) malaise and fever 2 to 3 days after beginning initial therapy

(B) lymphadenopathy

(C) depressed CH50 level

(D) positive C1q binding assay

(E) fever

**VII-21.** Each of the following agents has been demonstrated to alter the course of rheumatoid arthritis EXCEPT

(A) gold

(B) omega-3 fatty acids

(C) methotrexate

(D) D-penicillamine

(E) hydroxychloroquine

**VII-22.** Which of the following is the LEAST common immunologic manifestation of HIV infection?

(A) Cutaneous reactions to drugs

(B) Anaphylactic reactions to drugs

(C) Anticardiolipin antibodies

(D) Oligoarticular arthritis

(E) Fibromyalgia

**VII-23.** A woman who has rheumatoid arthritis suddenly develops pain and swelling in the right calf. The most likely diagnosis is

(A) ruptured plantaris tendon
(B) pes anserinus bursitis
(C) ruptured popliteal cyst
(D) thrombophlebitis
(E) Achilles tendonitis

**VII-24.** A 70-year-old woman presents with blurring of her vision in the left eye since waking earlier in the morning. She reports two months of fevers, sweats, anorexia, and a 10-pound weight loss. She also reports increasingly severe left temporal headaches over the same time period. Her physical exam reveals scalp tenderness over the left temporal region. Her laboratories reveal a normochromic, normocytic anemia, mildly elevated alkaline phosphatase, and an erythrocyte sedimentation rate of 92. Appropriate action includes

(A) obtaining an emergent MRI/MRA of her head
(B) referring the patient for a biopsy of her temporal artery, but abstaining from initiating therapy until the biopsy results are available
(C) initiating high-dose glucocorticoid therapy and referring the patient for a temporal artery biopsy
(D) obtaining a head CT to rule out metastatic disease and scheduling a colonoscopy
(E) performing a lumbar puncture to rule out meningitis

**VII-25.** Which histologic subtype of lymphoma occurs most commonly in patients infected with HIV?

(A) Immunoblastic (large cell) lymphoma
(B) Small, noncleaved (Burkitt's) lymphoma
(C) Small, cleaved (follicular) lymphoma
(D) Primary central nervous system lymphoma
(E) Hodgkin's disease, mixed cellularity

**VII-26.** A 68-year-old woman presents to her internist for a routine checkup. Her physical examination is normal and routine laboratory evaluation is also normal except for an elevated total protein of 90 g/L (9.0 g/dL). Further work-up includes the following: serum protein electrophoresis that reveals an M spike (proved to be IgG-κ on immuno-electrophoresis) of 19 g/L (1.9 g/dL), an unremarkable urine protein electrophoresis, bone marrow aspirate and biopsy that discloses normal hematopoiesis and 3 percent bone marrow plasma cells, and a negative skeletal survey. The proper course of action at this point is to

(A) obtain quantitative immunoglobulin levels
(B) obtain beta-microglobulin level
(C) begin therapy with melphalan and prednisone
(D) begin therapy with high-dose prednisone
(E) reassure the patient; no additional action is required at this time

**VII-27.** Which of the following systemic manifestations is LEAST characteristic of early adult rheumatoid arthritis?

(A) High fever
(B) Weight loss
(C) Muscle wasting
(D) Vague musculoskeletal symptoms
(E) Fatigue

**VII-28.** Which of the following conditions is LEAST likely to occur in late extraarticular seropositive rheumatoid arthritis?

(A) Neutropenia
(B) Dry eyes
(C) Leg ulcers
(D) Sensorimotor polyneuropathy
(E) Hepatitis

**VII-29.** Within minutes after injection of radiocontrast at the time of abdominal CT, a patient develops urticaria, flushing, and congestion of tongue and larynx. Respiratory stridor develops and intubation is emergently required. The mechanism of this event is

(A) direct activation of mediator release from mast cells or basophils or both
(B) IgE-mediated reaction against protein-hapten conjugates
(C) IgE-mediated reaction against native proteins
(D) deficiency of C1 esterase inhibitor
(E) inherited inability to normally catabolize the radiocontrast agent

**VII-30.** A 35-year-old woman relates a 1-year history of recurrent crops of small, reddish-brown pruritic skin bumps. She also notes facial flushing, lightheadedness, and lower abdominal pain. Pressure on one of these skin lesions results in increased itching and redness. Some attacks are brought on by the use of alcohol or non-steroidal anti-inflammatory agents. An upper GI series reveals an ulcer crater in the duodenal bulb. Skin biopsy would reveal

(A) aggregates of neutrophils in small venules
(B) mast cell infiltration
(C) hyperkeratosis and infiltration of lymphocytes into the dermis
(D) malignant-appearing neovascularization
(E) normal findings

**VII-31.** In which of the following clinical situations would a diagnosis of ankylosing spondylitis most likely be correct?

(A) For the last 10 years, a 28-year-old man has had low back pain and stiffness, worse at night and relieved with activity

(B) For the last 5 years, a 32-year-old man has had low back pain made worse with activity but improved with bed rest

(C) For the last 10 years, a 34-year-old man has had intermittent bouts of mild low back pain; now, however, he suddenly is unable to dorsi-flex his right great toe

(D) For the last 10 years, a 65-year-old man has had low back pain radiating down both poste-rior thighs to the knees

(E) For the last 15 years, a 72-year-old man has had progressive low back pain made worse with walking but improved with rest and lean-ing forward

**VII-32.** Arthritis associated with psoriasis can be manifest in several different ways. Each of the following is char-acteristic of psoriatic arthritis EXCEPT

(A) asymmetric oligoarticular arthritis

(B) rheumatoid factor-positive symmetric polyarthritis

(C) arthritis of distal interphalangeal joints

(D) severe destructive polyarthritis (arthritis mutilans)

(E) spondylitis and sacroiliitis with or without peripheral arthritis

**VII-33.** A 26-year-old woman with systemic lupus erythema-tosus (SLE) is noted to have a prolonged partial thrombo-plastin time. This abnormality is associated with

(A) leukopenia

(B) drug-induced lupus

(C) central nervous system vasculitis

(D) central nervous system hemorrhage

(E) deep venous thrombosis

**VII-34.** A patient with diffuse cutaneous scleroderma (sys-temic sclerosis) who had been stable for several years is recently noted to have hypertension. This patient is at significant risk of dying from

(A) thrombotic stroke

(B) central nervous system hemorrhage

(C) renal failure

(D) pulmonary hypertension

(E) pulmonary fibrosis

**VII-35.** For the last two years, a 27-year-old man has had recurrent episodes of asymmetric inflammatory oligo-articular arthritis involving his knees, ankles, and elbows lasting from 2 to 4 weeks. He also states he has had recurrent, painful "canker sores" in his mouth for the last 10 years. Now, he presents with fever, arthritis, mild ab-dominal pain, severe headache, and superficial thrombo-phlebitis in the left leg. The most likely diagnosis in this man is

(A) regional enteritis

(B) systemic lupus erythematosus

(C) Behçet's syndrome

(D) Whipple's disease

(E) ulcerative colitis

**VII-36.** A 37-year-old woman with Raynaud's phenome-non complains of progressive weakness with inability to arise out of a sitting position without assistance. On examination, the patient has swollen "sausage-like" fin-gers, alopecia, erythematous patches on the knuckles, facial telangiectasias, and proximal muscle weakness. Laboratory evaluation includes a normal CBC and serum chemistries, except for creatine phosphokinase 4.5 μkat/L (270 U/L) and aldolase 500 nkat/L (30 U/L). The following serologic profile is found: rheumatoid fac-tor is positive at 1:1600; ANA is also positive at 1:1600 with a speckled pattern and very high titers of antibodies against the ribonuclease-sensitive ribonucleoprotein component of extractable nuclear antigen. This patient probably has

(A) early rheumatoid arthritis

(B) systemic sclerosis

(C) systemic lupus erythematosus

(D) dermatomyositis

(E) mixed connective-tissue disease

**VII-37.** An 18-year-old man presents with abdominal pain, nausea, and vomiting. He also notes the onset of a rash and painful joints. Physical examination is remarkable for the presence of palpable purpura distributed over the buttocks and lower extremities as well as guaiac-positive stool. Laboratory evaluation is remarkable for urinalysis that discloses mild proteinuria and red blood cell casts. Other serum studies are normal. Skin biopsy would likely reveal

(A) necrotizing angiitis

(B) eosinophilic angiitis

(C) leukocytoclastic vasculitis

(D) extravasated red blood cells without vasculitis

(E) mast cell infiltration

**VII-38.** All the following physical findings may be seen in osteoarthritis EXCEPT

(A) Heberden's nodes
(B) Bouchard's nodes
(C) bony crepitus on joint movement
(D) boutonniere deformity
(E) positive "shrug" sign

**VII-39.** A 50-year-old woman has had Raynaud's phenomenon of the hands for 15 years. The condition has become worse during the last year, and she has developed arthralgias and arthritis involving the hands and wrists as well as mild sclerodactyly and difficulty swallowing solid foods. Laboratory studies reveal a positive serum antinuclear antibody assay at a dilution of 1:160. Anticentromere antibodies are present in high titers; antiribonucleoprotein antibodies are not detectable. The most likely diagnosis of this woman's disorder is

(A) systemic sclerosis
(B) mixed connective-tissue disease
(C) overlap syndrome
(D) dermatomyositis
(E) systemic lupus erythematosus

**VII-40.** A 62-year-old man complains of several weeks of progressive difficulty descending stairs or rising from a sitting position. He has also noted weakness in his upper body such that he has difficulty getting objects down from shelves above shoulder height. More recently, he has noted dysphagia. He denies pain or muscle soreness. He notes recent development of a rash over his forehead, cheeks, eyelids, chest, elbows, and knuckles. Examination reveals a violaceous rash on the eyelids and a maculopapular eruption in the previously cited areas. There is significant weakness of the proximal muscles in the hips, thighs, and shoulder girdle. Initial laboratories reveal elevated creatine phosphokinase, aldolase SGPT, and LDH. Complete blood count is normal. Electromyography reveals motor unit action potentials which are of low amplitude, polyphasic, and have abnormally early recruitment. Each of the following are true statements EXCEPT

(A) a muscle biopsy is likely to show evidence of an inflammatory cell infiltrate, muscle fiber degeneration, and capillary loss
(B) a workup for malignancy is warranted
(C) high dose glucocorticoids are the treatment of choice
(D) despite therapy, most patients will experience disease progression
(E) this condition may be associated with various connective tissue diseases

**VII-41.** True statements about human T cells include which of the following?

(A) They are the principal cells in the cortical "germinal centers" and medullary cords of lymph nodes
(B) They carry membrane-bound IgD on their surface
(C) They constitute 70 to 80 percent of circulating blood lymphocytes
(D) They arise from stem cells in the thymus
(E) They are the main effectors of antibody-dependent, cell-mediated cytotoxicity

**VII-42.** A 27-year-old woman with systemic lupus erythematosus is in remission; current treatment is azathioprine, 75 mg/d, and prednisone, 5 mg/d. Last year she had a life-threatening exacerbation of her disease. She now strongly desires to become pregnant. Which of the following is the LEAST appropriate action?

(A) Advise her that the risk of spontaneous abortion is high
(B) Warn her that exacerbations can occur in the first trimester and in the postpartum period
(C) Tell her it is unlikely a newborn will have lupus
(D) Advise that fetal loss rates are higher if anticardiolipin antibodies are detected in her serum
(E) Stop the prednisone just before she attempts to become pregnant

**VII-43.** Human immunoglobulin A (IgA) can be described by which of the following statements?

(A) It is the predominant immunoglobulin in plasma
(B) It exists in four subclasses, of which IgA2 is predominant
(C) It can prevent attachment of microorganisms to epithelial cell membranes
(D) It is prominent early in the immune response and is the major class of antibody in cold agglutinins
(E) It has the shortest half-life of the five classes of immunoglobulin

**VII-44.** Which of the following is LEAST likely to be seen in Sjögren's syndrome?

(A) Dental caries
(B) Corneal ulceration
(C) Renal tubular acidosis
(D) Lymphoma
(E) Cardiac fibrosis

**VII-45.** A 34-year-old man with AIDS complains of general malaise, low grade fevers, and diffuse myalgias of one month duration. His medications include only zidovudine and zalcitabine which he has been taking for eight months. Physical examination is remarkable for oral thrush, diffuse lymphadenopathy, and generalized muscle tenderness and weakness. The remainder of his examination is normal. Complete blood count reveals a hematocrit of 27 percent, WBC 2900/μL with 60 percent neutrophils, 30 percent lymphocytes, and 10 percent monocytes. Creatine phosphokinase is 6000 U/L. Which of the following is most likely to yield the diagnosis?

(A) Blood cultures
(B) Lymph node biopsy
(C) Electromyography
(D) Discontinuing the zidovudine
(E) Muscle biopsy

**VII-46.** Each of the following disorders is associated with neuropathic joint disease EXCEPT

(A) meningomyelocele
(B) acromegaly
(C) diabetes mellitus
(D) intraarticular glucocorticoid injections
(E) amyloidosis

**VII-47.** Each of the following may cause hyperuricemia and thereby may provoke an attack of gouty arthritis EXCEPT

(A) thiazide diuretics
(B) exercise
(C) hospitalization
(D) cyclosporine
(E) ascorbic acid

**VII-48.** Each of the following agents may be useful in the treatment of acute gouty arthritis EXCEPT

(A) indomethacin
(B) oral colchicine
(C) intravenous colchicine
(D) allopurinol
(E) intraarticular glucocorticoids

**VII-49.** All of the following are true of Marfan syndrome EXCEPT

(A) cardiovascular abnormalities are the major source of morbidity and mortality
(B) all patients should have a slit-lamp examination
(C) striae may occur over the shoulders and buttocks
(D) most patients have mutation in a gene coding for fibrillin
(E) the disorder is generally inherited as an autosomal recessive disorder

**VII-50.** Each of the following may be seen in Alport syndrome EXCEPT

(A) hematuria
(B) X-linked association
(C) leiomyomatosis
(D) blue sclerae
(E) deafness

**VII-51.** Each of the following statements regarding infections in prosthetic joints is true EXCEPT

(A) the majority of infections are acquired intraoperatively or immediately postoperatively
(B) prosthetic joint sepsis is invariably heralded by joint pain, swelling erythema, and warmth
(C) diagnosis is best made by needle aspiration of the joint
(D) successful treatment usually requires complete removal of the prosthesis
(E) the risk of infection is increased in patients undergoing a repeat total joint replacement

**VII-52.** Each of the following statements about fibromyalgia is true EXCEPT

(A) the condition is found predominantly in women
(B) disturbed sleep has been implicated as a factor in the pathogenesis
(C) many patients have psychological abnormalities
(D) joint examination yields normal findings
(E) low-dose glucocorticoids are often beneficial

**DIRECTIONS:** Each question below contains five suggested responses. For **each** of the five responses listed with every question, you are to respond either YES (Y) or NO (N). In a given item **all, some, or none** of the alternatives may be correct.

**VII-53.** A physician working on a Hopi Indian reservation in New Mexico develops a flu-like illness with the additional features of cough; conjunctivitis; painful, red lesions on his legs; and a painful, swollen right knee. Correct statements regarding this patient's arthritis include

(A) culturing the joint fluid will probably yield the diagnosis

(B) serology may be helpful in establishing the diagnosis

(C) the arthritis could have arisen from hematogenous seeding

(D) the arthritis could be a sterile manifestation of acute hypersensitivity

(E) the arthritis could have arisen from adjacent osteomyelitis

**VII-54.** Correct statements regarding T-cell immunophenotype include which of the following?

(A) The T-cell antigen receptor is the earliest surface marker of T-cell lineage.

(B) The expressions of CD4 (T4) and CD8 (T8) surface antigens are mutually exclusive.

(C) The T-cell adhesion molecule, CD2 (T11), accounts for the ability of T cells to form rosettes with sheep red blood cells.

(D) The T-cell antigen receptor complex consists of a signal-transducing moiety and an antigen-recognition moiety.

(E) Mature T cells display surface proteins that are members of the immunoglobulin gene super-family.

**VII-55.** Correct statements about isolated immunoglobulin A deficiency include which of the following?

(A) The incidence of atopic disease is high.

(B) The risk of adverse reactions to transfusions is increased.

(C) The incidence of autoimmune disease is increased.

(D) Secretory IgA levels usually are normal.

(E) The reduced number of IgA-bearing B cells accounts for the reduced serum IgA levels.

**VII-56.** True statements regarding immune-complex disease include which of the following?

(A) Normally, most immune complexes are removed by the reticuloendothelial system.

(B) Signs and symptoms stem from the deposition of immune complexes in tissues other than those of the reticuloendothelial system.

(C) Persistence of immune complexes in the circulation seems to be a requirement for the development of renal manifestations.

(D) Renal lesions depend on antigen-antibody combinations in which antigen is in slight excess.

(E) The rash of cutaneous necrotizing vasculitis may be an example of immune-complex disease.

**VII-57.** True statements regarding HLA class I molecules include which of the following?

(A) They consist of four polypeptide chains

(B) They consist of $\beta_2$-microglobulin subunit

(C) They share less than 25 percent homology with one another

(D) They are distributed unevenly from one racial group to another

(E) They are expressed on all cells except mature red blood cells

**VII-58.** A 63-year-old woman with a history of rheumatoid arthritis since age 42 is seen for the first time by a new physician. The patient has been doing poorly of late. Though her joint disease has not been a problem, she has lost weight and has been plagued by chronic foul-smelling diarrhea, easy bruising, profound fatigue, and peripheral edema. On examination she has waxy skin plaques clustered in the axillary folds, a large tongue, a quiet precordium, hepatosplenomegaly, guaiac-positive stool, and peripheral neuropathy. Laboratory evaluation includes the findings of proteinuria (5 g/d), normal serum chemistry except slightly low albumin and slightly elevated alkaline phosphatase, and low-voltage QRS complexes on electrocardiography. In order to expeditiously diagnose the problem, one could

(A) perform a bone marrow aspirate and biopsy

(B) obtain three serial sputum samples for acid-fast bacillus (AFB) culture

(C) perform an abdominal CT examination

(D) obtain an abdominal subcutaneous fat pad aspirate

(E) perform a rectal biopsy

**VII-59.** Drug-induced systemic lupus erythematosus (SLE) can be characterized by which of the following statements?

(A) Twenty percent of patients receiving procainamide develop drug-induced lupus

(B) Nephritis is a frequent consequence of hydralazine-induced lupus

(C) Most patients on hydralazine develop a positive antinuclear antibody (ANA) test; however, only 10 percent suffer from lupuslike symptoms

(D) If patients with drug-induced lupus fail to respond within several weeks of discontinuing the offending agent, a trial of corticosteroids is indicated

(E) If a patient with drug-induced lupus has persistent symptoms for longer than 6 months, an anti-ds antibody and CH50 levels should be drawn

**VII-60.** Correct statements concerning the use of nonsteroidal anti-inflammatory drugs (NSAIDs) in the treatment of rheumatoid arthritis include which of the following?

(A) The mechanism of action of NSAIDs is the blockade of 5-lipoxygenase

(B) The newer NSAIDs are more efficacious than aspirin

(C) The newer NSAIDs induce platelet dysfunction

(D) NSAIDs can exacerbate allergic rhinitis and asthma

(E) The mechanism of NSAID-induced azotemia is unrelated to these drugs' ability to disrupt arachidonic acid metabolism

**VII-61.** True statements about sarcoidosis include which of the following?

(A) Accumulation of suppressor-cytotoxic T lymphocytes occurs in sites of disease activity

(B) The ratio of black to white patients in the United States may exceed 10:1

(C) Chest radiography and pulmonary function testing are sensitive means of evaluating the intensity of pulmonary inflammation

(D) Transbronchial biopsy may reveal granulomata in a high percentage of patients and is a useful means of diagnosis

(E) Asymptomatic hilar adenopathy accounts for 10 to 20 percent of cases of sarcoidosis in the United States

**VII-62.** Accurate statements about rheumatoid factors include which of the following?

(A) They are antibodies to the Fc fragment of immunoglobulin G

(B) They are associated with several conditions in which there is chronic antigenic stimulation

(C) Their presence in the serum of persons with rheumatoid arthritis correlates with a worse prognosis than that for persons with seronegative disease

(D) Their presence correlates with articular manifestations of rheumatoid arthritis

(E) They frequently do not appear in the serum of persons with rheumatoid arthritis until late in the course of the illness

**VII-63.** The diagnosis of many rheumatic diseases, including rheumatoid arthritis, is based entirely on clinical grounds. Clinical characteristics associated with rheumatoid arthritis include

(A) prolonged morning stiffness

(B) migratory polyarthritis

(C) arthritis involving the distal interphalangeal joints

(D) arthritis of the cervical spine

(E) carpal tunnel syndrome

**VII-64.** A 27-year-old man presents because of a painful, swollen knee and ankle of 2 weeks' duration. He has never had joint disease prior to this time. The patient also complains of low back pain and a recent history of clear penile discharge. On examination he has vesicles (some of which have crusted over) on the palms, soles, and glans penis; injected conjunctivae; a swollen right index finger; and arthritis of the right knee and left ankle. Correct statements regarding this patient include

(A) he will probably benefit from indomethacin

(B) his joint disease will probably improve after a course of tetracycline

(C) he is probably HLA-B27-positive

(D) x-ray of the pelvis would probably demonstrate blurring of the sacroiliac joint

(E) his erythrocyte sedimentation rate is likely to be elevated

**VII-65.** A 40-year-old woman presents with purulent nasal discharge, cough, hemoptysis, and dyspnea. Chest x-ray reveals bilateral nodules; creatinine and erythrocyte sedimentation are elevated; urinalysis reveals hematuria and proteinuria. Accurate statements regarding this woman's condition include

(A) she probably has circulating anti-basement membrane antibodies

(B) she probably has circulating antineutrophil antibodies

(C) necrotizing granulomatous vasculitis would probably be found if a lung biopsy was carried out

(D) glucocorticoids and cyclophosphamide should be administered

(E) even with appropriate therapy, her prognosis is poor

**VII-66.** Acute sarcoidosis is characterized by which of the following syndromes?

(A) Cough, hemoptysis, and interstitial pulmonary involvement

(B) Myopathy, keratotic skin lesions on the palms and soles, and arthralgias

(C) Fever, pulmonary stenotic murmur, and nailbed lesions

(D) Erythema nodosum, arthralgias, and hilar adenopathy

(E) Fever, parotid enlargement, uveitis, and facial nerve palsy

**VII-67.** A 52-year-old woman presents with nasal discharge and stuffiness, difficulty in breathing through the nose, and sinus pain. ENT examination reveals ulcers on the nasal septum and perforation of the soft palate. There is no history of prior illness or drug abuse. Biopsy of involved material under anesthesia reveals noncaseating granulomatous inflammation with necrotic debris. No malignant cells, vasculitis, or microorganisms are noted. Correct statements concerning this patient's condition include which of the following?

(A) The history and findings are consistent with Wegener's granulomatosis

(B) If she is not appropriately treated, the disease will probably be fatal

(C) The treatment of choice is radiation therapy

(D) The disease, if unchecked, can progress to involve the mediastinum and lungs

(E) Optimal treatment should involve surgical debridement

**DIRECTIONS:** The group of questions below consists of five lettered headings followed by a set of numbered items. For each numbered item select the one lettered heading with which it is most closely associated. Each lettered heading may be used once, more than once, or not at all.

**Questions VII-68–VII-71.**

For each diagnosis that follows, select the synovial fluid findings with which it is most likely to be associated.

   (A) Fluid, clear and viscous; white blood cell count, 400/$\mu$L; no crystals

   (B) Fluid, cloudy and watery; white blood cell count, 8000/$\mu$L; no crystals

   (C) Fluid, dark brown and viscous; white blood cell count, 1200/$\mu$L; no crystals

   (D) Fluid, cloudy and watery; white blood cell count, 12,000/$\mu$L; crystals, needle-like and strongly negatively birefringent

   (E) Fluid, cloudy and watery; white blood cell count, 4800/$\mu$L; crystals, rhomboidal and weakly positively birefringent

**VII-68.** Pigmented villonodular synovitis

**VII-69.** Calcium pyrophosphate deposition disease

**VII-70.** Gout

**VII-71.** Degenerative joint disease

# VII. IMMUNOLOGIC, ALLERIGIC, AND RHEUMATIC DISORDERS

## ANSWERS

**VII-1. The answer is D.** *(Chap. 305)* Lymphoid cells, including both T and B lymphocytes, arise from hematopoietic stem cells. Those cells destined to enter the B-cell lineage arise continuously in the bone marrow. The earliest cells destined to become B cells express surface CD10 (CALLA, J-5) protein, an endopeptidase thought to inactivate certain peptide hormones. These pre-B cells are large lymphoid cells containing cytoplasmic $\mu$ chains, the heavy chain of immunoglobulin M (IgM), as detected by immunofluorescence. Cytoplasmic light chains are not present, and pre-B cells lack membrane-bound IgM or immunoglobulin of any other class. In the process of B-cell maturation, smaller lymphoid cells will appear that bear a narrow rim of cytoplasmic IgM; later, cells with membrane-bound IgM develop.

**VII-2. The answer is E.** *(Chap. 305. Frank, N Engl J Med 316:1525–1530, 1987.)* Complement activity, resulting from the sequential interaction of a large number of plasma and cell-membrane proteins, plays an important role in the inflammatory response. The classical pathway of complement activation is initiated by an antibody-antigen interaction. The first complement component (C1, a complex composed of three proteins) binds to immune complexes with activation mediated by C1q. Active C1 then initiates the cleavage and concomitant activation of components C4 and C2. The activated C1 is destroyed by a plasma protease inhibitor termed C1 esterase inhibitor. This molecule also regulates clotting factors XI and kallikrein. Patients with deficiency of C1 esterase inhibitor may develop angioedema, sometimes leading to death via asphyxia. Attacks may be precipitated by stress or trauma. In addition to low antigenic or functional levels of C1 esterase inhibitor, patients with this autosomal dominant condition may have normal levels of C1 and C3, but low levels of C4 and C2. Danazol therapy produces a striking increase in the level of this important inhibitor and alleviates symptoms in many patients. An acquired form of angioedema due to C1 esterase inhibitor deficiency has been described in patients with autoimmune or malignant disease.

**VII-3. The answer is D.** *(Chap. 310)* Urticaria and angioedema are common disorders, affecting approximately 20 percent of the population. In acute urticarial angioedema, attacks of swelling are of less than 6 weeks' duration; chronic urticarial angioedema is by definition more long-standing. Urticaria usually is pruritic and affects the trunk and proximal extremities. Angioedema is generally less pruritic and affects the hands, feet, genitalia, and face. The woman described in the question has chronic urticaria, which probably is due to a cutaneous necrotizing vasculitis. The clues to the diagnosis are the arthralgias, presence of residual skin discoloration, and elevated sedimentation rate—these would be uncharacteristic of other urticarial diseases. Diagnosis can be confirmed by skin biopsy. Chronic urticaria is rarely of allergic cause; hence, allergy skin tests and measurement of total immunoglobulin E levels are not helpful. Measurement of C1 esterase inhibitor activity is useful in diagnosing hereditary angioedema, a disease not associated with urticaria. Patch tests are used to diagnose contact dermatitis.

**VII-4. The answer is D.** *(Chap. 310. Naclerio, N Engl J Med 325:860–869, 1991.)* Allergic rhinitis can be either seasonal as a result of pollen exposure or perennial as a result of exposure to dust or mold spores (or both). In these IgE-mediated reactions to inhaled foreign substances, nasal eosinophilia is common. Vasomotor rhinitis is a chronic, non-allergic condition in which vasomotor control in the nasal membranes is altered. Irritating stimuli, such as odors, fumes, and changes in humidity and barometric pressure, can cause nasal obstruction and discharge in affected persons, and nasal eosinophilia is not noted. Because the man described in the question has either perennial allergic rhinitis due to dust or mold-spore allergy or eosinophilic nonallergic rhinitis, skin testing for responses to suspected allergens should be diagnostic. Though total serum IgE may be elevated, demonstration of specificity is critical. Specificity can be demonstrated by binding to a solid-phase antigen and detected by uptake of radiolabeled anti-IgE (radioallergosorbent technique; RAST). RAST is more difficult than skin testing due to the requirement for defined antigens and standardization. Pollen skin tests are unlikely to be helpful because of the perennial nature of the condition described. An elimination diet can be used diagnostically or therapeutically in persons with suspected food allergy; however, food allergy rarely causes rhinitis. Sinus x-rays, whether positive or negative, would not reveal the underlying cause of the rhinitis.

**VII-5.    The answer is C.** *(Chap. 305)* Reactions are initiated by mononuclear leukocytes and require 48 to 72 h to evidence a response after antigen exposure. Such delayed-type hypersensitivity reactions are best exemplified by local reactions to skin challenge in persons previously exposed to the test antigen. The cellular events resulting in such hypersensitivity responses are centered around T cells (particularly lymphokine-secreting TH-1-helper T cells) and macrophages. Antigen processed by monocytes-macrophages is presented to specific T cells. Macrophages secrete interleukin 1 and interleukin 6 to clonally amplify the specific T cell and also secrete lymphokines such as IL-2 and interferon-γ to recruit additional T cells and macrophages to participate in the inflammatory response. Macrophages recruited in this fashion may undergo epithelioid cell transformation to form giant cells, perhaps in response to IL-4 and interferon-γ. In addition to mycobacterial infections, diseases in which delayed-type hypersensitivity is important include histoplasmosis, chlamydial infections, schistosomiasis, and berylliosis.

**VII-6.    The answer is D.** *(Chap. 114)* Plasma cell diseases are a group of conditions in which a clone of cells capable of synthesizing and secreting immunoglobulins, or the heavy- or light-chain component of these molecules, proliferates abnormally. IgG immunoglobulins are the most common class produced in such diseases. Also, free light chains usually are produced in excess and are detected in urine as Bence-Jones protein. Multiple myeloma is the most common plasma cell neoplasm. Its classic presentation includes bone pain, anemia, hypercalcemia, renal failure, and recurrent infections in an elderly person. Diagnosis is best made by looking for a homogeneous globulin peak on electrophoresis of serum, urine, or both. Waldenstrom's macroglobulinemia is a related condition in which the monoclonal immunoglobulin is of the IgM class. Because IgM is so large (it circulates as a pentamer), it is restricted to the bloodstream and in high concentrations tends to cause hyperviscosity of the blood. Other features differentiating Waldenstrom's macroglobulinemia from multiple myeloma are enlargement of lymph nodes and spleen and occasional transformation to chronic lymphocytic leukemia or lymphocytic lymphoma.

**VII-7.    The answer is D.** *(Chap. 319)* Polyarteritis nodosa is a vasculitis of medium-sized vessels. Early systemic features include fever, weakness, anorexia, weight loss, myalgias, and arthralgias (although severe and persistent arthritis is uncommon). Pericarditis and pleuritis also can occur. Mononeuritis multiplex develops because of involvement of the vasa vasorum; it is reflected in the man described by the sudden loss of the ability to dorsiflex his right great toe. Abdominal pain occurs in 60 to 70 percent of affected persons and is related to disease involvement of mesenteric arteries. Hypertension develops from arterial occlusion and occurs before renal involvement. Laboratory findings of elevated erythrocyte sedimentation rate, anemia of chronic disease, and polymorphonuclear leukocytosis all occur with polyarteritis nodosa. Pulmonary involvement is unusual and serves to distinguish this entity clinically from allergic granulomatosis and Wegener's granulomatosis. Hypersensitivity vasculitis is a term applied to small-vessel vasculitides associated with a range of findings from purely cutaneous disease to minimal skin disease but life-threatening involvement of major organs. Giant cell arteritis involves the aorta and other great vessels, producing constitutional symptoms and large-vessel occlusion in young women (Takayasu's disease) and in the elderly (temporal arteritis, polymyalgia rheumatica).

**VII-8.    The answer is C.** *(Chap. 312. Balow, Ann Intern Med 106:79, 1987.)*    Renal disease is clinically evident in about half those persons with systemic lupus erythematosus (SLE). However, nearly all persons with SLE have some evidence of renal disease on renal biopsy. Renal disease associated with SLE includes both glomerulonephritis and interstitial nephritis. Glomerular disease has been classified into membranous nephritis and mesangial, focal, and diffuse glomerulonephritis. Immune-complex interstitial nephritis occurs most commonly in persons who have diffuse glomerulonephritis. Urinalysis performed for persons with active renal disease usually reveals microscopic hematuria, red cell casts, and proteinuria; the exception is membranous lupus nephritis, in which proteinuria is the dominant finding. Drug-induced lupus rarely leads to renal disease. Anti-dsDNA antibodies at high titer are associated with severe nephritis. Renal biopsy is not necessary in SLE patients whose renal function is rapidly deteriorating when they have an active sediment. If such patients fail to respond to the prompt initiation of glucocorticoid therapy demanded in such a situation, then biopsy should be undertaken. Patients with mild clinical disease should have a biopsy to determine if they have active, severe, inflammatory lesions, which might respond to therapy.

**VII-9.    The answer is C.** *(Chap. 207. Sneller, Ann Intern Med 118:720–730, 1993.)*    Common variable immunodeficiency represents a heterogeneous group of adults who have in common deficiencies of all major immunoglobulin classes. The defect is believed to be due to an abnormality in B-cell maturation, though most of these patients tend to have normal levels of clonally diverse B lymphocytes. The B cells can recognize antigen and proliferate, but fail to differentiate to the immunoglobulin-secreting stage. Associated with this abnormality is nodular lymphoid hyperplasia in various organs (including the gut) and splenomegaly. This panhypogammaglobulinemic disorder should be suspected in adults with chronic pulmonary infections, unexplained bronchiectasis (like the case presented in this example), chronic giardiasis, malabsorption, and atrophic gastritis. Patients develop intestinal neoplasms at increased frequency. They also develop autoimmune conditions, such as Coombs-positive hemolytic anemia and idiopathic thrombocytopenic purpura. There is some suggestion that, in addition to failure of B cells to secrete immunoglobulin, T cells have an impaired ability to release lymphokines. The mainstay of therapy for common variable immunodeficiency is to increase the antibody content by administration of intravenous immunoglobulin concentrates. The goal is to increase the IgG level to 5 g/L, which can generally be accomplished by monthly administration of 200 to 400 mg/kg of intravenous immunoglobulin. True anaphylactic reactions to immunoglobulin treatment are rare.

**VII-10.    The answer is B.** *(Chap. 308)*    Among U.S. cases of AIDS, male-to-male sexual contact represents the most frequently reported mode of HIV transmission among persons with AIDS. However, over the past few years, the number of newly reported cases of AIDS among other groups, including IV drug users and heterosexuals, from certain large cities have surpassed the number of newly reported cases among men who had sex with men. The proportion of new cases attributed to IV drug use and heterosexual sex has increased dramatically over the past ten years. There is a small but existent occupational risk of HIV transmission. Large, multi-institutional studies have indicated the risk of a penetrating injury, such as a needlestick from an HIV-infected person, to be approximately 0.3 percent. Risk posed by a mucocutaneous exposure is probably closer to 0.1 percent. Current measures used to screen donors now include p24 antigen testing which has resulted in a further decrease in the risk of being infected from a unit of blood to at most 1 in 450,000 to 1 in 660,000. Pediatric AIDS arises mainly from infants born to mothers who are HIV-infected. The remainder are generally exposed via blood transfusions. Although HIV can be rarely isolated from saliva, there is no convincing evidence that saliva can transmit HIV infection, either through kissing or other exposures, such as occupationally to health care workers.

**VII-11.** **The answer is B.** *(Chap. 308. Carpenter, JAMA 276:146–154, 1996.)* Zidovudine (ZDV) was the first antiretroviral agent proven to be effective in the treatment of HIV-infected patients. While zidovudine monotherapy was shown to be effective in symptomatic disease and in asymptomatic patients with CD4+ cell counts <500/μL, several trials have shown improvement of combinations of two nucleoside analogues for initial therapy based on laboratory indices or clinical measures. Three trials compare combination therapy with zidovudine and didanosine or zidovudine and zalcitabine with monotherapy regimens. In these trials, didanosine monotherapy was as effective as the combinations and both were superior to zidovudine monotherapy. In other studies, initial combination treatment with zidovudine and lamivudine (3TC) reduced plasma HIV RNA levels and raised CD4+ cell counts more than either drug alone. Combinations of nucleoside analogues appear to have more potent antiretroviral activity than zidovudine alone and may also delay or prevent the emergence of drug resistance.

**VII-12.** **The answer is A.** *(Chap. 306)* The major histocompatibility gene complex (MHC), located on the short arm of chromosome 6, contains genes involved in the recognition of self, antigen presentation to T and B cells, and the rejection of tissue allografts. Ubiquitously expressed class I molecules are the products of the HLA-A, -B, and -C genes. Also in the MHC, the HLA-D region, separated from the ABC genes by an area responsible for certain complement components (C2, C4B, Bf, C4A) and tumor necrosis factor, codes for class II molecules, which are only expressed on T cells, B cells, and monocytes (and their derivatives, such as Langerhans' skin cells). Class I molecules are responsible for the mixed lymphocyte reaction (MLR), which is important in determining compatibility of donor and host tissues in a potential transplant situation. Because the ABC and D regions are closely linked, recombination between these two areas is uncommon (approximately 2 percent). Thus, an ABC-matched sibling is usually, but not always, matched at the D locus as well. In addition to a recombination event, another reason for a positive MLR in an HLA-ABC matched sibling pair is histoincompatibility at minor loci, which are located throughout the genome.

**VII-13.** **The answer is A.** *(Chap. 308)* The standard serologic test for HIV infection, the enzyme-linked immunosorbent assay (ELISA), has a sensitivity of over 99.5 percent. However, this test is not particularly specific in that low-risk patients are subject to a false-positive rate of over 10 percent. If the ELISA test is indeterminate or positive, the test should be repeated. If the repeat is positive or indeterminate, one should proceed to the next step, which is a western blot test. If the repeat ELISA is negative, then the person can be assumed not to have HIV infection. A western blot test involves the reaction of the serum with a strip impregnated with HIV-1 antigens. Binding of antibodies in the patient's serum to the antigens on the strip is detected with an enzyme-conjugated anti-human antibody. A positive western blot test requires the detection of antibodies to several HIV-1 gene products. If the western blot is indeterminate, perhaps due to infection in evolution or due to cross-reacting antibodies in the patient's serum, one should proceed to a PCR test and repeat the western blot in 1 month. If the PCR is negative and there is no progression on the western blot, the diagnosis of HIV infection is ruled out. The PCR test is extraordinarily sensitive, but the false-positive rate would be too high for use as a cost-efficient screening test. A DNA PCR test for HIV involves the isolation of DNA from blood mononuclear cells and incubation with primers from both the gag and LTR regions, followed by amplification and hybridization to detect HIV proviral DNA. An RNA PCR test can be used to monitor the level of HIV genome present in plasma (i.e., before cell entry and reverse transcription of the RNA genome).

**VII-14.  The answer is D.**  *(Chap. 308. Carpenter, JAMA 276:146–154, 1996.)*  Saquinavir, the first approved protease inhibitor is well tolerated, but has poor bioavailability (and therefore potency) in its currently available formulation. A new formulation with improved bioavailability is under study. Ritonavir has more frequent side effects than either of the other protease inhibitors; such effects include gastrointestinal disturbance (20 to 25 percent of patients), hepatotoxicity, and headache. Ritonavir is a potent inhibitor of cytochrome P450 which complicates its use with other drugs metabolized by this pathway. This may be particularly troublesome in patients with HIV, in whom some of these drugs are commonly used. Indinavir is very potent and well tolerated. The main side effects of indinavir are nephrolithiasis (4 percent of patients) and asymptomatic hyperbilirubinemia (seen in 10 percent of patients). This hyperbilirubinemia is not an indication to discontinue the drug. With all of the protease inhibitors, care should be taken to maintain continuous drug administration at the optimal dosage levels, because dose reduction will contribute to the development of resistance to these drugs.

**VII-15.  The answer is B.**  *(Chap. 307. Rosen, N Engl J Med 311:235, 300, 1984.)*  Ataxia-telangiectasia is an autosomal recessive primary immunodeficiency disorder associated with abnormal thymic development, progressive cerebellar ataxia, and oculocutaneous telangiectasia. The responsible gene, located on chromosome 11, leads to a generalized defect in the ability to repair damage to DNA. Such a defect accounts for the frequent occurrence of malignancies, particularly lymphomas, and the exquisite sensitivity to therapeutic irradiation. There is evidence for both humoral and cellular immunodeficiency; most patients have depressed IgA and IgE levels as well as cutaneous anergy. Sinopulmonary infections are common with severe resultant respiratory insufficiency, often associated with bronchiectasis. Adenosine deaminase deficiency is associated not with ataxia-telangiectasia but with severe combined immunodeficiency.

**VII-16.  The answer is B.**  *(Chap. 308)*  AIDS Clinical Trial Group 076 demonstrated that ZDV (AZT) administration to women reduced the rate of HIV transmission in neonates from 25 percent in the placebo group to 8 percent in ZDV recipients. Postnatal transmission of HIV from mother to infant via breast feeding has been clearly documented. A meta-analysis of several prospective trials indicated a risk of 7 to 22 percent. Certainly, in developed countries, breast feeding by an infected mother should be avoided. There is, however, disagreement regarding this recommendation in developing countries where breast milk is the only source of adequate nutrition for the infant. Plasma HIV RNA assays provide precise and compelling data on the relative magnitude and durability of antiretroviral therapy. Most authorities recommend the use of HIV RNA assays (viral load) and CD4+ counts to guide decisions regarding antiretroviral therapy. While zidovudine has proven benefit in patients with <500 CD4+ lymphocytes, its use as monotherapy is suboptimal and should be reevaluated in any patient receiving it. Rifabutin and macrolides have both demonstrated marked efficacy in the primary prophylaxis against *Mycobacterium avium* with a concomitant decrease in bacteremia and improvement in survival.

**VII-17.  The answer is A.**  *(Chap. 308)*  Most patients with HIV infection evidence clinical disease of the central nervous system (CNS) at some point in their course. Cerebrospinal fluid findings are abnormal in approximately 90 percent of patients, even during asymptomatic states of infection. Such abnormalities include pleocytosis, isolation of virus and antiviral antibodies, and elevated CSF protein. The most common CNS disease in HIV-infected persons is the AIDS dementia complex, which refers to a syndrome of signs and symptoms that generally occurs late in the course of disease. In addition to dementia, patients may have various additional problems such as unsteady gait and poor balance or behavior problems such as apathy and lack of initiative. The precise cause of the AIDS dementia complex is unclear, but it is probably due to direct effects of HIV infection in the CNS. Eighty to ninety percent of patients with HIV infection can be shown to have some degree of histologic evidence of CNS involvement. The radiologic correlate of AIDS dementia complex is general atrophy, ventricular dilation, and bright spots on T2-weighted MRI images. The ring-enhancing lesions in toxoplasmosis are seen in about 15 percent of all HIV-infected patients with CNS disease and are the second most common cause of seizures after the AIDS dementia complex. The third most common cause of seizures is cryptococcal meningitis. Progressive multifocal leukoencephalopathy is relatively unusual and produces multiple white-matter lesions on T2-weighted MR images. Neurosyphilis, CNS lymphoma, and tuberculous meningitis are other less common CNS diseases in patients with HIV infection. Antiretroviral treatment has been associated with some improvement in patients with the AIDS dementia complex and therefore merits a therapeutic trial in patients so afflicted.

**VII-18.  The answer is B.**  *(Chap. 308)*   Kaposi's sarcoma (KS) is a neoplasm consisting of multiple vascular nodules in the skin, mucous membranes, and viscera. The course ranges from indolent with only minor skin or lymph node involvement to fulminant with extensive visceral involvement. Generally, the tumor respects tissue planes and is rarely invasive. Unlike many other tumors, lymph node involvement may occur early and is of no special clinical significance. The chest x-ray in pulmonary KS characteristically shows bilateral lower-lobe infiltrates that obscure the margins of the mediastinum and diaphragm. Pleural effusions are seen in 70 percent of cases. Treatment may consist of local therapy with radiation, intralesional chemotherapy, cryotherapy, systemic chemotherapy, or interferon. The response to interferon is most dependent upon the CD4+ count with response rates of 80 percent in patients with CD4+ cells > 600/µL and less than 10 percent in patients with CD4+ cells < 150/µL. Interestingly, the incidence of KS is declining. A growing body of epidemiologic and virologic data points to the likelihood that a sexually transmitted cofactor plays an important role in the development of KS. Human herpesvirus-8 has been strongly implicated as this cofactor. As safer sexual practices are employed, the risk of transmission of this cofactor and thus the risk of KS has decreased.

**VII-19.  The answer is C.**   *(Chap. 308)*   Based on the expanded definition of AIDS to include any HIV-infected person whose CD4+ T-cell count is <200/µL, the clinical situation suggests the diagnosis of the acquired immunodeficiency syndrome (AIDS). *M. pneumoniae*, while a frequent cause of mild community-acquired pneumonia in the otherwise normal host, is not commonly associated with AIDS. *P. carinii*, a protozoal pathogen, is the most frequent cause of respiratory disease in the AIDS patient; it affects approximately 60 percent of such patients some time during the course of their illness. Both cytomegalovirus and *C. neoformans* are less common but significant respiratory pathogens in this patient population. Tuberculosis must always be considered in an AIDS patient with pulmonary symptoms. Tuberculous dissemination occurs frequently.

**VII-20.  The answer is A.**  *(Chap. 305. Lawly, N Engl J Med 311:1407, 1984.)*   The administration of horse antithymocyte globulin (ATG) to patients with aplastic anemia or as an immunosuppressant after bone marrow transplant can lead to a clinical syndrome identical to that of classic serum sickness and one that approximates animal models of immune complex disease. Eight to thirteen days after beginning therapy with ATG, the clinical features begin with fever, malaise, rash (often urticarial), arthralgias, nausea, melena, lymphadenopathy, and proteinuria. There are high levels of circulating immune complexes; more precise quantitation rests on one of a number of generally inconclusive assays, including the Raji cell assay (lymphoblastoid line that binds to C3) and C1q binding assay (first complement subcomponent). With all these circulating immune complexes containing their Fc receptors, the complement system is overactivated, so there are accompanying decreases in C3, C4, and CH50.

**VII-21.  The answer is B.**  *(Chap. 313)*  Medical management of rheumatoid arthritis involves the use of nonsteroidal anti-inflammatory drugs to control the symptoms and signs of the local inflammatory process. These agents have little or no effect on progression of the disease. Systemic glucocorticoids also suppress signs and symptoms of inflammation. Recent evidence, however, suggests that low-dose glucocorticoids may also retard the development and progression of bony erosions. A third line of agents includes a variety of drugs categorized as disease modifying or slow-acting anti-rheumatic drugs. These drugs decrease elevated levels of the acute phase reactants and are thought to modify the destructive capacity of the disease. These agents include gold compounds, D-penicillamine, antimalarials, sulfasalazine, and methotrexate. Other useful agents include immunosuppressive and cytotoxic drugs, such as azathioprine and cyclophosphamide, which have been shown to ameliorate the disease process in some patients. Substitution of omega-3 fatty acids found in certain fish oils or dietary omega-6 essential fatty acids has been shown to provide symptomatic improvement in patients with rheumatoid arthritis, but has not been shown to alter the disease process.

**VII-22.  The answer is B.**  *(Chap. 308. Kaye, Ann Intern Med 11:158, 1989.)*  In contrast to the profound immunodeficiency that characterizes most manifestations of AIDS, a host of immunologic and rheumatologic disorders are common in patients with HIV infection. Certainly the most common such reaction is cutaneously manifested sensitivity to the antibiotics required for treatment of the secondary infections so common in these patients. Sixty-five percent of patients who receive trimethoprim-sulfamethoxazole develop an erythematous morbilliform pruritic eruption. Fortunately, anaphylaxis is very rare, and desensitization is possible. Patients infected with HIV may develop diseases that resemble classic autoimmune diseases in non-HIV-infected persons. A variant of Sjögren's syndrome characterized by dry eyes, dry mouth, and lymphocytic infiltrates of the salivary gland and lung may be seen. HIV-associated arthropathy is characterized by a nonerosive oligoarticular arthritis that generally involves the large joints. Widespread musculoskeletal pain of at least 3 months' duration with tender points, typical of fibromyalgia, may occur in up to 10 percent of HIV-infected IV drug abusers. Reactive arthritides, such as Reiter's syndrome or psoriatic arthritis, have also been described.

**VII-23.  The answer is C.**  *(Chap. 313)*  Persons who have rheumatoid arthritis can develop popliteal cysts as a complication of synovitis of the knee. Popliteal cysts can expand upward into the thigh or downward into the calf. Rupture of a popliteal cyst produces sudden pain and swelling; because these symptoms resemble those of thrombophlebitis—though perhaps more dramatic in onset—an arthrogram may be needed to confirm the diagnosis. Although rupture of the plantaris tendon can occur in persons exposed to mechanical trauma, it would not be the most likely diagnosis for the woman described in the question. The anserine bursa is located on the medial aspect of the knee joint and not in the calf. Achilles tendonitis should not cause pain and swelling of the calf.

**VII-24.  The answer is C.**  *(Chap. 319)*  This patient has symptoms and laboratory values characteristic of temporal arteritis. The disease classically presents with fever, anemia, elevated erythrocyte sedimentation rate (ESR), and headaches in an elderly patient. Other manifestations include fatigue, malaise, sweats, anorexia, weight loss, and arthralgias. Scalp tenderness and jaw claudication may occur as well. Laboratory findings include an elevated ESR and normochromic or slightly hypochromic anemia. Liver function abnormalities are common, particularly increased alkaline phosphatase levels. A catastrophic potential complication, particularly in untreated patients, is ocular involvement due to ischemic optic neuritis which may lead to sudden and irreversible blindness. The diagnosis is often made clinically and confirmed by temporal artery biopsy. A temporal artery biopsy should be obtained as quickly as possible and, in the setting of ocular symptoms, therapy should not be delayed pending a biopsy. Therapy consists of high-dose glucocorticoids to which the disease is quite responsive. MRI/MRA cannot establish the diagnosis and hence are not warranted. This patient's presentation is classic for TA and would be unusual for either metastatic colon cancer or meningitis.

VII-25.   **The answer is A.**   *(Chap. 308)*   Lymphoma generally does not occur until the CD4+ T-lymphocyte count falls beneath 200/μL. This contrasts with Kaposi's sarcoma, which occurs at a relatively constant rate throughout the course of the illness. The lymphomas are generally B cell in origin, may contain Epstein-Barr virus DNA in the malignant cell genome, and may be either monoclonal or oligoclonal. Intermediate to high-grade lymphomas account for 80 percent of lymphomas in patients with AIDS. Three-fourths of these are either large cell or immunoblastic lymphomas. The remainder of systemic high-grade lymphomas are small, noncleaved cell (Burkitt's) lymphomas, which demonstrate the characteristic translocation between chromosome 8 and chromosome 14 or 22. Primary CNS lymphoma accounts for about 20 percent of lymphomas in HIV-infected patients. CNS lymphomas tend to occur at an even lower CD4+ T-cell count than do the aforementioned peripheral lymphomas. Primary CNS lymphoma may present with focal neurologic deficits; radiologic evaluation may reveal up to three 5-cm lesions. Results with the multiagent chemotherapy used to treat similar lymphomas in non-HIV-infected persons have been quite disappointing. The median survival is 10 months for systemic HIV-related lymphoma and 2 to 4 months for those with primary CNS lymphoma. Hodgkin's disease, particularly the mixed cellularity or lymphocyte-depleted subtypes, may also occur, and, unlike the high cure rates for patients with Hodgkin's disease in general, the median survival for those with HIV infection and Hodgkin's disease is only 12 to 15 months.

VII-26.   **The answer is E.**   *(Chap. 114. Barlogie, Blood 73:865, 1989.)*   The diagnosis of multiple myeloma rests on bone marrow plasmacytosis (greater than 10 percent of the cells should be malignant-appearing plasma cells), lytic bone lesions, and a serum or urine M component. The M component represents either complete or partial antibody molecules synthesized by a monoclonal proliferation of plasma cells. Patients with myeloma may have a host of clinical problems related to the plasma cell neoplasm and its secreted products. Skeletal destruction can produce hypercalcemia, pathologic fractures, spinal cord compression, bone pain, and lytic bone lesions. Renal failure is common and may be due to light-chain deposition in renal tubules, amyloidosis, or calcium or urate nephropathy. Cytopenias due to bone marrow infiltration are typical. Infection with encapsulated microorganisms occurs because of associated hypogammaglobulinemia, believed to be due to B-cell dysregulation. However, certain patients have a serum M spike but no such clinical problems and do not have an excessive number of bone marrow plasma cells. These individuals have benign monoclonal gammopathy, also called monoclonal gammopathy of uncertain significance (MGUS). MGUS patients are generally over age 50. Their M spike is less than 20 g/L (2.0 g/dL) and they do not have Bence-Jones proteinuria. These patients require no therapy and should merely be followed over time since only about 11 percent go on to develop frank myeloma.

VII-27.   **The answer is A.**   *(Chap. 313)*   Systemic manifestations in early rheumatoid arthritis may be severe, but are frequently nonspecific. Such nonspecific constitutional symptoms require a period of observation before synovitis supervenes and the diagnosis becomes clear. Weight loss and muscle wasting may be as severe as in persons who have a malignancy or primary muscle disease. In about 10 percent of patients, the disease begins in a more fulminant fashion with the rapid onset of polyarthritis associated with fever, lymphadenopathy, and splenomegaly.

VII-28.   **The answer is E.**   *(Chap. 313)*   Many of the systemic manifestations of late rheumatoid arthritis are related to the presence of rheumatoid factors in high titer in the serum. Joint disease, paradoxically, may not be active during this stage of the illness. Nail-fold thrombi, leg ulcers, and sensorimotor polyneuropathy are all manifestations of rheumatoid vasculitis and presumably are related to the effect of immune complexes containing rheumatoid factors. High levels of immune complexes are detected by immune-complex assays done at this stage of disease. Felty's syndrome, characterized by neutropenia and splenomegaly, occurs late in the course of rheumatoid arthritis and is related to the presence of high titers of rheumatoid factors. Many affected persons also have rheumatoid vasculitis. Fifteen to twenty percent of patients with rheumatoid arthritis develop Sjögren's syndrome with associated dry eyes. Hepatitis is not a common feature of late extraarticular seropositive rheumatoid arthritis.

**VII-29.** **The answer is A.** *(Chap. 310. Bochner, N Engl J Med 324:1785–1790, 1991.)* Anaphylaxis is the word used to describe the rapid and generalized immunologically mediated events characterized clinically by cutaneous wheals and upper or lower airway obstruction (or both) after exposure to a specific antigen. The angioedema and urticaria that occur during anaphylaxis are believed to be due to the release of mast cell (and possibly basophil) mediators (histamine and serum proteases from preformed granules, arachidonic acid metabolites such as leukotrienes, and cytokines including, but not limited to, tumor necrosis factor-$\alpha$, interferon-$\gamma$, and interleukin 1). The mechanism of this release depends on the inciting agent. For example, anaphylaxis in response to bee stings, foods, and heterologous serum (e.g., tetanus antitoxin) is believed to be on the basis of IgE-mediated reaction against the relevant protein. On the other hand, anaphylaxis to penicillin and other antibiotics is due to IgE recognition of protein-hapten conjugants. Dialysis-induced anaphylaxis is due to complement activation. Finally, radiocontrast media directly activate mast cells or basophils or both to release the mediators of anaphylaxis.

**VII-30.** **The answer is B.** *(Chap. 310)* Most patients with systemic mastocytosis have an indolent syndrome characterized by mast cell infiltration of the skin, gastrointestinal mucosa, liver, and spleen. Cutaneous manifestations include the small, reddish-brown macules or papules, termed urticaria pigmentosa, which would be characterized histopathologically as having excess numbers of mast cells. These lesions are associated with Darier's sign, in which urticaria and erythema develop in response to trauma. Histamine-mediated hypersecretion of gastric acid accounts for an increased incidence of gastritis and peptic ulcers in patients with systemic mastocytosis. Bone pain, organomegaly, or lymphadenopathy may also be seen. In addition to documentation of mast cells in various organs, biochemical confirmation can be made by urine collection for histamine metabolites or by measuring increased blood levels of histamine or mast cell-derived neutral protease tryptase. The spectrum of mast cell disease ranges from indolent to more aggressive varieties characterized by mast cell infiltration of liver and spleen and in some cases the invariably fatal development of mast cell leukemia.

**VII-31.** **The answer is A.** *(Chap. 317)* The diagnosis of ankylosing spondylitis is made on clinical grounds. Historical features suggesting inflammatory back disease include pain and prolonged stiffness that are worse at night and during rest periods and characteristically relieved with activity. In contrast, mechanical low back pain usually is eased with bed rest and made worse with activity, such as sitting, standing, walking, and lifting. Signs of nerve-root compression are not part of the clinical spectrum of ankylosing spondylitis. Ankylosing spondylitis usually presents before the age of 40 years; on the other hand, degenerative joint disease and degenerative disk disease are common causes of back pain in the elderly. Back pain made worse with walking and improved with rest and lumbar flexion is characteristic of the pseudoclaudication syndrome associated with lumbar spinal stenosis.

**VII-32.** **The answer is B.** *(Chap. 325)* Five different clinical syndromes of psoriatic arthritis have been described. The most common (70 percent of cases) is an asymmetric oligoarticular arthritis. A second group produces arthritis mainly in distal interphalangeal joints and is associated with severe psoriatic nail changes. Psoriatic spondylitis is similar to the spondylitis of Reiter's syndrome. Rheumatoid factor-negative symmetric polyarthritis also is associated with psoriasis, and this condition can look very much like rheumatoid arthritis. About 5 percent of patients with psoriatic arthritis have a destructive variety called "arthritis mutilans." Persons who have psoriasis and rheumatoid factor-positive symmetric polyarthritis are thought to have both psoriasis and rheumatoid arthritis.

**VII-33.** **The answer is E.** *(Chap. 312)* Patients with SLE may have a host of autoantibodies. Virtually all have antinuclear antibodies directed at multiple nuclear and cytoplasmic antigens. Approximately 50 percent have an anticardiolipin antibody, which is associated with a prolonged partial thromboplastin time and false-positive serologic tests for syphilis. This so-called lupus anticoagulant may be manifested by thrombocytopenia, venous or arterial clotting, recurrent fetal loss, and valvular heart disease. Though thrombotic problems are most common, if the antibody is associated with hypoprothrombinemia, severe thrombocytopenia, or antibodies to clotting factors (usually VIII or IX), bleeding may result. Confirmation that the partial thromboplastin time is prolonged on the basis of a lupus anticoagulant may be proved by failure of normal plasma to correct the defect.

**VII-34.** **The answer is C.** *(Chap. 312)* Patients with the more malignant variant of systemic sclerosis (scleroderma) have diffuse cutaneous disease characterized by skin thickening in the extremities, face, and trunk. It is this subset of patients, in contrast to those with limited cutaneous disease who often have the CREST syndrome, who are at risk for developing kidney and other visceral disease. Hypertension heralds the onset of a renal crisis manifested by malignant hypertension, encephalopathy, retinopathy, seizures, and left ventricular failure. The renin-angiotensin system is markedly activated; therefore, angiotensin-converting enzyme inhibitors are particularly effective. Even patients who require dialysis may reverse course and have a slow return of renal function after the passage of several months. Patients with systemic sclerosis may also develop esophageal dysfunction, hypomotility of the small intestine (which can produce pain and malabsorption), pulmonary fibrosis sometimes progressing to pulmonary hypertension, and heart failure due to myocardial fibrosis.

**VII-35.** **The answer is C.** *(Chap. 318)* Behçet's syndrome, a recurrent disease of unknown cause, is characterized by painful oral and genital ulcers, eye inflammation, arthritis, central nervous system symptoms, thrombophlebitis, fever, and abdominal symptoms. The combination of fever, aphthous ulcers, arthritis, and abdominal pain may mimic inflammatory bowel disease, although central nervous system involvement (e.g., severe headache) and thrombophlebitis would make this diagnosis less likely. Whipple's disease is associated with arthritis, abdominal pain, and central nervous system disease, but not with aphthous ulcers and thrombophlebitis; also, Whipple's disease usually affects middle-aged men. Fever, arthritis, abdominal pain, and headache would be compatible with a diagnosis of systemic lupus erythematosus. However, the mucosal lesions of lupus are painless and occur on the hard and soft palate, and thrombophlebitis is not a characteristic feature. The diagnosis of Behçet's disease now requires the presence of recurrent oral ulcers plus two of the following: recurrent genital ulcerations, eye lesions, skin lesions, or a positive pathergy test (inflammatory reactivity to scratches or intradermal saline).

**VII-36.** **The answer is E.** *(Chap. 314)* Mixed connective-tissue disease (MCTD) is a syndrome characterized by high titers of circulating antibodies to the ribonucleoprotein component of extractable nuclear antigen in association with clinical features similar to those of SLE, systemic sclerosis, polymyositis, and rheumatoid arthritis. The average patient with MCTD is a middle-aged woman with Raynaud's phenomenon who also has polyarthritis, sclerodactyly (including swollen hands), esophageal dysfunction, pulmonary fibrosis, and inflammatory myopathy. Cutaneous manifestations include telangiectasias on the face and hands, alopecia, a lupuslike heliotropic rash, and erythematous patches over the knuckles. Myopathy may involve severe weakness of proximal muscles associated with high levels of creatine phosphokinase and aldolase. Both pulmonary involvement and esophageal dysmotility are common, but frequently asymptomatic until quite advanced. Almost all patients have high titers of rheumatoid factor and antinuclear antibodies. Such antibodies are directed toward the ribonuclease-sensitive ribonucleoprotein component of extractable nuclear antigen.

**VII-37.    The answer is C.** *(Chap. 319)*    Hypersensitivity vasculitis refers to a group of disorders presumed to be associated with a reaction to an antigen such as an infectious agent or drug. The common denominator of this group is the involvement of small vessels, especially postcapillary venules. Vasculitis is leukocytoclastic, meaning that nuclear debris remaining from neutrophilic infiltration is present. In the subacute or chronic stages, mononuclear cells predominate. Henoch-Schonlein purpura is caused by immune complexes containing IgA antibody, which may be due to a reaction to drugs, certain foods, insect bites, or immunization. Such complexes are deposited in the skin, gastrointestinal mucosal vessels, and glomeruli. The disease is characterized by arthralgias, glomerulonephritis, and gastrointestinal signs and symptoms (particularly nausea, vomiting, diarrhea, constipation, or passage of blood and mucus per rectum). However, the most characteristic finding is palpable purpura on the buttocks and lower extremities. Though the disease is usually self-limited, it can progress to a chronic form. Patients occasionally require glucocorticoid therapy.

**VII-38.    The answer is D.** *(Chap. 322)*    Osteoarthritis, the most common joint disease, is diagnosed on the basis of clinical and laboratory features. One of the earliest x-ray findings is joint space narrowing as periarticular cartilage is lost. A joint involved with osteoarthritis may be tender or slightly swollen; significant effusions are rare. The sensation of bone rubbing against bone (bony crepitus) may be elicited upon movement of an affected joint. Bony prominences on both the distal interphalangeal joints (Heberden's nodes) and the proximal interphalangeal joints (Bouchard's nodes) are commonly seen. Osteoarthritis in the patellofemoral joint may manifest as a positive "shrug" sign, i.e., pain when the patella is manually compressed against the femur when the quadriceps contracts. In contrast, rheumatoid arthritis (RA) commonly involves the proximal interphalangeal joint. Moreover, destruction of ligaments and tendons seen in RA may result in characteristic hand changes such as hyperextension of the proximal interphalangeal joints with compensatory flexion of the distal interphalangeal joints (swan-neck deformity) or flexion deformity of the proximal interphalangeals and extension of the distal interphalangeals (boutonniere deformity).

**VII-39.    The answer is A.** *(Chap. 314)*    Systemic sclerosis can be classified into two variants depending on whether scleroderma is present only in the fingers (sclerodactyly) or whether it is also present proximal to the metacarpophalangeal joints. The former disorder is associated with a constellation of findings labeled the CREST syndrome: calcinosis, Raynaud's phenomenon, esophageal dysmotility, sclerodactyly, and telangiectasia. Although once thought not to be associated with significant internal organ involvement, the CREST variant of systemic sclerosis has occurred in association with the development of pulmonary arterial hypertension or biliary cirrhosis. The fluorescent antinuclear antibody (ANA) test is positive in 40 to 80 percent of persons with systemic sclerosis. Antibodies are produced to deoxyribonucleoprotein, nucleolar, centromere, and topoisomerase 1 antigens. Mixed connective-tissue disease is the overlap of three rheumatic disease syndromes: systemic lupus erythematosus (SLE), polymyositis, and the CREST variant of systemic sclerosis. It is associated with high titers of antinuclear antibodies directed against the extractable nuclear antigen ribonucleoprotein. Arthritis and a positive ANA are not sufficient to make a diagnosis of SLE. Overlap syndromes are diseases that fulfill diagnostic criteria for two rheumatic diseases. In the case described, symptoms and signs were insufficient to fulfill the diagnostic criteria for more than one rheumatic syndrome.

**VII-40.    The answer is D.** *(Chap. 315)*    The clinical picture of skin rash and proximal or diffuse muscle weakness has few causes other than dermatomyositis. The skin manifestations may precede or follow the development of muscle weakness. The rash may be a localized or diffuse erythema, maculopapular, scaling eczematoid, or rarely exfoliative dermatitis. The classic violaceous heliotrope rash is on the eyelids and may include the bridge of the nose, cheeks, forehead, elbows, knees, knuckles, and around the nailbeds and may be pruritic. The painless myopathy involves skeletal muscles and is noted initially in the proximal limb muscles. At presentation, 25 percent have dysphagia. Laboratory findings reveal elevation of the serum levels of the skeletal muscle enzymes. Electromyography reveals the typical myopathic triad of motor unit action potentials which are of low amplitude and polyphasic, and have abnormally early recruitment. Muscle biopsy shows an inflammatory cell infiltrate with muscle fiber degeneration and regeneration. Vasculitis is also seen in dermatomyositis associated with connective tissue disorders. The incidence of malignancy is higher in patients over the age of 60, the most common types being lung, ovarian, breast, gastrointestinal, and lymphoproliferative tumors. A limited workup for malignancy is warranted in older patients with dermatomyositis. Dermatomyositis may be associated with various connective tissue disorders, including systemic sclerosis, rheumatoid arthritis, lupus erythematosus, or mixed connective tissue disorder. High-dose glucocorticoids are the accepted treatment for dermatomyositis. Cytotoxic drugs should be used if response to glucocorticoids is inadequate. About half of patients recover and can discontinue therapy within 5 years, 20 percent still have active disease requiring continued therapy. The remaining 30 percent have inactive disease but residual muscle weakness.

**VII-41.    The answer is C.**    *(Chap. 305)*    T lymphocytes are the principal mediators of cellular immunity and also serve important helper and suppressor functions in the regulation of antibody synthesis by B lymphocytes. In humans, they have the property of forming rosettes with sheep erythrocytes (E-rosettes), and they lack readily detectable immunoglobulin of any class on their membranes. Although the maturation of T cells is thymus-dependent, the cells arise from precursors in bone marrow. T cells constitute about 70 to 80 percent of blood lymphocytes; they comprise greater than three-quarters of thymus lymphocytes but less than one-quarter of bone marrow lymphocytes. In lymph nodes, they are found in paracortical areas. Specific monoclonal antibodies have been developed to characterize various subsets of T cells—cells that carry a CD4+ surface antigen are helper cells, and those with a CD8+ antigen function as cytotoxic-suppressor cells. Antibody-dependent cell-mediated cytotoxicity is a property of a class of non-B, non-T lymphocytes called large granular lymphocytes (LGL cells). Antibody-dependent cell-mediated cytotoxicity can also be mediated by monocyte-macrophages and neutrophils.

**VII-42.    The answer is C.**    *(Chap. 312)*    Although most clinicians believe that women with systemic lupus erythematosus should not become pregnant if they have active disease or advanced renal or cardiac disease, the presence of SLE itself is not an absolute contraindication to pregnancy. The outcome of pregnancy is best for those women in remission at the time of conception. Even in women with quiescent disease, exacerbations may occur (usually in the first trimester and in the immediate postpartum period), and 25 to 40 percent of pregnancies end in spontaneous abortion. Fetal loss rates are higher in patients with lupus anticoagulant or anticardiolipin antibodies. Flare-ups should be anticipated and vigorously treated with steroids. Steroids given throughout pregnancy also usually have no adverse effects on the child. In the case presented, the fact that the woman had a life-threatening bout of disease a year ago would argue against stopping her drugs at this time. Neonatal lupus, which is manifested by thrombocytopenia, rash, and heart block, is rare but can occur in mothers with anti-Ro antibodies.

**VII-43.    The answer is C.**    *(Chap. 305)*    Immunoglobulin A is the predominant immunoglobulin in body secretions (IgG is predominant in serum). Each secretory IgA molecule is a dimer consisting of a secretory component and a J chain. The secretory component, a protein of molecular weight 70,000, is synthesized by epithelial cells and facilitates IgA transport across mucosal tissues. The J chain is a small glycopeptide that aids the polymerization of immunoglobulins. IgA exists as two subclasses: IgA1 (75 percent of the total) and IgA2 (25 percent but more prevalent in secretions). IgA provides defense against local infections in the respiratory, gastrointestinal, and genitourinary tracts, and prevents access of foreign substances to the general systemic immune system. It also can prevent virus binding to epithelial cells. IgM, not IgA, is the principal immuno-globulin in the primary immune response and is the usual antibody in cold agglutinins. The half-life of IgA is about 6 days; IgE has the shortest half-life, approximately 2 to 2.5 days.

**VII-44.** **The answer is E.** *(Chap. 316)* Sjögren's syndrome, an autoimmune destruction of the exocrine glands, can be primary or it can occur in association with rheumatoid arthritis, SLE, or systemic sclerosis. A mononuclear cell infiltrate, which can be seen in virtually any organ, is pathognomonic if found in the salivary gland in association with keratoconjunctivitis sicca (conjunctival and corneal dryness) and xerostomia (lack of salivation). Since minor salivary glands will be obtained in a lip biopsy, such a procedure can be diagnostic. Severe dryness of the mouth can lead to an increased incidence of dental caries. Corneal dryness may be severe enough to result in ulceration. The most common form of renal involvement (seen in 40 percent of patients with primary Sjögren's) is an interstitial nephritis resulting in renal tubular acidosis. Hypersensitivity vasculitis, manifested by palpable purpura of the lower extremities, is not uncommon. Sensory neuropathies, interstitial pneumonitis, and autoimmune thyroid disease may also accompany primary Sjögren's syndrome. Finally, pseudolymphoma, characterized by lymphadenopathy and enlargement of the parotid gland, and frank non-Hodgkin's lymphoma may occur. Cardiac disease is very rare in Sjögren's syndrome.

**VII-45.** **The answer is E.** *(Chaps. 308, 315, and 319)* The differential diagnosis of myopathy in an AIDS patient is vast and includes infection, zidovudine-induced myositis, vasculitis, and polymyositis. Electromyography would likely show similar findings in all of these conditions. Blood cultures may be useful if the etiology is infectious, but generally are of little benefit in further narrowing the differential diagnosis. Similarly, lymph node biopsy may detect specific infections or malignant processes, but will not necessarily determine the etiology of the myopathy. Discontinuing the zidovudine, a drug which can cause myositis, will aid in determining the diagnosis only in zidovudine-induced myopathy. Muscle biopsy is the procedure best suited to establish a definitive diagnosis.

**VII-46.** **The answer is B.** *(Chap. 323)* Neuropathic joint disease, also known as Charcot's joint, is a severe form of osteoarthritis associated with loss of pain sensation, proprioception, or both. Normal muscle reflexes that modulate joint movement are diminished. Without these protective mechanisms, joints are subjected to repeated trauma resulting in progressive damage to cartilage. The underlying neurologic disorder determines which joints are affected. For example, the tarsal and tarsometatarsal joints are primarily affected in diabetes mellitus. Repeated intraarticular glucocorticoid injections are thought to predispose to neuropathic joint disease by an analgesic effect on overused joints, leading to further overuse of a damaged joint; this results in accelerated cartilage destruction. Other potential causes include leprosy, tabes dorsalis, syringomyelia, and congenital indifference to pain. The excessive production of growth hormone characteristic of acromegaly stimulates proliferation of cartilage, periarticular connective tissue, and bone which may result in musculoskeletal abnormalities including osteoarthritis, but not to neuropathic joint disease.

**VII-47.** **The answer is E.** *(Chap. 344)* Hyperuricemia may be caused by increased production and/or decreased excretion. Strenuous exercise may result in hyperuricemia from excessive degradation of skeletal muscle ATP. Acute gouty attacks occur in 20 to 86 percent of individuals with a prior history of gout during hospitalization for medical or surgical reasons. The stress of illness, shifts in fluid status or electrolytes, and general anesthesia probably contribute. Thiazides decrease urate clearance and excretion probably due to increased reabsorption secondary to extracellular volume depletion. Cyclosporine also causes a decrease in urate clearance, increasing the incidence of gout in transplant patients receiving this immunosuppressive agent. Ascorbic acid is uricosuric and thus does not cause hyperuricemia.

**VII-48.    The answer is D.**    *(Chap. 344)*    Nonsteroidal anti-inflammatory drugs, colchicine, or intraarticular glucocorticoids may all be used in the treatment of an acute flare of gouty arthritis. Colchicine inhibits neutrophil activation by inhibiting crystal-induced protein tyrosine phosphorylation. Oral colchicine is not tolerated by most patients because of the gastrointestinal side effects. Colchicine may be given intravenously, but administration by this route is potentially dangerous and should be used with caution. Depressed bone marrow function, renal or liver disease, and sepsis are contraindications to intravenous colchicine. Allopurinol should not be used in an acute flare of gouty arthritis as it may prolong the attack.

**VII-49.    The answer is E.**    *(Chap. 348)*    Marfan syndrome is caused by a mutation in the gene for fibrillin. Severe disease is characterized by the triad of: (1) long thin extremities frequently associated with other skeletal changes; (2) ectopia lentis; (3) aortic aneurysms. Milder forms of the disorder may be more difficult to diagnose. Cardiovascular abnormalities are the major source of morbidity and mortality. Mitral valve prolapse is common and progresses to regurgitation in one-quarter of patients. Dilatation of the aortic root can progress to cause aortic regurgitation, aortic dissection, or frank rupture. All patients should have a slit-lamp examination to check for lens dislocation. Striae may occur over the shoulders and buttocks, but otherwise the skin is normal. The disorder is generally inherited as an autosomal dominant trait, but approximately one-fourth of cases are probably new mutations.

**VII-50.    The answer is D.**    *(Chap. 348)*    Alport syndrome is an inherited disorder associated with hematuria that exists in four forms. Classic Alport syndrome is inherited as an X-linked disorder with hematuria, sensorineural deafness, and conical deformation of the anterior surface of the lens (lenticonus). A second X-linked form is associated with leiomyomatosis. Autosomal recessive and autosomal dominant also exist. These autosomal forms can cause renal disease without deafness or lenticonus. Blue sclerae, which may be present in other inherited disorders of connective tissue, such as osteogenesis imperfecta or Type VI Ehlers-Danlos syndrome, are not seen in Alport syndrome.

**VII-51.    The answer is B.**    *(Chap. 324)*    The majority of infections are acquired intraoperatively or perioperatively as a result of wound breakdown or infection. The presentation may be acute with dramatic signs of inflammation including joint pain, swelling, erythema, and warmth. Alternatively, infection may be more indolent and persist for months or even years. The presentation depends primarily on the virulence of the infecting organism. Joint aspiration is the most efficacious method of diagnosis. Successful treatment generally requires removal of prosthetic material and antimicrobial therapy. Simple surgical drainage and antimicrobial therapy results in an 80 percent failure rate. The risk of infection is increased in repeat total joint replacements as well as any factor or event that delays wound healing (e.g., steroid use, diabetes mellitus, poor nutrition, etc.).

**VII-52.    The answer is E.**    *(Chap. 326)*    Fibromyalgia is characterized by widespread musculoskeletal pain, stiffness, paresthesias, nonrestorative sleep, and easy fatigability associated with multiple tender points which are widely and symmetrically distributed. Fibromyalgia is more prevalent in women. Several causative mechanisms for fibromyalgia have been postulated. Disturbed sleep has been implicated as a factor in the pathogenesis. Many patients fit a psychiatric diagnosis, the most common being depression, anxiety, somatization, and hypochondriases. There is disagreement about whether some of these abnormalities may represent reactions to chronic pain or if fibromyalgia is a reflection of psychiatric disturbance. However, fibromyalgia also occurs in patients without psychiatric diagnoses. Patients may complain of joint pain and perceive their joints are swollen; however, joint examination is normal. Glucocorticoids have little benefit and should not be used. Other therapies include local measures, biofeedback, anxiolytics, and antidepressants.

**VII-53.   The answer is A-N, B-Y, C-Y, D-Y, E-Y.** *(Chaps. 324, 204)*   The patient has desert fever, a syndrome caused by coccidioidomycosis infection, which is endemic in the southwest United States. This syndrome is largely an acute hypersensitivity reaction to the primary pulmonary infection, which is symptomatic in only 40 percent of affected persons. Manifestations of hypersensitivity may include erythema nodosum, erythema multiforme, arthralgia, arthritis, conjunctivitis, and episcleritis. However, disseminated coccidioidomycosis may occur during the primary infection and could result in osteomyelitis (which may seed an adjacent synovium directly), fungal arthritis, skin lesions, or CNS disease. Even in the case of hematogenously derived joint infection, synovial fluid cultures will rarely be positive; synovial biopsy for culture and histology may be required. Serologic tests, while possibly acutely negative in a patient with primary pulmonary infection only, can be quite helpful, particularly when there is disseminated involvement.

**VII-54.   The answer is A-N, B-N, C-Y, D-Y, E-Y.** *(Chap. 305)*   T-cell precursors leave the yolk sac, fetal liver, or bone marrow and migrate to the thymus, where they undergo further maturation. Even before T-cell receptor gene rearrangements occur, pre-T cells express the CD7 antigen, the earliest marker of T-cell lineage. After the CD2 adhesion molecule, which functions as the receptor for sheep red blood cells, is expressed on the cell surface, assembly of the T-cell receptor complex begins. This complex consists of the five proteins that make up the CD3 signal transduction moiety plus the two antigen-recognizing heterodimer molecules that form the actual T-cell antigen receptor. The proteins that can function as part of the T-cell antigen receptor all have a variable (produced by V-J recombination) and constant region and bear homology to the immunoglobulin heavy and light chains. Along with the histocompatibility proteins and the CD2, CD4, and CD8 molecules, the T-cell antigen receptor chains are members of the immunoglobulin gene superfamily, which provides the immunologic diversity required to distinguish self from nonself and recognize an inordinate number of foreign antigens. After CD3 T-cell receptor expression, but before suppressor or helper phenotype is determined, there is a thymic stage wherein both CD4 and CD8 antigens are expressed. Some lymphoblastic lymphomas arise at this stage of T-cell development.

**VII-55.   The answer is A-Y, B-Y, C-Y, D-N, E-N.** *(Chap. 307. Buckley, N Engl J Med 325:110, 1991.)*   Isolated IgA deficiency is the most common immunodeficiency disorder, with an incidence between 1:600 and 1:800. Affected persons have a normal or reduced number of B cells with surface IgA, but seem to have overabundant immature cells that coexpress IgA and IgM, suggesting a block in B-cell terminal differentiation. This presumption is substantiated by in vitro studies showing that lymphocytes from IgA-deficient persons can synthesize but are unable to secrete IgA. Both serum IgA and secretory IgA usually are reduced. Although IgA deficiency need not be associated with clinical disease, it frequently is. Recurrent sinopulmonary infection is most common. Allergy occurs with an incidence of 1:200 to 1:400, compared with 1:600 to 1:800 in the general population. Approximately 30 to 40 percent of IgA-deficient persons have antibodies directed against IgA, thus predisposing them to anaphylactoid reactions following the infusion of blood products unless the blood is obtained from IgA-deficient donors. Persons with isolated IgA deficiency are also at greater risk for developing autoimmune diseases, including lupus and rheumatoid arthritis. Immunoglobulin treatment will not restore IgA levels to normal and is of little value in this condition.

**VII-56.   The answer is A-Y, B-Y, C-Y, D-Y, E-Y.** *(Chap. 305)*   Most antigen-antibody complexes are cleared by cells of the reticuloendothelial system. It appears that in some conditions the reticuloendothelial system can be overwhelmed by immune complexes, thereby impeding the removal and leading to the deposition of immune complexes. Deposition of these complexes in tissues other than those of the reticuloendothelial system is responsible for the signs and symptoms of immune-complex disease. In animal models, the persistence of complexes is necessary for the development of renal disease; also, slight antigen excess has been found to predispose to the formation of antigen-antibody complexes, which persist in the circulation and lead to inflammatory illness. Immune complex-mediated vascular damage can lead to cutaneous necrotizing vasculitis. Electron microscopy reveals subendothelial immune complexes that presumably incite an array of inflammatory cells to migrate toward the vessel.

**VII-57.** **The answer is A-N, B-Y, C-N, D-Y, E-Y.** *(Chap. 306)* Class I HLA antigens are encoded at the A, B, and C loci of the human major histocompatibility complex on chromosome 6. Each such antigen consists of an 11.5-kilodalton (kDa) $\beta_2$-microglobulin subunit (also encoded in the HLA region) and a 44-kDa chain with three separate domains that contain the antigenic specificity. Only certain areas of the heavy chain are diverse, so individual molecules share greater than 80 percent sequence homology. Class I molecules are expressed on all cells except mature red blood cells. These antigens are defined serologically and are useful in predicting results for organ transplants. Because class I antigens are not distributed evenly from one racial group to another, it can be more difficult for a person of African descent, for example, to procure a bone marrow donor from a registry where most of the potential donors descend from Northern Europe.

**VII-58.** **The answer is A-N, B-N, C-N, D-Y, E-Y.** *(Chap. 309)* This patient has many of the hallmarks of systemic amyloidosis. An abdominal fat pad aspirate or a rectal biopsy is the best way to make the diagnosis, although biopsy of any affected organ may be carried out. A positive Congo red histologic stain helps to establish the diagnosis. The classification of amyloid protein fibrils that are deposited in the tissues is based on their biochemical type. AL amyloid residues bear homology to immunoglobulin light chains and are seen in de novo or myeloma-associated disease. The AA type of amyloid, made up of a protein of 76 amino acids, is seen secondary to a host of chronic inflammatory conditions, including long-standing rheumatoid arthritis, tuberculosis, bronchiectasis, familial Mediterranean fever, and leprosy. Other types of amyloid proteins are seen in familial amyloid polyneuropathy, medullary carcinoma of the thyroid, and Alzheimer's disease (the beta, or A4, protein). Amyloidosis should be suspected in any patient with an underlying chronic inflammatory disease who develops hepatomegaly, splenomegaly, malabsorption, cardiac disease, or proteinuria. Cardiac disease usually consists of congestive heart failure with low QRS-complex voltage, arrhythmias, and exquisite sensitivity to digitalis. Waxy papules or plaques in the axillary folds may signal the deposition of amyloid in the skin; purpura after minor trauma is not uncommon. Gastrointestinal problems caused by amyloid include macroglossia, malabsorption, and bleeding. In addition to amyloid-induced synovitis, peripheral neuropathy and carpal tunnel syndrome may be seen.

**VII-59.** **The answer is A-Y, B-N, C-N, D-Y, E-Y.** *(Chap. 312)* The most common cause of drug-induced SLE is procainamide, which produces a positive ANA in 75 percent of those who take it and a 20 percent incidence of clinical lupus. In contrast, hydralazine induces an ANA in 25 percent and a clinical lupus syndrome in 10 percent. Slow acetylators seem to have more problems with drug-induced autoimmune phenomena. Though up to 50 percent of those with drug-induced lupus have arthralgias, pleuropericarditis, or both, renal disease is rare. In an effort to distinguish drug-induced lupus (which should last less than 6 months) from de novo lupus (a disease uniquely positive for anti-dsDNA and anti-Sm), a complete ANA panel should be sent. Most patients will respond initially to withdrawal of the offending drug; if not, then a brief trial of steroids is indicated.

**VII-60.** **The answer is A-N, B-N, C-Y, D-Y, E-N.** *(Chap. 313. Brooks, N Engl J Med 324:1716–1725, 1991)* NSAIDs, including aspirin, are effective agents in the treatment of symptomatic rheumatoid arthritis. However, none of the newer agents have been shown to be more effective than aspirin, though some do have fewer gastrointestinal side effects. All of these agents induce platelet dysfunction. Their mechanism of action is the blockage of the activity of the enzyme cyclooxygenase, which converts arachidonic acid into the inflammation-mediating prostaglandins. 5-Lipoxygenase, which is not inhibited by most NSAIDs, converts arachidonic acid into leukotrienes. It may be the dysregulation of normal arachidonic acid metabolism that leads to the occasional NSAID-induced worsening of allergic rhinitis and asthma. The absence of renal vasodilatory prostaglandins normally produced by the action of cyclooxygenase can lead to renal insufficiency, particularly in those with underlying renal vascular disease.

**VII-61.**   **The answer is A-N, B-Y, C-N, D-Y, E-Y.**   *(Chap. 320)*   Sarcoidosis is a systemic granulomatous inflammatory disorder that frequently involves the lungs, where it causes a typical interstitial lung disease that may be asymptomatic, may cause transient respiratory difficulties with or without hilar adenopathy, or may progress to end-stage pulmonary fibrosis. Extrapulmonary sarcoidosis may involve the eyes, skin, liver, bones, gastrointestinal tract, kidneys, nervous system, and heart. In the United States, 10 to 20 percent of cases consist of asymptomatic hilar adenopathy detected on chest radiographs taken for other reasons; these cases may constitute a higher fraction of the total in other countries where routine preemployment chest radiography is more widely practiced. The disease occurs more frequently among blacks than whites by a substantial margin. At sites of disease activity, such as the lung, there is an accumulation of activated helper-inducer (CD4+) lymphocytes, with release of immunologic mediators such as interleukin 2 and gamma-interferon, and resultant granuloma formation. In contrast to other interstitial lung diseases, the diagnosis may frequently be made by the demonstration of the characteristic granulomatous inflammation in tissue obtained by transbronchial biopsy. Prognosis depends on the risk of progression to advanced pulmonary fibrosis, and those persons with intense pulmonary inflammation may benefit from treatment with corticosteroids. Chest radiography and pulmonary function testing cannot distinguish accurately between active inflammation and established fibrosis; hence, most clinicians familiar with the disease utilize procedures such as bronchoalveolar lavage or gallium-67 scanning, or both, to assess the intensity of the alveolitis present. These procedures may be performed serially during the course of the patient's illness to follow the progress of the disease and response to therapy.

**VII-62.**   **The answer is A-Y, B-Y, C-Y, D-N, E-N.**   *(Chap. 313)*   Rheumatoid factors are antibodies to the Fc fragment of immunoglobulin G. They may be of the IgG, IgA, or IgM class; the widely used latex and sheep-cell agglutination tests detect rheumatoid factors primarily of the IgM class. Chronic antigenic stimulation is one of the processes important in the production of rheumatoid factors. Rheumatoid factors are associated not only with rheumatoid arthritis and other autoimmune diseases but also with lymphoreticular malignancies and chronic infections, such as subacute bacterial endocarditis. Rheumatoid factors are usually present within the first year of onset of rheumatoid arthritis; their presence correlates with the extraarticular manifestations of the disease. Patients with rheumatoid arthritis who have positive serologic tests for IgM rheumatoid factor have a worse prognosis than those who are seronegative.

**VII-63.**   **The answer is A-Y, B-N, C-N, D-Y, E-Y.**   *(Chap. 313)*   Joint stiffness in the morning or after periods of inactivity lasting more than 1 h is characteristic of inflammatory rheumatic disease. Arthritis characteristic of rheumatoid arthritis is persistent, remaining in the same joints for months. Migratory arthritis, in which short-lived arthritis symptoms in one joint subside as symptoms begin in another joint, is not characteristic of rheumatoid arthritis. Persons who have rheumatoid arthritis can have involvement of the cervical spine, the wrist joints, and all the small joints of the hand except the distal interphalangeal joints. Wrist-joint arthritis can lead to median-nerve entrapment (carpal tunnel syndrome).

**VII-64. The answer is A-Y, B-N, C-Y, D-N, E-Y.** *(Chap. 317)* This patient has an acute inflammatory asymmetric polyarthritis associated with ocular (conjunctivitis, occasionally anterior uveitis) and cutaneous (keratoderma blennorhagicum on palms and soles; circinate balanitis on the glans penis) disease. Moreover, he has had a recent episode of urethritis, possibly caused by chlamydia. He therefore has so-called reactive arthritis, also known as Reiter's syndrome. This entity can follow certain infectious illnesses, most notably dysentery or venereal disease usually in patients who are HLA-B27-positive. The constitutional symptoms associated with the acute illness can be severe. The erythrocyte sedimentation rate is frequently elevated. Sacroiliitis and spondyloarthropathy may be seen as late sequelae. Patients will respond to nonsteroidal agents, but there is little evidence to support the benefit of antibiotics, other than in eradicating chlamydia, if present.

**VII-65. The answer is A-N, B-Y, C-Y, D-Y, E-N.** *(Chap. 319. Hoffman, Ann Intern Med 116:488–498, 1992.)* This patient presents with findings characteristic of Wegener's granulomatosis. Sinus disease (manifested by bloody or purulent nasal discharge), pulmonary disease, and glomerulonephritis are seen in greater than 80 percent of affected patients. Sinus involvement would be unlikely in Goodpasture's syndrome, which is associated with anti-basement membrane antibodies. Other findings characteristic of Wegener's include ocular involvement, skin lesions, and nervous system manifestations (including cranial neuritis or mononeuritis multiplex), as well as elevated ESR, anemia, leukocytosis, and hypergammaglobulinemia. The diagnosis can be made by finding necrotizing granulomatous vasculitis in an involved site. Although the immunopathogenesis of this entity is unclear, antibodies to a neutrophil protein (found in the azurophilic granules) can be frequently found. The disease can be successfully treated in over 90 percent of patients with the use of glucocorticoids and cyclophosphamide. The glucocorticoids are gradually tapered and the cyclophosphamide, the mainstay of treatment, should be continued for about 1 year after complete remission.

**VII-66. The answer is A-N, B-N, C-N, D-Y, E-Y.** *(Chap. 320)* While 10 to 20 percent of patients with sarcoidosis present with asymptomatic disease found incidentally on chest x-ray and 40 to 70 percent have the characteristic insidious development of disease, the remainder present over the span of a few weeks. Constitutional and respiratory symptoms dominate the acute presentation. Two distinct patterns of acute sarcoidosis are recognized. Lofgren's syndrome, seen in Scandinavian, Irish, and Puerto Rican females, is characterized by erythema nodosum, arthralgias, and bilateral hilar lymphadenopathy. The constellation of findings in the Heerfordt-Waldenstrom syndrome consists of fever, parotid enlargement, anterior uveitis, and facial nerve palsy. Interstitial pulmonary involvement would be rare in acute sarcoidosis. Myopathy and skin lesions are most consistent with dermatomyositis. Although 5 percent of patients with sarcoidosis have cardiac abnormalities, valvular heart disease—other than occasional instances of papillary muscle dysfunction—is rare.

**VII-67. The answer is A-N, B-Y, C-Y, D-N, E-N.** *(Chap. 319)* Patients with midline granuloma, characterized by local inflammation and destructive mutilation of head and neck tissues, may present with nasal and sinus symptoms. Ulcerations of the nasal septum and soft and hard palates are harbingers of very destructive processes in any area in the neck or above. Granulomatous infiltration and necrosis will be noted on pathologic examination of the involved areas. Radiation therapy is the treatment of choice and is successful in averting the almost certainly fatal course in untreated patients. Midline granuloma can be difficult to distinguish from cocaine-induced septal perforation, malignant lymphoma, and a host of chronic infections including histoplasmosis, blastomycosis, coccidioidomycosis, leprosy, tuberculosis, syphilis, and leishmaniasis. While Wegener's granulomatosis is associated with similar upper airway findings, the absence of vasculitis on biopsy, the absence of pulmonary and renal disease, and the presence of palatal perforation make the diagnosis of midline granuloma much more likely. Midline granuloma never involves structures below the neck.

**VII-68–VII-71.   The answers are 68.-C, 69.-E, 70.-D, 71.-A.**   *(Chaps. 321, 326. Baker, N Engl J Med 329:1013–1020, 1993.)*   The analysis of synovial fluid begins at the bedside. When fluid is withdrawn from a joint into a syringe, its clarity and color should be assessed. Cloudiness or turbidity is caused by the scattering of light as it is reflected off particles in the fluid; these particles are usually white blood cells, although crystals may also be present. The viscosity of synovial fluid is due to its hyaluronate content. In inflammatory joint disease, synovial fluid contains enzymes that break down hyaluronate and reduce fluid viscosity. In contrast, synovial fluid taken from a joint in a person with degenerative joint disease, a noninflammatory condition, would be expected to be clear and have good viscosity. The color of the fluid can indicate recent or old hemorrhage into the joint space. Pigmented villonodular synovitis is associated with noninflammatory fluid that is dark brown in color ("crankcase oil") as a result of repeated hemorrhage into the joint. Gout and calcium pyrophosphate deposition disease produce inflammatory synovial effusions, which are cloudy and watery. In addition, these disorders may be diagnosed by identification of crystals in the fluid—sodium urate crystals of gout are needle-like and strongly negatively birefringent, whereas calcium pyrophosphate crystals are rhomboidal and weakly positively birefringent.

# VIII. DISORDERS OF THE ALIMENTARY TRACT AND HEPATOBILIARY SYSTEM

## QUESTIONS

**DIRECTIONS:** Each question below contains five suggested responses. Choose the **one best** response to each question.

**VIII-1.** A 56-year-old woman has had profuse watery diarrhea for 3 months. Laboratory studies of fecal water show the following:

Sodium: 39 mmol/L
Potassium: 96 mmol/L
Chloride: 15 mmol/L
Bicarbonate: 40 mmol/L
Osmolality: 270 mosmol/kg $H_2O$ (serum osmolality: 280 mosmol/kg $H_2O$)

The most likely diagnosis is

(A) villous adenoma
(B) lactose intolerance
(C) laxative abuse
(D) pancreatic insufficiency
(E) nontropical sprue

**VIII-2.** A 56-year-old man presents to his internist with jaundice. The patient is receiving no medication, and his only symptomatic complaint is mild fatigue over the past 2 months. Physical examination is remarkable only for the presence of scleral icterus. The patient has no significant past medical history. Analysis of serum chemistry reveals the following:

SGOT: 0.58 μkat/L (35 U/L)
SGPT: 0.58 μkat/L (35 U/L)
Total bilirubin: 91.7 μmol/L (7 mg/dL)
Direct bilirubin: 85.5 μmol/L (5 mg/dL)
Alkaline phosphatase: 12 μkat/L (720 U/L)

Which of the following is the next most appropriate diagnostic step?

(A) CT of the abdomen
(B) Liver biopsy
(C) Review of peripheral blood smear
(D) Endoscopic retrograde cholangiopancreatography (ERCP)
(E) No further evaluation necessary; the patient has Dubin-Johnson syndrome

**VIII-3.** A 24-year-old patient known to be infected with type 1 human immunodeficiency virus (HIV-1) presents with a 2-week history of intermittent bloody diarrhea, urgency, abdominal pain, and malaise. Stool culture for enteropathogenic organisms is negative, and analysis for ova and parasites is similarly unrevealing. The patient is taking no medication. The diarrheal symptoms do not respond to a course of trimethoprim-sulfamethoxazole. Colonoscopic examination reveals multiple areas of ulceration and mucosal erosion. Biopsy reveals the presence of cells containing a large, densely staining nucleus and abundant intracytoplasmic inclusions. The most appropriate therapy for this patient is

(A) pentamidine
(B) pyrimethamine
(C) ganciclovir
(D) acyclovir
(E) isoniazid

**VIII-4.** All the following can inhibit the secretion of gastric acid EXCEPT

(A) reduction of the intragastric pH below 3.0
(B) somatostatin
(C) secretin
(D) histamine
(E) presence of fat in the duodenum

**VIII-5.** A 45-year-old man says that for the past year he occasionally has regurgitated food particles eaten several days earlier. His wife complains that his breath has been foul-smelling. He has had occasional dysphagia for solid foods. The most likely diagnosis is

(A) gastric outlet obstruction
(B) scleroderma
(C) achalasia
(D) Zenker's diverticulum
(E) diabetic gastroparesis

**VIII-6.** A 57-year-old man seeks attention in the emergency department for weakness and melena, which he has had for 3 days. He says he has not had significant abdominal pain and had no prior gastrointestinal bleeding. On examination he is disheveled and unshaven, appears older than his stated age, and has a 20 mmHg orthostatic drop in blood pressure. Findings include bilateral temporal wasting, anicteric and pale conjunctivae, spider angiomas on his upper torso, muscle wasting, hepatosplenomegaly, and hyperactive bowel sounds without abdominal tenderness to palpation. Stool is melenic. Nasogastric aspiration reveals "coffee-grounds" material, which quickly clears with lavage. Hematocrit is 30 percent, and mean corpuscular volume is 105 fL. Saline gastric lavage is initiated. The appropriate next step in the management of this man's illness would be to

(A) perform gastroscopy
(B) pass a Sengstaken-Blakemore tube and begin an intravenous infusion of vasopressin (Pitressin)
(C) order an upper gastrointestinal series
(D) order immediate visceral angiography
(E) insert a large-bore intravenous line and type and cross-match the man's blood

**VIII-7.** A 42-year-old woman presents with a complaint of watery diarrhea and abdominal pain that has occurred intermittently over the past 4 years. After the passage of three or four loose stools in the morning, she feels well for the rest of the day and never has nocturnal diarrhea. Physical examination reveals an anxious woman with a tender left lower abdominal quadrant and no fecal material in the rectum; the results are otherwise normal. Sigmoidoscopic examination discloses excess mucus, but the mucosa appears normal. Barium enema is normal except for sigmoid spasticity, and examination of a stool specimen reveals well-formed feces that are negative for blood, pathogenic bacteria, and parasites. Results of thyroid studies are normal. A trial of milk restriction results in no change in symptoms. At this point the physician should

(A) consider a trial of diphenoxylate or loperamide to control symptomatic diarrhea
(B) tell the patient that her symptoms are largely emotional in origin
(C) consider a trial of psyllium to increase stool bulk
(D) obtain stool electrolytes and osmolality
(E) perform a jejunal aspirate and analyze the fluid for parasites

**VIII-8.** All the following statements about achalasia are true EXCEPT

(A) the underlying abnormality appears to be defective innervation of the esophageal body and lower esophageal sphincter
(B) dysphagia, chest pain, and regurgitation are the predominant symptoms
(C) chest x-rays often reveal a large gastric air bubble
(D) manometry reveals a normal or elevated pressure of the lower esophageal sphincter
(E) nifedipine is effective in controlling the symptoms in many patients

**VIII-9.** A 45-year-old man presents with sharp epigastric pain relieved by antacids and food. Barium study of the upper gastrointestinal tract reveals a crater in the proximal portion of the duodenal bulb. Which of the following statements concerning therapeutic alternatives is correct?

(A) Atropine or related anticholinergic agents are effective in improving the symptoms
(B) Sucralfate is effective in eradicating *Helicobacter pylori* colonization
(C) Cimetidine or other $H_2$-receptor antagonists are more effective than sucralfate in promoting healing
(D) Sucralfate can significantly reduce the bioavailability of fluoroquinolone antibiotics
(E) Omeprazole, a specific inhibitor of parietal cell $H^+$, $K^+$-ATPase, is contraindicated in routine situations because of its carcinogenic potential

**VIII-10.** A 75-year-old woman with a history of aspirin-induced gastritis 5 years ago now has severe knee and hip pain that is thought to be due to osteoarthritis. She requires treatment with nonsteroidal anti-inflammatory agents. Which of the following agents would be most helpful for prophylaxis against recurrent gastrointestinal bleeding?

(A) Omeprazole
(B) Misoprostol
(C) Nizatidine
(D) Sucralfate
(E) Atropine

**VIII-11.** Four months ago, a 36-year-old man with a peptic ulcer underwent a Billroth II anastomosis, antrectomy, vagotomy, and gastrojejunostomy. He now returns for evaluation of a stomal (anastomotic) ulcer. Fasting serum gastrin level is 350 ng/L; 5 min after the intravenous infusion of secretin the serum gastrin level is 200 ng/L. The man should be advised that the most appropriate treatment for his condition is

(A) total vagotomy
(B) total gastrectomy
(C) resection of the distal antrum attached to the duodenal stump
(D) laparotomy to search for a gastrin-producing tumor
(E) medical therapy with liquid antacids

**VIII-12.** All the following statements regarding eosinophilic enteritis are true EXCEPT

(A) peripheral blood eosinophilia is present
(B) it may affect the stomach, small intestine, and colon
(C) the majority of patients have a history of food allergies or asthma
(D) treatment with corticosteroids is often effective
(E) it may be difficult to distinguish from regional enteritis

**VIII-13.** Which of the following diagnostic studies for malabsorption is usually normal in persons who have bacterial overgrowth syndrome?

(A) Fecal fat quantitation (24 h)
(B) Stage II Schilling test (intrinsic factor given with vitamin $B_{12}$)
(C) D-Xylose absorption test
(D) Lactulose breath test
(E) Quantitative cultures of jejunal aspirates

**VIII-14.** A 30-year-old man complains of abdominal cramps, bloating, and diarrhea. He believes that these symptoms are exacerbated after the ingestion of dairy products. He is otherwise well and has no abnormalities on physical or laboratory examination. Which is the most specific and sensitive measurement to diagnose this patient's condition?

(A) Breath hydrogen after ingestion of 50 g lactose
(B) Blood glucose after ingestion of 100 g lactose
(C) Breath labeled carbon dioxide after ingestion of oral glycine-1-[$^{14}$C] glycocholate
(D) Urine xylose after ingestion of 25 g D-xylose
(E) Vitamin A serum level

**VIII-15.** A 72-year-old woman with known mitral stenosis and atrial fibrillation presents with severe abdominal pain. The pain began fairly suddenly 24 h ago and was located in the periumbilical region; however, today the pain is present throughout the abdomen. Other than the aforementioned cardiac disease, the past medical history is unremarkable. Her only medication is digoxin 0.25 mg/d. Physical examination reveals an anxious patient with a temperature of 38.3°C (101°F) orally, blood pressure of 100/60, pulse of 120, and respiratory rate of 26. Her skin is cold and clammy. The oral mucosa is dry. Cardiac auscultation is remarkable for a grade 2/4 diastolic rumble. Bowel sounds are normal. There is mild abdominal distention and tenderness without rebound. Stool is guaiac-positive but not grossly bloody or melenic. Initial laboratory evaluation reveals a WBC of 16,000/μL with a differential of 75 percent neutrophils, 10 percent bands, 10 percent lymphocytes, and 5 percent monocytes; hematocrit of 42 percent; and platelet count of 522,000/mL. Plain film of the abdomen reveals air-fluid levels. The most appropriate diagnostic maneuver at this time is

(A) exploratory laparotomy
(B) laparoscopy
(C) angiography
(D) CT of the abdomen
(E) upper GI series with small bowel follow-through

**VIII-16.** For the last 6 months a 50-year-old man has had diarrhea and migratory arthralgias and has lost 9.1 kg (20 lb). An upper gastrointestinal barium study shows a malabsorption pattern in the small bowel. Stool fat content is 35 g per 24 h. After oral administration of 25 g of D-xylose, a 5-h urine collection contains 0.8 g of D-xylose. A peroral small-bowel biopsy reveals subtotal villus atrophy, dilated lymphatics, and infiltration of the lamina propria with macrophages that stain positively with periodic acid Schiff (PAS) stain. The man's physician should now

(A) start him on a gluten-free diet
(B) prescribe prednisone, 60 mg/d and tapered over 2 months
(C) prescribe prednisone, 60 mg/d indefinitely
(D) prescribe trimethoprim-sulfamethoxazole for at least 1 year
(E) recommend an exploratory laparotomy with splenectomy and biopsy of retroperitoneal nodes

**VIII-17.**   A 70-year-old Irish consular official seeks local medical attention for diarrhea and weight loss, which have been present for 2 years. He says he has always been in good health "even though I'm the runt of the litter" (he is the smallest of eight siblings). Laboratory studies include normal complete blood cell count and serum electrolyte concentrations. Serum D-xylose concentration is 0.76 mmol/L (15 mg/dL) 2 h after an oral challenge, and 24-h fecal fat determination is 12 g on a 100-g fat diet. A representative biopsy specimen of his jejunum is shown below. Which of the following statements about the man's illness is correct?

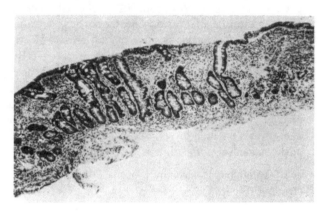

(A)   This condition is believed to be due to a gram-negative bacillus

(B)   Abdominal pain, arthralgia, low-grade fever, and lymphadenopathy are frequently present

(C)   Corticosteroid therapy is the treatment of choice

(D)   Adherence to a strict gluten-free diet usually results in normalization of malabsorption tests and reversal of jejunal pathology

(E)   A rebiopsy after gluten challenge is indicated at this time

**VIII-18.**   A 28-year-old man has had diarrhea and crampy abdominal pain of the right lower quadrant for the last 4 weeks. During the last 10 days he also has had episodic low-grade fever, abdominal distention, and anorexia without vomiting but leading to a weight loss of 3.2 kg (7 lb). On examination, he is mildly uncomfortable. Vital signs are temperature 37.8°C (100.1°F), pulse 100 beats per minute, and blood pressure 110/60 mmHg. His sclerae are anicteric, and there is no palpable lymphadenopathy. A tender, indistinct fullness is palpable in the right lower quadrant of the abdomen, but otherwise the abdomen is soft and without rebound tenderness or palpable hepatosplenomegaly. Rectal examination reveals no masses or focal tenderness, but the stool is guaiac-positive. Laboratory values include a hematocrit of 30 percent and a white blood cell count of 11,300/μL with a shift to the left. Flat-plate and upright x-rays of the abdomen show some air-filled loops of small bowel but no air-fluid levels. Sigmoidoscopy is unremarkable. On barium enema examination, barium fails to reflux into the terminal ileum, but the colon is otherwise normal. A representative film from a small-bowel barium examination is shown below. Which of the following disorders is most consistent with the clinical picture described?

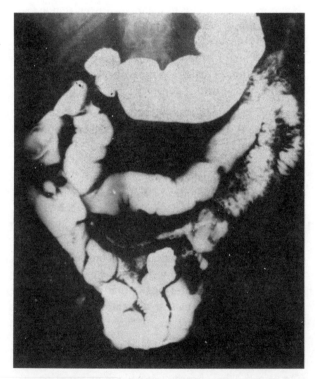

(A)   Perforated appendix with appendiceal abscess

(B)   Whipple's disease

(C)   Regional enteritis

(D)   Adenocarcinoma of the small intestine

(E)   Lymphoma of the small intestine

**VIII-19.** A 20-year-old man was found to have ulcerative proctitis 2 years ago. Mild rectal bleeding was well controlled on daily steroid enemas, which were discontinued a year ago. For the last 3 months he has had increasingly frequent bloody diarrhea (now 6 to 10 times a day), lower abdominal cramps, low-grade fever, anorexia, and a 5-kg (11-lb) weight loss. Physical examination of this thin, pale young man, who appears acutely ill, reveals these vital signs: temperature 37.8°C (100°F), pulse 110 beats per minute, and blood pressure 120/70 mmHg. The lower abdomen is mildly and diffusely tender, but there is no rebound tenderness and bowel sounds are active. Stool is grossly bloody. Sigmoidoscopy, limited to 10 cm because of discomfort, shows marked mucosal erythema and friability; diffuse ulceration is present, and an exudate contains pus and blood.

Three hours after a barium enema, which shows ulcerations throughout the colon, the man's abdominal pain worsens markedly. Vital signs now are temperature 39.6°C (103.2°F), pulse 130 beats per minute, and blood pressure 90/60 mmHg. On examination the abdomen is distended and diffusely tender with rebound; bowel sounds are infrequent. An abdominal flat-plate x-ray is pictured below.

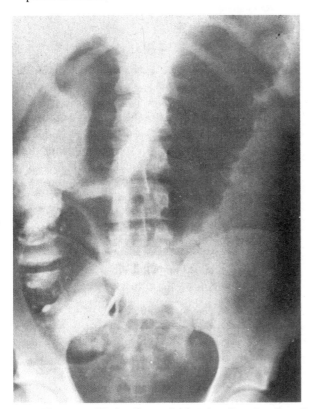

The most likely diagnosis for the disorder described above is

(A) acute colonic perforation
(B) inferior mesenteric artery occlusion
(C) nonthrombotic mesenteric ischemia
(D) volvulus
(E) toxic megacolon

**VIII-20.** As a consequence of severe liver damage, hepatic amino acid handling is deranged. In this situation, plasma levels of which of the following are likely to be lower than normal?

(A) Ammonia ($NH_3$)
(B) Ammonium ($NH_4^+$)
(C) Alanine
(D) Urea
(E) Glycine

**VIII-21.** Which of the following drugs will be less potent in the presence of severe liver disease?

(A) Phenytoin
(B) Lidocaine
(C) Tetracycline
(D) Imipramine
(E) Propranolol

**VIII-22.** All the following statements regarding primary biliary cirrhosis (PBC) are true EXCEPT

(A) a positive antimitochondrial antibody test is present in more than 90 percent of these patients
(B) ursodial treatment is helpful
(C) the majority of these patients are women
(D) administration of D-penicillamine appears to be an effective treatment
(E) rheumatoid arthritis, CRST syndrome, and scleroderma occur with increased frequency in patients with PBC

CREST : Calcinosis - Raynauds - Oesophageal - Systemic - Telangiect
Motility at Sclerosis

**VIII-23.** A 19-year-old female exchange student from London has had bouts of jaundice, fever, malaise, arthralgias, and marked elevation of hepatic transaminases over the last 6 months. The patient was not exposed to hepatotoxic drugs. Hypergammaglobulinemia has been noted. Serologic evaluation for infection with hepatitis A, B, and C has been negative, as have tests for systemic lupus. Liver biopsy now reveals bridging necrosis. Which of the following tests will be most helpful in confirming the diagnosis?

(A) Rheumatoid factor
(B) Hemoglobin electrophoresis
(C) Antibodies to liver and kidney microsomal antigens
(D) Antibodies to hepatitis D virus
(E) Antibodies to hepatitis E virus

**VIII-24.**   Which of the following is an important physiologic function of bile acids?

(A)   Conjugation with toxic substances, thus allowing their excretion

(B)   Allowing the excretion of hemoglobin breakdown products

(C)   Aiding the absorption of vitamin $B_{12}$

(D)   Facilitating absorption of dietary fats

(E)   Maintaining appropriate intestinal pH

**VIII-25.**   A 37-year-old man with chronic alcoholism is admitted to the hospital with acute pancreatitis. On the third hospital day sudden, complete blindness develops in the left eye. The most likely explanation is

(A)   alcohol withdrawal symptoms

(B)   transient ischemic attack (transient monocular blindness)

(C)   occlusion of the retinal vein

(D)   acute glaucoma

(E)   Purtscher's retinopathy

**VIII-26.**   In which one of the following situations would therapy with oral chenodeoxycholic acid be most effective in dissolving gallstone(s)?

(A)   A 27-year-old Asian woman with thalassemia

(B)   A 49-year-old woman with two 2-cm stones

(C)   A 60-year-old man with gallstones visible on chest x-ray

(D)   A 45-year-old woman with a history of gallstone pancreatitis and a residual 1-cm radiolucent gallstone

(E)   A 55-year-old man with a history of biliary colic, several small gallstones seen on ultrasonography, and a poorly opacified gallbladder after oral cholecystography

**VIII-27.**   Which of the following could falsely depress the serum amylase level in a patient suspected of having acute pancreatitis?

(A)   Hypertriglyceridemia

(B)   Hypercholesterolemia

(C)   Hypocalcemia

(D)   Associated pleural effusion

(E)   Associated intestinal infarction

**VIII-28.**   Mechanical obstruction of the colon is most commonly caused by

(A)   adhesions

(B)   carcinoma

(C)   volvulus

(D)   hernia

(E)   sigmoid diverticulitis

**VIII-29.**   In which of the following causes of fatty liver is microvesicular fat seen in biopsy specimens of liver?

(A)   Jejunoileal bypass for morbid obesity

(B)   Acute fatty liver of pregnancy

(C)   Total parenteral nutrition

(D)   Prolonged intravenous hyperalimentation

(E)   Carbon tetrachloride poisoning

**VIII-30.**   Of the following agents that can account for drug-induced hepatitis, which one produces liver injury in a predictable and dose-dependent fashion?

(A)   Halothane

(B)   Chlorpromazine

(C)   Methyldopa

(D)   Acetaminophen

(E)   Erythromycin

**VIII-31.**   In a patient with hepatic cirrhosis, hepatic encephalopathy can be precipitated by all the following factors EXCEPT

(A)   gastrointestinal bleeding

(B)   metabolic acidosis

(C)   renal insufficiency

(D)   vomiting

(E)   viral hepatitis

**VIII-32.**   One month ago, a 21-year-old woman was begun on daily isoniazid therapy because of a positive tuberculin skin test. She now feels well, and her physical examination is unremarkable. Routine laboratory data include the following: serum alanine aminotransferase (ALT) 2.5 μkat/L (150 Karmen units/mL), total bilirubin 17 μmol/L (1.0 mg/dL), and alkaline phosphatase 25 units. The most appropriate action by the woman's physician would be to order

(A)   another antituberculous drug

(B)   corticosteroids

(C)   a liver biopsy

(D)   an ultrasound of the gallbladder

(E)   continuation of isoniazid therapy

**VIII-33.** A 45-year-old man with Laennec's cirrhosis and a history of hepatic encephalopathy comes to the local emergency room because of alcoholic intoxication. Physical examination is remarkable for palmar erythema, spider angiomas, and bilateral gynecomastia. Liver span is 8 cm, and the edge cannot be felt; a spleen tip, however, is palpable. Stool is guaiac-negative. He has no asterixis. Laboratory studies include the following:

Hematocrit: 38 percent
Mean corpuscular volume: 104 fL
White blood cell count: 4000/μL
Platelet count: 97,000/μL
Prothrombin time: 17.5 s
Total serum bilirubin: 14 μmol/L (0.8 mg/dL)
Serum aspartate aminotransferase (AST): 0.5 μkat/L (30 U/L)
Serum alkaline phosphatase: 1.0 μkat/L (60 U/L)

The man is given intravenous hydration and vitamin and mineral supplements, including folic acid (1 mg), thiamine (100 mg), magnesium (2 g), and vitamin K (10 mg). After spending the night in the hospital's detoxification unit, he awakens sober and alert. Repeat prothrombin time is 12 s. The most likely explanation for the elevation in the man's initial prothrombin time is

(A) alcoholic hepatitis
(B) folate deficiency
(C) intestinal malabsorption
(D) disseminated intravascular coagulation
(E) laboratory error

**VIII-34.** A 67-year-old woman who has previously been healthy undergoes emergency surgery for a ruptured abdominal aortic aneurysm. Intraoperatively she requires 8 units of packed red blood cells to maintain her blood pressure and hematocrit. After surgery she is hemodynamically stable. On the third postoperative day she appears jaundiced, but abdominal examination is unremarkable and she is afebrile. Total serum bilirubin concentration at this time is 141 μmol/L (8.3 mg/dL) [direct, 107 μmol/L (6.3 mg/dL)]. Serum alkaline phosphatase level is 6 μkat/L (360 U/L), and serum AST level is 0.85 μkat/L (51 Karmen units/mL). The most likely explanation for the woman's jaundice is

(A) a stone in the common bile duct
(B) halothane hepatitis
(C) posttransfusion hepatitis
(D) acute hepatic infarct
(E) benign intrahepatic cholestasis

**VIII-35.** A 35-year-old former hemodialysis nurse is seen because of a 6-month history of fatigue and amenorrhea. On examination she has scleral icterus, a mildly tender liver, and a tibial rash consistent with erythema nodosum. ALT and AST levels are both in the range of 1.5 μkat/L (100 U/L) and bilirubin is 51.3 μmol/L (3 mg/dL), while alkaline phosphatase and serum albumin levels are normal. Hepatitis serologic testing detects HBsAg and IgG anti-HBcAg. Liver biopsy discloses a mononuclear cell portal infiltrate and hepatocyte destruction at the periphery of lobules. Which of the following therapeutic strategies is best?

(A) Administration of low-dose cyclophosphamide, 50 mg/d for 2 months
(B) Administration of prednisone, 20 to 40 mg/d for 2 months and then a taper based on the response
(C) Administration of prednisone, 10 mg every other day for 3 months
(D) Administration of acyclovir, 400 mg every 6 h for 2 weeks
(E) Administration of interferon-α, 10 million units three times per week for 4 months

**VIII-36.** Chronic active hepatitis is most reliably distinguished from chronic persistent hepatitis by the presence of

(A) extrahepatic manifestations
(B) hepatitis B surface antigen in the serum
(C) antibody to hepatitis B core antigen in the serum
(D) a significant titer of anti-smooth-muscle antibody
(E) characteristic liver histology

**VIII-37.** A 52-year-old woman is hospitalized for medical management of severe alcoholic hepatitis. On the ninth hospital day she develops a temperature of 38.3°C (101°F) and generalized abdominal discomfort. Abdominal examination reveals a fluid wave and significant and diffuse abdominal tenderness without guarding; hepatosplenomegaly is present but is unchanged from the admission examination. Rectal and pelvic examinations reveal no area of localized tenderness; stool guaiac testing is positive. Hematocrit is 27 percent, white blood cell count is 12,000/μL, and liver function tests are unchanged from admission: total serum bilirubin 214 μmol/L (12.5 mg/dL), serum AST 2.5 μkat/L (150 Karmen units/mL), and serum alkaline phosphatase 3.0 μkat/L (180 U/L).

The procedure most likely to yield diagnostic information in this case would be

(A) serum amylase determination
(B) blood culture
(C) supine and upright x-rays of the abdomen
(D) abdominal sonography
(E) paracentesis

**VIII-38.** A 64-year-old man with insulin-dependent adult-onset diabetes mellitus seeks emergency medical treatment after 2 days of increasingly severe abdominal pain in the right upper quadrant that has spread over the entire abdomen and is associated with nausea, vomiting, fever, and chills. On examination, he is alert and oriented but appears to be quite acutely distressed. Vital signs are temperature 39.4°C (103°F), pulse 140 beats per minute, and blood pressure 100/60 mmHg. His sclerae are mildly icteric. His abdomen is diffusely tender with marked guarding in the right upper quadrant; there is no palpable hepatosplenomegaly, and there are no audible bowel sounds. Rectal examination reveals no focal tenderness; stool is guaiac-negative. Laboratory values are as follows:

Hematocrit: 34 percent
White blood cell count: 22,500/μL with a marked left
   shift
Plasma glucose: 17.8 mmol/L (325 mg/dL)
Blood urea nitrogen: 10.5 μmol/L (30 mg/dL)
Serum AST: 2.1 μkat/L (125 Karmen units/mL)
Serum alkaline phosphatase: 210 units
Serum amylase: 3.3 μkat/L (200 U/dL)

His abdominal flat-plate x-ray is shown below. During the first 4 h of hospitalization the man's condition is stabilized somewhat by the administration of intravenous fluids and insulin. A nasogastric tube is inserted, blood cultures are drawn, and he is begun on broad-spectrum antibiotics.

The most appropriate management at this point would be to order

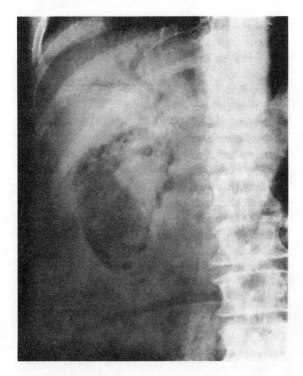

(A) conservative medical measures only for the next 48 to 72 h
(B) an abdominal ultrasound examination
(C) an upper gastrointestinal examination with Gastrografin dye
(D) endoscopic retrograde cholangiopancreatography
(E) preparations for an emergency laparotomy

**VIII-39.** All the following conditions are known to predispose to the formation of cholesterol gallstones EXCEPT

(A) obesity
(B) hypercholesterolemia
(C) clofibrate therapy
(D) oral contraceptive therapy
(E) surgical resection of the ileum

**VIII-40.** A 58-year-old man with biopsy-proven hepatic cirrhosis is hospitalized because of massive ascites and pedal edema. There is no evidence of respiratory compromise or hepatic encephalopathy. Initial laboratory values are as follows:

Serum electrolytes (mmol/L): $Na^+$ 130; $K^+$ 3.6; $Cl^-$
   85; $HCO_3^-$ 30
Serum creatinine: 88 μmol/L (1.0 mg/dL)
Blood urea nitrogen: 6.4 μmol/L (18 mg/dL)

Bed rest, sodium and water restriction, and the administration of spironolactone (50 mg/d) produce no significant weight change after 5 days. Which of the following therapeutic measures would be most appropriate at this time?

(A) Intravenous furosemide, 80 mg now
(B) Oral spironolactone, 100 mg/d
(C) Oral acetazolamide, 250 mg/d
(D) Placement of a peritoneovenous shunt
(E) Therapeutic paracentesis

**VIII-41.** Administration of which of the following drugs or classes of drugs has been shown to prolong survival in persons with acute pancreatitis?

(A) Cimetidine
(B) Aprotinin (Trasylol)
(C) Antibiotics
(D) Anticholinergics
(E) None of the above

**VIII-42.** Complications of chronic pancreatitis include all the following EXCEPT

(A) gastric varices
(B) erythema nodosum
(C) vitamin $B_{12}$ malabsorption
(D) pleural effusion
(E) jaundice

**VIII-43.**   All the following factors portend a poor survival rate during an attack of acute pancreatitis EXCEPT

(A)  hyperbilirubinemia
(B)  hypoalbuminemia
(C)  hypocalcemia
(D)  hypoxemia
(E)  discolored peritoneal fluid

**VIII-44.**   A 52-year-old woman has hepatomegaly. Percutaneous liver biopsy reveals "adenocarcinoma," but the woman refuses further evaluation or treatment. A year later she presents with weight loss [13.6 kg (30 lb)] and a skin rash that has waxed and waned. Examination shows angular stomatitis and a firm, enlarged liver. An erythematous, bullous, necrotic skin rash (Plate A) is present on the face, perineum, and legs. Sonography reveals an enlarged pancreas. Hematologic testing shows that the woman is anemic. The diagnostic test of choice would be

(A)  serum amylase determination
(B)  plasma glucagon determination
(C)  plasma vasoactive intestinal polypeptide (VIP) determination
(D)  plasma gastrin determination
(E)  pancreatic arteriography

**VIII-45.**   A 35-year-old woman with a history of acute lymphoblastic leukemia is seen 7 weeks after receiving an allogeneic bone marrow transplant. Routine prophylaxis for graft-versus-host disease with corticosteroids and methotrexate is being administered. She complains of midsternal pain upon swallowing. Biopsy of one of the lesions noted on endoscopy (Plate B) would reveal

(A)  lymphoblasts on a Wright's-stained smear
(B)  multinucleated giant cells on Wright's staining
(C)  hyphal forms on silver staining
(D)  small cysts on silver staining
(E)  overgrowth of bacteria on Gram's stain

**VIII-46.**   Chronic reflux esophagitis is LEAST likely to result in the development of

(A)  gastrointestinal bleeding
(B)  an esophageal peptic stricture
(C)  a lower esophageal ring
(D)  Barrett's esophagus (esophagus lined by columnar epithelium)
(E)  adenocarcinoma

**VIII-47.**   A patient with scleral icterus and a positive reaction for bilirubin by urine dipstick testing could have which of the following disorders?

(A)  Autoimmune hemolytic anemia
(B)  Dubin-Johnson syndrome
(C)  Crigler-Najjar type II disorder
(D)  Thalassemia intermedia
(E)  Gilbert's syndrome

**VIII-48.**   Which one of these extraintestinal complications of inflammatory bowel disease is LEAST likely to be associated with ulcerative colitis?

(A)  Pericholangitis
(B)  Pyoderma gangrenosum
(C)  Arthritis
(D)  Uveitis
(E)  Oxalate kidney stones

**VIII-49.**   All the following statements describing Meckel's diverticulum are true EXCEPT

(A)  it is the most common congenital anomaly of the digestive tract
(B)  mechanical obstruction resulting from intussusception may occur
(C)  in young adults inflammatory complications may produce a clinical syndrome indistinguishable from acute appendicitis
(D)  it is usually present in the jejunum
(E)  technetium scans are valuable in the diagnosis of diverticula associated with gastrointestinal bleeding

**VIII-50.**   Which one of the following statements about hepatitis B *e* antigen (HBeAg) is LEAST accurate?

(A)  HBeAg can be detected transiently in the sera of patients ill with acute hepatitis B infection
(B)  The presence of HBeAg in the serum is correlated with infectiousness
(C)  The absence of HBeAg in the serum rules out chronic infection caused by the hepatitis B virus
(D)  HBeAg is immunologically distinct from HBsAg but is genetically related to HBcAg
(E)  The disappearance of HBeAg from the serum may be a harbinger of resolution of acute hepatitis B infection

**VIII-51.** Which of the following statements regarding delta hepatitis virus (HDV) is correct?

(A) HDV is a defective DNA virus

(B) HDV can infect only persons infected with HBV

(C) The HDV genome is partially homologous with hepatitis B virus (HBV) DNA

(D) HDV infection has been found only in limited areas of the world

(E) Simultaneous infection with HDV and HBV results in an increased risk of the development of chronic hepatitis

**VIII-52.** All the following statements about the management of variceal hemorrhage are true EXCEPT

(A) Because of the risk of perforation, endoscopic sclerotherapy should be reserved for patients who rebleed after surgery

(B) Peripheral vein infusion of vasopressin is as effective as superior mesenteric artery infusion in controlling variceal hemorrhage

(C) Propranolol reduces the risk of bleeding in patients with large varices

(D) Elective portacaval shunt surgery prevents recurrent variceal hemorrhage but does not improve life expectancy

(E) The selective distal splenorenal shunt appears to be associated with a lower incidence of postoperative hepatic encephalopathy than is the portacaval shunt

**VIII-53.** Which of the followng statements regarding the prophylaxis of viral hepatitis is true?

(A) Although immune globulin (IG) is effective in preventing clinically apparent type A hepatitis, not all IG preparations have adequate anti-HAV titers to be protective

(B) If given soon enough after exposure to hepatitis B, hepatitis immune globulin (HBIG) is effective in preventing infection

(C) HBIG and hepatitis B vaccine can be effectively administered simultaneously

(D) Hepatitis B vaccine is ineffective in preventing delta hepatitis infection in persons who are not HBsAg carriers

(E) IG prophylaxis after needle-stick, sexual, or perinatal exposure to hepatitis C is effective in preventing infection

**VIII-54.** All the following antiemetics will act on the chemoreceptor trigger zone in the brain EXCEPT

(A) ondansetron

(B) metoclopramide

(C) prochlorperazine

(D) haloperidol

(E) diphenhydramine

**VIII-55.** The medical therapy for Crohn's disease can be described by all the following statements EXCEPT

(A) Metronidazole is useful if the perineal area is involved

(B) Azathioprine may reduce steroid requirements

(C) The frequency of recurrence is not altered by prophylactic therapy with steroids

(D) The frequency of recurrence is not altered by prophylactic therapy with sulfasalazine

(E) Sulfasalazine is contraindicated in the treatment of pregnant women who have Crohn's disease

**VIII-56.** A 40-year-old man has a history of ulcerative colitis. Features of his illness that would contribute to an increased risk of developing colon cancer include which of the following?

(A) Disease duration of less than 10 years

(B) History of toxic megacolon

(C) Presence of pancolitis (total colonic involvement)

(D) Presence of pseudopolyps on colonoscopy

(E) High steroid requirements

**VIII-57.** Subacute ischemic colitis can be described by all the following statements EXCEPT

(A) cobblestoning is noted on contrast studies

(B) rectal bleeding may be the presenting symptom

(C) involvement of the rectum is uncommon

(D) symptoms and signs of nonocclusive ischemic colitis resolve in 2 to 4 weeks

(E) angiography is the definitive diagnostic procedure

**VIII-58.** True statements regarding acute bleeding from colonic diverticula include all the following EXCEPT

(A) diverticulitis usually is present

(B) the source of hemorrhage is more likely to be on the right side than on the left side of the colon

(C) bleeding usually abates spontaneously

(D) angiographic detection of bleeding usually is helpful

(E) it is the most common cause of acute lower GI bleeding in the elderly

**VIII-59.** Percutaneous needle liver biopsy would be indicated in a diagnostic workup in all the following situations EXCEPT

(A) unexplained hepatosplenomegaly
(B) persistently abnormal liver function tests
(C) suspected hepatic angioma
(D) suspected miliary tuberculosis
(E) intrahepatic cholestasis of uncertain course

**VIII-60.** All the following conditions probably would be associated with the set of serum values presented below EXCEPT

Total bilirubin: 34 μmol/L (2 mg/dL)
AST: 1.0 μkat/L (60 U/L)
Alkaline phosphatase: 8.0 μkat/L (480 U/L)

(A) primary biliary cirrhosis
(B) stricture of the common bile duct
(C) sarcoidosis
(D) acetaminophen overdose
(E) chlorpromazine therapy

**VIII-61.** An 18-year-old man is evaluated because of weight loss and diarrhea. On examination he is found to have pedal edema and decreased breath sounds at the right lung base. A thoracentesis reveals milky fluid. Subsequent laboratory workup reveals lymphocytopenia, hypoproteinemia, and hypogammaglobulinemia. All the following features would also be expected with this condition EXCEPT

(A) abnormal peripheral lymphatics
(B) dilated and telangiectatic lymphatic vessels in the lamina propria on small-bowel biopsy
(C) hypogammaglobulinemia
(D) response to a low-fat diet supplemented by medium-chain triglycerides
(E) 1 g D-xylose in 5-h urine collection after 25 g oral D-xylose

**VIII-62.** A patient with newly diagnosed tropical sprue could have all the following extragastrointestinal manifestations of malabsorption EXCEPT

(A) megaloblastic anemia
(B) night blindness
(C) purpura
(D) tetany
(E) pyoderma gangrenosum

**VIII-63.** A patient undergoes a liver biopsy for chronic abnormalities on liver function tests. On pathologic review, multiple granulomas are found. All the following statements concerning this patient's condition are true EXCEPT

(A) an empirical trial of steroids should be instituted
(B) sarcoidosis is a possible etiology
(C) a careful drug-exposure history should be obtained
(D) schistosomiasis is a possible etiology
(E) *Mycobacterium avium-intracellulare* is the most common cause of this finding in patients with AIDS

**VIII-64.** A 45-year-old man presents with a history of crushing nonradiational chest pain. Electrocardiography and exercise stress testing reveal no evidence of cardiac edema. A more detailed history is taken, and the patient states that he has had a sensation of sticking after swallowing. He notes this sensation equally whether he is eating solids or liquids. The diagnosis that would most likely account for these symptoms is

(A) achalasia
(B) diffuse esophageal spasm
(C) lower esophageal (Schatzki) ring
(D) esophageal carcinoma
(E) Zenker's diverticulum

**VIII-65.** A 35-year-old woman presents to the emergency room because of acute pain in the left upper quadrant after eating a meal. The pain radiates to the left side of the chest and has been relieved by the expulsion of flatus. The electrocardiogram is normal, as are routine blood tests, including liver function studies. The most likely diagnosis in this case is

(A) magenblase syndrome
(B) splenic flexure syndrome
(C) ingestion of beans
(D) peptic ulcer disease
(E) *Giardia* infection

**VIII-66.** Each of the following represents a correct mechanism of action for the laxative noted EXCEPT

(A) psyllium increases stool bulk
(B) docusate salts lower the surface tension of stool
(C) sorbitol stimulates colonic motor activity
(D) cisapride enhances intestinal transit
(E) castor oil stimulates intestinal secretion

**VIII-67.** All the following conditions may cause secretory diarrhea EXCEPT

(A) medullary carcinoma of the thyroid
(B) resection of the distal ileum
(C) Zollinger-Ellison syndrome
(D) somatostatinoma
(E) carcinoid tumor

**VIII-68.** A 65-year-old woman complains of a 20-lb weight loss over the last 6 months. She is of average build and has not been on a diet. She states that she has just not been very hungry. Physical examination is unrevealing. Complete blood count is normal, as is urinalysis, multiphased chemical screen, thyroid-stimulating hormone, chest x-ray, and stool for blood. The next most appropriate study would be

(A) abdominal CT
(B) serum protein electrophoresis
(C) colonoscopy
(D) blood cultures
(E) short ACTH test

**VIII-69.** All the following can be causes of a false-positive card test for occult lower GI bleeding EXCEPT

(A) ingestion of undercooked meat
(B) ingestion of dietary peroxidases
(C) use of nonsteroidal anti-inflammatory agents
(D) use of aspirin for rheumatoid arthritis
(E) ingestion of vitamin C

**VIII-70.** All the following features are more commonly associated with Crohn's disease than with ulcerative colitis EXCEPT

(A) fistulas
(B) rectal bleeding
(C) segmental involvement
(D) an abdominal mass
(E) mesenteric lymph node involvement

**VIII-71.** A 25-year-old Sephardic Jew from Israel presents with pleuritic chest pain, left knee pain, diffuse abdominal pain, and fever. Physical examination reveals an acutely ill individual with a temperature of 40°C (104°F). The abdomen is distended and rigid. He has had a history of similar painful attacks that last for about a day every month since he was an early teenager. Laboratory exam is remarkable for an elevated erythrocyte sedimentation rate and a white cell count of 25,000/μL with a left-shifted differential. The best therapy to prevent further attacks is

(A) appendectomy
(B) sulfasalazine
(C) prednisone
(D) colchicine
(E) azathioprine

**VIII-72.** Gastrointestinal complaints are common in clinical practice. All the following complaints are suggestive of a functional disorder EXCEPT

(A) diarrhea only during the daytime
(B) crampy abdominal pain, relieved by defecation
(C) pellet-like stools
(D) change in stool diameter
(E) alternating periods of diarrhea and constipation

**VIII-73.** A 55-year-old man who has complained of heartburn over the last 10 years undergoes endoscopy. The endoscopist notes a change in the appearance of the epithelium in the distal esophagus. Biopsy reveals erosion of the squamous mucosa and replacement with metaplastic columbar epithelium. Which of the following steps should be taken?

(A) Repeat endoscopy and biopsy in 12 months
(B) Resection of the distal esophagus
(C) Esophageal dilation
(D) Treatment with a beta blocker
(E) Elevation of the head of the patient's bed

**VIII-74.** A 37-year-old woman presents for evaluation because of recurrent abdominal pain. The pain is cramping in nature and is relieved by defecation. Physical examination is unremarkable. The patient is taking enalapril for hypertension. Laboratory studies reveal normal CBC and liver function tests, except that the total serum bilirubin level is 2.5 μmol/L (42 mm/L); the direct fraction is 0.2 mg/dL (3.7 μmol/L). The most important next step is

(A) examination of the peripheral blood smear
(B) computed tomography of the abdomen
(C) endoscopic retrograde pancreaticoduodenography
(D) urine dipstick test
(E) reassurance

**VIII-75.** A 45-year-old man presents with heartburn and morning hoarseness. All the following are appropriate therapeutic measures for this patient EXCEPT

(A) ranitidine, 150 mg at bedtime
(B) metaclopramide, 10 mg 30 min before meals and at bedtime
(C) sleeping with the head elevated
(D) omeprazole, 20 mg daily
(E) avoidance of fatty foods

**VIII-76.** All the following statements concerning gastrinoma are correct EXCEPT

(A) most are malignant
(B) most are multiple
(C) they are associated with multiple endocrine neoplasia syndrome type II
(D) they usually secrete multiple hormones
(E) the secretin injection test is the most valuable provocative diagnostic test

**VIII-77.** Which of the following statements concerning the relationship of duodenal ulcer and *H. pylori* infection is correct?

(A) Virtually all patients with a duodenal ulcer harbor *H. pylori*
(B) Most patients infected with *H. pylori* will develop an ulcer
(C) *H. pylori* invades the gastric mucosa
(D) The demonstration of *H. pylori* as a causative feature in a given patient with a duodenal ulcer requires biopsy
(E) The relapse rate for duodenal ulcer is equivalent whether *H. pylori* eradication therapy or $H_2$-receptor antagonists are used

**VIII-78.** Atrophic gastritis is associated with all the following EXCEPT

(A) elevated MCV
(B) anti-parietal-cell antibodies
(C) carcinoid tumors
(D) antral predominance
(E) *H. pylori* infections

**VIII-79.** A 25-year-old male intravenous drug abuser presents with 1 week of a flu-like syndrome and 2 days of tenderness in the right upper quadrant. Examination at the time of presentation was remarkable for a fever of 38.3°C (101°F), normal vital signs, scleral icterus, and right upper quadrant pain. Laboratory examination was most notable for aminotransferases in the 3000 IU/μl range and a serum bilirubin of 178 mM/L (10 mg/dL), 50 percent of which was direct. During the first 3 hospital days the patient has intermittent nausea and vomiting and poor oral intake. Serologic studies reveal the presence of HBsAg and anti-HBc IgM. On the fourth hospital day the patient becomes confused. Neurologic examination is nonfocal, though the patient exhibits asterixis. He is noted to have bleeding from intravenous sites and a diminution in the size of his previously enlarged liver. His prothrombin time is 20 s and his bilirubin is now up to 510 mM/L (30 mg/dL).

In addition to supportive care, the most appropriate therapy for this patient is

(A) interferon-α
(B) plasmapharesis
(C) intravenous gammaglobulin
(D) liver transplantation
(E) total parenteral nutrition

**VIII-80.** All the following represent pathologic changes resulting from drug-induced hepatic injury EXCEPT

(A) carbon tetrachloride causes necrosis and fatty infiltration
(B) acetaminophen causes panlobular infiltration with mononuclear cells and hepatic cell necrosis
(C) isoniazid causes panlobular infiltration with mononuclear cells and diffuse necrosis
(D) chlorpromazine causes cholestasis with portal inflammation
(E) oral contraceptive agents cause cholestastis without portal inflammation

**VIII-81.** A 35-year-old woman with known hepatitis C virus infection has persistently elevated hepatic transaminases and chronic fatigue as well as intermittent fever. Liver biopsy reveals a dense mononuclear infiltrate along the portal tracts with destruction of the hepatocytes at the periphery of lobules. Some hepatocellular dropout is noted to span lobules. The patient's serum contains antibodies against liver, kidney, and muscle antigens. Which of the following statements concerning the patient's treatment is correct?

(A) She should receive glucocorticoids

(B) A successful response to interferon will be accompanied by a transient elevation in aminotransferase activity

(C) A good response to therapy is associated with a relatively low burden of hepatitis C virus

(D) Therapy may be deferred because progression to cirrhosis is unlikely

(E) The presence of antiliver antibodies suggests that an autoimmune process has supervened

**VIII-82.** A 55-year-old male alcoholic has recurrent attacks of severe mid-epigastric pain after eating. Serum amylase determinations after such attacks have been in the normal range. The examination reveals mild cachexia but is otherwise unremarkable. On further questioning, the patient states that he has been sober for the past 10 years but prior to that time had multiple episodes of alcohol-induced pancreatitis. He is currently taking pancreatic replacement enzymes by mouth. An ERCP reveals a stricture of the pancreatic duct but is otherwise unremarkable. Computed tomography of the abdomen reveals calcifications in the pancreas but does not show any evidence of malignancy. The patient is taking 30 mg of continuous-release morphine sulfate twice a day. The best strategy at this point would be to

(A) double the dose of morphine

(B) double the dose of pancreatic replacement enzymes

(C) resect the head of the pancreas

(D) institute a low-fat diet

(E) begin a continuous search for other causes of abdominal pain

**VIII-83.** The secretin-choleycystokinin test is useful in the evaluation of patients with suspected chronic pancreatitis. All the following statements regarding this test are correct EXCEPT

(A) those with chronic pancreatitis usually have a low bicarbonate output after stimulation

(B) secretion of pancreatic enzymes may be measured

(C) in patients with early chronic pancreatitis, enzyme output is relatively more deranged than failure to achieve an adequate bicarbonate concentration

(D) the volume of duodenal contents after stimulation is an end-point of the test

(E) the test cannot distinguish between chronic pancreatitis and pancreatic carcinoma

**VIII-84.** A 53-year-old woman with hypertension and hypercholestremia presents with right upper quadrant pain and fever. Examination reveals a moderately ill-apppearing woman who has a temperature of 39°C (103°F), blood pressure of 110/70, pulse of 110, and respiratory rate of 25. The rest of the physical examination is remarkable for scleral icterus and right upper quadrant rebound tenderness. Laboratory examination reveals a white blood cell count of 18,000 with 70 percent neutrophils, 10 percent band forms, 10 percent monocytes, and 10 percent lymphs; a hematocrit of 36.2 percent; and a platelet count of 522,000/μl. Serum chemistries are remarkable for a total bilirubin of 6 mg/dL and a direct bilirubin of 4 mg/dL; serum aminotransferases are mildly elevated, and alkaline phosphatase is two times normal. Computed tomography of the abdomen reveals dilation of the common bile duct and no other abnormalities. The next most appropriate diagnostic study is

(A) magnetic resonance imaging

(B) ultrasonography

(C) liver biopsy

(D) intravenous cholangiography

(E) exploratory laparotomy

**DIRECTIONS:** The question below contains five suggested responses. For **each** of the five responses, you are to respond either YES (Y) or NO (N). In this item **all, some,** or **none** of the alternatives may be correct.

**VIII-85.** Which of the following serologic patterns would be consistent with acute hepatitis B infection?

|       | HBsAg | Anti-HBs | Anti-HBc | HBeAg | Anti-HBeAg |
|-------|-------|----------|----------|-------|------------|
| (A)   | +     | −        | IgM      | +     | −          |
| (B)   | +     | −        | IgG      | +     | −          |
| (C)   | −     | −        | IgM      | −     | −          |
| (D)   | +     | −        | IgG      | −     | +          |
| (E)   | −     | +        | IgG      | −     | −          |

**VIII-1.** **The answer is A.** *(Chap. 42. Donowitz, N Engl J Med 322:725, 1995.)* In the case described, the osmolality of fecal water is approximately equal to serum osmolality. Furthermore, there is no osmotic "gap" in the fecal water; the osmolality of the fecal water can be accounted for by the stool electrolyte composition: $\{2 \times [(Na^+) + (K^+)]\} = [2 \times (39 + 96)] = 270$. A villous adenoma of the colon typically produces a secretory diarrhea. Lactose intolerance, nontropical sprue, and excessive use of milk of magnesia produce osmotic diarrheas with osmotic "gaps" caused by lactose, carbohydrates, and magnesium, respectively. Pancreatic insufficiency causes steatorrhea, not watery diarrhea.

**VIII-2.** **The answer is A.** *(Chaps. 45, 292, 294. Frank, JAMA 262:3031, 1989.)* Initial considerations in evaluating a patient with jaundice require a determination of whether the patient has primarily unconjugated hyperbilirubinemia or conjugated hyperbilirubinemia, in which case more than 50 percent of the serum bilirubin is direct-reacting. Since this patient has clear-cut conjugated hyperbilirubinemia, he may have the (solubilized) bilirubin detectable in the urine. The major differential diagnosis in this case is between impaired hepatocyte bilirubin excretion and extrahepatic biliary obstruction. In the former case, interference with the biliary excretion of bilirubin that has been previously conjugated by hepatocytes leads to the entry of this pigment into the systemic circulation. Such intrahepatic obstruction may occur in drug reactions, alcoholic hepatitis, the third trimester of pregnancy, the postoperative state, and viral or autoimmune hepatitis. In the case of the Dubin-Johnson and Rotor syndromes, the conjugated hyperbilirubinemia is due to a congenital defect in bilirubin excretion and generally is not associated with abnormalities of alkaline phosphatase or hepatic aminotransferases. Patients who have conjugated hyperbilirubinemia and abnormal liver enzymes generally fall into two groups: those whose aminotransferase elevation is dominant and who are suspected of having a hepatocellular disorder and those who have primary elevation of alkaline phosphatase and are likely to have either intra- or extrahepatic biliary obstruction. In the latter group of patients, it is imperative to rule out extrahepatic obstruction by means of ultrasonography of the right upper quadrant or abdominal CT. If the biliary ducts are not dilated on radiologic evaluation, the next most appropriate procedure would be percutaneous transhepatic cholangiogram or endoscopic retrograde cholangiopancreatography.

**VIII-3.** **The answer is C.** *(Chaps. 42, 187, 308. Goodgame, Ann Intern Med 119:924, 1993.)* Diarrhea in patients with AIDS may be due to many microbiologic agents. Patients infected with HIV-1 are at risk of infection with nonopportunistic pathogens such as *Salmonella, Shigella, Campylobacter, Entamoeba, Chlamydia, Neisseria gonorrhoeae, Treponema pallidum,* and *Giardia lamblia* and are also at risk for infections that occur in the presence of immunodeficiency. Infectious agents in the latter category include protozoa such as *Cryptosporidium, Isospora belli,* and *Blastocystis;* bacteria such as *Mycobacterium avium-intracellulare;* and viral pathogens such as cytomegalovirus (CMV), herpes simplex virus, adenovirus, and HIV itself. CMV infection of the gastrointestinal tract may present with upper GI symptoms, nausea, vomiting, abdominal pain, or symptoms of ulcerative colitis such as bloody diarrhea. A diagnosis of CMV infection, which almost certainly represents reinfection or reactivation since affected persons are virtually always previously exposed to CMV, can be made by finding typical cytomegalic cells on histopathologic analysis. Such cells, which provide evidence of the CMV-mediated cytopathic effect, are characterized by being large (25 to 35 μm) with a basophilic internuclear inclusion (sometimes surrounded by a clear halo—the "owl's eye" effect) and frequently are associated with clusters of intracytoplasmic inclusions. Serious CMV-mediated gastroenteritis should be treated with ganciclovir, which may result in weight gain and improved quality of life. Foscarnet, an inhibitor of viral DNA polymerase, may be useful in cases of ganciclovir failure or intolerance. Antibacterial antibiotics, antifungal agents, antituberculous drugs, and acyclovir play no role in treating histologically proven CMV colitis.

**VIII-4. The answer is D.** *(Chap. 284)* Physiologic feedback loops mediate the inhibition of gastrin release, thus inhibiting secretion of acid in the stomach; the two most important are acidic gastric pH and the presence of fat or hypertonic fluids in the duodenum. Acid-induced release of somatostatin by antral endocrine cells may mediate, in a paracrine fashion, the inhibition of secretion of gastrin and the activity of parietal cells. Secretin is released in the presence of acid in the upper small intestine and also can inhibit the secretion of gastric acid, although it stimulates the secretion of pepsinogen, a precursor to the low-pH active enzymes which are important in the pathophysiology of peptic ulcers. Other peptides found in the small intestine that may play a role in the inhibition of secretion of gastric acid include gastric inhibitory peptide, vasoactive intestinal peptide, enteroglucagon, neurotensin, peptide YY, and urogastrone. Histamine, presumably released by the mast cells lying adjacent to the acid secretory parietal cells in the gastric mucosa, acts together with gastrin and acetylcholine to stimulate the release of acid.

**VIII-5. The answer is D.** *(Chaps. 31, 283)* A Zenker's diverticulum typically causes halitosis and regurgitation of saliva and food particles consumed several days earlier. When a Zenker's diverticulum fills with food, it may produce dysphagia by compressing the esophagus. Gastric outlet obstruction can cause bloating and regurgitation of newly ingested food. Gastrointestinal disorders associated with scleroderma include esophageal reflux, the development of wide-mouthed colonic diverticula, and stasis with bacterial overgrowth. Achalasia typically presents with dysphagia for both solids and liquids. Gastric retention caused by the autonomic neuropathy of diabetes mellitus usually results in postprandial epigastric discomfort and bloating.

**VIII-6. The answer is E.** *(Chaps. 44, 299)* The presence of coffee-grounds material in a nasogastric aspirate from a person with melena indicates recent bleeding of the upper gastrointestinal tract. In a patient with obvious signs of cirrhosis, esophageal varices must be considered in the differential diagnosis of upper gastrointestinal bleeding; other possible diagnoses include peptic ulcer, gastroduodenitis, esophagitis, and a Mallory-Weiss tear. Before diagnostic procedures such as endoscopy and an upper gastrointestinal series are undertaken, the placement of a large-bore intravenous line and commencement of volume replacement therapy are mandatory to prevent hypotension. Moreover, blood should be typed and cross-matched in case of further bleeding. Diagnostic angiography is indicated only when brisk bleeding prevents diagnosis by endoscopy or barium study. Specific therapy for variceal bleeding—i.e., passage of a Sengstaken-Blakemore tube and intravenous infusion of vasopressin, banding, or endoscopic sclerotherapy—should be considered if diagnostic studies reveal bleeding varices.

**VIII-7. The answer is A.** *(Chap. 287. Lynn, Med Clin North Am 79:373, 1995.)* This presentation is classic for one of the three clinical variants of the irritable bowel syndrome, each of which is associated with abnormal colonic motility and increased visceral perception. Other groups have chronic abdominal pain and constipation or alternating constipation and diarrhea. The chronic nature of the condition and the presence of formed stool argue against a workup for secretory or osmotic diarrhea. Giardiasis, while typically occult and requiring jejunal sampling for diagnosis, usually presents with belching and pain, not diarrhea of 4 years' duration. The absence of discernible significant organic pathology should not prompt a discussion with the patient that centers on a psychogenic cause of her problem; such an approach frequently leads to alienation of the patient. Instead, an effort to effect safe symptomatic improvement of the diarrhea with antispasmodics is worthwhile. Psyllium to increase stool bulk is a good choice for patients with irritable bowel syndrome who complain of constipation.

**VIII-8.**    **The answer is C.**  *(Chap. 283)*  Achalasia is a motor disorder of esophageal smooth muscle in which the lower esophageal sphincter (LES) does not relax properly in response to swallowing and normal esophageal peristalsis is replaced by abnormal contractions. Manometry reveals a normal or elevated LES pressure and reduced or absent swallow-induced relaxation. A decreased number of ganglion cells are noted in the esophageal body and LES of patients with achalasia, suggesting that defective innervation of these areas is the underlying abnormality. Dysphagia, chest pain, and regurgitation are the predominant symptoms. The chest x-ray often reveals absence of the gastric air bubble, and the barium swallow reveals a dilated esophagus. Calcium channel antagonists such as nifedipine relax smooth muscle and have been effective in treating some patients. However, the mainstay of therapy remains pneumatic dilation.

**VIII-9.**    **The answer is D.**  *(Chap. 284. Fendrick AM, Ann Intern Med 123:260, 1995.)*  A physician has many alternatives in deciding on a therapeutic course in a patient with a radiographically or endoscopically proven duodenal ulcer. Therapy is based on neutralization of gastric acids by antacids, inhibition of gastric acid secretion by antisecretory agents such as $H_2$-receptor antagonists, prostaglandins ($PGE_1$, $PGE_2$), and proton pump inhibitors (e.g., omeprazole). Drugs such as sucralfate act locally by impeding diffusion of hydrogen ions to the base of the ulcer and by binding other injurious molecules. Colloidal bismuth stimulates gastric mucosal secretion of prostaglandins and glycoprotein mucus and may eradicate *H. pylori* colonization. All patients should receive therapy to eradicate *H. pylori*. Treatment for 4 to 6 weeks with any individual member of any of the above classes probably will be sufficient to induce healing in most patients. For the average patient, maintenance therapy is not required. While there is no evidence that dietary changes are important, elimination of cigarette smoking should be undertaken. There is no evidence, for example, that cimetidine or any other related $H_2$-receptor antagonist is superior to sucralfate in promoting ulcer healing. Side effects among the various drug classes differ. Sucralfate is associated with a very low rate of side effects; however, it can reduce the bioavailability of the fluoroquinolone antibiotics, and so these drugs should not be used concomitantly.

**VIII-10.**    **The answer is B.**  *(Chap. 284. Silverstein, Ann Intern Med 123:241, 1995.)*  Gastric mucosal injury, potentially resulting in ulcers and erosive gastritis, may be produced by aspirin and nonsteroidal anti-inflammatory agents, including indomethacin, ibuprofen, and naproxen. These agents may be directly toxic to the gastric mucosa by depleting protective endogenous mucosal prostaglandins. Moreover, they more directly interrupt the mucosal barrier, allowing back-diffusion of hydrogen ions as well as reducing gastric mucus secretion and increasing gastric acid secretion. The prostaglandin $E_1$ analogue misoprostol is effective in preventing ulcers and gastritis caused by nonsteroidal anti-inflammatory drugs. Its mechanism of action is believed to be stimulation of gastric mucus and duodenal bicarbonate secretion as well as the maintenance of the gastric mucosal barrier via epithelial cell restitution.

**VIII-11.**    **The answer is C.**  *(Chap. 284)*  The causes of stomal (anastomotic) ulceration after peptic ulcer surgery include incomplete vagotomy, retained gastric antrum, the Zollinger-Ellison syndrome (gastrinoma), poor gastric emptying, ingestion of ulcerogenic drugs, and especially persistent *H. pylori* infection. In the case presented, if the previous antrectomy had been complete, the serum gastrin level should not be elevated. An elevated serum gastrin level that declines after intravenous administration of secretin is characteristic of a retained gastric antrum attached to the duodenal stump. Neither frequent antacid therapy nor a total vagotomy is effective in healing a stomal ulcer; thus, resection of the retained antrum is indicated. In the Zollinger-Ellison syndrome, the serum gastrin level paradoxically increases after the intravenous infusion of secretin.

**VIII-12.   The answer is C.**   *(Chap. 285)*   Eosinophilic enteritis is a disorder of the stomach, small intestine, colon, or all three in which some part of the gut wall is infiltrated by eosinophils. The diagnosis also requires the presence of peripheral blood eosinophilia. Although early reports emphasized the presence of food allergies, less than half these patients have a history of food allergies or asthma. The presence of anemia, Hemoccult-positive stools, abnormalities of the ileum and cecum on barium radiographic studies, and a favorable response to the administration of steroids may make eosinophilic enteritis difficult to distinguish from Crohn's disease. Although no controlled trials of corticosteroid therapy have been performed, the symptoms usually respond to short-term corticosteroid therapy.

**VIII-13.   The answer is C.**   *(Chap. 285)*   Malabsorption caused by bacterial overgrowth results from bacterial utilization of ingested vitamins and the deconjugation of bile salts by bacteria in the proximal jejunum. Deconjugated bile salts do not form micelles in the jejunum, and long-chain fatty acids cannot be absorbed. The bacteria also separate ingested vitamin $B_{12}$ from intrinsic factor, thus interfering with its absorption from the ileum. The absorption of simple carbohydrates generally is not impaired, though complex carbohydrates may be metabolized by bacteria. Thus, persons with bacterial overgrowth have steatorrhea, an abnormal Schilling test (even with the administration of intrinsic factor), increased metabolism of nonabsorbable carbohydrates (e.g., lactulose), and increased bacterial concentrations in jejunal aspirates. Absorption of D-xylose, a simple carbohydrate, is often normal.

**VIII-14.   The answer is A.**   *(Chap. 285)*   The incidence of isolated lactase deficiency is about 10 percent in the adult white population but higher in black Americans and Asians. Patients with acquired lactase deficiency have failure of normal hydrolysis of disaccharides in the brush border of intestinal epithelial cells. Common symptoms include abdominal cramps, bloating, and diarrhea after the ingestion of milk or dairy products. Since the lactose is not hydrolyzed and absorbed, an osmotic effect shifts fluid into the lumen. The symptoms are not due to an allergic reaction. Blood glucose fails to rise normally after the ingestion of an oral dose of lactose. However, this test is plagued by frequent false-positive and false-negative results. Measurement of hydrogen released after the ingestion of 50 g lactose is more sensitive and specific. Hydrogen release resulting from the action of colonic bacteria on unabsorbed lactose causes a rapid rise in breath hydrogen, indicative of a failure to absorb the disaccharide. Interestingly, patients with lactase deficiency may tolerate yogurt because of the presence of bacterial-derived lactases.

**VIII-15.   The answer is C.**   *(Chap. 288)*   Occlusive acute ischemia of the small intestine may result from an arterial thrombus or embolus in the celiac or superior mesenteric arteries and occurs most commonly in patients with atrial fibrillation, artificial heart valves, or valvular heart disease. Arterial thrombosis is associated with extensive atherosclerosis, low cardiac output, or both. Acute mesenteric ischemia, such as might be caused by an embolus originating in the dilated left atrium of a patient with rheumatic valvular disease, produces colicky periumbilical pain that changes to diffuse and constant discomfort. Vomiting and diarrhea also may occur. Abdominal examination reveals mild tenderness and distention but often is not dramatic even in the face of intestinal necrosis. Mild gastrointestinal bleeding, rather than massive hemorrhage, is the rule. Abdominal films disclose air-fluid levels and distention. Barium study, if undertaken, will reveal nonspecific dilation, poor motility, and thick mucosal folds ("thumb printing") of the small intestine. Gangrene may occur with more dramatic manifestations of peritonitis, sepsis, and shock 24 to 72 h after the initial insult. When acute mesenteric ischemia is suspected, patients should undergo immediate celiac and mesenteric angiography to localize the embolus, and then embolectomy should be performed. However, in many cases the ischemic duration has been prolonged, and at the time of surgery, resection of a segment of small bowel may be necessary. Moreover, many patients who require surgery to correct the complications of acute mesenteric ischemia are poor operative risks because of age, dehydration, sepsis, and comorbid disease.

**VIII-16.    The answer is D.**    *(Chap. 285. Relman, N Engl J Med 327:293–301, 1992.)*    The man described in the question has Whipple's disease, a bowel disorder associated with dilated gut lymphatics and characterized by weight loss, abdominal pain, diarrhea, malabsorption, central nervous system manifestations, and arthralgias. Electron microscopy has revealed the presence of bacilliform bodies in the lamina propria; these rod-shaped structures, which are located within or adjacent to macrophages that contain PAS-positive granules, have been identified as the gram-negative actinomycete *Tropheryma whippelii*. The treatment of choice is at least 1 year of therapy with antibiotics; trimethoprim-sulfamethoxazole is the first-line therapy. Clinical recovery is accompanied by the disappearance of the bacilliform bodies.

**VIII-17.    The answer is D.**    *(Chap. 285. Trier, N Engl J Med 325:1709–1719, 1991.)*    The histologic specimen pictured in the question shows villous atrophy, crypt hyperplasia, and inflammation typical of intestinal changes in nontropical sprue (celiac disease), an illness with a high incidence in Ireland. The disease, which is caused by gluten (water-insoluble wheat protein)-mediated intestinal damage, is associated with an increased incidence of histocompatibility antigens HLA-DR3 and HLA-DQw2. Although two-thirds of symptomatic cases present in childhood, the onset of the clinical symptoms of malabsorption may occur at any age. Persons with subclinical sprue during adolescence may have mild growth retardation and may be smaller than their siblings. Because the villous absorptive surface is markedly reduced in affected persons, an acquired lactase deficiency is often present and causes symptoms of milk intolerance. A strict gluten-free diet or the use of corticosteroids in patients with refractory disease usually relieves the symptoms and signs of malabsorption and promotes the restoration of normal jejunal histology. Failure to respond to a gluten-free diet suggests alternative diagnoses such as intestinal lymphoma, and gluten challenge followed by biopsy is indicated. A malabsorptive syndrome associated with abdominal pain, arthralgias, low-grade fever, and lymphadenopathy is not typical of celiac disease and should suggest another diagnosis, such as Whipple's disease or intestinal lymphoma.

**VIII-18.    The answer is C.**    *(Chap. 286)*    Radiographic demonstration of luminal narrowing, mucosal ulceration, and cobblestoning in the ileum is compatible with a diagnosis of regional enteritis. In Whipple's disease, x-rays characteristically show marked thickening of mucosal folds in the duodenum and jejunum. On barium enema, an appendiceal abscess usually presents as a mass indenting the cecal tip. Adenocarcinoma of the small bowel usually occurs as an ulcerated mass lesion in the duodenum. Infiltrating lymphomas of the distal bowel may be difficult to distinguish from regional enteritis radiographically, but stenotic bowel segments would not suggest lymphoma.

**VIII-19.    The answer is E.**    *(Chap. 286)*    The clinical history and x-ray presented in the question are consistent with toxic megacolon in association with severe ulcerative colitis. Toxic megacolon is most likely to occur when hypomotility agents such as diphenoxylate and loperamide are given to persons with severe colitis or when such persons undergo a barium enema radiographic procedure. In the case presented, a barium enema was not only dangerous but in fact unnecessary, because the presence of diarrhea and signs of systemic illness indicated that the disease no longer was limited to the rectum.

Colonic perforation also may be associated with severe ulcerative colitis; the presence of subdiaphragmatic air on abdominal x-rays would be suggestive.

**VIII-20.** **The answer is D.** *(Chap. 293)* Amino acids (except for the branched-chain amino acids leucine, isoleucine, and valine) are taken up by the liver via the portal circulation and are metabolized to urea. Severe liver damage disrupts normal amino acid metabolism and is reflected in elevated serum levels of non-branched-chain amino acids. Since urea cannot be produced, ammonia cannot be handled. Elevated levels of serum ammonia certainly play a large role in the development of hepatic encephalopathy in patients with liver failure and portal hypertension. Therefore, levels of ammonia and, in the case of alkylosis, ammonium ion rise at the expense of urea. Other mechanisms leading to increased blood ammonia levels include excessive amounts of intestinal nitrogen (e.g., resulting from bleeding); decreased intestinal motility allowing greater bacterial deamination of amino acids; depressed renal function leading to an increase in blood urea nitrogen and a greater opportunity for bacterial urease to convert this to ammonia; alkalosis, which will preferentially lead the $NH_4^+/NH_3$ equilibrium in favor of ammonia; and portal hypertension, which will allow ammonia from the gut to bypass hepatic detoxification.

**VIII-21.** **The answer is D.** *(Chap. 293)* Hepatic enzymes play a critical role in the metabolism of many drugs and hormones. So-called phase I reactions result in modification of reactive groups by oxidation, reduction, hydroxylation, sulfoxidation, deamination, dealkylation, or methylation. The microsomal P450 system is an example of an enzymatic system that carries out some of these reactions, usually leading to drug inactivation. Therefore, in the case of severe liver disease and suppressed availability of such detoxifying enzymes, drug clearance will decrease. The following drugs require dosage adjustments in patients with liver disease: phenytoin, phenobarbital, acetaminophen, glucocorticoids, lidocaine, quinidine, propranolol, nafcillin, chloramphenicol, tetracycline, trimethoprim, and rifampin. By contrast, certain drugs, such as cyclophosphamide and the antidepressant imipramine, require conversion to their active moieties by this enzyme system. Phase II reactions, generally resulting in a more soluble compound that allows biliary or renal excretion, include conversion of substances to their glucuronide or sulfate derivatives.

**VIII-22.** **The answer is D.** *(Chap. 298. Poupon, N Engl J Med 330:1342, 1994.)* Primary biliary cirrhosis (PBC) is a disease of unknown etiology, but its frequent association with autoimmune disorders such as rheumatoid arthritis, CRST syndrome, scleroderma, and sicca syndrome has suggested that an abnormal immune response plays an etiologic role. The disease typically affects middle-aged women and runs a slowly progressive course, with death resulting from hepatic insufficiency occurring within 10 years of diagnosis. A positive antimitochondrial antibody test is relatively sensitive and specific for PBC, occurring in over 90 percent of patients. Other serum abnormalities include increased alkaline phosphatase and 5'-nucleotidase activities and the presence of cryoproteins. Treatment is entirely supportive, although ursodiol may be helpful and live transplantation must be considered in severe cases. Neither corticosteroids nor D-penicillamine has proved to be effective. Colchicine, methotrexate, ursodiol, and cyclosporine may each play a role in slowing the progression of disease. Ursodiol treatment leads to symptomatic improvement but may not prevent progression to cirrhosis. Impaired bile excretion may lead to sequelae associated with malabsorption of the fat-soluble vitamins A, D, E, and K.

**VIII-23.** **The answer is C.** *(Chap. 297. Krawitt, N Engl J Med 334:897, 1996.)* Autoimmune hepatitis is a serious disorder characterized by progressive hepatic inflammation with a 6-month mortality of 40 percent. Typical cases have features of autoimmunity such as arthritis, vasculitis, and sicca syndrome. Serologic correlates include hypergammaglobulinemia (generally >2.5 g/dL), rheumatoid factor, and circulating autoantibodies (i.e., antinuclear, smooth muscle, and thyroid). There are several variants: (1) type 1, the classic syndrome seen in young women with lupoid features and circulating ANA; (2) type

2a, also seen in young women (mainly from western Europe) but associated with high titers of antibodies to liver and kidney microsomal antigens (LKM-1) and responsive to corticosteroids; (3) type 2b, which occurs in older (Mediterranean) men and is associated with low LKM-1 levels and interferon responsiveness; and (4) type 3, seen in patients who lack ANA and anti-LKM but have circulating antibodies to soluble live antigens. Rheumatoid factor elevation is nonspecific and is not helpful in establishing the diagnosis. Hepatitis D infection would require prior infection with hepatitis B. Hepatitis E is rare in western Europe and never progresses to chronicity.

**VIII-24.** **The answer is D.** *(Chap. 302)* Synthesized from hepatic cholesterol, the primary bile acids cholic acid and chenodeoxycholic acid are conjugated with glycine or taurine and excreted into the bile. Other secondary bile acids may be formed in the intestine by the action of colonic bacteria. One of the most important characteristics of bile acids is their detergent properties, which allow them to form molecular aggregates with cholesterol that are termed *micelles*. Cholesterol is poorly soluble in water; its solubility in bile is dependent on both the lipid concentration and the relevant amount of bile acids and lecithin. Bile acids also are required for the normal intestinal absorption of dietary fats by a similar micellar transport mechanism. Finally, bile acids are important in facilitating water and electrolyte transport in the intestine. To maintain the reusable pool of bile acids, the molecules are actively reabsorbed in the distal ileum, taken up in the portal bloodstream, and returned to hepatocytes for reconjugation and resecretion. Compared with a normal-size bile acid pool of 2 to 4 g, the daily fecal loss of bile acids is only in the range of 0.5 g.

**VIII-25.** **The answer is E.** *(Chap. 304)* Purtscher's retinopathy is a relatively rare but devastating complication of acute pancreatitis. It is characterized by sudden loss of vision and the presence of cotton-wool spots and hemorrhages in the area of the optic disc and macula. The cause is thought to be occlusion of the posterior retinal artery by aggregated granulocytes.

**VIII-26.** **The answer is D.** *(Chap. 302. Johnston, N Engl J Med 328:412, 1993.)* Selected patients with gallstones may respond well to treatment with oral chenodeoxycholic acid, its related molecule ursodeoxycholic acid, or both. Patients who are candidates for such therapy must have either cholesterol (rather than pigments, as in thalassemia) or mixed radiolucent gallstones. Second, gallstones greater than 1.5 cm in diameter and those in gallbladders that fail to opacify after oral cholecystography will be very unlikely to respond to dissolution therapy. Chenodeoxycholic acid is thought to work by decreasing HMG-CoA reductase activity and thus hepatically secreted cholesterol. Deoxycholic acid works by a similar mechanism as well as by retarding cholesterol crystal nucleation. Up to 2 years of therapy with these agents often is required to dissolve a gallstone; after withdrawal, there is a recurrence rate of up to 30 to 50 percent. The same group of patients who are candidates for medical therapy to dissolve gallstones are also generally the patients who are candidates for gallstone lithotripsy, a method of fragmenting stones by extracorporeal shock waves.

**VIII-27.** **The answer is A.** *(Chaps. 303, 306)* Serum amylase is an effective screening test for acute pancreatitis. Levels greater than 300 U/dL make the diagnosis extremely likely, especially if intestinal perforation and infarction are excluded (both of these conditions can raise serum amylase). In all but 15 percent of patients with acute pancreatitis, the serum amylase level is elevated within 24 h and begins to decline by 3 to 5 days in the absence of extensive pancreatic necrosis, partial infarction, or pseudocyst formation. Reasons for normal values could be a delay in obtaining the blood test, the presence of chronic rather than acute pancreatitis, and the presence of hypertriglyceridemia. Both serum amylase and lipase (perhaps the single best enzyme to diagnose acute pancreatitis) will be falsely low in patients with hypertriglyceridemia. Serum trypsinogen may have theoretical advantages over amylase and lipase insofar as the pancreas is the only source of this enzyme.

**VIII-28.** **The answer is B.** *(Chap. 289)* Carcinoma of the colon is the most common cause of mechanical obstruction of the colon and is followed in frequency by sigmoid diverticulitis and volvulus. These three causes account for 90 percent of cases of colonic obstruction. Adhesions and hernias cause about 75 percent of cases of small-intestine obstruction but are uncommon causes of colonic obstruction.

**VIII-29.** **The answer is B.** *(Chap. 300)* Fatty liver refers to the infiltration of hepatocytes by triglyceride. Typically, the fat accumulates in large cytoplasmic droplets. However, in acute fatty liver of pregnancy and in Reye's syndrome (fatty liver with encephalopathy, thought to be caused by viruses or drugs), the fat is contained in small vacuoles and is termed microvesicular fat. The reason for the specific morphologic appearance of fat in these two disorders is unknown, but it provides a useful histologic differential point.

**VIII-30.** **The answer is D.** *(Chap. 295. Snilkstein, N Engl J Med 319:1557, 1988.)* Acetaminophen hepatotoxicity is mediated by a toxic metabolite formed by the hepatic cytochrome P450 system. Glutathione is responsible for detoxifying the metabolite, but when stores of this scavenger are depleted, hepatocyte necrosis may ensue. Thus, acetaminophen is a direct hepatotoxin; a single dose of 10 to 15 g will produce evidence of liver injury, and doses above 25 g can be fatal. Such injury can be ameliorated somewhat by timely administration (<24 h after overdose) of a glutathione-restoring sulfhydryl compound such as *N*-acetylcysteine. Many other agents produce hepatic injury in an idiosyncratic fashion as a result of apparent hypersensitivity (halothane, methyldopa, chlorpromazine), genetic variations in the handling of drug metabolites (isoniazid, diphenylhydantoin), or unknown mechanisms.

**VIII-31.** **The answer is B.** *(Chaps. 294, 299)* Gastrointestinal bleeding, which causes an increase in the production of ammonia and other nitrogenous substances in the colon, is a common predisposing factor to hepatic encephalopathy in persons with cirrhosis. Hypokalemic alkalosis, which is caused by excessive diuresis or vomiting, may precipitate hepatic encephalopathy by increasing the ratio of ammonia to ammonium; gut and renal absorption of ammonia increases, and more ammonia enters the brain. Acidosis has the opposite effect. Deterioration of liver function, such as that seen in viral hepatitis, can precipitate encephalopathy in cirrhotic persons. If worsening renal function produces an increase in blood urea nitrogen, there is additional availability for $NH_3$ production via the action of gut bacterial urease on urea.

**VIII-32.** **The answer is E.** *(Chap. 295)* About 10 percent of persons treated with isoniazid develop mild elevations of serum aminotransferase levels during the first few weeks of therapy. These levels usually return to normal despite continued use of isoniazid. About 1 percent of persons with elevated aminotransferase levels develop symptoms of hepatitis and are at high risk for developing fatal hepatic failure. The older the patient, the higher the risk of isoniazid hepatitis; thus, because the patient described in this question is young and asymptomatic, isoniazid can safely be continued as long as she is watched for symptoms of hepatitis. A liver biopsy would not be indicated at this time.

**VIII-33.** **The answer is C.** *(Chaps. 298, 299)* Alcohol produces impairment in the absorption of many nutrients, including vitamin K. (The use of neomycin in the treatment of hepatic encephalopathy also can lead to a decrease in vitamin K.) When hypoprothrombinemia in a person with liver disease is easily corrected by parenteral vitamin K administration, decreased intestinal absorption of vitamin K should be suspected. Coagulopathy resulting from impaired hepatic function, as is seen in alcoholic hepatitis, is unlikely to be corrected by exogenous vitamin K. Although the patient discussed in the question is probably deficient in folate, as evidenced by the high mean corpuscular volume, folic acid administration has no effect on prothrombin time. Exogenous vitamin K would not correct the hypoprothrombinemia associated with disseminated intravascular coagulation.

**VIII-34.   The answer is E.** *(Chap. 294)* Benign postoperative intrahepatic cholestasis can develop as a consequence of major surgery for a catastrophic event in which hypotension, extensive blood loss into tissues, and massive blood replacement are notable. Factors contributing to jaundice include the pigment load from transfusions, decreased liver function resulting from hypotension, and decreased renal bilirubin excretion caused by tubular necrosis. Jaundice becomes evident on the second or third postoperative day, with bilirubin levels (mainly levels of conjugated bilirubin) peaking by the tenth day. Serum alkaline phosphatase concentration may be elevated up to tenfold, but aspartate aminotransferase (AST) levels are only mildly elevated. Hepatitis, choledocholithiasis, and hepatic infarct are unlikely diagnoses in the absence of abdominal tenderness, fever, or a significant rise in AST levels. The incubation period of posttransfusion hepatitis is 7 weeks, making this diagnosis unlikely.

**VIII-35.   The answer is E.** *(Chap. 297. Niederau, N Engl J Med 334:1422, 1996.)* Glucocorticoid therapy has been shown to prolong survival in patients with chronic active hepatitis of nonviral etiology. This patient, who has evidence of chronic hepatitis B infection as the cause of her chronic active hepatitis (this diagnosis has been made because of piecemeal necrosis on liver biopsy), would not benefit from the administration of steroids. Although many agents have been tried in chronic active viral hepatitis, none have been shown to be effective in the majority of patients. A 4-month course of interferon-α is associated with a 40 percent seroconversion rate from HBeAg positivity to detectable levels of anti-HBe. Interferon therapy is also beneficial in patients with chronic hepatitis C infection.

**VIII-36.   The answer is E.** *(Chap. 297)* Although chronic active hepatitis may be associated with extraintestinal manifestations (e.g., arthritis) and the presence in the serum of autoantibodies (e.g., anti-smooth-muscle antibody), these factors are not invariably present. The distinction between chronic active and chronic persistent hepatitis can be established only by liver biopsy. In chronic active hepatitis there is piecemeal necrosis (erosion of the limiting plate of hepatocytes surrounding the portal triads), hepatocellular regeneration, and extension of inflammation into the liver lobule; these features are not seen in chronic persistent hepatitis. Both diseases may be associated with serologic evidence of hepatitis B infection.

**VIII-37.   The answer is E.** *(Chap. 299. Rolachon, Hepatology 22:1171, 1995.)* Persons who have cirrhosis, particularly alcoholic cirrhosis and ascites, may develop acute bacterial peritonitis without a clearly definable precipitating event. The clinical presentation of spontaneous bacterial peritonitis may be subtle, such as fever of unknown origin and mild abdominal pain, and may be attributed to other causes. Diagnosis is based on a careful examination of ascitic fluid obtained by paracentesis and should include cell count, Gram's stain, and culture. The most common organisms causing this syndrome are enteric gram-negative bacilli, with pneumococci and other gram-positive rods being less likely. Empiric therapy with cefatoxime or ampicillin and an aminoglycoside is appropriate. Recurrence is common; quinolone prophylaxis is helpful.

**VIII-38.   The answer is E.** *(Chap. 302)* The radiograph reproduced in the question shows emphysematous cholecystitis, a form of acute cholecystitis in which the gallbladder, its wall, and sometimes even the bile ducts contain gas secondary to infection by gas-producing bacteria. This condition occurs most frequently in elderly men and diabetic persons. The morbidity and mortality associated with emphysematous cholecystitis exceed those of acute cholecystitis. Once preoperative preparations are complete, laparotomy and cholecystectomy should be performed promptly.

**VIII-39.   The answer is B.** *(Chap. 302)* Obesity, clofibrate therapy, age, and oral contraceptive therapy predispose to gallstone formation by increasing biliary cholesterol excretion. Extensive ileal resection leads to malabsorption of bile salts, depletion of the bile acid pool, and an inability to micellize cholesterol, resulting in an increased risk of gallstone formation. No correlation exists between serum cholesterol concentration and biliary cholesterol secretion; consequently, hypercholesterolemia per se does not predispose to cholelithiasis. Other important predisposing factors to the formation of cholesterol gallstones include gallbladder hypomotility resulting from prolonged parenteral nutrition, fasting, or pregnancy.    *Hyperlipidoemia type IV - ↑TG (VLDL)*

**VIII-40.  The answer is E.**  *(Chap. 299. Ochs, N Engl J Med 332:1192, 1995.)*  If fluid and sodium restriction is unsuccessful in the mobilization of ascitic fluid, cautious diuresis is indicated; spironolactone, rather than furosemide or acetazolamide, would be the drug of choice. Aggressive diuretic therapy can lead to volume depletion, azotemia, electrolyte disturbances, and hepatic encephalopathy. Therapeutic paracentesis (4 to 6 L) is now felt to be effective, especially if albumin is infused to avoid exacerbation of intravascular depletion. The peritoneovenous (LeVeen) shunt (such a shunt may now be placed by the transjugular route) should be reserved for cases of intractable ascites; its use is accompanied by significant complications, including infection and disseminated intravascular coagulation.

**VIII-41.  The answer is E.**  *(Chap. 304. Steinberg, N Engl J Med 330:1198, 1994.)*  Conventional therapy for acute pancreatitis includes analgesia, intravenous volume replacement, and abstinence from oral intake to "rest" the pancreas. Controlled trials have not demonstrated any benefit in regard to symptomatic recovery or survival rate from the administration of cimetidine, aprotinin (an inhibitor of pancreatic enzyme release), antibiotics, or glucagon. However, antibiotics are beneficial when secondary infection supervenes (e.g., abscess, phlegmon, or ascending cholangitis). Anticholinergic agents have not been shown to be beneficial and may worsen tachycardia, bowel hypomotility, and oliguria.

**VIII-42.  The answer is B.**  *(Chap. 304)*  Vitamin $B_{12}$ (cobalamin) malabsorption is commonly associated with chronic pancreatitis. The mechanism of vitamin $B_{12}$ malabsorption is thought to be excessive binding of the vitamin by non-intrinsic-factor binding proteins, which normally are destroyed by pancreatic proteases. Consequently, the condition is corrected by the administration of pancreatic enzymes. Gastric varices, which may bleed, are caused by splenic vein thrombosis that results from inflammation of the tail of the pancreas. Pleural effusions, most notably left-sided, can result from leaking pseudocysts or a pancreatic-pleural fistula; effusion fluid has a high amylase content. Jaundice results from compression of the common bile duct caused by edema or inflammation in the head of the pancreas. Although persons with chronic pancreatitis may develop tender red nodules on the legs, those nodules are due to subcutaneous fat necrosis, not to erythema nodosum.

**VIII-43.  The answer is A.**  *(Chap. 304. Agarwal, Am J Gastroenterol 86:1385, 1991.)*  Serum bilirubin elevations >68 μmol/L (>4.0 mg/dL) occur in about 10 percent of patients with acute pancreatitis, are usually transient, and do not portend a poor prognosis unless they are accompanied by very high levels of serum lactic dehydrogenase. The finding of hypoxemia, often heralding the development of the adult respiratory distress syndrome, is ominous. Hypocalcemia [<1.96 mmol/L (<8 mg/dL)], which possibly indicates interperitoneal fatty acid saponification of calcium, is also a grave prognostic sign. Hypoalbuminemia and a massive requirement for colloid replacement suggest profound peripancreatic disease, as does the presence of discolored or hemorrhagic fluid obtained at paracentesis. Other risk factors for high mortality during an attack of acute pancreatitis include older age, hypotension, leukocytosis, hyperglycemia, a fall in hematocrit, and azotemia.

**VIII-44.  The answer is B.**  *(Chap. 95)*  The combination of weight loss, anemia, and a bullous skin eruption in a patient with hepatic metastases and evidence of a pancreatic lesion is highly suggestive of a glucagonoma. This tumor of pancreatic alpha cells is usually malignant, metastasizes early, often occurs in middle-aged women, and is accompanied by hyperglycemia, painful stomatitis and cheilosis, hypoaminoacidemia, and a characteristic skin rash—necrolytic migratory erythema. With appropriate histologic techniques, the diagnosis of a pancreatic alpha-cell tumor can be established by liver biopsy, but marked plasma hyperglucagonemia is pathognomonic. Arteriography may demonstrate a pancreatic tumor but is not diagnostic. Treatment consists of early surgical removal; chemotherapy of metastatic disease is usually ineffective.

**VIII-45.   The answer is C.** *(Chaps. 282, 283)*   Though candidal infection is a common cause of esophagitis, typically manifested by dysphagia, it may be seen with immunodeficiency states such as AIDS, with the use of immunosuppressive agents including glucocorticoids, and with the use of broad-spectrum antibiotics. Esophagitis also may be seen in diabetics, patients with systemic lupus erythematosus, and those who have experienced a corrosive esophageal injury. Oral thrush is a helpful but not invariant coexisting finding. Candidal esophagitis may be complicated by bleeding, perforation, stricture, or systemic invasion. Upper gastrointestinal radiography may reveal multiple nodular filling defects. Endoscopic evaluation typically reveals a whitish exudate in the setting of underlying erythematous mucosa. The definitive diagnosis would require the demonstration of yeast or hyphal forms on Gram's, periodic acid Schiff, or silver stain. Uncomplicated cases of candidal esophagitis respond well to fluconazole, which is preferred to ketoconazole because of reduced bioavailability of ketoconazole at increased gastric pH.

**VIII-46.   The answer is C.** *(Chap. 283)*   Chronic acid-induced (reflux) esophagitis may cause bleeding from diffuse erosions or discrete ulcerations. Peptic damage to the submucosa can result in fibrosis and subsequent stricture. Barrett's esophagus is formed as destroyed squamous epithelium is replaced by columnar epithelium, usually similar to that of the adjacent gastric mucosa. Adenocarcinoma may develop in 2 to 5 percent of persons with a Barrett's esophagus. A lower esophageal ring is a structural lesion that is not related to reflux esophagitis.

**VIII-47.   The answer is B.** *(Chaps. 45, 294)*   A simple and important method to determine whether the cause of jaundice is conjugated or unconjugated hyperbilirubinemia is measurement of the urinary excretion of bilirubin. Under normal circumstances the urine contains no bilirubin since the unconjugated, water-soluble bilirubin, which accounts for 96 percent of the bilirubin in serum, is tightly bound to albumin and is not filtered by the glomeruli. Even in cases of unconjugated hyperbilirubinemia resulting from overproduction (as in hemolysis and the ineffective erythropoiesis characteristic of certain hemoglobinopathies) or decreased conjugation, there is no urinary excretion of bilirubin. Congenital deficiencies of the glucuronyl transferase enzyme responsible for converting bilirubin into its soluble form include Gilbert's syndrome and Crigler-Najjar disorder types I and II (in type I disease, the transferase enzyme is totally absent). In cases of conjugated hyperbilirubinemia, in which more than 50 percent of the serum bilirubin is composed of the conjugated type, enough bilirubin remains unbound that filtration of this substance occurs and the urine dipstick becomes positive. In addition to extrahepatic obstruction, causes of conjugated hyperbilirubinemia include defects in hepatic excretion of a congenital (e.g., Dubin-Johnson or Rotor syndrome) or an acquired (hepatocellular disease or estrogen use) nature.

**VIII-48.   The answer is E.** *(Chap. 286)*   Most extraintestinal disorders of inflammatory bowel disease are associated with both Crohn's disease and ulcerative colitis, including pericholangitis, uveitis, and a variety of skin and joint manifestations. Complications that are unique to Crohn's disease because of inflammation of the terminal ileum include hypocalcemia, which is caused by malabsorption of vitamin D, and the formation of urinary oxalate stones, which results from increased colonic absorption of dietary oxalate. Owing to bile-salt malabsorption caused by ileal disease, cholesterol gallstones tend to form in persons with regional enteritis.

**VIII-49.   The answer is D.** *(Chap. 288)*   Meckel's diverticulum is the most commonly occurring congenital anomaly of the gastrointestinal tract and is found in 2 percent of adult autopsies. The diverticulum may contain ectopic gastric mucosa, and local acid secretion may produce ileal ulceration and lower gastrointestinal bleeding. In young adults Meckel's diverticulitis can mimic acute appendicitis. Technetium, taken up by diverticular gastric mucosa, can detect the lesion, which is easily missed on conventional barium x-rays. Gastrointestinal obstruction may occur if the diverticulum intussuscepts or twists on a fibrous remnant of the omphalomesenteric duct. Surgical excision is the treatment for any significant complication of a Meckel's diverticulum.

**VIII-50.** **The answer is C.** *(Chap. 295)* Hepatitis B *e* antigen (HBeAg) is a protein that is associated with the HBV core particle. HBeAg is a soluble protein found only in HBsAg-positive serum and is immunologically distinct from HBsAg as well as from intact HBcAg, an antigen expressed on the hepatitis B virus nucleocapsid core. Interestingly, both HBcAg and HBeAg are encoded on the so-called C-gene of the hepatitis B genome. Owing to the close association of HBeAg and HBsAg, the presence of HBeAg in the serum is linked with infectiousness, and the antigen is present during the viremic period of acute hepatitis B. HBeAg correlates well with viral replication, and detection of HBeAg persistence predicts for the subsequent development of chronic hepatitis B infection; however, the absence of HBeAg in serum does not preclude the development of chronic hepatitis B infection. In acute hepatitis B, the disappearance of HBeAg from serum often presages resolution of the acute infection; however, HBeAg-negative persons should be considered infectious until antibody to HBsAg is no longer detected in the serum.

**VIII-51.** **The answer is B.** *(Chap. 295. Hoofnagle, JAMA 261:1321, 1989.)* The delta agent hepatitis D virus (HDV) is a recently recognized defective RNA virus that coinfects with and requires the helper function of HBV for its replication and expression. Therefore, the duration of HDV infection is determined by and limited to the duration of HBV infection. Although the delta core is encapsulated by an outer coat of HBsAg, the delta antigen has no antigenic similarity to that of any of the HBV antigens, and the RNA genome is not homologous with HBV DNA. HDV infection has a worldwide distribution and exists in two epidemiologic patterns: endemic and epidemic. In endemic areas (Mediterranean countries) HDV infection is found among those with HBV infection and is transmitted predominantly by nonpercutaneous routes, such as close personal contact. In nonendemic areas such as the United States and northern Europe, HDV infection is limited to persons with frequent exposure to blood products, such as intravenous drug addicts and hemophiliacs. In general, patients with simultaneous HBV and HDV infections do not have an increased risk of developing chronic hepatitis compared with patients with acute HBV infection alone. HDV superinfection of patients with chronic HBV infection carries an increased risk of fulminant hepatitis and death.

**VIII-52.** **The answer is A.** *(Chaps. 44, 299. Planas, Hepatology 20:370, 1994.)* Peripheral (intravenous) and central (superior mesenteric artery) infusions of vasopressin are equally effective in temporarily controlling variceal hemorrhage. For more permanent hemostasis, surgery may be required. Elective portacaval shunt surgery can prevent recurrent variceal bleeding, although the overall survival rate is not improved. Compared with the portacaval shunt, the distal splenorenal shunt appears to have a lower incidence of postoperative encephalopathy; for either procedure, however, the presence of jaundice, ascites, or encephalopathy portends a less favorable operative outlook. Sclerotherapy and esophageal variceal banding are therapies which should be employed before surgery. Beta blockade with propranolol at doses sufficient to lower the resting heart rate by 25 percent appears to reduce the incidence of recurrent variceal bleeding and may be an effective prophylactic agent in those who have large varices but have not yet bled. Systemic somatostatin or its analogue, octreotide, may help control bleeding without the peripheral vasoconstriction associated with the use of vasopressin.

**VIII-53.** **The answer is C.** *(Chap. 295)* The prevention of viral hepatitis is of particular importance because of the limited therapeutic options. The prophylactic approach varies with the type of hepatitis. All preparations of immune globulin (IG) contain sufficient titers of anti-HAV to prevent clinically apparent type A hepatitis. If they are given early enough, infection will be prevented in approximately 80 percent of patients. For intimate contacts, 0.02 mL/kg of IG is recommended as soon as possible after exposure. An inactivated HAV vaccine is the preferred approach to preexposure (before travel to an endemic area) prophylaxis. The prevention of hepatitis B is based on passive immunoprophylaxis with both hepatitis B immune globulin (HBIG) and hepatitis B vaccine. HBIG appears to be effective in reducing clinically apparent illness but does not appear to prevent infection. Hepatitis B vaccine has been shown to be highly effective in preventing HBV infection. Because only persons with HBV infection are susceptible to delta hepatitis, hepatitis B vaccine is effective in preventing delta infection in persons who are not carriers of HBsAg. There is no effective prophylaxis of HDV infection in patients who are already HBsAg carriers. Postexposure prophylaxis of hepatitis C with IG is not effective.

**VIII-54.  The answer is E.**  *(Chap. 41. Grunberg, N Engl J Med 329:1790, 1993.)*   Two areas in the central nervous system control the act of vomiting. The vomiting center in the lateral reticular formation in the medulla receives input from both the gastrointestinal tract and higher centers in the brain and controls outflow to the phrenic nerve, spinal nerve, and vagus, each of which innervates muscles involved in retching. The chemoreceptor trigger zone located near the floor of the fourth ventricle can be activated by a host of stimuli or drugs, including opiates, dopaminergics, and digitalis; radiation; and varied metabolic toxins and abnormalities (e.g., uremia). Pathways emanating from the chemoreceptor trigger zone lead to the vomiting center, which directly controls the act of vomiting. Dopaminergic inhibitors such as haloperidol and the phenothiazine derivative prochlorperazine inhibit the dopamine receptors in the chemoreceptor trigger zone, thus suppressing vomiting. Phenothiazine derivatives frequently are associated with troublesome anticholinergic side effects, such as sedation, dry mouth, and hypotension. Metoclopramide is another dopamine antagonist that can affect central pathways, but it has the added benefit of a cholinergic effect that enhances gastric emptying. Cisapride is an agent that has marked peripheral effects and the sometimes troublesome central nervous system side effects (drowsiness, anxiety, and confusion) seen with metaclopramide. Antihistamines such as diphenhydramine and anticholinergics such as scopolamine do not act on the chemoreceptor trigger zone but can be helpful in the control of vomiting caused by dysfunction of the inner ear. Ondansetron and granisetron are particularly effective in the treatment of chemotherapy-induced nausea and vomiting. These relatively new agents are serotonin antagonists that block $HT_3$ receptors in the chemoreceptor trigger zone and gut.

**VIII-55.  The answer is E.**  *(Chap. 286. Peppercorn, Ann Intern Med 112:50–60, 1990.)*  Among the findings of the National Cooperative Crohn's Disease Study in 1979 were that corticosteroids are more efficacious in the treatment of Crohn's disease of the small intestine than in the treatment of Crohn's disease of the colon. However, steroids can mask a septic deterioration and must be used cautiously. Azathioprine and mercaptopurine may be useful corticosteroid-sparing agents. Sulfasalazine was found to be effective in therapy for active colonic disease, but neither sulfasalazine nor corticosteroids decrease the frequency of recurrence once remission has been achieved. Both drugs may be used safely in treating pregnant women. In more recent studies, metronidazole, which is not useful in ulcerative colitis, has been reported to be useful in the treatment of the perineal and colitic manifestations of Crohn's disease.

**VIII-56.  The answer is C.**  *(Chap. 286)*   Risk factors for the development of colon carcinoma in persons who have ulcerative colitis include the presence of the disease for more than 10 years, extensive mucosal involvement (pancolitis), and a family history of carcinoma of the colon. The risk of cancer in persons with pancolitis is estimated to be 12 percent at 15 years, 23 percent at 20 years, and 42 percent at 24 years. Neither a history of toxic megacolon nor the prolonged use of high-dose steroids increases the risk of cancer. Pseudo-polyps, although frequently associated with severe disease, are not precancerous lesions.

**VIII-57.    The answer is E.** *(Chap. 288)*    Ischemic colitis most often occurs in elderly persons who have vascular disease. Areas of the colon with extensive collateral circulation, such as the rectum, usually are spared. Angiography of arteries and veins rarely is indicated for diagnosis or therapy because vessel occlusions are almost never detected. Barium studies reveal edema, cobblestoning, thumbprinting, and ulceration. Even though acute ischemic colitis may present with rectal bleeding and lower abdominal pain, most cases do not present with the severity of signs and symptoms suggestive of an acute abdomen. This disease usually does not recur, and symptoms tend to resolve in 2 to 4 weeks. Ischemic colitis sometimes is diagnosed retrospectively as the cause of a colonic stricture.

**VIII-58.    The answer is A.** *(Chap. 288)*    Acute hemorrhage from colonic diverticula is the most common cause of lower gastrointestinal bleeding among elderly persons. Although diverticula are more common on the left side of the colon, bleeding tends to originate from the ascending (right) colon. Bleeding usually stops with bed rest and transfusion; however, when conservative measures fail to curb hemorrhage, intraarterial infusion of vasoconstrictive medications introduced during angiography can be effective. Although acute diverticulitis may be associated with occult bleeding, gross hemorrhage rarely occurs.

**VIII-59.    The answer is C.** *(Chap. 292)*    Unexplained hepatosplenomegaly and unexplained persistence of elevated liver function tests are the principal indications for percutaneous needle liver biopsy. The presence of these phenomena suggests a diagnosis of diffuse parenchymal disease of the liver, which occurs with drug reactions and metabolic liver disease, or multiple focal lesions, which are caused by granulomatous or metastatic disease. The diagnosis of miliary tuberculosis, for example, often can be made by liver biopsy (more than 40 percent of all these patients have a positive liver biopsy). A focal defect identified on a liver scan also can be evaluated by percutaneous liver biopsy, often with sonographic guidance of the needle. A percutaneous liver biopsy should never be performed, however, when a vascular lesion of the liver, such as an angioma, is suspected. Other contraindications include coagulopathies, septic cholangitis, and suspected echinococcal cyst. Although liver biopsy can confirm the presence of suspected biliary obstruction, ultrasonography, computed tomography, and transhepatic or endoscopic cholangiography are better techniques for determining the cause of common bile duct obstruction.

**VIII-60.    The answer is D.** *(Chap. 292)*    Elevated levels of serum alkaline phosphatase (of hepatic origin) generally reflect impaired hepatic excretory function. Thus, the concentration of this enzyme may be elevated in persons with infiltrative diseases of the liver (leukemia, sarcoid, tuberculosis), incomplete extrahepatic biliary obstruction (e.g., bile duct stricture), or intrahepatic cholestasis (e.g., chlorpromazine-induced cholestasis or early primary biliary cirrhosis); in all three of these examples, serum bilirubin concentration is only slightly elevated. Both acute viral hepatitis and acetaminophen hepatotoxicity are associated with extensive hepatocellular damage and frequently produce peak serum aspartate aminotransferase levels above 8.33 μkat/L (500 U/L).

**VIII-61.    The answer is E.** *(Chap. 285)*    Patients with intestinal lymphangiectasia—characterized by protein-losing enteropathy, hypoproteinemia, hypogammaglobulinemia, edema, chylous effusions, fat malabsorption, and lymphocytopenia—typically present in childhood or young adulthood. The generalized congenital disorder of lymphatic development includes the dilated lymph vessels typically seen on small-bowel biopsy. The abnormal lymphatics are presumed to rupture into the bowel lumen, leading directly to hypoproteinemia and steatorrhea. Absorption of carbohydrates such as D-xylose and lactose that are not dependent on lymphatics typically is preserved. The decreased lymph flow associated with a low-fat diet supplemented by medium-chain triglycerides (transported by the portal vein rather than the lymph) results in significant clinical improvement. Despite hypogammaglobulinemia, infections with encapsulated organisms are not increased.

**VIII-62.   The answer is E.**   *(Chap. 285)*   Tropical sprue is a malabsorptive disease of unclear etiology that may be due to a nutritional deficiency, a microorganism, or a toxin elaborated by a microorganism. Malabsorption of at least two nutrients is the rule. Patients commonly malabsorb iron, vitamin $B_{12}$, xylose (carbohydrates), and fat. Consequently, megaloblastic anemia and problems associated with the absorption of the fat-soluble vitamins A (night blindness), D (hypocalcemia possibly with tetany), and K (hypoprothrombinemia and purpura) may be seen. In the setting of prolonged calorie malnutrition, a state of secondary hypopituitarism may be manifested by decreased libido. The diagnosis of tropical sprue is supported by a jejunal biopsy that discloses shortened and thickened villi, increased crypt height, and infiltration of mononuclear cells in the lamina propria. In addition to a trial of antibiotic therapy (sulfonamide or tetracycline), treatment with vitamin $B_{12}$, folate, and antibiotics should be undertaken. Pyoderma gangrenosum is an ulcerative skin lesion found in patients with inflammatory bowel disease.

**VIII-63.   The answer is A.**   *(Chap. 300)*   Granulomas can be found on liver biopsy in patients with fever of unknown origin or during evaluation of patients who have abnormalities of unclear etiology on liver function tests. Although mild transaminase abnormalities may occur, hepatic dysfunction usually is restricted to mild elevations of alkaline phosphatase. In approximately 20 percent of cases it is not possible to identify a systemic cause of the hepatic granulomas. In such a situation, and only if a diagnosis of miliary tuberculosis is rigorously excluded (even including an initial empirical trial of antituberculous therapy), a trial of steroids could be considered. Although tuberculosis is the etiology in the majority of cases when caseating lesions are present, the absence of caseating granulomas does not exclude tuberculosis. Systemic granulomatous diseases other than tuberculosis that may involve the liver include schistosomiasis, histoplasmosis, brucellosis, berylliosis, sarcoidosis, and drug reactions. Granulomatous hepatitis is relatively common in patients with MDS. *Mycobacterium avium-intracellulare* is the most cause, but sulfuramides, CMV, and fungal infections also can lead to pathologic findings.

**VIII-64.   The answer is B.**   *(Chaps. 40, 283)*   "Sticking" during the passage of food through the mouth, pharynx, or esophagus is almost always associated with a significant pathologic problem. The history can provide the correct diagnosis in over three-fourths of patients with dysphagia. Motor dysphagias, such as those caused by achalasia and diffuse esophageal spasm, are equally affected by solids and liquids from the onset. Patients with an esophageal carcinoma typically initially have problems swallowing solid food, but with progression of the cancer, difficulty with liquids also is encountered. Since this patient has dysphagia with both solids and liquids and has severe chest pain, diffuse esophageal spasm is the likely diagnosis. Diagnostic studies would include both barium swallow esophagastroscopy and upper endoscopy to exclude an associated structural abnormality.

**VIII-65.   The answer is B.**   *(Chap. 41)*   A host of gastrointestinal complaints are commonly described by patients as indigestion. Among them are abdominal pain, nonulcer dyspepsia (symptoms suggesting a diagnosis of peptic ulcer despite the absence of a documented ulcer), heartburn, food intolerance, aerophagia, and gaseousness-bloating-flatulence. Many patients have chronic, repetitive eructation (belching) that can result from air swallowing rather than excessive gas production in the stomach or intestine. Accumulation of swallowed air in the stomach may lead to postprandial fullness and the finding of a large amount of air in the gastric fundus on x-ray, the so-called magenblase (i.e., gastric bubble) syndrome. In this situation, the patient experiences discomfort when lying supine after a large meal, allowing air to be "trapped" below the gastroesophageal junction without the ability to be eructated. If the swallowed air can successfully pass the stomach, diffuse abdominal distention may occur or the air may be trapped in the splenic flexure of the colon. Such trapping can lead to the so-called splenic flexure syndrome, which is characterized by left upper quadrant fullness with radiation to the left side of the chest. Relief occurs after defecation or expulsion of flatus. The splenic flexure syndrome is associated with increased tympany in the left lateral abdomen with a large amount of splenic flexure air on plain abdominal radiography. Bloating and excess flatulence caused by excessive air production in the intestine often occur after the ingestion of certain foods. For example, beans contain oligosaccharides (stachyose and raffinose) that cannot be split by intestinal mucosal enzymes but are metabolized by colonic bacteria. The ingestion of fructose or sorbitol and infection with the protozoal organism *Giardia lamblia* also may lead to excessive production of intestinal gas and a sensation of bloating. Gallstone-associated pain would be most likely to be localized to the epigastrium or the right upper quadrant.

**VIII-66.  The answer is C.**  *(Chap. 42)*  Constipation, which is defined as fewer than three defacatory episodes per week, is a common complaint in clinical practice. It is important to consider serious causes such as obstruction resulting from colonic neoplasms or strictures and pathologic states of disturbed colonic motility such as multiple sclerosis, central nervous system lesions, and Chagas' disease. Other causes of constipation include drugs such as anticholinergics, narcotics, iron supplements, and calcium channel blockers; endocrinopathies such as hypothyroidism and diabetes; and collagen vascular diseases such as progressive systemic sclerosis. In most patients, however, constipation has no clear-cut cause and is due to either irritable bowel syndrome or other functional-psychological causes. Treatment of constipation must be individualized. Fiber supplementation with agents such as psyllium may increase stool bulk and is appropriate for many patients. Emollients such as mineral oil and docusate salts soften and lower the surface tension of the stool by allowing the mixing of aqueous and fatty substances. Hypertonic agents such as lactulose and sorbitol cause an osmotic impetus to diarrhea. Stimulants include castor oil, senna, and phenolphthalein bisacodyl, which enhance intestinal secretion and motility. Cispride is prokinetic and promotes intestinal transit through the proximal colon; its role in the treatment of constipation remains unclear.

**VIII-67.  The answer is D.**  *(Chap. 42)*  Diarrhea, which is defined as an increase in daily stool volume above 200 g, can be classified into acute and chronic forms. By far the most common causes of acute diarrhea are infectious agents. Diarrhea that persists for weeks or months and is considered chronic may be due to inflammation or an orally ingested nonabsorbed solute such as a maldigested or malabsorbed nutrient that exerts osmotic force and thus draws fluid into the intestinal lumen, altered intestinal motility (usually associated with neurologic diseases), or intestinal secretion by which abnormal fluid transport occurs (not usually related to the ingestion of food). Secretory diarrhea usually persists despite fasting. The best example of secretory diarrheas are those caused by abnormal hormonal secretion, such as metastatic carcinoid, in which a variety of vasoactive substances, including serotonin, histamine, and prostaglandin, are secreted by the tumor. Zollinger-Ellison syndrome, which is due to a gastrin-producing tumor, causes diarrhea in one-third of affected patients as a result of both high volumes of secreted hydrochloric acid and the maldigestion of fat caused by inactivation of pancreatic lipase. Other examples of secretory diarrheas include those caused by neoplasms such as pancreatic adenomas, villous adenomas, and medullary carcinoma of the thyroid. Systemic mastocytosis, which is seen with skin lesions typical of urticaria pigmentosa, is associated with diarrhea caused by histamine release from mast cells which have infiltrated the small intestine. The absence of a terminal ileum as a result of surgery or severe disease also causes secretory diarrhea through stimulation of colonic secretion by bile salts that have escaped absorption in a dysfunctional or absent terminal ileum. Somatostatinoma, a rare pancreatic tumor, causes steatorrhea, not intestinal secretion.

**VIII-68.**    **The answer is A.**  *(Chap. 43)*   Involuntary weight loss is almost always due to a serious condition. The three mechanisms of weight loss are increased energy expenditure (relatively rare), loss of energy in stool or urine, and decreased food intake. In young persons the most likely causes of weight loss are diabetes, hyperthyroidism, anorexia nervosa, and infection (particularly with human immunodeficiency virus). In older persons cancer is the most likely cause of weight loss, with psychiatric illness, including Alzheimer's disease and depression, being the second most important cause. A simple round of screening tests is recommended during the initial evaluation of a patient with significant weight loss. In the current case, the normal CBC and negative stool for occult blood loss suggest that upper or lower gastrointestinal endoscopy probably would not be useful. Since this patient has normal electrolytes, Addison's disease is also less likely, making the short ACTH test an inappropriate initial diagnostic study. Since the patient has no fever, blood cultures or bone marrow biopsy cultures are not likely to be revealing. Serum protein electrophoresis would be appropriate in the setting of anemia or abnormal protein excretion on urinalysis. An abdominal CT, which will provide a reasonable initial screen for pancreatic or gynecologic malignancies, is probably the best initial test in the case of occult weight loss in an older individual.

**VIII-69.**    **The answer is E.**  *(Chap. 41)*   Patients over age 50 should have an annual stool sample subjected to testing for hemoglobin peroxidase on a card test. A positive test and a subsequent workup could potentially detect colonic neoplasia at a curable stage. Multiple stools should be tested each year, ideally two samples from three stools. In addition to any cause of upper or lower GI bleeding, a false-positive test result can be due to the ingestion of dietary peroxidases, undercooked meat, or nonsteroidal anti-inflammatory agents or high doses of aspirin. The ingestion of over 500 mg of vitamin C may result in a false-negative test. The daily low dose of aspirin used to prevent cardiovascular disease generally does not lead to false-positive results.

**VIII-70.**    **The answer is B.**  *(Chap. 286)*   There are many similar manifestations of Crohn's disease (CD) and ulcerative colitis (UC). However, UC almost always displays continuous rather than the more segmental involvement characteristic of CD. UC rarely involves the entire bowel wall, whereas such transmural disease in CD can lead to abdominal masses, mesenteric node inflammation, and fistula formation. Since CD is much less likely to involve the rectum, hematochezia is less common than it is in UC. Extraintestinal manifestations, colonic malignancy, and toxic megalcolon can occur with either entity; a distinction between the two diseases can be made in about 80 percent of cases.

**VIII-71.**    **The answer is D.**  *(Chap. 288. Pras, N Engl J Med 326:1509, 1992.)*   Familial Mediterranean fever (FMF) is an inherited disorder linked to chromosome 16 and predominately occurring in Arabs, Armenians, and Sephardic Jews. The disease is characterized by recurrent episodes of fever, peritonitis, and/or pleuritis. Arthritis, skin lesions, and amyloidosis also are seen. An initial attack, especially if it is manifested by fever alone, can present a diagnostic dilemma; recurrent attacks in a person in the appropriate ethnic group make the diagnosis more straightforward. The greatest hazard is prolonged hospitalization with unnecessary tests. Chronic administration of colchicine reduces the number of attacks.

**VIII-72.**    **The answer is D.**  *(Chap. 281)*   As in most of internal medicine, a thorough clinical history is likely to yield important, if not essential, clues regarding the primary pathologic abnormality. Complaints of abdominal pain, distention, and stool frequency and type are very common. Abdominal pain is likely to be more serious if it is acute rather than chronic. The character of the pain, its location, and the exacerbating factors (especially those related to eating) must be elicited carefully. If a patient complains of diarrhea only during the day, it is much more likely to be functional than it would be if the diarrhea occurred at night or during both the day and the night. Blood loss is almost always suggestive of an organic cause, as is fever or weight loss. Crampy abdominal pain is relieved by defecation; it may well be due to a functional bowel syndrome. Either pellet-like stools or alternation of diarrhea and constipation is similarly compatible with functional bowel syndrome. However, a definite change in stool diameter suggests a colonic neoplasm. Stool characteristics also may be helpful historic features. For example, a pungent stool odor with the presence of undigested meat in the bowel movement may be suggestive of pancreatic insufficiency. White-colored stool signifies cholestasis or steatorrhea. Mucus mixed in with the stool is also suggestive of functional bowel syndromes, whereas pus is more likely to be found in association with an infection or inflammation.

**VIII-73.    The answer is A.**    *(Chap. 283)*    Although not every patient with heartburn requires upper endoscopy, indications include dysphagia, a structural mass or ulcer on contrast radiograph, and prolonged or persistent symptoms. This patient underwent appropriate esophagoscopy and was found to have Barrett's esophagus, a replacement of the distal squamous mucosa with columnar epithelium which is similar to the stomach lining both morphologically and functionally, being more resistant to digestion in a low-pH environment. This metaplastic epithelium is more likely to undergo malignant transformation and should be surveyed by repeat studies with biopsy every 12 to 24 months, particularly if dysplasia is present. Dilation would be appropriate if a benign stricture were noted.

**VIII-74.    The answer is E.**    *(Chap. 45)*    The patient's complaints are most likely not related to the abnormality in bilirubin metabolism suggested by the elevated concentration of total bilirubin. The patient has an elevation in the unconjugated, relatively water-insoluble albumin-bound form of bilirubin. The urine dipstick test would almost certainly be negative because bilirubin is excreted into the urine only in the conjugated form. For the unconjugated bilirubin level to rise, there must be either an overproduction of bilirubin, as in the case of hemolysis, or ineffective marrow production, impaired hepatic uptake of bilirubin, or impaired conjugation with glucuronide to allow for excretion. Given that the patient's CBC is normal, there is no evidence that she has hemolysis to account for overproduction. Moreover, the LDH and SGOT are normal, further supporting the lack of ongoing red cell destruction. Rare cases of drug-induced jaundice may be due to impaired hepatic uptake of bilirubin, but the remaining patients have impaired glucuronide conjugation resulting from a hereditary deficiency of the glucuronosyl enzyme. Neonatal jaundice, which occurs between the second and fifth days of life, is in fact due to a relatively low level of glucuronosyl transferase activity. There are three inherited deficiencies of this enzyme which can result in elevations of unconjugated serum bilirubin. This patient most likely has Gilbert's syndrome, which is associated with a mild decrease in enzyme activity and produces asymptomatic elevations in unconjugated hyperbilirubin. In Crigler-Najjar syndromes types II and I the enzyme is moderately diminished or totally absent. In the type I disorder childhood mortality from profound kernicterus-induced central nervous system dysfunction occurs. While impairments in glucuronosyl transferase activity also may be acquired, in most liver diseases bilirubin excretion is impaired to a greater degree than is bilirubin conjugation, leading primarily to conjugated hyperbilirubinemia. Therefore, in this patient's case no further testing is necessary.

**VIII-75.    The answer is D.**    *(Chap. 283. Klingenberg-Knoll, Ann Intern Med 121:161, 1994.)* The history is strongly suggestive of reflux esophagitis, given the heartburn and morning hoarseness. Patients also often complain of laryngitis and a bitter taste in the mouth. For mild cases a complete diagnostic workup which could include barium studies, esophagoscopy, and manometry usually is not required. Measures which help decrease reflux in uncomplicated patients include weight reduction, sleeping with the head of the bed elevated, and elimination of fatty foods, coffee, chocolate, alcohol, mint, orange juice, anticholinergic drugs, calcium channel blockers, and smooth muscle relaxants. Large quantities of fluids with meals should be avoided. In mild cases $H_2$-receptor antagonists such as cimetidine, ranitidine, and famotidine may suffice. Metaclopramide or cisapride, both of which are prokinetic agents, may be taken 30 min before meals and at bedtime. These drugs raise sphincter pressure and aid gastric emptying to provide esophageal clearance. In refractory cases, inhibiting the parietal cell pump responsible for acid secretion with omeprazole may be highly effective; the use of omeprazole should, however, be reserved until after the failure of more conservative measures.

**VIII-76.   The answer is C.** *(Chap. 284. Jensen, JAMA 271:1429, 1994.)* Zollinger-Ellison syndrome consists of ulcerative disease of the upper GI tract, marked increases in gastric acid secretion, and nonbeta islet cell tumors of the pancreas (gastrinomas). Gastrinomas generally occur as multiple tumors in the pancreatic head and are usually malignant, with one-third of these patients presenting with metastatic disease. Metastasis is most commonly found in the regional lymph nodes and liver. In 20 to 60 percent of those with Zollinger-Ellison syndrome the gastrinoma is a component of the multiple endocrine neoplasia syndrome type I. This is an autosomal dominant disorder which is linked to chromosomes 11 (q11 through q13). Patients with MEN type I have neoplasms of the parathyroid glands, pancreatic islets, and pituitary. In addition to gastrin, most gastrinomas secrete other hormones, including ACTH, glucagon, and vasoactive intestinal peptide. Clinical features of Zollinger-Ellison syndrome include persistent ulcers and elevated basal-acid output, often leading to diarrhea. The diagnosis of gastrinoma requires a demonstration of increased serum gastrin levels, which, if not above 1000 ng/L, may require a provocative test to demonstrate hypersecretion. In normal patients, secretin infusions would produce either no change or small reductions in the serum gastrin levels; however, Zollinger-Ellison patients routinely display a marked and prompt increase in serum gastrin after secretin injection.

**VIII-77.   The answer is A.** *(Chap. 284. Walsh, N Engl J Med 338:984, 1995.)* Although only 15 to 20 percent of people infected with the spiral-shaped gram-negative bacillus *H. pylori* will develop an ulcer, 95 to 100 percent of those with a documented duodenal ulcer can be shown to have *H. pylori* infection. Typically, the organism is found in the deep portion of the mucus gel; although bacteria may adhere to the luminal surfaces of the gastric epithelial cells, they do not invade the muscosa. It appears that the bacteria activate inflammatory cells which produce mucosal damage and release enzymes, such as proteases and phospholipases, which degrade the mucus gel layer. The prevalence of gastric colonization with *H. pylori* increases with age and with lower socioeconomic status. There are multiple ways to diagnose *H. pylori* infection, including histologic examination, culture, measurement of urease activity, and serologic studies. The most effective way to decrease the relapse rate for duodenal ulcer is to institute therapy that successfully eradicates *H. pylori*. The relapse rate is much higher if $H_2$-receptor antagonists are used alone. The most effective regimen for eradicating *H. pylori* is so-called triple therapy with bismuth, metronidazole, and either amoxicillin or tetracycline.

**VIII-78.   The answer is D.** *(Chap. 284)* The type of gastritis associated with pernicious anemia usually involves the fundus and the body of the stomach with relative sparing of the antrum. Patients with this type of gastritis typically have antibodies to parietal cells as well as thyroid antigens, hypoparathyroidism, Addison's disease, and vitiligo. Autoimmune features, however, are not invariably present, and some cases are associated with *H. pylori* infection. In this type of gastritis the reduction in gastric acid secretion is profound and results in a marked elevation in serum gastrin levels since the antrum, which has many gastrin-containing cells, is relatively spared. Given the pronounced hypergastrinemia in this syndrome, carcinoid tumors may develop.

**VIII-79.   The answer is D.** *(Chaps. 295, 301. Samuel, N Engl J Med 329:1842, 1993.)* Although most patients with acute viral hepatitis recover completely and a smaller proportion develop chronic hepatitis, death may occur in up to 2 to 3 percent because of fulminant hepatitis. This catastrophic event is seen primarily in patients affected with hepatitis B and/or D as well as hepatitis E. In addition to confusion, disorientation, and edema indicative of hepatic failure with encephalopathy, the liver usually shrinks and the prothrombin time is prolonged by a profound shutdown of hepatic protein synthesis. Since the mortality is high (over 80 percent in those who develop hepatic coma) yet all the extrahepatic manifestations are essentially reversible, liver transplantation may be lifesaving in the few patients for whom a suitable donor can be found in a timely fashion. If cerebral edema has already ensued, liver transplantation is probably inappropriate. Long-term prophylaxis with hepatitis B immunoglobulin (HBIG) is associated with a significant lowering of the risk of reinfection. Since long-term HBIG prophylaxis is cumbersome and expensive, alternatives are being explored, particularly the use of nucleoside analogues such as famcyclovir and lamivudine.

**VIII-80.  The answer is B.**  *(Chap. 296. Lee, N Engl J Med 333:1118, 1995.)*  Since the liver is responsible for the detoxification of numerous substances, it is not surprising that drug administration frequently results in hepatic abnormalities if not frank dysfunction. There are certain well-recognized patterns of hepatic damage secondary to therapeutic agents. For example, large doses of acetaminophen cause direct hepatotoxicity that is manifested pathologically by the development of central lobular necrosis. Isoniazid frequently causes a hypersensitivity-type liver pathology with findings similar to those seen in viral hepatitis; that is, there is often a mononuclear cell infiltrate. This pattern of injury also is seen with halothane, methyldopa, and a host of additional medicines. Fatty liver may occur in individuals taking tetracycline, sodium valproate, asparaginase, or alcohol. A cholestatic picture is seen with many different types of steroids, particularly oral contraceptive agents, and major tranquilizers such as chlorpromazine. Chlorpromazine causes cholestasis with portal inflammation, but this response is not seen with oral contraceptive use.

**VIII-81.  The answer is C.**  *(Chap. 297. Tong, N Engl J Med 332:1463, 1995.)*  Chronic hepatitis follows acute hepatitis C in 50 to 70 percent of cases. Many such cases are asymptomatic; however, this patient has symptoms including fatigue and pathologic findings of active disease that include bridging necrosis, both clearly risk factors for the eventual development of cirrhosis. Chronic hepatitis C tends to be very slowly and insidiously progressive in most patients. The course is worse in those who have a high level of hepatitis C as assessed by sensitive PCR-based detection methods. Curiously, patients with chronic hepatitis C often have autoantibodies to liver and muscle antigens, as is typical of patients with autoimmune hepatitis. Glucocorticoids are ineffective in treating chronic hepatitis C. As is the case for chronic hepatitis B infection, interferon-α is the treatment of choice. With prolonged treatment, a biochemical response is likely. In chronic hepatitis B patients treated with interferon there is often a transient elevation in aminotransferase activity; however, with chronic hepatitis C, transaminase levels drop precipitously. Responses occur within the first 3 months of therapy. Asymptomatic hepatitis C carriers with normal enzyme levels need not be treated.

**VIII-82.  The answer is C.**  *(Chap. 304. Steer, N Engl J Med 332:1482, 1995.)*  This patient has chronic pancreatitis requiring narcotic analgesia, based on historical features and CT revealing calcifications in the pancreas. Pain management for patients with chronic pancreatitis is fraught with the problems of chronic narcotic use. The attacks of abdominal pain in patients with chronic pancreatitis should be treated similarly to those of patients with acute pancreatitis. Alcohol should be avoided completely, as should large meals rich in fat. If a stricture of the pancreatic duct is demonstrated on ERCP, local resection may ameliorate the pain. Although such a finding is unusual, dealing in an anatomic fashion with patients who have such ductal obstruction can lead to long-term pain relief in about 50 percent. In some patients resection of most of the pancreas is required. Such radical surgery is contraindicated in those who are depressed or continue to drink alcohol. Furthermore, the cost of the pain relief achieved by surgery is pancreatic endocrine and exocrine insufficiency. Nonsurgical anatomic approaches such as sphincterotomy, dilatation of strictures, removal of calculi, and extension of the ventral or dorsal pancreatic duct are associated with significant complications and have not yet been shown to be definitively effective. Nonanatomic approaches include pancreatic enzyme treatment, diet restriction (moderate fat, high protein and carbohydrate, restriction of long-chain triglycerides), and non-narcotic analgesics. Although the cost of chronic pancreatitis to society is great, most patients do well with vigorous enzyme replacement therapy and abstention from alcohol.

**VIII-83.** **The answer is C.** *(Chap. 303)* The secretin test may be used to detect diffuse pancreatic disease. The secretin response of the pancreas is directly related to the functional mass of pancreatic tissue; therefore, failure to secrete adequate amounts of bicarbonate-containing fluid and/or pancreatic enzymes indicates some degree of pancreatic insufficiency. In patients with early chronic pancreatitis the bicarbonate output is usually low, without a concomitant severe drop in enzyme levels. The test involves the administration of secretin and cholecystokinin, followed by the collection and measurement of duodenal contents. The contents are assayed for the volume of output and bicarbonate content as well as for pancreatic amylase, lipase, trypsin, and chymotrypsin. The pancreas has a great reserve of enzyme secretion ability; intraluminal lipolytic and other digestive functions require only small amounts of enzymes. Consequently, patients with chronic pancreatitis often have low outputs of bicarbonate after secretin while still having normal fecal fat excretion. Steatorrhea occurs only in the setting of markedly low intraluminal levels of pancreatic lipase. Since the normal secretin-CCK test permits only the identification of chronic pancreatic damage, it cannot distinguish between chronic pancreatitis and pancreatic carcinoma, which usually does not produce a major loss of exocrine pancreatic function.

**VIII-84.** **The answer is D.** *(Chap. 302)* Complications of gallstones include acute cholecystitis, biliary colic, gallstone ileus, fistula formation, porcelain gallbladder caused by calcium and salt deposition in the wall, and stones in the common bile duct, which occur in 10 to 15 percent of these patients. Occult duct stones remain behind after approximately 1 to 5 percent of cholecystectomies. Occasionally, primary stones can arise in the ducts in the setting of pigment stones or congenital abnormalities.

Patients with acute cholangitis have biliary colic, jaundice, and spiking fevers with chills (so-called Charcot's triad). Many patients with this condition respond rapidly to supportive measures, including antibiotics; however, in the case of supperative acute cholangitis a completely obstructive ductal system can lead to profound illness, including circulatory collapse. Since most patients who have biliary obstruction caused by duct stones have associated chronic cholecystitis, the gallbladder is relatively indistensible. Therefore, the presence of a palpable gallbladder (Courvoisier's sign) suggests carcinoma of the pancreas. The most appropriate diagnostic study for choledocholithiasis is cholangiography, usually by preoperative ERCP with endoscopic papillotomy and stone extraction, which is now considered the preferred approach compared with laparotomy. Laparascopic cholestectomy can be combined with ERCP to treat the entire problem and reduce the incidence of complicated biliary tract disease with the need for choledocholithotomy and T-tube drainage.

**VIII-85.** **The answer is A-Y, B-N, C-Y, D-Y, E-N.** *(Chap. 295)* The diagnosis of acute hepatitis B infection can be made through the detection of HBsAg in serum unless there is the simultaneous presence of anti-HBc IgG, which indicates chronic infection. The only exception to the latter rule is in the case of late acute (or early chronic) infection when anti-HBe is present as well as HBsAg and the anti-HBcAg has already been converted from IgM to IgG. HBeAg is a marker of infectivity in acute or chronic infection. Positivity for both IgG anti-HBcAg and anti-HBsAg indicates recovery from prior infection (anti-HBeAg may be positive or negative in this case). An additional caveat is the relatively uncommon situation during acute infection when the level of HBsAg is too low to be detected but the presence of anti-HBcAg IgM establishes the diagnosis (the "anti-HBc window"). Recovery from prior infection is denoted by the appearance of anti-HBs (also seen after vaccination).

# IX. HEMATOPOIETIC DISORDERS AND NEOPLASIA

## *QUESTIONS*

**DIRECTIONS:** Each question below contains five suggested responses. Choose the **one best** response to each question.

**IX-1.** All the following conditions impair the release of oxygen to body tissues EXCEPT

(A) methemoglobinemia
(B) carbon monoxide poisoning
(C) hyperventilation
(D) hypothermia
(E) acidosis

**IX-2.** A 70-year-old man of Irish descent returns to his physician for a routine check of his blood pressure. He is a vigorous, retired executive who except for mild hypertension is healthy. After his examination, as he is getting dressed, he states that his wife has been nagging him to mention a spot on his nose (as shown in Plate C). He is certain that this lesion, which has been present for several years, is of no significance. The most likely diagnosis for this lesion is

(A) dermal nevus
(B) sebaceous hyperplasia
(C) clear cell acanthoma
(D) xanthoma
(E) basal cell carcinoma

**IX-3.** A 52-year-old woman sees her physician for an "insurance physical." Physical examination reveals only a pigmented lesion (as shown in Plate D) present on one foot. The woman states that the lesion apparently was present at birth and does not itch or bleed; it is, however, not as homogeneous in color as it used to be. Which of the following statements about the condition described is true?

(A) Bleeding and tenderness would be the first signs of malignant degeneration
(B) It is unlikely that the lesion, present since birth, is malignant
(C) The diagnostic procedure of choice is an incisional biopsy of this lesion
(D) Change in color of the lesion is a suspicious sign for potential malignancy
(E) Early diagnosis of this lesion would not affect prognosis

**IX-4.** A 58-year-old man presents with fatigue. His physical examination is normal except for the presence of splenomegaly. CBC discloses hematocrit, 29 percent; platelet count, 90,000/$\mu$L; WBC, 2700/$\mu$L; and an essentially normal red cell morphology (differential 12 percent monocytes, 12 percent granulocytes, and 76 percent lymphocytes). A bone marrow aspirate and biopsy were performed. The aspirate was dry and the biopsy is pending. Based on the available information, the most likely diagnosis in this case is

(A) chronic lymphocytic leukemia
(B) hairy cell leukemia
(C) chronic myeloid leukemia
(D) myelofibrosis
(E) multiple myeloma

**IX-5.** A 58-year-old chronic alcoholic and heavy smoker presents with a 3-cm, firm, right midcervical neck mass. An excisional biopsy reveals squamous cell carcinoma. Which of the following is the most appropriate approach at this time?

(A) Bronchoscopy, esophagoscopy, and laryngoscopy
(B) CT of the neck
(C) CT of the brain
(D) Neck dissection
(E) Radiation therapy

**IX-6.** A 28-year-old man with newly diagnosed acute myelogenous leukemia spikes a temperature to 38.7°C (101.7°F) on the sixth day of induction therapy. He feels well and has no physical complaints. His only medicine is intravenous cytosine arabinoside, 140 mg every 12 h. Physical examination is unrevealing. His white blood count is 900/μL, of which 10 percent are granulocytes and the rest mostly lymphocytes; platelet count is 24,000/μL. Findings on chest x-ray and urinalysis are normal.

After obtaining appropriate cultures, the man's physician should

(A) observe closely for the development of a clinically evident source of fever
(B) begin antibiotic therapy with gentamicin and mezlocillin
(C) begin granulocyte transfusion and antibiotic therapy with gentamicin and mezlocillin
(D) begin gammaglobulin treatment and antibiotic therapy with gentamicin and mezlocillin
(E) begin antibiotic therapy with amphotericin, gentamicin, and mezlocillin

**IX-7.** Coumarin-induced skin necrosis is occasionally associated with the institution of oral anticoagulants in patients with

(A) antithrombin III deficiency
(B) protein C deficiency
(C) factor VIII deficiency
(D) plasminogen deficiency
(E) dysfibrinogenemias

**IX-8.** A 55-year-old woman presents to the emergency department because her family notes that she has yellow skin. The patient has lost 15 lbs over the past 3 months, but states that this is because she has been dieting in preparation for her daughter's wedding. Her past medical history is significant only for vitiligo. Her physical examination is unremarkable except for the presence of scleral icterus and a yellow tinge to the skin. Laboratory evaluation reveals hematocrit of 17 percent, WBC count of 2500/μL, and platelet count of 70,000/μL. Serum chemistries are normal except for direct bilirubin of 51 μmol/L (3 mg/dL) and indirect bilirubin of 12 μmol/L (0.7 mg/dL). The patient's reticulocyte count is 3 percent. MCV is 108 fL. Which one of the following additional laboratory findings would most likely be associated with this patient's clinical syndrome?

(A) Clonal chromosomal abnormalities on karyotypic analysis of the bone marrow
(B) Positive direct Coombs' test
(C) Extrahepatic biliary obstruction
(D) Decreased gastric fluid pH
(E) Antiparietal cell antibody

**IX-9.** All the following hereditary syndromes are associated with the development of malignancies EXCEPT

(A) neurofibromatosis
(B) chronic granulomatous disease of childhood
(C) ataxia-telangiectasia
(D) familial polyposis coli
(E) Fanconi's anemia

**IX-10.** A 27-year-old woman presents with stage II (breast and lymph node involvement) right breast cancer. Her family history is markedly positive for other tumors. One of her sisters developed an osteogenic sarcoma at age 17, her brother was diagnosed with acute leukemia at age 5, her mother died of breast cancer, and she has two uncles with soft-tissue sarcomas, both developing this disease when in their thirties. This patient's peripheral blood lymphocytes would be most likely to reveal which of the following abnormalities?

(A) Retinoblastoma gene mutation
(B) p53 gene mutation
(C) Translocation between chromosomes 9 and 22
(D) Translocation between chromosomes 8 and 14
(E) Mutations of epidermal growth factor receptor gene

**IX-11.** A patient with a myelodysplastic syndrome (subtype, refractory anemia with ringed sideroblasts) has been transfusion-dependent for the past 2 years. The patient has received a total of 50 units of packed red blood cells. His physical examination is normal except for hyperpigmentation. Laboratory evaluation reveals mild glucose intolerance. A trial of erythropoietin was unsuccessful. Which of the following would be the most important therapeutic approach at this time?

(A) Granulocyte colony-stimulating factor
(B) Phlebotomy
(C) Ascorbic acid
(D) Desferrioxamine
(E) Hypertransfusion (maintain hematocrit at 40 percent)

**IX-12.** A 26-year-old woman has painful mouth ulcers. Six weeks ago, she was started on propylthiouracil for hyperthyroidism. She is afebrile, and physical examination is unremarkable except for several small oral aphthous ulcers. White blood cell count is 200/μL (15 percent neutrophils, 80 percent lymphocytes, 5 percent monocytes); hemoglobin concentration, hematocrit, and platelet count are normal. The woman's physician should stop the propylthiouracil and

(A) schedule a follow-up outpatient appointment
(B) arrange for HLA typing of her siblings in preparation for bone marrow transplantation
(C) prescribe oral prednisone, 1 mg/kg
(D) hospitalize her for broad-spectrum antibiotic therapy
(E) hospitalize her for white blood cell transfusion

**IX-13.** An 18-year-old black man undergoing a physical examination prior to playing college sports is found to have a normal CBC except that the MCV is 72 fL. Subsequent testing reveals a normal metabisulfite test and a normal hemoglobin electrophoresis. Which of the following conditions most likely accounts for these findings?

(A) Hemoglobin E trait
(B) Sickle C disease
(C) Sickle β thalassemia
(D) β-thalassemia trait
(E) α-thalassemia trait

**IX-14.** A 30-year-old black woman with long-standing sickle cell anemia presents with severe pain in the chest and abdomen approximately 1 week after having an upper respiratory infection. No intrathoracic or intra-abdominal pathology was immediately obvious on routine physical examination and laboratory evaluation. The most appropriate therapeutic intervention at this point is

(A) hypertransfusion
(B) hydration and narcotic analgesia
(C) hydroxyurea
(D) broad-spectrum antibiotics
(E) exploratory laparotomy

**IX-15.** In persons who have chronic myelogenous leukemia, the translocation that accounts for the Philadelphia chromosome most commonly is found in

(A) all cells of the body
(B) all three hematopoietic cell lines but not in nonhematopoietic cells
(C) all cells of the granulocytic cell line but not in nongranulocytic cells
(D) all bone marrow stem cells but not in mature cells
(E) all bone marrow stem cells and certain mature granulocytes

**IX-16.** Which of the following statements describes the relationship between testicular tumors and serum markers?

(A) Pure seminomas produce α-fetoprotein (AFP) or β-human chorionic gonadotropin (β-hCG) in more than 90 percent of cases
(B) More than 40 percent of nonseminomatous germ cell tumors produce no cell markers
(C) Both β-hCG and AFP should be measured in following the progress of a tumor
(D) Measurement of tumor markers the day following surgery for localized disease is useful in determining completeness of the resection
(E) β-hCG is limited in its usefulness as a marker, because it is identical to human luteinizing hormone

**IX-17.** A 45-year-old man presents with fatigue. Two years ago the patient received six cycles of combination chemotherapy (each cycle consisted of cyclophosphamide, doxorubicin, vincristine, and prednisone) for non-Hodgkin's lymphoma in chest and abdominal sites. The patient entered complete remission and has been followed expectantly since that point. His last prior visit was 3 months ago at which time he had no evidence of recurrent lymphoma, felt well, and had a normal laboratory examination. At this time his physical examination is remarkable for a purple discoloration of the fingertips, ears, and nose. The patient is somewhat pale. There is no evidence for peripheral lymphadenopathy. Laboratory studies include the following: white count 10,000/μL (differential 60 percent neutrophils, 10 percent bands, 10 percent lymphocytes, 10 percent monocytes, 3 percent eosinophils, 1 percent basophils, 2 percent metamyelocytes, 1 percent myelocytes, and 1 percent nucleated red blood cell), hematocrit 28 percent, and platelet count 300,000/μL. The following results are also found: MCV 98 fL, lactic dehydrogenase 6.8 μkat/L (400 U/L), total bilirubin 51 μmol/L (3.0 mg/dL), and direct bilirubin 5.1 μmol/L (0.3 mg/dL). Review of the peripheral blood smear reveals clumped red cells. A routine direct Coombs' test is negative. Additional laboratory testing would most likely reveal

(A) positive direct Coombs' test (using anti-IgG antisera) if specimen is processed without allowing cooling
(B) positive indirect Coombs' test detected with anti-IgG antibodies
(C) circulating antibodies against Epstein-Barr virus
(D) circulating antibodies against fetal red blood cells
(E) circulating antibodies against *Mycoplasma pneumoniae*

**IX-18.** A 50-year-old woman presents with bleeding gums. Other than petechiae, her physical examination is normal. She has not had any recent infections, nor has she been exposed to any drugs or industrial solvents. Hematologic laboratory values are as follows: hemoglobin 80 g/L (8 g/dL), hematocrit 24 percent, mean corpuscular volume (MCV) 101 fL, reticulocyte count 0.5 percent, WBC count 1500/μL (10 percent neutrophils), and platelet count 18,000/μL. Bone marrow examination is remarkable for a dry aspirate and a biopsy that discloses a severely hypocellular marrow with 90 percent fat infiltration. The remaining scant hematopoietic elements do not appear to be dysplastic. Further laboratory studies reveal the lack of antinuclear antibodies, normal sugar water and acid hemolysis tests, normal vitamin B$_{12}$ levels, normal serum folate levels, and no evidence of antibodies to HIV.

The patient is placed on nandrolone decanoate for a period of 6 months without response. Which of the following is the most appropriate therapeutic approach at this time?

(A) Plasmapheresis
(B) Splenectomy
(C) Equine antithymocyte serum
(D) Erythropoietin
(E) Daunorubicin and cytosine arabinoside combination chemotherapy

**IX-19.** A 25-year-old, previously healthy woman presents with jaundice, confusion, and fever. Initial physical examination is unremarkable except for scattered petechiae on the lower extremities, scleral icterus, and disorientation on mental status examination. Laboratory examination discloses the following: hematocrit, 27 percent; white cell count, 12,000/μL; platelet count, 10,000/μL; bilirubin, 85 μmol/L (5 mg/dL); direct bilirubin, 10 μmol/L (0.6 mg/dL); urea nitrogen, 21 mmol/L (60 mg/dL); creatinine, 400 μmol/L (4.5 mg/dL). Red blood cell smear discloses fragmented red blood cells and nucleated red blood cells. Prothrombin, thrombin, and partial thromboplastin times are all normal.

The most effective and appropriate therapeutic maneuver is likely to be

(A) plasmapheresis
(B) administration of aspirin
(C) administration of high-dose glucocorticoids
(D) administration of high-dose glucocorticoids plus cyclophosphamide
(E) splenectomy

**IX-20.** A 38-year-old woman presents with redness and burning in the distal extremities. She has no other complaints. She has never been pregnant. Physical examination is normal except for redness of the fingertips and splenomegaly. Laboratory examination reveals hematocrit 40 percent, WBC count 9000 with a normal differential, and platelet count of 950,000/μL. Other laboratory studies include reticulocyte count of 1 percent, bone marrow examination that discloses a hypercellular marrow with megakaryocytic hyperplasia and hyperlobated megakaryocytes, absent collagen deposition, and the presence of normal amounts of bone marrow iron. Cytogenetic studies reveal a normal female karyotype. A red cell mass study is normal. Which of the following statements concerning the patient's condition is true?

(A) Observation is indicated
(B) Splenectomy should be performed
(C) Oral administration of chlorambucil, 0.4 mg/kg daily for 5 days, should begin
(D) Aspirin, 2 tablets every 6 h, should be administered
(E) Hydroxyurea, 1000 mg daily orally, is indicated

**IX-21.** A 42-year-old woman presents with epistaxis and gum bleeding. Physical examination is remarkable for a temperature of 38°C (100.4°F) and petechiae on the lower extremities. Laboratory evaluation includes a hematocrit of 29 percent, platelet count of 15,000/μL, and WBC of 2100/μL (differential including 22 percent blasts, 30 percent promyelocytes, 20 percent lymphocytes, 10 percent monocytes, 2 percent myelocytes and 3 percent metamyelocytes). PT is 15 s and PTT is 55 s. Bone marrow examination discloses a hypercellular marrow infiltrated with myeloblasts and heavily granulated promyelocytes. Myeloperoxidase stain of a bone marrow aspirate smear is markedly positive and demonstrates numerous intracellular rodlike forms. The patient is begun on all-*trans* retinoic acid. Which of the following is the most likely complication of this therapy?

(A) Worsening of disseminated intravascular coagulopathy
(B) Infection during neutropenia
(C) Respiratory distress
(D) Uric acid nephropathy
(E) Mucositis

**IX-22.** All the following statements regarding toxic effects of chemotherapy are correct EXCEPT

(A) of all the antineoplastic agents, anthracyclines suppress bone marrow stem cells to the greatest degree
(B) vincristine is a relatively weak myelosuppressive agent and can be administered during periods of low blood counts
(C) cisplatin-induced nausea and vomiting can usually be controlled by metoclopramide or dexamethasone or both
(D) the use of melphalan (phenylalanine mustard) has been associated with secondary leukemia
(E) cisplatin can produce hypocalcemia by inducing renal electrolyte wasting

**IX-23.** A 45-year-old man develops leukocytosis and fatigue. Workup reveals infiltration of the bone marrow with lymphoblasts. A sample of bone marrow is also sent for immunologic and cytogenetic analysis. Which of the following findings would be associated with the best prognosis?

(A) Common acute lymphocytic leukemia antigen (CALLA) CD10 positivity, normal cytogenetics
(B) CALLA CD10 positivity, t(9;22)
(C) Surface immunoglobulin positivity, t(8;14)
(D) My10 (CD34) positivity, normal cytogenetics
(E) My7 (CD13) positivity, t(4;11) translocation

**IX-24.** Two years ago a 68-year-old man was found to have a prostate nodule on routine examination. Biopsy revealed poorly differentiated prostatic adenocarcinoma; staging studies failed to reveal any evidence of extraprostatic spread. Because of a desire to maintain potency, the patient opted for radiation therapy as primary treatment. Except for requiring lower extremity revascularization for intractable claudication, he did well until recently, when he developed pain in his right hip. Prostate specific antigen was elevated. Bone scan revealed areas of positive uptake in the pelvis and ribs (not present on the original staging study). The patient expresses a desire not to have a bilateral orchiectomy, "unless it would significantly improve my quality of life or survival compared with other therapies."

The most appropriate strategy at this point is to

(A) biopsy one of the bony lesions
(B) administer cisplatin and 5-fluorouracil
(C) administer leuprolide and flutamide
(D) administer diethylstilbestrol (DES) at low dose
(E) perform an orchiectomy

**IX-25.** All of the following findings would help to distinguish β-thalassemia trait from iron deficiency EXCEPT

(A) microcytic red blood cells
(B) presence of anemia
(C) elevated hemoglobin A2 level
(D) normal transferrin saturation
(E) normal serum ferritin concentration

**IX-26.** Adhesion of platelets to walls of injured blood vessels involves all of the following EXCEPT

(A) collagen
(B) platelet glycoprotein Ia-IIa
(C) platelet glycoprotein Ib-IX
(D) platelet glycoprotein IIb-IIIa
(E) von Willebrand factor

**IX-27.** A patient being treated for refractory anemia has required monthly transfusions of 2 units of packed red blood cells over the past several months. Three days after receiving 2 units of packed red blood cells for a hematocrit of 22 percent, the patient's hematocrit was 27 percent. One week after the transfusion the hematocrit is 22 percent; the patient feels ill, has a low-grade fever, and is mildly jaundiced. Which of the following statements about this situation is incorrect?

(A) This problem is probably due to alloantibodies
(B) Intravascular hemolysis has probably occurred
(C) The Rh status of donor and recipient should be rechecked
(D) If the patient is Rh-negative, one should look for anti-Kell or anti-Duffy antibodies in the patient's serum
(E) A positive direct Coombs' test is likely

**IX-28.** True statements regarding both hemophilia A (factor VIII deficiency) and hemophilia B (factor IX deficiency) include all of the following EXCEPT

(A) the defective gene is located on the X chromosome
(B) the affected factors require vitamin K for biologic activity
(C) the partial thromboplastin time is elevated, but the prothrombin time is normal
(D) joint bleeding is common
(E) the optimal therapy is replacement with recombinant factors

**IX-29.** True statements regarding ovarian cancer include all of the following EXCEPT

(A) most patients require a surgical debulking procedure
(B) nulliparity is a risk factor
(C) a history of breast cancer is a risk factor
(D) stromal cell and germ cell tumors of the ovary are the most common histologic subtypes
(E) histologic grade is an important prognostic factor

**IX-30.** All of the following factors will influence the frequency of dissemination of cutaneous malignant melanoma EXCEPT

(A) primary tumor site
(B) dermatologic level of invasion
(C) thickness of the primary lesion
(D) geographic area of residence
(E) presence of microscopic tumor satellites

**IX-31.** Correct statements regarding carcinoma of the prostate include all of the following EXCEPT

(A) histologic grade is an important prognostic indicator
(B) most prostate cancers arise from the transitional cell epithelium
(C) cancer of the prostate is the most common malignancy in men
(D) cancer of the prostate may spread hematogenously, via lymphatics, or by direct extension
(E) most cases are clinically occult

**IX-32.** Stable-phase chronic myelogenous leukemia (CML) is associated with all of the following EXCEPT

(A) splenomegaly
(B) basophilia
(C) low leukocyte alkaline phosphatase
(D) diagnostic bone marrow findings
(E) favorable response to interferon-α

**IX-33.** Characteristics of dysplastic nevi include all of the following EXCEPT

(A) dysplastic nevi serve only as markers for the risk of melanoma; melanomas arise only in apparently normal skin
(B) dysplastic nevi tend to have a varied appearance in a given individual
(C) dysplastic nevi are usually more than 6 mm in diameter
(D) if two family members have melanoma, there is a 50 percent risk of developing melanoma in the patient with dysplastic nevi
(E) patients commonly have nevi on areas not exposed to the sun

**IX-34.** Correct statements concerning the hereditary polyposis syndromes include all the following EXCEPT

(A) Gardner's syndrome is characterized by multiple hamartomatous polyps in the large and small intestines

(B) in Peutz-Jeghers syndrome adenomatous polyps in the large and small intestine have a low rate of malignant degeneration

(C) Turcot's syndrome is similar to familial colonic polyposis except that malignant brain tumors frequently accompany the polyposis

(D) familial colonic polyposis is inherited in an autosomal dominant fashion

(E) patients with familial colonic polyposis have a 100 percent incidence of colon cancer by age 40

**IX-35.** Each condition listed below is associated with an increased risk of cancer of the esophagus. Which one is most closely linked to adenocarcinoma of the esophagus?

(A) Achalasia

(B) Smoking

(C) Barrett's esophagus

(D) Tylosis

(E) Alcoholism

**IX-36.** A 59-year-old man presents with fatigue, epigastric pain, early satiety, and iron-deficiency anemia. Upper gastrointestinal endoscopy reveals diffuse thickening throughout the stomach with some extension into the duodenum. Biopsy is undertaken. Review of the specimen reveals infiltration with malignant-appearing lymphocytes. Which of the following statements concerning the current situation is correct?

(A) The patient has a greater than average likelihood of having blood group A

(B) The patient should receive combination chemotherapy with 5-fluorouracil, doxorubicin, and mitomycin C

(C) The prognosis would have been better if the biopsy had revealed neoplastic signet-ring cells

(D) Chemotherapy is absolutely contraindicated because of the risk of bleeding and perforation

(E) Immunoperoxidase studies probably would reveal evidence of B-cell derivation

**IX-37.** Which of the following statements concerning screening for colorectal cancer is correct?

(A) Patients who have a positive fecal Hemoccult test while on a low-meat diet are likely to have colorectal carcinoma

(B) The vast majority of patients with documented colorectal cancers have a positive fecal Hemoccult test

(C) No randomized studies of Hemoccult screening have documented a significant reduction in mortality from colorectal cancer in annually screened persons

(D) Present American Cancer Society recommendations include Hemoccult screening beginning at age 50 and sigmoidoscopic examination every 3 to 5 years beginning at age 50 for persons at average risk

(E) Rehydration of Hemoccult slides has no effect on the positivity rate

**IX-38.** A 53-year-old man with rectal bleeding was found to have adenocarcinoma 2 cm below the peritoneal reflection. After a negative metastatic workup, the patient underwent resection of the tumor with primary reanastomosis. Pathologic examination revealed a moderately well-differentiated adenocarcinoma of the rectum with 2 of 10 adjacent lymph nodes that contained cancer. The patient has no other medical problems. Optimal therapy at this point should include

(A) pelvic radiation therapy alone

(B) a chemotherapy regimen containing 5-fluorouracil

(C) a combination of pelvic irradiation and a chemotherapy regimen containing 5-fluorouracil

(D) a chemotherapy regimen containing 5-fluorouracil plus levamisole

(E) observation alone

**IX-39.** All the following are risk factors for the development of cancer of the colon EXCEPT

(A) Crohn's colitis

(B) adenomatous polyps

(C) uterosigmoidostomy

(D) ulcerative colitis

(E) juvenile polyposis

**IX-40.** A 50-year-old man with a history of organomegaly and an elevated hematocrit without an apparent secondary cause was well until the sudden onset of pain in the right upper quadrant. On examination the patient is afebrile and has clear lungs, normal cardiac function, an abdominal fluid wave, splenomegaly, and a markedly enlarged liver with a palpable, very tender edge. Liver function tests are normal except for mild elevation of hepatic transaminases. Which of the following is the most appropriate procedure for the purposes of establishing a diagnosis?

(A) CT scan of the liver
(B) Abdominal ultrasound
(C) Radionuclide liver-spleen scan
(D) Hepatic venography
(E) Paracentesis

**IX-41.** A 65-year-old man with long-standing, stable biopsy-proven postnecrotic cirrhosis develops abdominal pain in the right upper quadrant and abdominal swelling. He is afebrile. Palmar erythema, spider telangiectasias, and mild jaundice are noted on physical examination. His abdomen is distended, shifting dullness is present, a tender, firm liver edge is felt 3 fingerbreadths below the right costal margin, and a spleen tip is palpable. A faint bruit is heard over the liver. Laboratory values include the following:

Hematocrit: 34 percent
White blood cell count: 4300/$\mu$L
Platelet count: 104,000/$\mu$L
Serum albumin: 26 g/L (2.6 g/dL)
Serum globulins: 46 g/L (4.6 g/dL)
Alkaline phosphatase: 8.0 $\mu$kat/L (480 U/L)

Paracentesis reveals blood-tinged fluid. The serum marker most specifically associated with this man's condition is

(A) antinuclear antibody
(B) alpha fetoprotein
(C) antimitochondrial antibody
(D) 5'-nucleotidase
(E) chorionic gonadotropin

**IX-42.** A 53-year-old black female presents with fatigue. Her CBC reveals a hematocrit of 30 percent, white count of 4,000/$\mu$L with a normal differential, and platelet count of 190,000. Her MCV is 89 and her reticulocyte count is 1.2 percent. Physical examination is unremarkable; specifically, occult blood testing on her stool is negative on several occasions. Iron studies are normal. Examination of the peripheral blood smear is essentially unremarkable. Bone marrow examination discloses infiltration with plasma cells which account for about 30 percent of the total nucleated cells. All of the following tests represent reasonable additional studies to be done at this time EXCEPT

(A) $\beta_2$-microglobulin
(B) 24-h urine protein determination
(C) bone scan
(D) serum protein electrophoresis
(E) skeletal survey

**IX-43.** A 73-year-old female with known myelodysplastic syndrome and chronic anemia has required multiple transfusions over the past several months. She now presents with profound fatigue and a hematocrit of 20 percent. Two units of blood are ordered, but the blood component lab informs you that they expect at least a day before a product will be ready for the patient. The most likely explanation for this problem in finding appropriate blood for transfusional therapy in this patient is

(A) presence of allo-antibodies in the patient's serum
(B) presence of autoantibodies in the patient's serum
(C) rare blood group
(D) careful screening necessary in myelodysplasia patients to prevent blood-born infection.
(E) anti-HLA antibodies in the patient's serum

**IX-44.** A 35-year-old female develops hirsutism, deepening voice, and clitorimegaly. A pelvic examination reveals a left ovarian mass. Assuming appropriate diagnostic and staging tests are performed, given this clinical presentation, if the patient requires chemotherapy she should be treated in a fashion analogous to the management of

(A) epithelial ovarian cancer
(B) lymphoma
(C) testicular cancer
(D) soft tissue sarcoma
(E) carcinoid tumor

**IX-45.** A 65-year-old female presents with severe pelvic pain with radiation down both legs. There is no evidence of a sensory level. Physical examination is unremarkable except for a colostomy in the right lower quadrant. There is a history of an abdominal-perineal resection for rectal cancer three years ago. Post-operatively she received pelvic irradiation and adjuvant chemotherapy with 5-FU. The most likely cause for this patient's pain is

(A) pelvic recurrence of rectal cancer
(B) bony metastasis
(C) secondary leukemia with bone pain
(D) post-radiation radiculitis
(E) sciatic nerve inflammation

**IX-46.** All of the following are distinguishing features of small cell lung cancer compared to non-small cell lung cancer EXCEPT

(A) small cell lung cancer is more radiosensitive
(B) small cell lung cancer is more chemosensitive
(C) small cell lung cancer is more likely to present peripherally in the lung
(D) small cell lung cancer is derived from neuro-endocrine tissues
(E) for patients who are being treated with curative intent, small cell lung cancer patients virtually always require radiation therapy

**IX-47.** A 43-year-old female presents with an hematocrit of 25 percent, an MCV of 101, reticulocyte count of 1.2 percent, platelet count of 25,000/$\mu$L, and white count of 2300/$\mu$L with 25 percent neutrophils.

Non-Hodgkin's lymphoma was diagnosed six years ago. At that time she presented with diffuse large cell lymphoma in abdominal and cervical lymph nodes. She underwent six cycles of cyclophosphamide, doxorubicin, vincristine, and prednisone chemotherapy followed by a disease-free interval of six months at which point she relapsed. She then received three additional cycles of identical chemotherapy. Because of persistent abnormal nodes, she then received four cycles of chemotherapy consisting of etoposide, ara-C, cisplatin, and methylprednisolone. She achieved a remission followed by consolidation therapy with high-dose cyclophosphamide and total body radiation with autologous marrow. She tolerated the transplant well (which was carried out approximately two years ago) and was working until her current presentation with fatigue. Serum chemistries at this time are normal. Her blood smear reveals a dimorphic population of red cells, diminished numbers of platelets, and a paucity of white cells; some of the neutrophils are bi-lobed. A bone marrow examination is performed. Given the above facts, which of the following is the most likely result?

(A) Hypolobated megakaryocytes, megaloblastic erythroid precursors, and excessive number of immature myeloid cells
(B) A marked increase in the ratio of fat to cells
(C) Foci of immature lymphoid cells
(D) Erythroid hypoplasia
(E) Normal-appearing bone marrow

**IX-48.** A 65-year-old male presents with cervical adenopathy and night sweats. Further work-up reveals a moderately large mediastinal mass and diffuse abdominal periaortic adenopathy on abdominal/pelvic computed tomogram. Bilateral bone marrow biopsies fail to disclose tumor. Cervical lymph node biopsy discloses infiltration with moderately immature-appearing lymphoid cells. Immunophenotypic studies performed on these cells obtained from the biopsied node reveals expression of the following antigens: CD19, CD20, and CD5, CD23 is absent. Cytogenetic studies showed a t(11;14) translocation. The patient's CBC is normal. The most likely diagnosis in this case is

(A) hairy cell leukemia
(B) small lymphocytic lymphoma
(C) diffuse large cell lymphoma
(D) mantle cell lymphoma
(E) acute lymphoblastic leukemia

**IX-49.** All of the following represent clinicopathologic associations EXCEPT

(A) acute monoblastic leukemia and gum infiltration

(B) acute promyelocytic leukemia and bleeding

(C) acute lymphoblastic leukemia (T-cell type) and mediastinal mass

(D) L3 acute lymphoblastic leukemia and CNS involvement

(E) acute megakaryoblastic leukemia and polyneuropathy

**IX-50.** A patient with stable phase chronic myeloid leukemia is being managed with α-interferon therapy. After having done well for two years, he now presents with an increasingly left shifted white cell differential on blood smear. Bone marrow examination shows a hypercellular marrow with increased numbers of basophils. Cytogenetic analysis reveals that there are two Philadelphia chromosomes per cell. The most likely explanation for this cytogenetic change is

(A) interferon effect

(B) accelerated or blastic phase

(C) diagnosis actually agnogenic myeloid metaplasia/myelofibrosis

(D) error in interpretation of cytogenetic result

(E) favorable prognostic sign

**IX-51.** The American Cancer Society recommends that men age 50 and over have prostate-specific antigen determination annually; however, the United States Preventative Services Task Force recommends against such studies. Each of the following statements represents a valid argument against annual prostate-specific antigen measurement EXCEPT

(A) Randomized studies have not yet shown a survival benefit for patients who are screened compared to those who are unscreened

(B) Early unimportant tumors may be detected in the screening group

(C) Screening may lead to net harm

(D) Most tumors are surgically incurable at the time of detection

(E) PSA screening may not lead to a change in the natural history of prostate cancer, but rather make it appear that life is prolonged after screening due to lead time bias

**IX-52.** A 68-year-old female with metastatic breast cancer with a pleural effusion and multiple bony metastases complains of moderately severe pain in the area of her left clavicle and right femur. She has already received radiation therapy to these areas, and plain x-ray of the leg reveals that there is little danger of a pathologic fracture. The patient's current medicines include amitriptyline, oxycodone 30 mg every 3 to 4 h, and acetaminophen 650 mg every 4 h. Which of the following is the best therapy at this point?

(A) Addition of morphine 30 mg every 4 h

(B) Morphine sulfate intravenous drip 1 mg/h

(C) Nerve block

(D) Substitute subcutaneous meperidine 50 mg every 3 h for the oxycodone

(E) Substitute controlled-release morphine 60 to 120 mg twice a day in place of the oxycodone

**IX-53.** Mutations in the retinoblastoma gene cause cancer by

(A) constitutively activating G proteins

(B) acting as a "turned-on" growth factor receptor

(C) constitutively activating tyrosine phosphorylation

(D) inability to initiate apoptosis

(E) failure to regulate transition from G1 to S phase

**IX-54.** A 30-year-old female with a very strong family history of breast cancer (breast cancer occurring at an early age in first-degree relatives) inquires about having her blood tested for a mutation in the BRCA-1 gene. All of the following are correct statements about this condition EXCEPT

(A) if a BRCA-1 mutation is detected, the patient has a very high risk of developing breast cancer

(B) if the BRCA-1 mutation is detected, the patient has a very high risk of developing ovarian cancer

(C) if a BRCA-1 mutation is detected, the patient's daughter will have a 50 percent chance of having a high risk of breast cancer

(D) unless the patient is an Ashkanazi Jew, BRCA-1 mutations may occur throughout the gene

(E) if the woman did not have a strong family history, she would have roughly a 1 in 50 chance of carrying a mutation of this gene

**IX-55.** A 42-year-old male is admitted to the hospital with a fever. Eight days ago he received his third cycle of cyclophosphamide, doxorubicin, vincristine, and prednisone chemotherapy to treat a diffuse large cell lymphoma that had presented in the right cervical area and in the mediastinum. After the first two cycles, the tumor had diminished markedly in size based on physical exam and chest radiography. At this time the patient appears mildly ill, has a temperature of 39°C (102°F) and a non-focal physical examination. His CBC reveals a hematocrit of 32 percent, white count of 1000 with 20 percent neutrophils, and a platelet count of 85,000/μL. The patient is treated with broad-spectrum antibacterial antibiotics, defervesces, and is released in eight days, at which time his neutrophil count exceeds 500/μL.

The most appropriate course of action would be to

(A) administer the same doses of chemotherapy used in the last cycle within one week; administer granulocyte colony-stimulating factor beginning the day after the chemotherapy is completed
(B) delay readministration of chemotherapy for two weeks
(C) decrease the dose of cyclophosphamide and doxorubicin by 25 percent; administer the chemotherapy within the next week
(D) change therapy to cyclophosphamide, vincristine, and prednisone
(E) change therapy to etoposide, methylprednisone, cytarabine, and cisplatin

**IX-56.** A 52-year-old male noted a pigmented lesion in the area of his left flank. Excisional biopsy revealed a malignant melanoma 2.5 mm in thickness. The patient then underwent a definitive resection of the tumor with 2-cm margins that were not involved. Chest x-ray and liver function tests are normal. The patient should receive

(A) interferon-α
(B) interleukin-2
(C) dacarbazine
(D) dacarbazine plus carmustine
(E) observation

**IX-57.** In which of the following neoplasms has neoadjuvant chemotherapy been demonstrated to be beneficial?

(A) Large primary infraglottic cancer with lymph node metastasis
(B) Large primary base of the tongue cancer
(C) Locally advanced laryngeal cancer
(D) Squamous carcinoma of the skin
(E) Locally advanced gastric cancer

**IX-58.** A 55-year-old female with a multiple myeloma is receiving chemotherapy. She currently has a serum IgG level of 5 gm/dL, mild anemia, and three osteolytic lesions on skull x-ray. Her serum calcium and creatinine are normal. All of the following are appropriate therapeutic approaches EXCEPT

(A) consolidation with high-dose chemotherapy with stem cell support if she has a good response to standard chemotherapy
(B) monthly pamidronate therapy
(C) high-dose dexamethasone to control disease
(D) monthly intravenous gammaglobulin
(E) plasmapheresis if she develops headache, fatigue, visual disturbances, and retinopathy

**IX-59.** A 23-year-old female underwent mantle irradiation for pathological stage 2A nodular sclerosis Hodgkin's disease 6 years ago. All of the following represent possible late complications EXCEPT

(A) increased incidence of breast cancer
(B) lower extremities paresthesia
(C) pneumonitis
(D) increased incidence of AML
(E) hypothyroidism

**IX-60.** Clinically important prognostic factors for patients with aggressive non-Hodgkin's lymphoma include all of the following EXCEPT

(A) age
(B) serum LDH
(C) performance status
(D) degree of extranodal involvement
(E) systemic symptoms

**IX-61.** A 35-year-old male with acute myeloid leukemia is 12 days status post receiving high-dose cytarabine for relapsed disease. He is complaining of severe right lower quadrant pain. His temperature is 39°C (103°F), blood pressure is 100/60, and heart rate is 110. He is moderately ill-appearing. His physical examination is remarkable for rebound tenderness in the right lower quadrant. Laboratory examination reveals a white count of 100/μL (differential: 0 polys and 100 lymphs), platelet count is 12,000/μL, hematocrit is 28.0 percent. Liver function tests are normal. KUB is unremarkable. CT scan of the abdomen shows a thickened proximal colonic wall due to a pericolonic mass or infiltrate. The most appropriate therapy or strategy at this time is

(A) exploratory laparotomy
(B) continued broad-spectrum antibiotics with good bowel organism coverage
(C) continued broad-spectrum antibiotics with good bowel organism coverage and do not allow the patient to eat
(D) administration of reinduction chemotherapy for the pericolonic chloroma
(E) placement of a CT-guided catheter for percutaneous drainage of the abdominal abscess

**IX-62.** A 70-year-old female presents to her internist for routine check-up. She has diabetes and hypertension, both of which are managed with oral therapy. She is chronically fatigued but has no specific complaints. Physical examination discloses several 1- to 2-cm nodes on both sides of the anterior neck and in the axilla. Routine blood counts reveal that her white count is 98,000 mainly due to preponderance of mature-appearing lymphs, hematocrit is 38.2 percent, and platelet count is 250,000/μL. Except for a mildly elevated LDH, her serum chemistries are normal. Serum protein electrophoresis reveals hypogammaglobulinemia. Flow cytometric analysis of the patient's peripheral blood reveals that most of the cells express the CD20, CD23, and CD5 antigens. A CT scan of the chest, abdomen, and the pelvis discloses multiple 1- to 2-cm lymph nodes in the peri-aortic area. The most appropriate therapy at this time is

(A) observation
(B) intravenous gammaglobulin
(C) chlorambucil
(D) chlorambucil and prednisone
(E) fludarabine

**IX-63.** A 65-year-old man presents because of fatigue. He has no other specific complaints except for mild left-sided abdominal pain. Physical exam is remarkable for a spleen tip which is palpable 7 finger breadths from the left costal margin. Serum chemistries are remarkable for an LDH which is elevated four-fold. Hematocrit is 26 percent, white count is 18,000/μL with 1 percent blasts, 5 percent promyelocytes, 4 percent myelocytes, 10 percent metamyelocytes, 10 percent band forms, 25 percent polys, 25 percent lymphs, 10 percent monocytes, and 10 percent nucleated red blood cells, and platelet count is 245,000/μL. The red cell smear discloses many tear drop–shaped red cells. A bone marrow examination is undertaken, but the bone marrow aspirate is impossible to obtain. The most likely finding on the bone marrow biopsy is

(A) myelofibrosis
(B) hairy cell leukemia
(C) acute myeloid leukemia
(D) aplastic anemia
(E) metastatic prostate cancer

**IX-64.** A 65-year-old former heavy smoker who was diagnosed with small cell cancer of the lung one year ago now presents with fever, chills, and cough. His disease originally presented with a right perihilar mass. After the histologic diagnosis was made and distant metastases were excluded, the patient received combination chemotherapy and radiation therapy to his right lung. At this time the patient looks mildly ill, has a temperature of 38°C (101°F), and decreased breath sounds at the right base. Chest x-ray shows tracheal deviation to the right, a question of a right lower lobe mass, and dense right lower lobe collapse or consolidation. There is a small right pleural effusion. Which of the following represents the most important next step in management?

(A) External beam radiation therapy
(B) Systemic chemotherapy
(C) Broad spectrum antibiotics
(D) External beam radiation therapy plus chemotherapy
(E) Bronchoscopy

**IX-65.** All of the following statements concerning chemotherapeutic agents are correct EXCEPT

(A) cytarabine is an S-phase specific antimetabolite
(B) doxorubicin inhibits DNA repair by interfering with the function of topoisomerase-II
(C) Taxol is a naturally derived substance that inhibits intracellular microtubular formation
(D) L-asparaginase is a bacterially derived protein that depletes lymphoblasts of a required nutrient
(E) irinotecan (CPT11) interferes with DNA repair by inhibiting topoisomerase-I

**IX-66.** A 72-year-old man who has become progressively more fatigued is found to be anemic. Hematologic laboratory values are as follows:

Hemoglobin: 100 g/L (10 g/dL)
Hematocrit: 27.5 percent
Mean corpuscular volume (MCV): 101 fL
Mean corpuscular hemoglobin (MCH): 30 pg
Mean corpuscular hemoglobin concentration (MCHC): 340 g/L (34 g/dL)
Reticulocyte count: 0.5 percent
White blood cell count: 7300/μL (65 percent neutrophils)
Platelet count: 210,000/μL

The most likely diagnosis is

(A) acute leukemia
(B) aplastic anemia
(C) autoimmune hemolytic anemia
(D) iron deficiency
(E) myelodysplastic syndrome

**IX-67.** Which of the following industrial toxins is associated with tumors of the liver?

(A) Asbestos
(B) Benzene
(C) Mustard
(D) Chromium
(E) Vinyl chloride

**IX-68.** A 59-year-old postmenopausal woman underwent radical mastectomy 3 years ago for carcinoma of the breast. All nodes biopsied were negative, and the estrogen receptor status of the tumor was positive at 150 fmol/mg of cytosol protein. No further therapy was ordered. Now the woman presents with right upper leg pain. Plain films reveal a 3-cm lytic lesion in the right upper femur with cortical erosion, and a bone scan shows not only the femoral lesion but also three separate lesions in her ribs, two in her skull, and one in her pelvis. Chest x-ray is unremarkable, and liver function tests are normal.

The most appropriate therapeutic option now would be

(A) tamoxifen, 10 mg twice daily
(B) tamoxifen, 10 mg twice daily, plus CMF combination chemotherapy (cyclophosphamide, methotrexate, and 5-fluorouracil)
(C) tamoxifen, 10 mg twice daily, plus external-beam radiation to the femoral lesion
(D) tamoxifen, 10 mg twice daily, plus prophylactic internal fixation of the right femur followed by external-beam radiation
(E) tamoxifen, 10 mg twice daily, plus both CMF and external-beam radiation to the femoral lesion

**IX-69.** A 65-year-old man develops superficial thrombophlebitis in multiple sites including the arms and chest. He has had several episodes in the past couple of months, each of which lasted a few days. Which of the following neoplasms is most closely associated with this patient's clinical problem?

(A) Prostate carcinoma
(B) Lung carcinoma
(C) Pancreatic carcinoma
(D) Acute promyelocytic leukemia
(E) Paroxysmal nocturnal hemoglobinuria

**IX-70.** Which of the following statements concerning the diagnosis of pernicious anemia is true?

(A) The presence of antiparietal-cell antibodies is diagnostic of pernicious anemia
(B) Hematologic response to folate therapy alone rules out pernicious anemia as the cause of megaloblastic anemia
(C) Hyperkalemia may be a consequence of vitamin $B_{12}$ therapy
(D) Bone marrow examination would be expected to reveal marked depletion of erythrocyte precursors in persons with untreated pernicious anemia
(E) Serum gastrin levels usually are elevated in persons with pernicious anemia

**IX-71.** A 65-year-old woman with myelodysplastic syndrome, subtype refractory anemia, has required platelet transfusional therapy intermittently for the past year. She normally receives one bag (approximately 6 units) of irradiated single donor platelets obtained by a pheresis. Her platelet count today is 6000 and she is receiving a bag of platelets. At the conclusion of the transfusion, she develops a temperature to 39°C (102.2°F) and has rigor. She has had several similar reactions in the past several weeks. Her platelet count drawn 1 h after the platelet transfusion is 36,000/μL. Assuming that blood and platelet culture results are negative, which of the following would be the best way to reduce the likelihood of such febrile reactions in the future?

(A) Premedicate the patient with acetaminophen and diphenhydramine
(B) Administer CMV-negative platelets
(C) Administer HLA-identical platelets
(D) Administer leukocyte-reduced platelets
(E) Administer platelets from the patient's sibling

**IX-72.** A 27-year-old man has a testicular mass. Chest x-ray reveals six discrete tumor nodules, and an abdominal CT scan shows enlarged paraaortic nodes. Serum α-fetoprotein level is elevated. He undergoes transinguinal orchiectomy, which reveals teratocarcinoma. Treatment is started with three cycles of combination chemotherapy consisting of bleomycin, etoposide, and cisplatin; he tolerates the chemotherapy well. Four of the six lung nodules resolve completely, the paraaortic nodes disappear, and α-fetoprotein levels return to normal. The two remaining pulmonary nodules, one in each lung, have diminished in size to about 2 cm. The man receives a fourth cycle of the same drugs with no change in his clinical status.

At this stage, his physician should

(A) continue the same chemotherapy for one more cycle but increase the dosage of drugs by 50 percent
(B) switch to a new drug regimen
(C) perform thoracotomy in order to biopsy and remove the nodule on one side
(D) administer low-dose, whole-lung radiation
(E) administer high-dose spot radiation to the individual lung nodules

**IX-73.** A 32-year-old man with acute myeloid leukemia in first remission undergoes an allogeneic bone marrow transplant with nonpurged marrow from his HLA-identical sister. Prior to the administration of his sister's marrow, the patient underwent preparation with high-dose cyclophosphamide and total body irradiation. About 6 days after the administration of the graft, the patient feels quite ill. He develops a fever to 39°C (102.2°F) and begins to note a maculopapular skin rash over the arms and back. He has severe diarrhea and intermittent abdominal pain. Results of his liver function tests are markedly abnormal with elevation of the serum bilirubin, SGOT, and alkaline phosphatase. The most likely cause for this clinical syndrome is

(A) graft-versus-host disease
(B) cytomegalovirus infection
(C) autoimmune transfusion reaction
(D) bacterial sepsis
(E) venoocclusive disease of the liver

**IX-74.** A 40-year-old woman undergoes her first mammogram. The study reveals a cluster of microcalcifications in the right breast. Needle biopsy reveals a focus of lobular carcinoma in situ (no invasion). At this point the patient should be offered

(A) quadrantectomy and lymph node dissection on the ipsilateral side
(B) quadrantectomy with irradiation
(C) right breast mastectomy with irradiation depending on lymph node status at the time of surgery
(D) irradiation therapy to the right breast
(E) resection followed by annual mammography and semiannual physical exam

**IX-75.** A 45-year-old woman with long-standing rheumatoid arthritis is diagnosed as having "anemia of chronic disease." The predominant mechanism causing this type of anemia in persons with chronic inflammatory disorders is

(A) defective porphyrin synthesis
(B) impaired incorporation of iron into porphyrin
(C) intravascular hemolysis
(D) depressed erythroid maturation due to decreased erythropoietin production
(E) impaired transfer of reticuloendothelial storage iron to marrow erythroid precursors

**IX-76.** Which of the following statements best characterizes the hemolysis associated with glucose-6-phosphate dehydrogenase (G6PD) deficiency?

(A) It is more severe in affected blacks than in affected persons of Mediterranean ancestry.
(B) It is more severe in females than in males.
(C) It causes the appearance of Heinz bodies on Wright staining of a peripheral smear.
(D) It most often is precipitated by infection.
(E) The best time to perform the diagnostic test is during a hemolytic crisis.

**IX-77.** A 65-year-old man with a benign past medical history presents to his internist for a routine medical checkup. His physical examination and laboratory studies are normal except for a serum prostate specific antigen value of 8 ng/mL (normal 0 to 3 ng/mL). Which of the following is a true statement about the man's condition?

(A) His likelihood of prostate cancer is 75 percent
(B) If he does have prostate cancer, the disease is likely confined to the gland.
(C) Assuming there is no evidence of metastatic spread, the patient should undergo a radical prostatectomy.
(D) Assuming there is no evidence of spread, the patient should receive radiation therapy to the prostate.
(E) The patient should receive therapy with leuprolide and flutamide.

**IX-78.** A 38-year-old premenopausal woman has a 3-cm mass in her left breast. Breast biopsy reveals infiltrating ductal carcinoma, and a left modified radical mastectomy is performed. The pathology report states that the primary tumor is estrogen-receptor-positive and that 4 of 28 lymph nodes identified are involved with tumor. Chest x-ray, bone scan, liver scan, and blood chemistries are all normal. The most appropriate next step in the management of this patient would be

(A) antiestrogen therapy (e.g., tamoxifen)
(B) appropriate combination chemotherapy
(C) postoperative radiation therapy to the left chest wall and axilla
(D) bilateral oophorectomy
(E) follow-up in 2 months

**IX-79.** A 55-year-old man complains of numbness in both legs and progressive inability to walk over the past 2 months. Physical examination is normal except for a decreased perception of light touch and pain in the lower extremities as well as bilateral leg weakness. There is no sensory level. Laboratory workup is remarkable for a hematocrit of 30 percent and elevated total protein. Serum protein electrophoresis reveals an M spike. The etiology of this patient's weakness is most likely

(A) necrosis of central nervous system gray and white matter
(B) inflammation of dorsal root ganglia
(C) loss of cerebellar Purkinje cells
(D) elaboration of tumor-associated protein that elicits an immune response that is cross-reactive with peripheral nerves
(E) tumor-elaborated immunoglobulin that is reacting with myelin components

**IX-80.** A 45-year-old woman presents with an axillary mass. She has no other complaints. Her past medical history is benign and she is taking no medication. Physical examination is unremarkable except for the presence of a firm, nonmoveable mass of 4 × 3 cm in the left axilla. Biopsy of the mass reveals poorly differentiated malignant neoplasm without gland formation. Immunoperoxidase staining of the tumor is negative for cytokeratin and positive for the leukocyte common antigen. The most appropriate next step for this patient is

(A) modified radical mastectomy with axillary radiation therapy
(B) axillary radiation therapy
(C) administration of cyclophosphamide, methotrexate, and 5-fluorouracil
(D) administration of tamoxifen
(E) chest and abdominal CT

**IX-81.** Evaluation of a person who has pure red blood cell aplasia would be expected to reveal

(A) markedly hypocellular bone marrow
(B) normochromic, normocytic red blood cells
(C) increased iron turnover on ferrokinetic studies
(D) a reticulocyte count greater than 2.0 percent
(E) decreased urinary erythropoietin content

**IX-82.** A 28-year-old man presents with chest pain. Chest x-ray reveals a large mediastinal mass. Abdominal CT reveals periaortic lymphadenopathy. Physical examination, including examination of the testes, is negative. Mediastinoscopic biopsy reveals poorly differentiated carcinoma. Which of the following laboratory tests would be most likely to be positive?

(A) Prostate specific antigen (PSA)
(B) Beta human chorionic gonadotropin (β-hCG)
(C) Carcinoembryonic antigen (CEA)
(D) CA-125
(E) CA19-9

**IX-83.** All the following are neoplasms of B-lymphocyte lineage EXCEPT

(A) chronic lymphocytic leukemia
(B) follicular lymphomas
(C) Burkitt's lymphoma
(D) mycosis fungoides
(E) small lymphocytic (well-differentiated) lymphomas

**IX-84.** Regarding local therapy of operable breast cancer, which of the following statements is accurate?

(A) Axillary radiation therapy should follow modified radical mastectomy.
(B) Radiation therapy administered following breast-conserving surgery has no effect on the local recurrence rate.
(C) Radiation therapy administered following breast-conserving surgery has no effect on the overall survival rate.
(D) All patients with a small tumor do equally well with either lumpectomy plus radiation or modified radical mastectomy.
(E) Node dissection should be performed in all patients in order to reduce the chance of local spread.

**IX-85.** A 21-year-old woman who has had severe menorrhagia is referred by her gynecologist for evaluation of a possible systemic coagulopathy. A younger sister has been noted to bleed excessively after trauma. She takes no medications; physical examination is unremarkable. Initial laboratory results include the following: platelet count, 252,000/μL; prothrombin time, 23.6 s (control 11.6 s); and partial thromboplastin time, 26.9 s (control 33.3 s). Further laboratory testing should include

(A) determination of alpha$_2$-antiplasmin level
(B) screening for inhibitors
(C) determination of bleeding time
(D) determination of factor VII level
(E) determination of factor VIII level

**IX-86.** Thrombocytosis would be LEAST likely to occur in persons who have

(A) polycythemia vera
(B) hemolytic-uremic syndrome
(C) sickle cell disease
(D) iron-deficiency anemia
(E) ulcerative colitis

**IX-87.** A 65-year-old woman with increasing abdominal pain is found to have a pelvic mass on physical examination. After appropriate staging studies she undergoes a laparotomy and is found to have serous carcinoma of the ovary with involvement of one ovary and several omental implants. She then undergoes a hysterectomy, bilateral salpingo-oophorectomy, liver biopsy, omentectomy, cytologic examination of abdominal washings, and extensive inspection. All evidence of disease is removed.

Assuming generally good health, an uneventful postoperative recovery, and lack of proximity to a center performing clinical trials, she should now receive

(A) no further therapy
(B) combination chemotherapy
(C) combination chemotherapy only if serum CA125 level is elevated
(D) intraperitoneal chemotherapy
(E) whole abdominal radiation therapy

**IX-88.** Which of the following clinical scenarios is LEAST likely to describe a paraneoplastic syndrome resulting from small cell tumors of the lung?

(A) Weakness and fatigability, primarily of proximal muscles; electromyographic results show increasing amplitude of contraction with repetitive stimulation
(B) Cerebellar ataxia, dysarthria, deafness, pleocytosis of cerebrospinal fluid, and cerebellar atrophy on CT scan of the brain
(C) Moon facies, truncal striae, hypertension, hypokalemia, and hyperglycemia
(D) Hypercalcemia, polydipsia, polyuria, and mental status changes in the absence of bony metastases
(E) Mental status changes, muscle weakness, hyponatremia, and decreased serum osmolality with inappropriately elevated urine osmolality

**IX-89.** A feature of idiopathic thrombocytopenic purpura common to both children and adults is

(A) occurrence after an antecedent viral illness
(B) presence of antibodies directed against target antigens on the glycoprotein IIb-IIIa complex
(C) absence of splenomegaly
(D) persistence of thrombocytopenia for more than 6 months
(E) necessity of splenectomy to ameliorate thrombocytopenia

**IX-90.** Persons with polycythemia vera and a hematocrit greater than 45 percent are most likely to display which of the following?

(A) Increased levels of urinary erythropoietin
(B) Increased bone marrow iron stores
(C) Decreased carotid blood flow
(D) Hypocellular bone marrow
(E) Myelophthisic changes in their peripheral blood smear, including teardrop-shaped red blood cells and normoblasts

**IX-91.** A young woman presents with bleeding after a dental extraction. She is found to have a bleeding time of greater than 20 min along with a normal prothrombin time and partial thromboplastin time. There is a familial history of bleeding, and the patient's laboratory evaluation reveals a normal platelet count. The factor VIII coagulant activity is 54 percent of normal, von Willebrand factor (vWF) antigen is 48 percent of normal, and ristocetin cofactor is 13 percent of normal. A normal spectrum of vWF multimers in the patient's plasma on SDS-agarose electrophoresis is noted. This patient's coagulopathy is primarily caused by

(A) defective release of vWF from endothelial cells
(B) inappropriate binding of vWF to platelets
(C) reduced synthesis of vWF by endothelial cells
(D) an inability to assemble high-molecular-weight multimers or premature catabolism of vWF
(E) an alteration in the platelet receptor for vWF

**IX-92.** A 1-year-old boy bleeds significantly after an inguinal hernia repair. The patient has no siblings, and there is no familial history of a bleeding diathesis. Platelet count, bleeding time, prothrombin time, and partial thromboplastin time are all normal. The most likely diagnosis is

(A) prekallikrein deficiency
(B) factor XII deficiency
(C) factor XIII deficiency
(D) thrombasthenia
(E) protein S deficiency

**IX-93.** The statements about doxorubicin (Adriamycin) cardiotoxicity are true EXCEPT

(A) acute cardiotoxicity, which is characterized by arrhythmias and other abnormal electrocardiographic changes, is brief and rarely serious

(B) chronic cardiotoxicity occurs in fewer than 3 percent of persons whose lifetime dose of doxorubicin is below 500 mg/m²

(C) weekly doxorubicin therapy is better tolerated than the same total dose given every 3 weeks

(D) doxorubicin cardiotoxicity and cytotoxicity occur via the same pathway

(E) previous cardiac irradiation and exposure to cyclophosphamide or anthracycline antibiotics other than doxorubicin increase the risk of cardiotoxicity

**IX-94.** Which statement regarding the treatment of patients with non-Hodgkin's lymphoma is true?

(A) Radiation therapy is curative for most patients with low-grade non-Hodgkin's lymphoma

(B) In those patients with low-grade lymphoma who require chemotherapy, only combinations of agents can change overall survival rate

(C) Over 75 percent of patients with intermediate-grade (e.g., diffuse large cell) lymphoma will achieve complete remission with combination chemotherapy

(D) Maintenance therapy (prolonged therapy after complete remission is achieved) improves survival in patients with diffuse large cell lymphoma

(E) Patients with non-Hodgkin's lymphoma who have AIDS have the same rate of response to chemotherapy as stage- and grade-matched patients without AIDS

**IX-95.** A 65-year-old man presents because his wife notes that his eyes are becoming yellow. On further questioning, the patient complains of epigastric discomfort, dark urine, light stools, and pruritus. Past medical history and physical examination are unremarkable. Laboratory tests confirm the clinical impression of an elevation in the serum level of conjugated bilirubin. Abdominal ultrasound demonstrates a mass in the head of the pancreas and enlargement of the common bile duct. Chest x-ray and abdominal-pelvic CT disclose no additional abnormalities. A CT-guided needle biopsy of the mass obtains tissue that on pathologic examination reveals neutrophils and fibrous elements. Which of the following procedures would be most reasonable at this point?

(A) Another attempt at CT-guided needle biopsy

(B) Radiation therapy

(C) Celiac angiography

(D) Repeat CT in 2 to 3 months

(E) Percutaneous placement of biliary stent

**IX-96.** In addition to a checkup including health counseling and examination of the oral cavity, thyroid gland, skin, lymph nodes, testes, and prostate, which, according to the American Cancer Society, of the following should be done annually after age 40 in the asymptomatic, average-risk man in order to promote the early detection of cancer?

(A) Colonoscopy

(B) Sigmoidoscopy

(C) Digital rectal examination with palpation of the prostate

(D) Digital rectal examination with palpation of the prostate and stool guaiac

(E) Digital rectal examination with palpation of the prostate, stool blood test, and chest x-ray

# IX. HEMATOPOIETIC DISORDERS AND NEOPLASIA

## ANSWERS

**IX-1. The answer is E.** *(Chaps. 36, 107)* The affinity of the hemoglobin molecule for oxygen is altered primarily by blood pH, temperature, red blood cell concentration of 2,3-bisphosphoglycerate (2,3-BPG), and arterial carbon dioxide tension. Increased affinity, such as is produced by a rise in pH or a drop in 2,3-BPG, temperature, or $P_{CO_2}$, inhibits the delivery of oxygen to body tissue. That is, under these conditions, at a given $P_{O_2}$ a greater percentage of hemoglobin will be saturated with oxygen and more oxygen can be carried by the blood but less $O_2$ is delivered to the tissue. Reduced affinity for oxygen occurs at lower pH (acidosis) and favors unloading of oxygen from the hemoglobin molecule to the tissues. Carbon monoxide exposure leading to the formation of carboxyhemoglobin shifts the oxygen dissociation curve to the left and thereby decreases oxygen release. Hyperventilation, by lowering $P_{CO_2}$ and raising pH, increases hemoglobin-oxygen affinity. Methemoglobin cannot carry oxygen, which results in a functional anemia and decreasing release of oxygen to the tissues.

**IX-2. The answer is E.** *(Chap. 88. Preston, N Engl J Med 327:1649, 1992.)* Basal cell carcinoma is the most common malignancy in the United States. The typical appearance is that of a slowly enlarging, pearly translucent papule with rolled borders and overlying telangiectasias. As the lesion enlarges, central ulceration may occur (rodent ulcer). Sun-exposed areas are most commonly involved—about 90 percent of tumors occur on the head and neck—and fair-skinned persons are at greatest risk. Dermal nevi, which occur commonly on the faces of adults, lack the translucency seen in basal cell carcinoma. Sebaceous hyperplasia usually is smaller and has a distinct yellowish color. Diagnosis of basal cell carcinoma is easily established by punch or incisional biopsy.

**IX-3. The answer is D.** *(Chap. 88. Koh, N Engl J Med 325:171, 1991.)* The characteristics that distinguish superficial spreading malignant melanoma from a normal mole include irregularity of its border and variegation of color. Instead of the homogeneous color and regular borders of a "normal" mole, the lesion shows disorderliness and irregularity. The first changes noted by persons who develop melanoma in a preexisting mole are a "darkening" in color or a change in the borders of the lesion. Irregularity of the borders in an expanding, darkening mole is melanoma until proved otherwise; excisional (not incisional) biopsy should be done promptly because early diagnosis and excision reduce the mortality. It is best not to cut into a lesion for which melanoma is in the differential diagnosis.

**IX-4. The answer is B.** *(Chap. 113. Saven, Ann Intern Med 120:169, 1994.)* Pancytopenia with a dry marrow aspirate argues against CLL and myeloma. Normal RBC morphology argues against myelofibrosis. The WBC count and differential count argue against CML. Hairy cell leukemia is a neoplasm of mature B lymphocytes typically presenting with pancytopenia, splenomegaly, and a dry bone marrow aspirate. Patients with hairy cell leukemia are prone to infections with unusual microorganisms, such as atypical mycobacteria; they tend to be granulocytopenic and have a preponderance of mature-appearing lymphocytes in the peripheral blood that have, on close inspection or on ultrastructural analysis, multiple hairlike projections. Bone marrow biopsies typically yield a "fried egg" appearance in that the cells appear to be separated from one another, due to these projections and fixation artifacts generated from them. Immunophenotypically, hairy cells are characterized by the presence of mature B cell markers as well as the CD25 antigen, which is the low affinity interleukin-2 receptor. Fortunately, there are many treatment modalities available for patients with hairy cell leukemia. The current treatment of choice is a 7-day intravenous infusion of 2-chlorodeoxyadenosine. This single course of treatment results in complete remissions in approximately 80 percent of patients. Other effective modalities include splenectomy, interferon-$\alpha$, or pentostatin (deoxycoformycin).

**IX-5.  The answer is A.** *(Chap. 89. Vokes, N Engl J Med 328:184–194, 1993.)*  Patients who are heavy smokers and drinkers are at increased risk to develop squamous cell carcinoma of the head and neck. In fact, the risk for those who both smoke and drink is multiplicatively increased compared with those who abuse just one of these substances. A firm neck mass in a patient with these habits should prompt an aggressive search for a primary lesion in the head and neck region and would include panendoscopy (laryngoscopy, esophagoscopy, and bronchoscopy) with biopsy of all suspicious areas. Squamous cell carcinoma in the midcervical chain in the presence of a normal physical examination (thereby excluding large tumors of the mouth or supraglottic region) could represent a metastasis from an infraglottic primary. Therefore, the best way to ascertain the diagnosis in this case is to perform a careful upper aerodigestive examination, which should begin with indirect laryngoscopy. CT of the neck, while helpful in delineating the extent of disease, would likely not reveal the primary. Treatment planning optimally requires delineation of the primary and definition of lymph node metastases. The standard approach to a primary head and neck squamous cell carcinoma with a large lymph node metastasis is radiation therapy or surgery or both. However, use of induction chemotherapy is being investigated as a possible means both to improve survival and to reduce the amount of disfiguring local therapy that would be required in such instances.

**IX-6.  The answer is B.** *(Chap. 87. Pizzo, N Engl J Med 328:1323, 1993.)*  If not attacked promptly, infection in neutropenic patients can be quickly fatal. Often, these patients display neither the signs nor the symptoms of infection. Fever should be regarded as an indication of infection, and antibiotic therapy should begin immediately after appropriate cultures are obtained. An effective initial antibiotic regimen would consist of an aminoglycoside antibiotic or third-generation cephalosporin and a semisynthetic antipseudomonal penicillin. Gammaglobulin is of little benefit in the treatment of granulocytopenic cancer patients. Granulocyte transfusions are of no benefit. Amphotericin B is appropriate if granulocytopenia persists and defervescence does not occur after 7 days of antibacterial antibiotics, or sooner, if clinical deterioration is noted.

**IX-7.  The answer is B.** *(Chap. 118)*  Several reports have described the association of coumarin-induced skin necrosis in patients with congenital protein C deficiency. The skin lesions occur on the breasts, buttocks, legs, and penis. They appear to be a result of diffuse thrombosis of the venules with interstitial bleeding. This condition is presumed to result from an imbalance in hemostatic mechanism activity favoring thrombosis during the early phases of coumarin administration. Protein C has a relatively short half-life within the circulation (about 14 h) compared with that of some of the vitamin K–dependent procoagulant clotting factors (factor X and prothrombin), and a rapid drop in its effective concentration could produce such a situation. However, only about ⅓ of cases of coumarin-induced skin necrosis are related to protein C deficiency.

**IX-8.  The answer is E.** *(Chaps. 59, 108. Stabler, Blood 76:871, 1990.)*  While pancytopenia is frequently due to an intrinsic bone marrow abnormality, vitamin B$_{12}$ and folate deficiency may also present with low blood counts. The elevated red cell volume coupled with a low reticulocyte index suggests a megaloblastic anemia. The history of vitiligo represents one of the several autoimmune-type diseases associated with pernicious anemia (PA). Other such immunologically mediated diseases include Graves' disease, myxedema, thyroiditis, idiopathic adrenocortical insufficiency, and hypoparathyroidism.

PA is a failure of gastric production of intrinsic factor due to autoimmune destruction of parietal cells, which prevents $B_{12}$ absorption in the distal ileum. Antibody-mediated destruction of parietal cells results in achlorhydria (an abnormally high gastric pH). The hematologic abnormalities of PA include elevated MCV, decreased reticulocyte count, hypersegmented neutrophil nuclei, and megaloblastic changes in the bone marrow that can, if severe, be confused with acute leukemia. Extramedullary manifestations of PA include neurologic abnormalities typified by demyelinization of the posterior and lateral spinal columns of the spinal cord, resulting in numbness and parasthesias, weakness, and ataxia. Patients with megaloblastic anemia on the basis of deficiency of intrinsic factor respond to cyanocobalamin injections within several days. Hypokalemia may complicate the recovery phase.

**IX-9.** **The answer is B.** *(Chap. 84)* Certain familial and genetic syndromes are associated with an increased propensity to development of malignant neoplasms. Ataxia-telangiectasia, an autosomal recessive condition characterized by abnormal cellular immunity, conjunctival telangiectasias, and progressive spinocerebellar atrophy, is also associated with lymphoma. Carcinoma of the colon develops in almost all persons with familial polyposis coli and is found at the time of initial diagnosis of the polyps in about 40 percent of cases. Fanconi's anemia is one of a group of familial disorders associated with cytogenetic abnormalities and an increased risk of development of cancer. Neurofibromas undergo sarcomatous change in approximately 10 percent of affected patients. Chronic granulomatous disease of childhood is a disorder of oxidative metabolism in phagocytes and is not associated with neoplasia.

**IX-10.** **The answer is B.** *(Chaps. 83, 84. Weinberg, Science 254:1138, 1991.)* The most common genetic alteration in human cancer is mutation or deletion of the p53 gene, which is found on the long arm of chromosome 17. Wild type p53 suppresses malignant transformation of cells in tissue culture. It appears to regulate cell cycle progression by holding cells at the G1 checkpoint. Like the retinoblastoma tumor suppressor gene, p53 may be activated by protein products of transforming viruses. A rare autosomal dominant cancer syndrome, the Li-Fraumeni syndrome, is characterized by families with a very high incidence of a diverse spectrum of childhood and adult tumors, including breast cancer, soft-tissue sarcomas, brain tumors, bone sarcomas, leukemia, and adrenocortical carcinoma. Germ line mutations in the p53 gene have been found in several of these families. Since an abnormality of one allele of p53 is inherited, these patients are at risk of developing homozygous p53 loss and a predisposition to neoplastic transformation. Mutations of the p53 gene are also very common in sporadic human tumors.

**IX-11.** **The answer is D.** *(Chap. 106)* Since each unit of transfused blood contains 200 to 250 mg of iron and normal iron excretion is only 1 mg/d, a patient receiving about 40 units of blood annually will accumulate about 8 g of iron, putting him or her at risk for problems related to transfusional iron overload. In addition to the requirement for many transfusions, the disorder must also have a long natural history to allow for the development of the clinical sequelae of chronic iron overload. Thalassemia major, myeloproliferative disorders, myelodysplastic syndromes (without excess myeloblasts), pure red cell aplasia, and moderately severe aplastic anemia are diseases that may be associated with transfusional iron overload. The spectrum of problems produced by iron deposition in tissues includes cardiac dysfunction (arrhythmias, conduction defects, and restrictive cardiomyopathy), hepatic cirrhosis, glucose intolerance, gonadal dysfunction, and hyperpigmentation due to increased melanin production secondary to dermal iron deposition. The only available treatment for transfusion-associated hemochromatosis (phlebotomy is not an option because of chronic anemia) is chelation with desferrioxamine, which must be given subcutaneously over 12 to 16 h/d by a portable pump. While oral ascorbic acid may enhance iron excretion in patients receiving desferrioxamine, it has no role as a monotherapy and may be associated with dangerous cardiac toxicity.

**IX-12.  The answer is A.**  *(Chaps. 62, 69)*   Severe neutropenia is a rare idiosyncratic reaction to certain drugs, including propylthiouracil. In addition to having sore throat and oral and anal mucosal ulcerations, affected persons are susceptible to overwhelming, life-threatening infections. However, in the absence of fever or clinical signs of infection, they should be followed as outpatients, saving them exposures to nosocomial pathogens in the hospital. Empirical use of broad-spectrum antibiotics without fever or other signs of infection is not advisable, and glucocorticoid therapy is not useful. White blood cell transfusion can be accompanied by serious morbidity (i.e., pulmonary leukostasis). Because severe drug-induced neutropenia is generally self-limited once use of the offending drug has been stopped, consideration of bone marrow transplantation is not justified.

**IX-13.  The answer is E.**  *(Chap. 107. Kazazian, Semin Hematol 27:209, 1990.)*   Hemoglobinopathies are a diverse group of congenital disorders characterized by one or more mutations in one of the genes coding for hemoglobin chains. The clinical consequences can range from no effect to incompatibility with life. Microcytosis occurs in these conditions except for the silent α-thalassemia carrier state in which only one of the four α-globin genes is deleted. Such persons have no hematologic abnormalities. Persons with deletion of two of the four alpha-chain genes (α-thalassemia trait) tend to have microcytic and slightly hypochromic red cells without significant hemolysis or anemia. Hemoglobin electrophoresis may be normal or may reveal a decreased amount of hemoglobin A2. Deletion of three of the four alpha-chain genes, so-called hemoglobin H disease, is associated with significant anemia and with a production of hemoglobin H (beta-chain tetramers) on hemoglobin electrophoresis. There are only two genes coding for the β-globin chain. Patients with abnormalities in one such chain have β-thalassemia trait characterized by microcytosis, abnormal-appearing red cells, and an elevated level of hemoglobin A2 or F or both on hemoglobin electrophoresis. Any patient who inherits at least one allele with a hemoglobin S mutation (sickle hemoglobin, valine to glutamic acid substitution at the sixth amino acid of the β-globin chain) will demonstrate red blood cell sickling under reduced oxygen tension, as is artificially produced by addition of an oxygen-consuming agent such as metabisulfite to the blood. Therefore, any patient with sickle cell trait, sickle cell anemia, or a compound heterozygote such as sickle β-thalassemia or sickle C will have a positive metabisulfite test (and would also have a positive hemoglobin electrophoresis). Hemoglobin E is a very common hemoglobin variant that is highly prevalent in Southeast Asia. Patients with this disorder have an abnormal hemoglobin electrophoresis, slightly macrocytic red cells, and target cells, but no anemia or other clinical manifestations unless they also inherit β thalassemia.

**IX-14.  The answer is B.**  *(Chap. 107. Wayne, Blood 81:1109–1123, 1993.)*   Most clinical problems arising in patients with sickle cell anemia are due to vasoocclusive phenomena caused by sickling of deoxygenated red blood cells in capillaries. Microinfarcts can occur suddenly and cause severe pain in almost any part of the body, although the abdomen, chest, back, and joints are most commonly affected. These crises may be precipitated by upper respiratory infection, cold weather, or dehydration. Unfortunately, it is often difficult to distinguish between a painful sickle abdominal crisis and an actual acute abdominal emergency. Pleuritic chest pain and fever may occur in the absence of an infiltrate. If an infiltrate does occur, distinguishing between pneumonia and pulmonary infarction is difficult, although culture and Gram stain of the sputum might be helpful in this regard. In addition to painful crises, microinfarcts can cause chronic damage in the lungs, kidneys, liver, skeleton, and skin. Painful crises should mandate the use of adequate analgesia, including narcotics, and hydration. Unfortunately, there is an increased risk of opiate addiction in this patient population. Oxygen is helpful if hypoxemia complicates a painful crisis. The role of transfusional therapy in sickle cell anemia is controversial. There is some evidence to suggest that use of aggressive transfusions may decrease the frequency of painful crises, but such an approach has little role in an ongoing crisis. Hydroxyurea therapy may reduce the incidence of sickle crises by increasing synthesis of fetal hemoglobin. Antibiotics should only be administered in the setting of documented infection.

**IX-15.  The answer is B.** *(Chap. 112)*   In about 95 percent of persons who have chronic myelogenous leukemia, material comprising approximately one-half of the long arm of chromosome 22 is translocated to the end of chromosome 9. This abnormality, called the Philadelphia chromosome, can be found in all hematopoietic cell lines. It is thought to represent an acquired somatic cell mutation in the bone marrow, with preferential survival and proliferation of the affected cell clone. The pathogenesis of chronic myelogenous leukemia is therefore a paradigm for all cancers that are believed to arise from a single cell that gives rise to the malignant clone. Normal stem cells exist in the marrow of patients with CML, but they are suppressed by the malignant cells.

**IX-16.  The answer is C.** *(Chap. 98)*   Ninety percent of persons with nonseminomatous germ cell tumors produce either α-fetoprotein (AFP) or β-hCG; in contrast, persons with pure seminomas usually produce neither. These tumor markers are present for some time after surgery—if the presurgical levels are high, 30 days or more may be required before meaningful postsurgical levels can be obtained. The half-lives of AFP and β-hCG are 6 days and 1 day, respectively. After treatment, unequal reduction of β-hCG and AFP may occur, suggesting that the two markers are synthesized by heterogeneous clones of cells within the tumor; thus, both markers should be followed. β-hCG is similar to luteinizing hormone except for its distinctive beta subunit.

**IX-17.  The answer is D.** *(Chap. 109)*   If patients develop circulating anti-IgM antibodies with specificity for polysaccharide antigens on red cell membranes, they may suffer from so-called cold-reactive hemolysis. The clinical manifestations of the presence of such antibodies are hemolysis, which is generally not severe, and a mild elevation of the reticulocyte count, agglutination of red cells, and an increased rate of hemolysis at temperatures below 37°C (98.6°F). A second clinical manifestation of cold hemolysis is the presence of acrocyanosis, characterized by marked purple discoloration of the extremities, ears, and nose during cooling. IgM antibodies may be missed if the blood is allowed to cool after it is drawn because of adsorption onto the patient's own red blood cells and subsequent removal as the blood clots. Therefore, the blood should be allowed to clot at a warm temperature. Serological analysis will reveal a positive direct Coombs' test if anti-C3 antisera is used. The activation of complement by the fixed IgM molecules results in the marked accumulation of the C3dg degradation product on the red cell surface, allowing detection in this fashion. The specificity of the cold agglutinin antibody may be helpful in that a reaction with adult red cells compared with fetal (cord) blood is more common in benign lymphoproliferative disorders. On the other hand, antibodies that react more strongly with fetal cells compared with adult cells are called anti-*i* and are generally seen in lymphomas and in infectious mononucleosis. The patient in this question may well have a recurrence of his lymphoma, which is presenting as a cold hemolytic disease because of the presence of monoclonal IgM antibody. This problem is best treated by successful anti-lymphoma therapy.

**IX-18.  The answer is C.** *(Chap. 110)*   Aplastic anemia may follow exposure to agents that are toxic to the bone marrow such as benzene, chloramphenicol, or gold, or it may occur in association with viral infections including hepatitis C, Epstein-Barr virus, and parvovirus, which may selectively impair erythroid maturation in patients with ongoing hemolysis. The course of the disease is determined by the severity of the aplasia. In this case the patient has anemia, severe thrombocytopenia, and neutropenia as well as a marrow that is almost totally infiltrated by fat. Vitamin deficiency, invasion of the bone marrow with a neoplasm, paroxysmal nocturnal hemoglobinuria, systemic lupus erythematosus, and AIDS have been appropriately ruled out. The best therapy for a patient with severe aplastic anemia is allogeneic bone marrow transplantation from a histocompatible donor, preferably a sibling. However, if the transplant option is not available, then in addition to receiving traditional use of blood products as part of a regimen of supportive care, patients with severe aplastic anemia should receive some form of immunosuppressive therapy, both because of the potential immune etiology of this disorder and the association of a 50 percent response rate with immunosuppressive agents. The most commonly used therapy is animal antisera to human lymphocytes. Such therapy may be complicated by serum sickness. High-dose glucocorticoids or cyclosporine may be associated with a similar response rate. Splenectomy has no role in the management of aplastic anemia and would be dangerous to perform in this pancytopenic patient. Insofar as aplastic anemia is not believed to be humorally mediated, plasmapheresis also has no role. The administration of chemotherapeutic agents to patients with limited marrow reserve is extremely dangerous and should not be considered. Androgens are no longer considered as first line therapy but a small fraction of patients unresponsive to immunosuppression may respond.

**IX-19.   The answer is A.**   *(Chap. 109. Thompson, Blood 80:1890, 1992.)*   This young woman is suffering from a combination of hemolytic anemia with fragmented red cells in the absence of disseminated intravascular coagulation (DIC), thrombocytopenia, fever, mental status changes, and renal dysfunction, which is essentially pathognomonic of thrombotic thrombocytopenic purpura (TTP). The etiology of TTP is unknown, though immunologic and primary vasculopathic phenomena have been associated with this disorder. Pathologically, arteriolar hyalinization, which is also seen in DIC, may be noted. Seventy percent of patients with TTP improve with exchange transfusion or plasmapheresis. Glucocorticoids, antiplatelet agents, splenectomy, and vincristine have been of benefit to subsets of patients, but each is less effective and probably associated with a greater risk than therapeutic plasmapheresis.

**IX-20.   The answer is E.**   *(Chap. 111)*   When a patient presents with thrombocytosis, it is important to determine if this abnormality is due to a myeloproliferative disorder or is reactive due to infection, malignancy, hemolytic anemia, the postoperative state, hemorrhage, iron deficiency, drug reaction, chronic inflammatory disease, response to exercise, recovery from myelosuppression, recovery from $B_{12}$ deficiency, or even myelodysplastic syndrome (either 5q-syndrome or rare cases of sideroblastic anemia). Once secondary causes of thrombocytosis have been satisfactorily excluded, then it is important to delineate the specific myeloproliferative disorder. The red cell mass virtually excludes polycythemia vera, and normal cytogenetics makes the diagnosis of chronic myelogenous leukemia most unlikely. Anemia, massive splenomegaly, teardrop red cell forms, or an elevated white count would advance consideration of agnogenic myeloid metaplasia/myelofibrosis. However, the bone marrow examination did not disclose excess collagen fibrosis. As such, the patient in this question has essential thrombocythemia. Patients with this disease may develop hemorrhage or thrombotic complications. Older patients have a higher risk of thrombosis; some younger patients can be observed. However, this patient is symptomatic due to erythromelalgia, the syndrome of redness and painful burning of the distal extremities caused by localized platelet aggregation. Chronic use of alkylating agents should be avoided due to the risk of leukemogenesis. Antiplatelet agents may protect against thrombosis but could lead to severe hemorrhage. Splenectomy would result in an even higher platelet count. The best treatment in this patient is probably the use of hydroxyurea at a dose titrated to lower the platelet count to below 500,000. Interferon-α may be a useful alternative for those patients unable to tolerate hydroxyurea. Anagrelide is also effective at lowering platelet counts, but it must be given continuously to maintain its effects.

**IX-21.   The answer is C.**   *(Chap. 112. Degos, Blood 85:2643, 1995.)*   Acute promyelocytic leukemia [M3 according to the FAB (French-American-British) classification system] is characterized by bone marrow infiltration with malignant-appearing promyelocytes. Distinctive features of this entity compared with other subtypes of de novo acute myeloid leukemia include the common presentation with leukopenia, the frequent development of disseminated intravascular coagulopathy (DIC) due to release of procoagulant granules from the promyelocytes, and the pathognomonic demonstration of a translocation between chromosomes 15 and 17 on cytogenetic analysis. This translocation juxtaposes sequences from the retinoic acid-receptor alpha gene on chromosome 17 with another DNA binding protein, called PML, on chromosome 17. The resultant fusion protein plays some role in preventing normal differentiation. Interestingly, even before the documentation of the genetic basis for this translocation, it was noted by investigators in China that the use of all-*trans* retinoic acid, an orally administered vitamin A derivative, led to complete remissions in the vast majority of patients with APML. The mechanism of action of this drug appears to be induction of differentiation of the malignant clone. As such, patients enter remission slowly over a period of 30 to 60 days. DIC, typically made worse by chemotherapy, is rapidly ameliorated by all-*trans* retinoic acid. Other cytotoxic effects of chemotherapy, such as mucositis and myelosuppression, do not occur with all-*trans* retinoic acid. Common side effects include dry skin and peeling at the corners of the mouth. A life-threatening complication, occurring in about 20 percent of patients treated with all-*trans* retinoic acid, is the so-called retinoic acid syndrome, manifested by pulmonary infiltrates and incipient respiratory failure, sometimes associated with a high white count. Glucocorticoids, leukopheresis, and hydroxyurea have each been associated with some improvement. Patients maintained on all-*trans* retinoic acid alone will eventually relapse, so initial induction therapy with all-*trans* retinoic acid should be combined with chemotherapy.

IX-22. **The answer is A.** *(Chap. 86)* The most prominent general side effects of chemotherapy relate to the effect of these drugs on dividing cells, including myelosuppression, stomatitis, and alopecia. Certain drugs, such as L-asparaginase and vincristine, can be administered during periods of low white blood cell count because they are relatively nonmyelosuppressive. Alkylating agents, such as melphalan, cyclophosphamide, and nitrogen mustard, damage bone marrow stem cells, an effect associated with the development of secondary myelodysplastic syndromes and acute leukemias. Anthracyclines are myelosuppressive, but they inhibit more committed hematopoietic cells than do the alkylating agents. Cisplatin is quite emetogenic; however, vomiting can be managed successfully with the use of a number of agents, including dexamethasone, ondausetron and metoclopramide. Massive losses of potassium and magnesium (in turn leading to hypocalcemia) must be anticipated with the use of cisplatin because of drug-induced renal tubular damage.

IX-23. **The answer is A.** *(Chap. 113)* Adults with acute lymphocytic leukemia (ALL) do not respond nearly as well to chemotherapeutic programs as do children with the same disease. The reason for the inferior results in adults is not poor tolerance of chemotherapy. Instead, adults with ALL are more likely to present with a disease typified by adverse prognostic factors, usually indicating derivation from a more primitive hematopoietic stem cell. For example, Philadelphia chromosome–positive ALL— t(9;22)—is much more common in adults than in children. Adults are also more likely to have leukemic cells that bear either myeloid antigens or immunophenotypic evidence of derivation from a primitive stem cell (CD34 positivity). Balanced translocations in ALL, such as the t(4;11) associated with biphenotypic leukemia, also portend a poor prognosis. The most favorable subtype of ALL is that derived from a pre-B cell—CALLA (CD10) or B4 (CD19) positivity—with normal cytogenetics. However, for reasons that remain unclear, even this "favorable" prognostic subgroup is not associated with the high cure rate characteristic of children with the same immunophenotype and cytogenetics.

IX-24. **The answer is C.** *(Chap. 97. Anonymous, Lancet 346:265, 1995.)* Given the poorly differentiated histology at presentation with the associated high risk of recurrence and the characteristic indicators of metastatic prostate cancer, biopsy is unnecessary. Since the patient has symptomatic disease, he should be started on androgen deprivation therapy, which is likely to cause a decrease in his pain. An equivalent response rate has been demonstrated with bilateral orchiectomy, diethylstilbestrol, and luteinizing hormone releasing hormone (LHRH) analogues such as leuprolide. Given his desire not to have an orchiectomy and his vascular disease, LHRH analogues would be the best approach. Though providing "total androgen blockade" may be beneficial, whether flutamide should be routinely combined with an LHRH agonist such as leuprolide is unclear. Prostatic carcinoma is poorly responsive to chemotherapy.

**IX-25. The answer is A.** *(Chaps. 106, 107)* Iron deficiency frequently is confused with thalassemia trait, both α and β, in that all three of these conditions are characterized by a microcytic anemia. Iron stores, as reflected by transferrin saturation, serum ferritin level, and bone marrow iron staining, are depleted in iron deficiency but normal in both types of thalassemia trait. Hemoglobin electrophoresis reveals an increased hemoglobin A2 level in β-thalassemia trait but subnormal levels in iron deficiency and α-thalassemia trait. (In the presence of concomitant iron deficiency, hemoglobin A2 levels may be normal in persons with β-thalassemia, but levels rise once iron stores are replenished.)

**IX-26. The answer is D.** *(Chaps. 60, 117)* The formation of a platelet plug at the site of vascular injury (i.e., primary hemostasis) requires adhesion of platelets, release of granules, and aggregation of platelets. The first of these three processes depends on the binding of platelets to deepithelialized vessel walls through an interaction between basement membrane collagen and the collagen receptor, composed of platelet glycoproteins Ia and IIa. This link is stabilized by the binding of von Willebrand factor, a multimeric adhesive glycoprotein, to platelet glycoprotein Ib-IX. The adherent platelets then release a host of mediators that serve to promote secretion of granules of platelets, aggregation of platelets, and activation of the coagulation cascade. Dense granules of platelets release adenosine diphosphate, which allows fibrinogen to serve as a bridge between platelets via platelet glycoprotein IIb-IIIa so that aggregation may occur. Thus, glycoprotein IIb-IIIa mediates interactions between platelets, not between platelets and vessel walls.

**IX-27. The answer is B.** *(Chap. 115)* The clinical scenario is consistent with a delayed transfusion reaction. Immediate transfusion reactions, which are most commonly due to ABO incompatibility and result from clerical error, are associated with intravascular hemolysis (anti-A and anti-B antibodies fix complement) manifested by lumbar pain, hemoglobinemia, and shock. Fever, malaise, and a drop in hematocrit with findings compatible with extravascular hemolysis (microspherocytes, indirect hyperbilirubinemia) 1 week after red cell transfusion are typical of a delayed transfusion reaction, which is usually mediated by antibodies to Rh (or if the recipient is Rh-negative, by anti-Duffy, anti-Kidd, or anti-Kell antibodies). A previous transfusion may have been the precursor of the clinically relevant anamnestic response. These antibodies likely coat the donor red cells, thereby producing a positive direct Coombs' test. Less commonly the donor's plasma could contain antibodies that would react with the recipient's cells. Sensitization to the alloantigens on donor leukocytes transfused along with the red cells could account for fever, but not hemolysis.

**IX-28. The answer is B.** *(Chap. 118)* Hemophilia A and B are clinically indistinguishable, X-linked disorders that cause bleeding into soft tissues, muscles, and weight-bearing joints. In both disorders, all tests of coagulation are normal except for an elevation of the partial thromboplastin time. Specific-factor assays are required to define a specific disorder. Factor VIII is a 265-kilodalton (kDa) protein that regulates the activation of factor X by intrinsic pathway proteases. Factor IX, which unlike factor VIII requires vitamin K–dependent, posttranslational modification, is a 55-kDa proenzyme converted to activated factor IXa by factor XIa. Factor IXa activates factor X with the participation of factor VIII. The distinction between these two entities is important because the therapy is different, since replacement factors for each have been produced by recombinant DNA technologist, thereby eliminating the risks of infection and transfusion or unwanted factors.

**IX-29. The answer is D.** *(Chap. 99)* Though the incidence of ovarian carcinoma is low, the propensity to present at an advanced stage (only 25 percent of patients have disease limited to one or both ovaries) helps to explain why this disease is the most common cause of death among all gynecologic malignancies. Due to the advanced stage at presentation, surgical debulking is the initial therapy for most patients. Only about 15 percent of ovarian cancers arise from nonepithelial elements. Epithelial tumors are most common in peri- or postmenopausal women, especially nulliparous women or those with few children. Prior breast cancer increases the risk of developing ovarian cancer by two- to fourfold. An advanced stage and a larger size of residual tumor after initial surgery carry an adverse prognosis, as do poorly differentiated ovarian carcinomas, which have a 5-year survival of well under 20 percent.

**IX-30.** **The answer is D.** *(Chap. 88)* Primary malignant melanoma of the skin is the leading cause of death among all diseases arising in the skin. A number of factors have been identified that correlate with increased or decreased likelihood of dissemination. The most common site for melanoma in males is the torso, and lesions occurring on the torso offer a worse prognosis than do those occurring on a lower extremity. Both dermatologic level of invasion and thickness of the primary lesion are predictive of dissemination and, hence, of survival. For example, melanomas less than 0.76 mm thick are almost always surgically cured; those that penetrate $\geq$ 3.65 mm have a 60 percent rate of distant metastases. While geographic area of residence is an important determinant of risk of development of melanoma, with incidence of disease higher in latitudes with greater sun exposure, it does not appear to affect risk of dissemination in those with clinically localized disease. The presence of an ulcer in the primary tumor, mitotic rate, and the demonstration of tumor satellites (microscopic foci of tumor distinct from the primary tumor in the reticular dermis or subcutaneous fat) are also prognostic factors.

**IX-31.** **The answer is B.** *(Chaps. 81, 97)* Foci of prostatic carcinoma are frequently noted at autopsy, but only about one-third of such cases are clinically apparent. Nonetheless, prostatic carcinoma is the most common cancer type in men and the second leading cause of male cancer deaths in those over age 75. Ninety-five percent of prostate cancers are adenocarcinomas. The grade of cellular differentiation is an extremely important prognostic variable; a higher Gleason grade (ranging from 2 to 10) indicates a biologically more aggressive tumor. Though the prostate capsule is a natural barrier to spread, dissemination may occur directly to the seminal vesicles and bladder floor, via lymphatics to the obturator, iliac, presacral, or paraaortic nodes, or hematogenously—usually to the bones, especially the pelvis and lumbar vertebrae. Staging consists of clinical examination of the prostate, pelvic CT or MRI, bone scan (with correlative x-rays for positive areas), and detection of the serum marker, prostate specific antigen (PSA). An elevated PSA is not pathognomonic for metastatic disease, but it is more common in those with spread to the bones. Though CT scans are helpful, the only certain way to determine local and regional lymph node spread is via surgical staging.

**IX-32.** **The answer is D.** *(Chap. 112. Wetzler, Am J Med 99:402, 1995.)* Chronic myelogenous leukemia (CML), a myeloproliferative disorder in which bone marrow stem cells are affected, can be diagnosed on clinical grounds alone. A bone marrow examination disclosing myeloid hyperplasia with basophilia would be supportive but not diagnostic. Every patient with CML has a Philadelphia chromosome (translocation between the long arms of chromosomes 22 and 9), which may be identified by either cytogenetic or molecular analysis. In addition to the cytogenetic abnormality, stable-phase CML is characterized by leukocytosis with a left shift, basophilia, splenomegaly, and a low leukocyte alkaline phosphatase (high in reactive leukocytosis and in agnogenic myeloid metaplasia). The duration of the stable phase is variable, but the disease always progresses on to blast crisis, unless interrupted by an allogeneic bone marrow transplant. The leukocytosis and metabolic symptoms of stable-phase CML can be controlled with a number of agents, including hydroxyurea, busulfan, and interferon-$\alpha$. Results with interferon-$\alpha$ treatment suggest that the percentage of cells containing the Philadelphia chromosome may be reduced and that long-term survival is improved compared with patients receiving hydroxyurea or busulfan.

**IX-33.   The answer is A.**   *(Chap. 88. Rigel, Cancer 63:386, 1989.)*   A distinctive pigmented lesion, the dysplastic nevus, occurs in families with a high incidence of melanoma, transmitted as an autosomal dominant trait and linked to chromosome 9q16. The recognition of this syndrome is important because the patient and family members can undergo intense dermatologic follow-up with early detection of malignant lesions. Patients with dysplastic nevi and two family members with melanoma have a 50 percent lifetime risk of developing melanoma. Dysplastic nevi tend to have irregular borders and be variable in color and shape on a given individual. They are usually large (minimum diameter of 6 mm) compared with benign nevi. The back is the most common site of dysplastic nevi, but they may also be seen on the scalp, buttocks, and breast. Though dysplastic nevi do serve as markers for the development of melanoma on normal skin, they also serve as precursor lesions, which makes it vital to watch each dysplastic nevus carefully.

**IX-34.   The answer is A.**   *(Chap. 92. Kinzler, Science 251:1366, 1991.)*   Familial polyposis of the colon is a rare condition that is inherited in an autosomal dominant fashion through loss of function of a tumor suppressor gene (APC) on the long arm of chromosome 5. It is characterized by adenomatous polyps throughout the colon. A total proctocolectomy can eliminate the certain risk of cancer by age 40. Peutz-Jeghers syndrome is characterized by hamartomatous polyps (without risk of malignant degeneration) in the stomach and all intestinal sites. In Gardner's syndrome adenomatous polyps line the large and small intestine; in addition to a high risk of colon cancer, such patients are plagued with multiple benign tumors, including osteomas, fibromas, and lipomas. Turcot's syndrome refers to the constellation of adenomatous colonic polyps and malignant brain tumors.

**IX-35.   The answer is C.**   *(Chap. 92)*   Squamous cell cancer of the esophagus accounts for approximately 10,000 deaths annually in the United States. Worldwide, incidences vary greatly, but it is particularly common in a belt from the Caspian Sea to northern China. In the United States, epidemiologic studies have linked smoking and alcohol to squamous cell cancer of the esophagus and may explain the association of this tumor with head and neck carcinoma. Exposure to agents that damage the mucosa (e.g., very hot tea, lye, radiation) or ingestion of carcinogens such as nitrites, smoked opiates, and fungal toxins is associated with an increased risk of esophageal carcinoma. The long-term stasis associated with achalasia leads to chronic irritation of the esophagus, which is thought to predispose to cancer formation. Tylosis is a genetically acquired disease characterized by thickening of the skin of the hands and feet and is associated with squamous cell cancer of the esophagus. Chronic gastric reflux (Barrett's esophagus) is associated with adenocarcinoma but not with squamous cell carcinoma of the esophagus.

**IX-36.   The answer is E.**   *(Chap. 92)*   Malignant neoplasms of the stomach typically present with epigastric pain, postprandial fullness, and weight loss or fatigue. Iron-deficiency anemia also may be seen. Histologically, 90 percent of stomach cancers are adenocarcinomas and 10 percent are due to non-Hodgkin's lymphomas or leiomyosarcomas. Risks for the development of gastric adenocarcinoma include decreased gastric acidity, prior antrectomy (latency period of 15 to 20 years), atrophic gastritis, and the presence of blood group A. These risk factors are not associated with the development of primary gastric lymphoma, which is a more treatable disease than adenocarcinoma. The only real chance for a cure with adenocarcinoma is complete surgical removal of the tumor and resection of the adjacent lymph nodes. The use of adjuvant chemotherapy, radiation therapy, or both after complete resections in patients with adenocarcinoma seems to offer some benefit compared with surgery alone. Moreover, the use of these modalities in cases where resection was only partial is controversial, although combination chemotherapy with a regimen such as 5-fluorouracil, doxorubicin, and mitomycin C will lead to partial responses in up to 50 percent of cases. However, complete removal of the tumor in patients with gastric lymphoma results in a 5-year survival rate of 40 to 60 percent (compared with 25 to 30 percent in adenocarcinoma). Combination chemotherapy may even be a useful adjunct in the postsurgical setting and may be able to substitute for surgery. The latter point is a subject of much debate; however, fears that presurgical chemotherapy would lead to an inordinant risk of bleeding or perforation seem unfounded on the basis of recent studies. Gastric lymphomas are nearly always of B cell origin.

**IX-37. The answer is D.** *(Chap. 92. Mandel, N Engl J Med 328:1365–1371, 1993.)* The goal of screening for colorectal cancer is to detect surgically curable neoplasms. Though rigid or flexible sigmoidoscopy clearly plays a role in early detection of distal colon cancers, the overall benefit or cost/benefit of routine screening in this fashion has not been established. Most efforts have been in the area of Hemoccult testing for occult fecal blood. The following features complicate the use of this modality: (1) Approximately 50 percent of those with documented colorectal cancers have a negative Hemoccult test; (2) asymptomatic cancers are found in only 10 percent of those who test positive (although benign polyps will be detected in an additional 20 to 30 percent); and (3) those with a positive test are subjected to additional uncomfortable and expensive procedures, including sigmoidoscopy, barium enema, and colonoscopy. Nonetheless, a study from the University of Minnesota documented a statistically significant reduction in mortality in a group of patients undergoing annual Hemoccult screening compared with a randomized control group that received routine care. A cost-effectiveness analysis of this study has not been performed. The present American Cancer Society recommendations are somewhat more aggressive than the available data would completely support: annual digital rectal examinations beginning at age 40, annual fecal Hemoccult screening beginning at age 50, and sigmoidoscopy (preferably flexible) every 3 to 5 years beginning at age 50 for asymptomatic persons at average risk. Of course, patients with a positive family history or other high-risk features in whom the probability of colorectal cancer is higher than that in the average population should be screened more aggressively.

**IX-38. The answer is C.** *(Chap. 289. Crook, N Engl J Med 324:709, 1991.)* Total resection of the primary tumor is the treatment of choice for both colon and rectal carcinoma. Assuming that metastases are ruled out, the presence or absence of extension into the muscularis mucosa or the presence of carcinoma in regional lymph nodes is an important prognostic feature. For example, those with regional lymph node involvement have 30 to 60 percent 5-year survival, whereas those whose cancer extends into the muscularis but not to the serosa and who do not have positive lymph nodes have 85 percent 5-year survival. 5-Fluorouracil (5-FU) is the most active single agent in treating advanced colorectal cancer, but adjuvant chemotherapy with 5-FU in high-risk (serosal or nodal involvement) patients has not shown a statistically meaningful reduction in the rate of recurrence. However, randomized trials have indicated a survival benefit if 5-FU is administered in combination with the antihelminthic agent levamisole in patients with node-positive tumors. Furthermore, radiation therapy to the pelvis can significantly lower the probability of local recurrence in patients with high-risk rectal carcinoma. Data from several controlled studies indicate that postoperative radiation therapy combined with chemotherapy (including 5-FU) appears to reduce the likelihood of local recurrences and increase the potential for long-term survival without recurrence. In this setting, chemotherapy may act as a radiation sensitizer.

**IX-39. The answer is E.** *(Chap. 92. Aaltonen, Science 260:812, 1993.)* The specific cause of colon cancer is unknown, although studies have revealed an excess of genetic allele loss in advanced colonic neoplasia. However, certain diseases are known to increase the risk of development of cancer of the colon. Crohn's colitis is associated with an increased risk of colon cancer, although the risk is less than that for patients with ulcerative colitis. Colon cancer has been observed to occur with increased frequency in

**322**                                     IX. HEMATOPOIETIC DISORDERS AND NEOPLASIA — ANSWERS

patients with uterine cancer. Patients with adenomatous polyps are at higher risk for the subsequent development of colon cancer than is the general population. Therefore, such patients should have periodic follow-up examinations. Up to 25 percent of patients with colorectal carcinoma have a family history of this disease; recent reports suggest the role of a gene on chromosome 2, which codes for a gene involved in DNA repair, in many of these cases. The polyps in juvenile polyposis are hamartomatous and have no malignant potential. Colonic neoplasms at a site distal to the ureteral implant have been noted to occur 15 to 30 years after uterosigmoidostomy.

**IX-40.  The answer is D.**  *(Chaps. 111, 118)*   Primary erythrocytosis with organomegaly strongly suggests the diagnosis of polycythemia rubra vera. One well-recognized complication of this condition is hypercoagulability, with a particular propensity toward hepatic vein thrombosis. Such an occlusion would lead to the Budd-Chiari syndrome, which is characterized by a grossly enlarged, tender liver with severe ascites. In addition to hepatic vein thrombosis secondary to a hypercoagulable state, such a syndrome could result from idiopathic causes, hepatic invasion by tumor, or the venoocclusive disease associated with chemotherapy or radiation. Once right-sided heart failure is excluded clinically, the diagnosis is best established by hepatic venography or liver biopsy showing sinusoidal dilatation.

**IX-41.  The answer is B.**  *(Chap. 93)*   The clinical constellation of tender hepatomegaly, a bruit in the right upper quadrant of the abdomen, bloody ascites, and very elevated alkaline phosphatase occurring in a patient with previously stable cirrhosis is characteristic of primary hepatocellular carcinoma. This disease typically is associated with very high levels of α-fetoprotein, a unique and specific fetal alpha$_1$ globulin. Rarely, ectopic hormones such as chorionic gonadotropin are found in the serum of patients with hepatocellular carcinoma. The enzyme 5′-nucleotidase may be elevated in a patient with any condition associated with hepatocellular damage. Antimitochondrial antibodies are found in primary biliary cirrhosis and are not typical of primary hepatocellular carcinoma.

**IX-42.  The answer is C.**  *(Chap. 114)*   Multiple myeloma, a disease characterized by the malignant proliferation of plasma cells, can present with unexplained normochromic normocytic anemia, hypercalcemia, bone pain, or infection. In this case the bone marrow examination showed a clear-cut excess of plasma cells which are almost certainly monoclonal. In addition to the problems arising directly from the proliferation of these cells, including myelosuppression and osteolytic lesions, the monoclonal protein excreted by these neoplastically proliferating cells can lead to a host of clinical problems, including "myeloma kidney," renal failure due to light-chain deposition in the renal tubules. Other causes of renal failure in multiple myeloma include uric acid necropathy, hypercalcemia, and infection. Patients with myeloma are prone to infections with encapsulated bacteria because of associated hypogammaglobulinemia, despite the usually elevated monoclonal protein spike characteristic of this disease. About 99 percent of patients with myeloma exhibit a monoclonal spike either in their serum and/or in their urine. The disease burden can be estimated by enumerating the number of osteolytic lesions on skeletal survey, the presence or absence of renal failure, the presence or absence of hypercalcemia, the height of the M-protein (or degree of urinary protein excretion), and the presence or absence of anemia. Another useful measure of disease in patients with myeloma is assessment of the serum β$_2$-microglobulin level. Since most bone lesions in patients with myeloma are osteolytic, radionuclide bone scanning, which detects lesions based on their blastic component, is not generally helpful in following patients with myeloma.

**IX-43.  The answer is A.**  *(Chap. 115)*   Although patients with myelodysplasia, especially those with normal cytogenetics and no excess myeloblasts in the marrow or blood, can be managed for long periods of time only with supportive care, including transfusion, limitations exist. Fortunately, given careful screening for blood-borne viral infections, the incidence of transfusion-associated infection is now rare. However, the need for chronic transfusional therapy may be associated with iron overload and the requirement to use an iron chelating agent such as desferrioxamine. Furthermore, either due to their disease and associated immune dysregulation or due to exposure to many different blood group antigens, chronically transfused patients, such as the one in question, frequently develop a large panel of serum allo-antibodies. The presence of these antibodies may make it very difficult to find blood which will be negative in a cross-match with the patient's serum. While the presence of these antibodies may or may not produce hemolysis if blood containing a potential target antigen is tranfused, blood bank practice requires a negative cross-match except in emergency situations.

**IX-44.   The answer is C.**   *(Chap. 99)*   Most ovarian neoplasms are epithelially derived. Typically, ovarian carcinoma presents in an indolent fashion with abdominal fullness at an advanced stage with extensive interperitoneal metastasis. However, a small subset of ovarian neoplasms are germ cell tumors which are capable of producing sex hormones such as the androgens, leading to virilization, as noted in this patient. Such ovarian germ cell tumors should be treated in an analogous fashion to testicular cancer in the male, since they are highly responsive to cisplatin and etoposide.

**IX-45.   The answer is A.**   *(Chap. 92)*   Invasive rectal cancer is generally treated with surgical resection followed by adjuvant chemotherapy and radiation therapy to decrease the risk of recurrence and metastasis. The use of combined modality therapy decreases the risk of recurrence in patients with rectal cancer whose primary lesions penetrate through the muscularis or into the surrounding lymph nodes. However, if rectal cancer recurs, it usually does so locally and can invade through tissue planes in the pelvis to create problematic pain due to nerve root invasion. Such patients typically have radicular-type pain due to local spread of their cancers. Bony metastases are uncommon. With the elimination of nitrosoureas from the adjuvant treatment regimen for rectal cancer patients, the likelihood of secondary leukemia (and concominant bone pain) is markedly diminished. Pelvic radiation therapy can contribute to adhesion, but would be an unlikely cause of chronic pelvic pain.

**IX-46.   The answer is C.**   *(Chap. 90)*   Approximately 20 percent of all lung cancers are small cell cancers. These tumors tend to present centrally, be derived from neuroendocrine tissues, and be much more chemo- and radiosensitive than non-small cell cancer. Histologic subtypes of non-small cell cancer include adenocarcinoma (which definitely does have a more peripheral presentation), large cell cancer, bronchoalveolar cell cancer, and squamous cell (or bronchogenic) lung cancer. All histologic types of lung cancer are associated with smoking. In the relatively uncommon patient who presents with a small non-small cell primary lesion and lymph node involvement, surgery alone may be curative. Patients with small cell lung cancer are divided into two staging groups: those with limited disease who have tumors generally confined to one hemithorax encompassable by a single radiation port and all others who are said to have extensive disease. About 20 percent of patients who present with limited stage small cell lung cancer are curable with a combination of radiation therapy and chemotherapy (cisplatin and etoposide being the two most active agents).

**IX-47.   The answer is A.**   *(Chap. 110. Stone, Blood 83:3437, 1994.)*   Myelodysplasia is a bone marrow stem cell disorder usually characterized by hypercellular marrows with peripheral blood cytopenias. Characteristic dysplastic changes seen in the bone marrow include hyperlobated megakaryocytes, megaloblastic nuclear maturation in the erythroid series, and dysplastic myeloid maturation including nuclear to cytoplasmic asynchrony and hyperlobated mature myeloid cells (Pelger-Huet anomaly). There may also be excessive numbers (greater than 5 percent) of bone marrow myeloblasts. Chromosomal changes frequently include abnormalities of the long arm of chromosome 5 and/or loss of chromosome 7. Myelodysplasia is a disease of the elderly, without a clear-cut etiologic predisposition; however, ionizing radiation, alkylating agent chemotherapy and industrial solvents are agents that can damage the bone marrow stem cell and lead to the clinical pathological syndrome of myelodysplasia. An unfortunate complication of autologous bone marrow transplantation for non-Hodgkin's lymphoma is the development of myelodysplastic syndrome. It is unclear whether the myelodysplasia occurs secondary to the preparative regimen, usually consisting of high-dose chemotherapy and total body radiation, or to the extensive therapy that many of these patients receive prior to the time of their transplant. Autologous bone marrow transplantation for non-Hodgkin's lymphoma is known to be potentially curative in patients who have entered into second remission or at least a minimal residual disease state. These patients were formerly considered incurable with additional standard chemotherapy. Therefore, despite the very serious problem of post-transplant myelodysplasia, for many patients autologous transplantation remains the best means to deal with relapsed non-Hodgkin's lymphoma. In this case, since there is no evidence of myelophthisis there is no reason to suspect infiltration of the marrow. Patients can develop the hemolytic uremic syndrome post-transplant and could have erythroid hyperplasia on that basis; but the presence of a normal blood smear mitigates against that diagnosis. While bone marrow aplasia could be a late complication of bone marrow transplantation, the presence of dysplastic cells in the peripheral blood argues against it.

**IX-48.    The answer is D.**  *(Chap. 113. Harris, Blood 84:1361, 1994.)*   Mantle cell lymphoma is a now well-recognized clinical entity that was formerly termed intermediate lymphoma. Cells typically are of intermediate differentiation, although a blastic variant also exists. Immunophenotypically, the cells express B-cell antigens such as CD19 and CD20 but also express the nominal T-cell antigen CD5. In addition to chronic lymphocytic leukemia, mantle cell lymphoma is one of the only B cell neoplasms that routinely expresses this antigen. It may be distinguished immunophenotypically from chronic lymphoid leukemia (or small lymphocytic lymphoma which is the lymph node predominant form) by the lack of CD23 expression. The t(11;14) brings cyclin $D_1$ under the influence of immunoglobulin heavy chain promoters and leads to cyclin $D_1$ overexpression. It is not clear how this contributes to lymphomagenesis. This translocation is nearly always associated with mantle cell lymphoma. The prognosis for patients with mantle cell lymphoma is poor. Although it is relatively chemotherapeutically resistant, as is the case with other low-grade lymphomas, the natural history is not nearly as indolent with median survival in the 2- to 3-year range.

**IX-49.    The answer is E.**  *(Chap. 112)*   The acute myeloid leukemias are subdivided, based on morphological, cytochemical, and immunophenotypical parameters, into eight subtypes according to the FAB classification. Certain subtypes have well-defined cytogenetic abnormalities and clinical findings. For example, acute promyelocytic leukemia (M3 AML) is associated with t(15;17) and commonly presents with a bleeding diathesis due to the disseminated intravascular coagulopathy engendered by the procoagulant-containing granules in the malignant promyelocytes. Acute myelomonocytic (M4) and acute monocytic leukemia (M5) have a higher likelihood than the other types of AML of presenting with extramedullary involvement, especially in the gums, skin, and central nervous system. Central nervous system involvement is also somewhat more likely in high-grade lymphoproliferative neoplasms, such as L3 (Burkitt's) and acute lymphoblastic leukemia. T-cell acute lymphoblastic leukemia typically presents in young adults with mediastinal masses and a high white count. M7 AML or acute megakaryocytic leukemia is difficult to diagnose because of the associated bone marrow fibrosis which makes bone marrow aspiration and therefore morphologic, immunophenotypic, and cytogenetic analysis difficult. M7 is not associated with polyneuropathy.

**IX-50.    The answer is B.**  *(Chap. 112)*   The Philadelphia chromosome is the diagnostic hallmark of chronic myeloid leukemia. This cytogenetic abnormality involves the translocation between the BCR gene on chromosome 22 and the c-*abl* pro-oncogene on chromosome 9. This results in hematopoiesis which is abnormally regulated. Patients with chronic myeloid leukemia typically experience a chronic phase which lasts for 3 to 4 years in which there is little clinical symptomatology. High platelet count, large spleen and the presence of excess basophils in the blood or bone marrow at the time of presentation suggest that the chronic phase may be relatively short. Nonetheless, the finding of any additional cytogenetic abnormalities during the course of treatment or follow-up during stable phase is an ominous sign. Specifically, it is likely that accelerated phase (or blast crisis) is impending. The most commonly observed second cytogenetic event is a duplicated Philadelphia chromosome.

**IX-51. The answer is D.** *(Chap. 82. Woolf, N Engl J Med 333:1401, 1995.)* In order to definitively prove that a screening test is worthwhile, a randomized controlled trial comparing screened and unscreened patients with cause-specific mortality as the endpoint is required. Any other endpoint, such as a reduction in the incidence of advanced stage disease, improved survival, or a stage shift, provides less clear-cut support of benefit. No such trials have been completed with regard to prostate-specific antigen screening. Moreover, screening for prostate-specific antigen is fraught with many potential biases. For example, the test may not lead to any change in the natural history of prostate-cancer (lead-time bias); the patient may be diagnosed at an earlier date and appear to survive longer, but life is not really prolonged. Second, length bias, which refers to the detection of slow-growing less aggressive cancers, is certainly a problem with prostate-specific antigen screening. It is highly likely that prostate-specific antigen screening will lead to over-diagnosis with many patients will be found to have prostate cancer in whom this disease never would have been a problem. It is not clear whether the most effective treatment for low-stage prostate cancer is radical prostatectomy, radiation therapy, observation, or possibly even early hormonal therapy. As such, treating low-stage prostate cancers will certainly cause excess morbidity, including impotence or urinary incontinence.

**IX-52. The answer is E.** *(Chap. 81. Levy, N Engl J Med 335:1124, 1996.)* Seventy-five percent of cancer patients with advanced disease experience pain which may be caused by tumor invasion, invasive surgical procedures, or radiation or chemotherapy injury. The vast majority of patients will experience pain relief with pharmacologic intervention. It is helpful to use the World Health Organization method for the rational titration of oral analgesia. The goal is to keep the patient ambulatory and pain-free. For mild pain patients should receive acetaminophen, aspirin, or a nonsteroidal adjuvant with or without an additional adjuvant such as glucocorticoid or antidepressant. The next step consists of adding an opioid such as codeine or hydrocodone. If pain persists despite these steps, the opioid should be replaced with a more potent drug, potentially at higher dose, such as immediate-release morphine 15 to 30 mg every 3 to 4 h, or controlled-release morphine, 60 mg twice a day (or higher).

**IX-53. The answer is E.** *(Chap. 83. Weinberg, Cell 81:323, 1995.)* Unbridled proliferation, one hallmark of cancer, may occur due to several mechanisms. Loss of normal control of movement through the cell cycle represents one group of such mechanisms. The G1-S transition (movement into DNA synthesis phase) and the G2-M transition (movement into mitotic phase) are tightly regulated. The G1-S transition is frequently disrupted in cancer. Cyclin/cyclin-dependent kinase (CdK) protein complexes are responsible for phosphorylating the retinoblastoma gene product, Rb, at ten different sites. Such modification alters the ability of this protein to associate with other cellular proteins such as E2F, a transcription factor that heterodimerizes with other transcription factors to active genes required to progress on to S phase. If an Rb mutation prevents normal association with E2F, the free E2F can act as a transcription factor and initiate S phase. Mutations in the retinoblastoma gene product are found in many tumors including osteosarcoma, retinoblastoma, breast cancer, and lung cancer.

**IX-54. The answer is E.** *(Chap. 84. Collins, N Engl J Med 334:186, 1996.)* While most patients with breast and ovarian cancer are not yet known to have a mutation in one of the high penetrance susceptibility genes so far identified (BRCA-1 and BRCA-2), for those 5 to 10 percent who do have a BRCA-1 mutation the lifetime risk of breast cancer is as high as 85 percent and of ovarian cancer is as high as 50 percent. The gene is inherited in an autosomal dominant fashion; therefore, the woman has a 50 percent chance of passing the risk of breast cancer on to her daughter. Roughly 1 in 500 women in this country carry a germ-line BRCA-1 mutation without a strong family history. BRCA-1 mutations may occur throughout the gene except in the Ashkanazi Jewish population where 1 in 100 individuals carries a two-base pair deletion in a specific location on the BRCA-1 gene. There are many additional complexities in genetic testing for cancer susceptibility. A major problem is what to do in cases where the test is positive. To definitively reduce a patient's risk in this situation, a bilateral mastectomy would be required. On the other hand, it could be quite reassuring to a given individual to know that she does not carry a BRCA-1 mutation. Most importantly, testing should not be undertaken without concomitant counseling to determine how the individual will handle a positive or a negative result.

**IX-55. The answer is A.** *(Chaps. 86, 105. American Society of Clinical Oncology, J Clin Onc 12:2471, 1994.)* Two hematopoietic growth factors are currently approved for use in the management of chemotherapy-induced neutropenia. Granulocyte macrophage colony-stimulating factor (GM-CSF) and granulocyte colony-stimulating factor (G-CSF) are now commonly used to ameliorate the myelosuppression associated with chemotherapy use. While the agents, particularly G-CSF, are well tolerated, their use is expensive and not appropriate for each cycle of chemotherapy. The American Society of Clinical Oncology has recommended that G-CSF be administered with the first cycle of planned chemotherapy only if the patient has a 40 percent or greater risk of experiencing fever and neutropenia. If the patient has experienced an episode of febrile neutropenia, then administration of the growth factor with a subsequent course is reasonable, especially if dose intensity is important. Clearly in the case of cyclophosphamide, doxorubicin, vincristine, and prednisone chemotherapy for early-stage large cell lymphoma, chemotherapy must be administered at full doses, on time, to ensure that cure is most likely. Consequently, since the patient has recovered within approximately two weeks after the administration of cycle three of chemotherapy, cycle four should be given on time, at full dose with granulocyte colony-stimulating factor support to limit the likelihood that the subsequent cycle would result in another hospitalization for febrile neutropenia. Since the tumor is responding well to chemotherapy, changing to an alternative regimen, particularly a less myelosuppressive one, would be inappropriate. Moreover, colony-stimulating factors are not recommended for routine use in either afebrile or febrile neutropenic patients unless factors predictive of deterioration are present.

**IX-56. The answer is A.** *(Chap. 88. Kirkwood, J Clin Oncol 14:7, 1996.)* The most important prognostic factor for outcome in malignant melanoma is the stage at presentation. Stages I and II refer to tumors in which there is no evidence, either clinically or pathologically, of disease in draining lymph nodes. For these patients, the risk of recurrence is critically dependent upon the depth of invasion; overall survival ranges from over 95 percent in those with primary lesions less than 0.75-mm thick to less than 50 percent in those whose primary lesion is greater than 4 mm in thickness. The presence of one or more pathologically involved lymph nodes is associated with a 45 percent or lower chance of long-term survival. Those with intermediate-risk local disease (lesions between 0.75 mm and 3.5 mm in thickness) may benefit from elective regional lymph node resection. Chemotherapeutic treatment for regional lymph node or distant metastasis is highly unsatisfactory. While dacarbazine and nitrosoureas are active agents, response rates of 20 percent or less make it unlikely that these agents would be useful in the adjuvant setting. However, clinical trials have suggested that adjuvant interferon-$\alpha$ can improve the disease-free and overall survival significantly in patients at extremely high risk for recurrence (those with deep lesions or with clinical or pathological evidence of nodal metastasis). A study performed by the Eastern Cooperative Oncology Group randomized patients to receive interferon-α 2B at a maintenance dose of 10 mU/m²/d twice weekly (after a higher induction dose) or observation for those with primary lesions greater than 4 mm in thickness and patients with clinical or pathological evidence of spread to regional nodes. There was a distinctly significant prolongation of both relapse-free and overall survival in the treated group. The effect was greatest in those patients with clinically palpable lymph nodes. Because the interferon was fairly toxic and was stopped in a significant portion of patients, ongoing studies are determining the minimum effective interferon dose.

**IX-57. The answer is C.** *(Chap. 89. Department of Veterans' Affairs. Laryngeal Cancer Study, N Engl J Med 324:1685, 1991.)* Locally advanced squamous cell carcinoma of the head and neck refers to disease that presents with either a large primary and/or lymph node metastases. Such extensive disease may be treated with curative intent with extensive surgery followed by postoperative radiation or radiation alone. Unfortunately, despite such aggressive local therapy, most patients die of their disease within two years. Since squamous cell carcinoma of the head and neck is a highly responsive tumor to chemotherapeutic agents such as cisplatin and 5-fluorouracil, numerous studies have addressed the issue of so-called "neoadjuvant chemotherapy." Unfortunately, several large studies which compared surgery/radiation therapy with chemotherapy followed by surgery/radiation therapy suggested no benefit in terms of survival for those receiving chemotherapy. The VA cooperative study clearly established that such "induction" chemotherapy can offer organ preservation in the case of advanced larynx cancer. The study showed no difference in survival for those patients with larynx cancer who received either surgery and radiation or chemotherapy and radiation; however, those who received chemotherapy were much more likely to have a preserved larynx.

**IX-58. The answer is D.** *(Chap. 114. Attal et al, N Engl J Med 335:91, 1996.)* Although about 10 percent of patients with multiple myeloma have indolent disease, the vast majority of patients with this disease require therapeutic intervention, either systemic chemotherapy to control the progression of the disease and/or symptomatic supportive care to prevent morbidity from the complications. While the standard approach is an alkylating agent such as melphalan plus prednisone, or VAD combination chemotherapy (vincristine via a 4-day continuous infusion, doxorubicin via a 4-day continuous infusion, and dexamethasone 40 mg/d for 4 days per week for 3 weeks), it appears likely that the most effective treatment is high-dose glucocorticoids. Maintenance therapy with interferon may prolong responses, but has not yet been shown to consistently prolong survival. A randomized trial compared conventional chemotherapy to high-dose therapy with autologous bone marrow transplantation and determined that patients randomly assigned to receive high-dose therapy experienced superior survival. Bisphosphonates such as pamidronate are useful not only in the treatment of hypercalcemia but also to reduce osteoclastic bone resorption, thereby preserving performance status and quality of life. Plasmapheresis is effective in clearing light chains if renal failure occurs and also is the treatment of choice for hyperviscosity. Neither routine use of prophylactic intravenous gammaglobulin nor oral antibiotics has been shown to be effective for those patients who have an increased likelihood of infection with bacterial pathogens such as *S. pneumoniae.*

**IX-59. The answer is D.** *(Chap. 113)* One of the reasons that there is a shift in the treatment of early stage Hodgkin's disease to abbreviated chemotherapy and limited radiation is the significant long-term side effects of mantle irradiation. Within months of mantle irradiation, about 15 percent develop lower extrimities paresthesia upon flexion of the neck (Lhermitte's sign), which does not appear to be associated with any late sequellae. Radiation pneumonitis occurs in less than 5 percent, with symptomatic pulmonary fibrosis being even more unusual. Other complications of late mantle radiation include pericardial effusion, frank myocardial injury, and a 3-fold increased risk for fatal coronary artery disease. Thyroid function tests need to be followed closely since hypothyroidism may occur in up to 80 percent of irradiated patients. Second solid tumors are common after radiation therapy, particularly breast cancer and lung cancer in smokers. Stomach, skin, soft tissue sarcomas, and primary bone tumors all occur in excess numbers in those who have received radiation. Secondary acute myeloid leukemias and myelodysplasias occur in patients treated with alkylating agent therapy for Hodgkin's disease; this potential complication may be enhanced by concomitant radiation therapy; however, mantle radiation therapy alone does not seem to impart a significant risk for secondary leukemia.

**IX-60.    The answer is E.**    *(Chap. 113. Shipp, Blood 83:1165, 1994.)*    Patients with intermediate grade non-Hodgkin's lymphoma may be cured with conventional (i.e. cyclophosphamide, vincristine, doxorubicin, prednisone) chemotherapy, but their likelihood of such a favorable outcome depends critically on a number of prognostic factors that can be easily determined at presentation. Patients' age (less than 60 vs greater than 60), serum LDH (normal vs abnormal), performance status (0 or 1 vs 2 to 4), stage (1 or 2, vs 3 or 4), and extranodal involvement (less than or equal to one site vs greater than one site) were independently prognostic for overall survival in an analysis of a large group of patients with diffuse large B-cell lymphomas. For example, those with only 0 or 1 of the aforementioned risk factors have a 73 percent 5-year survival rate with standard chemotherapy; those with 4 or 5 risk factors have a 26 percent 5-year survival rate. The ability to predict how patients will fare with standard chemotherapy can form the basis of clinical trials in which poor-prognosis patients are given higher-dose therapy either during initial therapy or after remission has been achieved. Patients with non-Hodgkin's lymphoma who relapse after initial remission and who then can be induced into a minimum residual disease state with additional chemotherapy can enjoy roughly a 40 percent chance of long-term disease-free survival if they receive myeloblative chemotherapy followed by rescue with autologous stem cells. Such patients have a very much smaller chance of long-term survival if they only receive standard chemotherapy after initial relapse. As such, it is possible that those patients who present with high-risk disease at presentation could be candidates for a primary high-dose approach.

**IX-61.    The answer is C.**    *(Chap. 87)*    Complications related to chemotherapy-induced myelosuppression and gastrointestinal epithelial dysfunction can be life-threatening. Bacteremias caused by enteric gram negative rods and gram positive cocci and disseminated Candidemia are common. Patients often experience painful mucositis and discomforting diarrhea as a consequence of antileukemic chemotherapy. One specific complication of chemotherapy is typhlitis, also called neutropenic enterocolitis, which refers to an inflammation of the bowel wall in the setting of profound neutropenia and gut denudation. Physical examination usually mimics an acute abdomen. CT typically discloses an inflammatory-type mass in the right lower quadrant and/or thickening of the cecal wall. Since the patient is profoundly neutropenic, there is no abscess to drain. Secondly, exploratory laporotomy would be prohibitively dangerous and not very effective in this setting. The most appropriate therapy is bowel rest, good antibiotic coverage for bowel flora, and waiting for time to elapse until the patient's neutrophils recover. Although very high mortality rates associated with typhlitis were originally reported, with a conservative management strategy most patients will recover assuming that their leukemia responds to therapy.

**IX-62.    The answer is A.**    *(Chap. 113)*    Chronic lymphocytic leukemia (CLL), the most common of the acute or chronic leukemias, is a malignancy of mature-appearing B lymphocytes which characteristically occurs in older adults. The diagnosis can be confirmed by flow cytometric means since CLL cells typically co-express B-cell antigens such as CD20 and CD23 as well as the nominal T-cell antigen, CD5. The prognosis of a patient with CLL is critically dependent on his or her stage: Rai stage 0 patients have lymphocytosis only, stage 1 patients have lymphocytosis plus lymphadopathy, stage 2 patients have splenomegaly, stage 3 patients have anemia (not due to autoimmune hemolysis), and stage 4 patients have thrombocytopenia. The expected length of survival for those with stage 0 CLL is similar to that of age-matched controls. The survival prognosis for those with stage I CLL is also favorable, with 7- to 10-year mean survival. As such there is no role for chemotherapy in this patient who is doing well, albeit with the knowledge that she does have a chronic malignancy. Although the patient is hypogammaglobulinemic, as is typical for patients with CLL, she has had no infection; it has been clearly shown that prophylactic intravenous gammaglobulin therapy for all patients with CLL is highly costly without clear-cut benefit. If a patient needs systemic therapy because of rapid doubling of the lymphocyte count, symptoms due to bulky nodes, or cytopenias, then fludarabine is often initially used because it offers the best response rate. The drug, however, is myelosuppressive and immunosuppressive and should be administered with caution. Given the indolent nature of the disease and advanced age of this patient, therapy is not warranted at this time.

**IX-63.** **The answer is A.** *(Chaps. 110, 111)* The myeloproliferative disorders are characterized by an overproduction of one or more cellular elements with, in general, normal morphologic appearance of the cells. In polycythemia vera the red cell mass is high, in essential thrombocytosis platelets are produced in far greater numbers than normal, and in chronic myeloid leukemia (CML) the white count is generally elevated. Patients with CML typically present with an elevated white count with a left-shifted differential, peripheral blood basophilia and/or eosinophilia and splenomegaly. However, the platelet count is usually elevated and the hematocrit is normal. The finding of a left-shifted white cell series, nucleated red blood cells, and tear drop–shaped red cells suggests a myelophthisic picture. Although myelophthisis could be due to infiltration with metastatic tumor, the splenomegaly in this case coupled with the dry bone marrow tap strongly suggests that this patient has idiopathic myelofibrosis (also termed agnogenic myeloid metaplasia). Median survival of patients with idiopathic myelofibrosis is approximately 5 years and is modified adversely by the size of the spleen, the patient's age, and particularly the degree of the anemia. Treatment is largely supportive, although splenectomy should be considered if symptoms of early satiety or intractable abdominal pain occur in the presence of refractory thrombocytopenia or the need for abundant red cell transfusions.

**IX-64.** **The answer is E.** *(Chap. 90)* Although patients with limited disease small cell carcinoma of the lung may be cured with a combination of chemotherapy and radiation therapy, most patients experience either local or systemic relapse. In this case, the patient is presenting with classic findings of post obstructive pneumonia due to an endobronchial lesion or due to bronchial compression from an extrinsic mass. Tracheal deviation, decreased breath sounds, and a collapsed lobe are all consistent with this diagnosis. While systemic antibiotics are generally administered, successful therapy critically depends on establishing a patent airway. Bronchoscopy can determine whether the lesion is intrinsic or extrinsic and whether laser cautery or brachytherapy (placing radiation seeds in the area of the tumor) could be helpful. It is unlikely that external beam radiation therapy could be delivered safely given the patient's prior extensive treatment for limited stage small cell lung cancer. Chemotherapy and even additional external beam radiation therapy might play a role in the management of this patient, but only after an attempt at an anatomic solution.

**IX-65.** **The answer is C.** *(Chap. 86)* Cancer chemotherapeutic agents are classified by various schemas, chief among them being intracellular mechanism of action and cell cycle phase of activity. An important class of chemotherapeutic agents are the antimetabolites, such as cytarabine, which generally are converted to molecules that serve as false substrates for nucleic acid biosynthesis. They are usually cell cycle active, S-phase specific agents. The antitumor antibiotics, exemplified by doxorubicin and other anthracyclines, were originally thought to exert cytotoxicity by intercalating between DNA bases; however, they actually stabilize the topoisomerase-II DNA complex. Topoisomerase-II and topoisomerase-I are critically important enzymes involved in DNA repair. An important new class of compounds, the camptothecins (irinotecan was the first such compound available for clinical use), inhibit topoisomerase-I. Vincristine, vinblastine, and taxol all interfere with the microtubular apparatus; taxol and the related taxotere actually stabilize formed microtubules, thereby preventing normal function. Vinblastine and vincristine inhibit microtubular formation. By virtue of depleting lymphoblasts of the L-asparagine they require, L-asparaginase has a unique mechanism of action.

**IX-66. The answer is E.** *(Chap. 110)* A slightly increased mean corpuscular volume and an inappropriately low reticulocyte count are characteristic of a macrocytic, hypoproliferative anemia. Iron-deficiency anemia is accompanied by microcytic red blood cell indices, and autoimmune hemolytic anemia typically is associated with reticulocytosis, unless a coexisting process, such as folate deficiency, interferes with the bone marrow erythropoietic response. Aplastic anemia and acute leukemia are unlikely diagnoses if white blood cell count and platelet count are normal. A macrocytic, hypoproliferative anemia in the older man described in the question would most likely be due to a myelodysplastic syndrome. A bone marrow examination with iron stain would be required to define the precise subtype of this heterogeneous disorder, which is characterized by a stem cell defect leading to disordered hematopoietic maturation. Given the normal platelet count and white blood cell count, either refractory anemia or refractory anemia with ringed sideroblasts is the most likely subtype.

**IX-67. The answer is E.** *(Chap. 82)* It is now well recognized that many environmental and industrial exposures are associated with an increased risk of neoplasia. For example, tobacco smoking is associated with an increased likelihood of developing cancer of the oral cavity, lung, esophagus, kidney, bladder, and pancreas. In fact, due to the increased frequency of cigarette smoking among American women after World War II, beginning in 1988 female deaths from lung cancer exceeded the deaths from breast cancer. Occupational causes of cancer include arsenic-induced lung cancer and skin cancer. Asbestos exposure is a well-recognized cause of mesothelioma of the lung, pleura, and peritoneum. Benzene and perhaps other industrial solvents are associated with an increased risk of leukemia. Chromium compounds and benzidine are industrial carcinogens associated with lung cancer and bladder cancer, respectively. The use of mustard gas in the workplace is associated with an increased incidence of lung and head and neck cancer. Finally, workers in the plastic industry exposed to vinyl chloride have been shown to develop angiosarcoma, a rare tumor of the liver.

**IX-68. The answer is D.** *(Chap. 91)* The appropriate systemic therapy for postmenopausal women with estrogen-receptor-positive breast cancer metastatic to bone is either tamoxifen, 10 mg twice daily. Radiation therapy can relieve bone pain and may prevent fractures if used prophylactically to treat lesions of weight-bearing bones. For lytic lesions greater than 2.5 cm in diameter in weight-bearing bones, prophylactic internal fixation followed by radiation therapy is the treatment of choice, especially if the lesions involve the cortex. Pamidronate may have a role in stabilizing the bone matrix to lessen the incidence of subsequent pathologic fracture.

**IX-69. The answer is C.** *(Chap. 118. Bick, Hematol Oncol Clin North Am 10:875, 1996.)* A unifying pathophysiologic explanation for the association between malignancy and thrombosis has not been developed; however, many factors may play a role in increasing the likelihood of abnormal clotting in cancer patients. Such factors include immobilization and bed rest, dysproteinemias producing hyperviscosity, abnormal platelet function in myeloproliferative disorders, tumor-associated low-grade DIC (disseminated intravascular coagulation), production of procoagulants by the tumor, and cancer-mediated thrombocytosis. Unlike the case for patients with coagulopathies, there is no useful laboratory test that will identify the hypercoagulable state. Different types of malignancies may be associated with specific thrombotic syndromes. For example, migratory superficial thrombophlebitis (Trousseau's syndrome) in the absence of apparent predisposing factors is most frequently associated with gastrointestinal malignancies, particularly pancreatic carcinoma. Hepatic vein thrombosis (Budd-Chiari syndrome) and portal vein thrombosis are associated with myeloproliferative disorders such as paroxysmal nocturnal hemoglobinuria, essential thrombocythemia, and polycythemia vera.

**IX-70. The answer is E.** *(Chap. 108)* Antiparietal-cell antibodies are detected in 90 percent of persons with pernicious anemia but also in persons with atrophic gastritis and 10 to 15 percent of an unselected patient population. Although folate in large doses can correct the megaloblastic anemia of pernicious anemia, it does not correct the neurologic abnormalities. Megaloblastic anemias are characterized by ineffective erythropoiesis and bone marrow erythroid hyperplasia. Hypergastrinemia accompanies the achlorhydria of pernicious anemia. Marrow morphology begins to improve within hours of parenteral $B_{12}$ therapy; reticulocytosis peaks in 1 week. Life-threatening hypokalemia may occur early in the course of therapy.

**IX-71. The answer is D.** *(Chap. 115. Heyman, Semin Oncol 17:198, 1990.)* Platelet transfusions are a mainstay of the therapy in the chronically thrombocytopenic patient. Automated platelet pheresis yields approximately 6 units of platelets (each unit is $6 \times 10^{10}$ platelets) from an individual donor, and these may be stored at room temperature for approximately 5 days. Each unit should raise the platelet count by at least 5000 cells/$\mu$L. Therefore, this patient has responded appropriately to her transfusion, although she has had a significant febrile reaction. It is important to rule out bacterial contamination of the transfused platelets, but this is a very rare complication. More commonly, febrile reactions after receiving platelets are due to reaction to HLA antigens to which the patient has been sensitized. While such reactions might be circumvented by administering platelets from an HLA-compatible donor or sibling, given the appropriate rise in the platelet count after the transfusion, the easiest way to approach the current problem would be to administer leukocyte-reduced platelets. Currently available filters can reduce the leukocyte content (and thereby diminish the exposure to sensitizing alloantigens) by more than 99.9 percent. Another advantage of leukocyte-reduced products is reduction of the risk of CMV transmission. Though transfusion-associated graft-versus-host disease is not eliminated by leukocyte reduction, since there are still a few remaining allogeneic lymphocytes in such products, this dreaded complication can be eliminated by irradiating all blood products at a dose of 25 Gy.

**IX-72. The answer is C.** *(Chap. 98. Roth, Semin Oncol 19:117, 1992.)* Persons with disseminated teratocarcinoma treated with combination chemotherapy achieve complete remission in more than 90 percent of cases. Occasionally, residual masses remain after chemotherapy and on biopsy prove to be benign mature teratomas rather than residual malignant disease. In these cases, partial responders can be converted to complete responders—and even cured—by surgical removal of residual masses. If viable cancer is detected in the surgical specimen, then additional chemotherapy should be administered.

**IX-73. The answer is A.** *(Chap. 116)* One of the most important complications of allogeneic bone marrow transplantation is acute graft-versus-host disease. This condition is believed to be due to a reaction by engrafted lymphoid cells, particularly T cells, against host tissues. Graft-versus-host disease is essentially not a complication of syngeneic (identical twin) or autologous transplants. Acute graft-versus-host disease typically involves the skin, gastrointestinal tract, and liver. Elevations of the alkaline phosphatase and jaundice are common. An isolated elevation of bilirubin and alkaline phosphatase and the onset of ascites would raise consideration of venoocclusive disease (VOD) of the liver. Such a problem would probably not be associated with a skin rash and diarrhea. Secondly, hepatic VOD is much more common when therapy with combined alkylating agents is used as the preparative regimen. Efforts to prevent acute graft-versus-host disease have centered upon the use of immunosuppressive agents including glucocorticoids, methotrexate, and cyclosporine. Another approach is the use of T cell-depleted donor marrows. However, while T cell-depleted donor marrows will reduce the risk of severe graft-versus-host disease, the rate of relapse may be lower in patients with graft-versus-host disease than in those without.

**IX-74.** **The answer is E.** *(Chap. 91. Harris, N Engl J Med 327:319–328, 390–398, 473–480, 1992.)* Given the increasing frequency of breast biopsy for patients with suspected breast cancer, the incidence of carcinoma in situ is increasing. There are two histologically distinct types of carcinoma in situ: ductal and lobular. Ductal carcinoma in situ may form palpable tumors and is frequently confined to one breast. This finding would be a marker for an increased risk of developing an invasive cancer. Although controversial, based on a recently published clinical trial, it appears that the optimal treatment for such patients is wide excision followed by radiation therapy. On the other hand, lobular carcinoma in situ does not form palpable tumors and tends to be a diffuse finding in both breasts. Without treatment the cumulative incidence of a breast cancer (in either breast) is about 25 percent with a latent period of 5 to 20 years. Most doctors recommend resection of the lesion with careful follow-up. Whether tamoxifen is of benefit is unknown. Molecular analysis may one day make it possible to predict which in situ cancers will become invasive. Women whose quality of life is lowered by the lingering risk may opt for bilateral prophylactic mastectomy.

**IX-75.** **The answer is E.** *(Chaps. 59, 106. Sears, Med Clin North Am 76:567, 1992.)* A mild-to-moderate degree of anemia often accompanies chronic infectious, inflammatory, or neoplastic diseases. Typically, the anemia of chronic disease is normochromic and normocytic. Bone marrow examination reveals normal erythroid maturation. Neither significant disturbance of hemoglobin synthesis nor hemolysis occurs in this type of anemia. Affected persons usually have a low serum iron concentration and a low total transferrin level (resulting in essentially normal or only slightly decreased transferrin saturation). Even though storage iron is abundant, there is a decreased amount of iron in erythroblasts, reflecting a defect in the transfer of reticuloendothelial iron to developing red blood cells.

**IX-76.** **The answer is D.** *(Chap. 109. Beutler, N Engl J Med 324:169, 1991.)* The gene for glucose-6-phosphate dehydrogenase (G6PD) is located on the X chromosome; thus, G6PD deficiency is a sex-linked trait. Hemolytic anemia occurs much more commonly in males than in heterozygote female carriers, who usually are asymptomatic. Of the more than 100 variants of G6PD, the most commonly encountered variant of clinical significance in the United States is the A-type, which is found in about 15 percent of black males. It generally causes less severe hemolysis than the Mediterranean variant. Hemolysis usually is precipitated by an environmental oxidant stress, most commonly viral or bacterial infection. Certain drugs, such as antimalarial agents, sulfonamides, phenacetin, and vitamin K, also can trigger hemolysis. These oxidant stresses cause precipitation of hemoglobin because affected persons are unable to maintain adequate intracellular levels of reduced glutathione. Precipitated hemoglobin forms Heinz bodies that are visualized only with supravital stains; these inclusions cause premature destruction of the red cells. The diagnosis should be considered in any person experiencing a hemolytic episode. However, since decreased G6PD levels are found mainly in older cells, a false-negative test may be obtained during a hemolytic crisis, and the test should be repeated upon recovery.

**IX-77.** **The answer is B.** *(Chap. 97. Andriole, J Clin Oncol 10:1205–1207, 1992.)* Prostate specific antigen (PSA) determinations are assuming an increasingly important role in the diagnosis, screening, and staging of men with prostate cancer. Patients with urinary symptoms found to have an elevated level of serum prostate specific antigen have a 60 percent likelihood of having prostate cancer. About 16 percent of patients with prostate cancer have an elevated level of serum PSA as their sole diagnostic abnormality. However, additional studies need to be done to precisely delineate the role of prostate specific antigen evaluation in screening. Fewer than 10 percent of ambulatory volunteers older than 50 years have elevated serum PSA values. A serum PSA between 4 and 10 ng/mL indicates that cancer is 25 percent likely, whereas values greater than 10 ng/mL increase the likelihood of cancer to about 60 percent. About 20 percent of those with an elevated PSA (alone) compared with 10 percent of those with a suspicious digital rectal examination (alone) will have prostate cancer. The vast majority of cancers that are detected by screening for prostate specific antigen are localized clinically and therefore have an excellent chance of being cured with either radiation or surgery. Moreover, few tumors detected by PSA screening are incidental since most have a high volume or a worrisome Gleason score (indicating a poor prognosis based on histologic grade). On the other hand, additional studies demonstrating a screening-induced decrease in cancer-related mortality are necessary in order to convince all that screening for prostate cancer with PSA determinations is beneficial. A clear use for serum PSA determination is in postoperative evaluation. If the postoperative serum PSA value is detectable, the presence of residual tumor is likely. A rising PSA value after definitive radiation therapy indicates a high likelihood of eventual metastatic spread. The use of systemic hormonal therapy for metastatic prostate cancer should be reserved for those patients with certain evidence of locally advanced or metastatic disease.

**IX-78.   The answer is B.**   *(Chap. 91. Early Breast Cancer Trialists' Collaborative Group, Lancet 339:71, 1992.)*   For premenopausal women who have stage II carcinoma of the breast (axillary metastases only), the drug regimen combining cyclophosphamide, methotrexate, and 5-fluorouracil (CMF), when employed as an adjuvant therapy, leads to a statistically significant reduction in the recurrence rate. It is the treatment of choice following mastectomy in this group of women. Mortality after 5 years is decreased approximately 30 percent in women treated with CMF. Median survival is prolonged by approximately 3 years with CMF treatment.

**IX-79.   The answer is E.**   *(Chaps. 103, 114. Posner, Neurol Clin 9:919, 1991.)*   A relatively common subtype of paraneoplastic neurologic syndromes is that which affects peripheral nerves. Subacute sensory neuronopathy, characterized by paresthesias and pain in the distal limbs with truncal sensory ataxia, is associated with axonal degeneration with relative myelin sparing. The most common type of paraneoplastic neuropathy is a mixed sensory and motor axonopathy. Symptoms may include muscle wasting, weakness, distal paresthesia, and occasionally pain. Pathologically, this disease is characterized by noninflammatory degeneration of axons with mild myelin loss and may be associated with small cell carcinoma of the lung, breast carcinoma, gastric carcinoma, Hodgkin's disease, lymphoma, and multiple myeloma. Another type of neuropathy associated with Waldenstrom's microglobulinemia or in certain patients with benign monoclonal gammopathy is the elaboration of IgM that reacts with a myelin-associated glycoprotein in peripheral nerves. Such an antibody tends to disrupt sensory rather than motor neurons. Another demyelinating neuropathy associated with IgG myeloma is predominantly motor, indolent, and not associated with an anti-myelin-associated glycoprotein antibody, although demyelinization is still the primary pathology. Patients with monoclonal gammopathies who develop neuropathy also include those with the POEMS syndrome, characterized by polyneuropathy, organomegaly, endocrinopathy, M-protein secretion, and skin changes. Any patient with a demyelinative myopathy secondary to monoclonal immunoglobulin protein may respond to immunosuppressive therapy.

**IX-80.   The answer is E.**   *(Chap. 101. Ellerbroek, Cancer 66:1461, 1990.)*   In general, women who present with an isolated axillary mass that proves to be adenocarcinoma or poorly differentiated carcinoma should receive treatment appropriate for stage II breast cancer. They should receive either a modified radical mastectomy or breast irradiation for purposes of decreasing local recurrence followed by adjuvant systemic therapy with chemotherapy or tamoxifen or both, depending on menopausal status and the hormone receptor status of the tumor. However, patients whose routine pathology reveals either poorly differentiated adenocarcinoma or poorly differentiated malignancy deserve a careful pathologic review to determine if there are any findings compatible with a specific organ of origin. In this case, the absence of cytokeratin filaments argues against the diagnosis of breast carcinoma; on the other hand, the leukocyte common antigen positivity is highly consistent with a lymphoid neoplasm. The patient would be expected to respond to therapy as if she had a more straightforward presentation of lymphoma. To determine the optimal therapy for such a patient, the disease should be staged as in any non-Hodgkin's lymphoma. Therefore, CT of the chest and abdomen should be performed to determine whether there are additional sites of disease.

**IX-81.    The answer is B.** *(Chaps. 59, 106, 110)*   Pure red blood cell aplasia is characterized by a normochromic, normocytic anemia and little production of reticulocytes. Erythroblasts are selectively absent from the bone marrow of affected persons. The production of white blood cells and platelets is preserved. In contrast to aplastic anemia, the bone marrow in persons with pure red blood cell aplasia is normocellular or even hypercellular. Iron kinetic studies reveal prolonged clearance of plasma iron and reduced turnover of iron. Levels of erythropoietin usually are markedly elevated.

**IX-82.    The answer is B.** *(Chap. 101. Hainsworth, N Engl J Med 329:257–263, 1993.)* Approximately 10 percent of all cancer patients present in such a manner that assignment of the organ of origin of the tumor is unclear. Most patients who present in this fashion will have neoplasms that are poorly responsive to systemic therapy. However, it is important to recognize certain subgroups in whom a specific approach to treatment might be beneficial or even associated with long-term disease-free survival. One such group has what has been termed the unrecognized extragonadal germ cell cancer syndrome. This includes those patients displaying one or more of the following features: age less than 50; tumor involving midline structures, lung, or parenchymal lymph nodes; an elevated serum alpha fetoprotein or βhCG level; or evidence of rapid tumor growth. If patients with these features do not have any histologic or immunohistochemical features suggesting a primary site, then strong consideration should be given to treatment with a cisplatin-based chemotherapy regimen (as would be used for germ cell cancer). Approximately 20 percent of patients presenting in this fashion may be cured with the use of cisplatin, bleomycin, and VP-16 chemotherapy.

**IX-83.    The answer is D.** *(Chap. 113)*   Lymphoid neoplasms may be classified as to their cell of origin by the use of antisera and monoclonal antibodies against certain cell surface phenotypic markers and, more recently, by the use of DNA probes for immunoglobulin genes and genes for the beta chain of the T-cell receptor. The malignant cell in chronic lymphocytic leukemia (CLL) is a morphologically normal but functionally abnormal B lymphocyte. Follicular lymphomas arise from the lymphoid follicle, while the diffuse, small lymphocytic lymphomas (identical to CLL) are derived from the secretory compartment of the medullary cords. The Burkitt's lymphoma cell is a malignant cell of B-lymphocyte lineage; in many cases it bears a characteristic chromosomal translocation—t(8;14). In contrast to these B-cell neoplasms, mycosis fungoides is a peripheral T-cell lymphoma in which helper-cell function and phenotype have been identified in some cases.

**IX-84.    The answer is C.** *(Chap. 91. Fisher, N Engl J Med 320:822, 1989.)*   Other than in the performance of early local therapy based on mammographic detection, no surgical or radiotherapeutic procedure has been shown to affect survival. In other words, survival is determined by the extent and response of systemic disease. The decision between lumpectomy plus radiation therapy and modified radical mastectomy therefore rests on which modality offers the best chance for local control. Although no survival benefit can be shown, radiation therapy should be administered along with lumpectomy because at least one study has documented a higher recurrence rate in those treated with lumpectomy alone (28 percent) compared with lumpectomy plus radiotherapy (5 percent). In most cases, local control can be achieved equally well with either approach. However, certain subgroups—especially those with extensive intraductal carcinoma or with positive lumpectomy resection margins—will experience a higher local recurrence rate if breast conservation is employed. Axillary lymph node dissection is appropriate in all patients for staging (in order to determine the appropriate systemic therapy), not therapeutic, purposes.

**IX-85.   The answer is D.** *(Chaps. 60, 118)*   A marked prolongation of the prothrombin time with a normal partial thromboplastin time localizes the hemostatic defect to the extrinsic limb of the coagulation cascade. Congenital factor VII deficiency is a rare, autosomal recessive disorder. Factor VIII deficiency and the presence of specific inhibitors directed toward a coagulation factor (most commonly factor VIII) would be associated with a prolongation of the partial thromboplastin time. Nonspecific inhibitors (lupus anticoagulants) most commonly are associated with prolongation of the partial thromboplastin time and occasionally with prolongation of the prothrombin time (particularly when hypoprothrombinemia is present). Patients with alpha$_2$-antiplasmin deficiency have a bleeding disorder associated with accelerated clot lysis. Both the prothrombin time and the partial thromboplastin time are normal in these persons.

**IX-86.   The answer is B.** *(Chaps. 117, 118)*   The hemolytic-uremic syndrome occurs predominantly in children and is related to thrombotic thrombocytopenic purpura. It is characterized by microangiopathic hemolytic anemia and thrombocytopenia. Polycythemia vera and the other myeloproliferative disorders often are associated with thrombocytosis. Thrombocytosis also is a long-term sequela of splenectomy or splenic infarction (e.g., in sickle cell disease) and chronic inflammatory states (e.g., inflammatory bowel disease). For reasons that are unclear, thrombocytosis frequently is associated with iron deficiency.

**IX-87.   The answer is B.** *(Chap. 99. Swenerton, J Clin Oncol 10:718, 1992.)*   The overall 5-year survival of those with disease that extends beyond the ovaries is 40 percent; however, some patients who are able to undergo complete or nearly complete initial cytoreductive surgery may be cured with combination chemotherapy. Presumably such therapy eradicates residual subclinical disease, which is invariably present despite the apparently complete resection. Effective drugs include taxol, cisplatin, cyclophosphamide, hexamethylmelamine, and doxorubicin. Paclitaxel plus cisplatin is the standard regimen. Since some patients may have recurrent disease without an elevation of CA125, which is a useful antigen in monitoring response to therapy in those who have elevated levels, the delay of therapy pending a rise in this level would not be prudent. Clear survival benefits have yet to be shown for the fairly toxic regimen of whole abdominal radiation therapy. Intraperitoneal chemotherapy holds promise in the eradication of minimal disease, but its role needs to be defined by further clinical trials.

**IX-88.   The answer is D.** *(Chaps. 102, 103)*   Small cell neoplasms of the lung are associated with a wide variety of paraneoplastic syndromes, some of which are humorally mediated, while others are of unknown pathophysiology. The Lambert-Eaton myasthenic syndrome, which is associated with proximal muscle weakness and characteristic electromyographic findings, is linked almost exclusively with small cell tumors. Subacute cortical cerebellar degeneration, as exemplified by the findings outlined in choice B, is associated with small cell tumors and some cases of ovarian cancer, carcinoma of the breast, and Hodgkin's disease. Cushing's syndrome (choice C) due to hypersecretion of glucocorticoids and the syndrome of inappropriate secretion of antidiuretic hormone (choice

E) are also associated with small cell lung tumors, in addition to other cancers. Hypercalcemia is infrequently associated with small cell neoplasms, but it is not an infrequent manifestation of squamous and large cell lung tumors, in which case it may be a result of secretion of substances with parathyroid hormone–like activity or of another factor associated with the humoral hypercalcemia of malignancy.

**IX-89.** **The answer is C.** *(Chap. 117)* The onset of severe thrombocytopenia after an antecedent viral illness is common in children with a diagnosis of idiopathic thrombocytopenic purpura (ITP). Unlike childhood ITP, adult ITP tends to be a chronic disease in which spontaneous remissions are rare, and a majority of patients will have a fall in their platelet count after the withdrawal of glucocorticoids, necessitating elective splenectomy. The presence of antibodies directed against target antigens on the glycoprotein IIb-IIIa or Ib-IX complex has been noted in some adults with chronic ITP but not in children. Splenomegaly is not a feature of ITP; it is a common finding in patients with secondary thrombocytopenia.

**IX-90.** **The answer is C.** *(Chap. 111)* Persons with polycythemia vera and a hematocrit greater than 45 percent usually have diminished cerebral blood flow and are particularly at risk for developing thrombotic complications. Functional platelet abnormalities may cause both thrombotic and bleeding problems (the gastrointestinal tract is a common site of bleeding), and affected persons frequently are iron-deficient even at the time of presentation. Erythropoietin production is suppressed in polycythemia vera, a disease characterized by loss of normal control of erythroid stem-cell proliferation. The bone marrow is hypercellular, with hyperplasia of all marrow elements. Therapy is aimed at reducing the hematocrit below 45 percent, usually with phlebotomy.

**IX-91.** **The answer is A.** *(Chap. 117)* Electrophoretic analysis has allowed the delineation of three major types of defects in von Willebrand's disease (vWD). The most common abnormality (type I disease) is characterized by a moderate decrease in the plasma level of von Willebrand factor (vWF antigen) resulting from defective release of the protein from endothelial cells. There are usually concordant reductions in antihemophilic factor or factor VIII coagulant activity as well as ristocetin cofactor activity.

The various forms of type II disease are characterized by normal or near normal levels of dysfunctional protein. In both types IIa and IIb, there is a loss of high-molecular-weight multimers on SDS-agarose electrophoresis. In type IIa patients, the pattern is caused by either an inability to assemble the larger multimers or by premature catabolism in the circulation. In contrast, patients with type IIb have inappropriate binding of the abnormal, larger vWF forms to platelets, which results in the formation of intravascular platelet aggregates. These are rapidly cleared from the circulation, which causes mild, cyclic thrombocytopenia.

A severe recessive form of vWD (type III disease) results from reduced synthesis of vWF by endothelial cells. A hyperactive platelet receptor (glycoprotein Ib) with increased affinity for larger vWF multimers is the defect in so-called platelet-type vWD, or pseudo-vWD. The gene encoding vWF has been cloned and localized to chromosome 12.

**IX-92.** **The answer is C.** *(Chap. 118)* Factor XIII deficiency may be inherited or acquired and frequently causes severe bleeding problems. In this disorder, the bleeding time, prothrombin time, and partial thromboplastin time (PTT) are all normal. The screening test for factor XIII deficiency is a clot solubility in urea assay. Persons with deficiencies of factor XII (Hageman factor) or prekallikrein often have dramatic prolongations of the PTT, but do not have bleeding problems even with surgery or trauma. The presence of a normal bleeding time excludes thrombasthenia, an inherited disorder in which there is defective-platelet aggregation in response to agonists that require fibrinogen binding, such as adenosine diphosphate, thrombin, or epinephrine. Protein S is a vitamin K-dependent plasma protein and a cofactor for the expression of the anticoagulant activity of activated protein C. Familial protein S deficiency is associated with a thrombotic diathesis.

IX-93. **The answer is D.** *(Chap. 86)* Two types of cardiotoxicity are associated with doxorubicin (Adriamycin) therapy. Acute cardiotoxicity produces electrocardiographic abnormalities, such as arrhythmias, but rarely is serious. Chronic cardiotoxicity, which rarely develops with total doxorubicin doses less than 500 mg/m$^2$, leads to congestive heart failure; it occurs with increased frequency in persons who also have received cardiac irradiation, cyclophosphamide, or anthracycline compounds other than doxorubicin. Up to half of all cases of cardiotoxicity occur 6 months or more after completion of therapy. Efforts to limit cardiotoxicity and thereby enable the administration of a higher total dose of anthracycline include weekly or continuous intravenous schedules, anthracycline analogues, and cardioprotective agents that limit free-radical-induced myocardial damage. While doxorubicin exerts its antineoplastic activity by inhibiting topoisomerase II function, cardiotoxicity appears to be due to oxidant-mediated damage. Dexrazoxone is a chelating agent that may prevent anthracycline-mediated cardiotoxicity.

IX-94. **The answer is C.** *(Chap. 113. Armitage, N Engl J Med 328:1023, 1993.)* Stage (extent of disease) and tumor grade (histologic appearance) are the most important factors for determining treatment of the non-Hodgkin's lymphomas. Since 80 to 90 percent of patients with low-grade lymphomas—small lymphocytic (diffuse, well-differentiated lymphocytic) or follicular, small cleaved cell (nodular, poorly differentiated lymphocytic)—present with disseminated disease, radiation therapy is rarely curative. On the other hand, such diseases behave in an indolent fashion and can be treated effectively in a palliative manner with single-agent alkylator therapy; the use of more aggressive combination regimens produces a higher complete response rate, but has never been conclusively shown to prolong survival. Most patients with diffuse large cell lymphoma, the most common intermediate-grade histology, achieve complete remission and many can be cured with combination chemotherapy regimens, including cyclophosphamide, doxorubicin, vincristine, and glucocorticoids (and possibly also etoposide or methotrexate, among others). Prolonged (greater than 1 year) maintenance therapy is of no value. A lymphoma presenting in a patient with AIDS has a much lower chance (less than 25 percent complete response rate) of responding to combination chemotherapy than does a lymphoma of similar histologic appearance in an immunocompetent patient, probably related to the heightened toxicity of treatment in AIDS patients rather than tumor drug resistance.

IX-95. **The answer is C.** *(Chap. 94. Warshaw, N Engl J Med 326:455–465, 1992.)* The clinical history is highly suggestive of carcinoma of the head of the pancreas. The failure to obtain diagnostic tissue at needle biopsy is not unusual because of surrounding inflammation, edema, and fibrosis. Even though well over 90 percent of patients with pancreatic cancer cannot be cured surgically, an attempt at such a procedure is appropriate, particularly for lesions in the pancreatic head, which tend to present earlier because they produce extrahepatic biliary obstruction and because of their frequent confusion with other, more curable lesions in this location (duodenal, ampullary, and distal bile duct tumors). Therefore, such a patient should undergo a preoperative celiac angiogram to rule out vascular invasion by tumor and ensure resectability. It would not be unreasonable to attempt a preoperative diagnosis via ERCP, although the yield would be small. Repeating a needle biopsy is unlikely to achieve diagnostic results. Neither watchful follow-up nor palliative biliary stent therapy is appropriate until a tissue diagnosis of cancer and a determination of unresectability have been made.

IX-96. **The answer is C.** *(Chap. 82)* Early detection of cancer is a major focus for the internist in evaluating his or her patients. Such detection depends on an awareness of the epidemiology of cancers and the sensitivity and specificity of any proposed test. It is recommended that each time a patient is seen by his or her physician, cancers of the oral cavity, thyroid, skin, lymph node, testes, and prostate be considered by performance of a careful physical examination. Between the ages of 20 and 39 the American Cancer Society recommends that such a physical examination be performed every 3 years. For men aged 40 to 49 a digital rectal examination with palpation of the prostate is recommended annually. For those aged 50 and older, the annual cancer-related checkup should include a digital rectal examination and palpation of the prostate as well as annual stool blood test plus sigmoidoscopy every 3 to 5 years. Screening for advanced prostate cancer by serologic measurement of the prostate specific antigen (PSA), while sometimes recommended for men over 50, remains controversial. It is important to recognize that for a screening test such as PSA to be effective, it must pick up disease in the curable stage. Chest radiography, for example, is not useful as a screening test for lung cancer in average-risk, asymptomatic patients because cancers that are picked up by this modality tend to be too far advanced for meaningful intervention. On the other hand, PSA detection might well pick up insignificant cancers that are unlikely to progress. Finally, it is important to recognize that a more aggressive approach to the detection of cancer is appropriate if a patient has a symptom, an abnormal physical examination, or a strong family history.

# X. DERMATOLOGIC DISORDERS

## *QUESTIONS*

**DIRECTIONS:** Each question below contains five suggested responses. Choose the **one best** response to each question.

**X-1.** A 7-year-old girl is brought to the local emergency room after having a generalized seizure during which she lost consciousness. No history of head trauma can be elicited from her family and friends. A paternal uncle is mentally retarded and has had seizures. On examination, numerous brown spots—each greater than 3 cm and similar to those in Plate F—are present on the torso and extremities; one spot is 5 cm in size. Many smaller lesions (1 mm or less) are noted, especially in the axillary areas. The most likely diagnosis is

(A) Peutz-Jeghers syndrome
(B) Gardner's syndrome
(C) neurofibromatosis
(D) xeroderma pigmentosum
(E) hemochromatosis

**X-2.** A 21-year-old woman is hospitalized for the treatment of a painful ulcer that has been present on her right lower leg for the last 4 weeks. The lesion began as a painful, reddish-purple nodule, then rapidly broke down and enlarged (see Plate G). Bacterial cultures did not yield a significant pathogen, and a 2-week course of oral dicloxacillin, 250 mg four times daily, was not helpful. The lesion border now is undermined with a violaceous rim; biopsy is consistent with pyoderma gangrenosum. The lesion described is associated with all the following disorders EXCEPT

(A) ulcerative colitis
(B) regional enteritis
(C) multiple myeloma
(D) rheumatoid arthritis
(E) pernicious anemia

**X-3.** A 55-year-old Japanese businessman visiting the United States has been in excellent health until 6 months ago, when he first noted mild upper abdominal fullness after meals. On examination the man is noted to have hyperpigmented, heaped-up velvety lesions (as shown in Plate H) confined to the neck, axillae, and groin. All the following conditions have been associated with the skin findings presented EXCEPT

(A) Cushing's syndrome
(B) massive obesity
(C) acromegaly
(D) adenocarcinoma of the stomach
(E) Addison's disease

**X-4.** A 43-year-old nurse whose job requires frequent hand washing has noted a small erosive skin lesion between the third interdigital web of the right hand (Plate I). The best therapy for this condition would be

(A) topical 5-fluorouracil
(B) topical clotrimazole
(C) oral griseofulvin
(D) topical hydrocortisone
(E) topical tar derivative

**X-5.** For the last 2 days, a 24-year-old woman has had fever and pain in the left wrist, right ankle, and left knee. Nine painful skin lesions are present on the distal extremities, predominantly about the joints (as shown in Plate K). The most likely diagnosis is

(A) herpes simplex
(B) meningococcemia
(C) gonococcemia
(D) erythema multiforme
(E) anthrax

**X-6.** A 26-year-old man from Cape Cod sees his physician because of a 3-week history of an expanding, slightly burning ring of redness (as shown in Plate J) that first surrounded a red papule on the posterior neck. He complains of headaches, generalized muscle aches, anorexia, and malaise. On examination, he is noted to be febrile (38.3°C [101°F]); his rash is slightly raised and slightly tender and displays central clearing but no scaling, even after vigorous scraping. Which of the following vectors has been strongly associated with the type of rash described above?

(A) Kissing bug
(B) Spider
(C) Flea
(D) Tick
(E) Housefly

**X-7.** A 35-year-old previously healthy female was given a 10-day course of erythromycin for a nonproductive cough, diffuse interstitial infiltrates, and a presumptive diagnosis of mycoplasma pneumonia. She now has a well-demarcated rash on her fingers (Plate L). She also has fever and severe erosions on the buccal mucous membranes. The most likely diagnosis is

(A) hypersensitivity vasculitis
(B) polyarteritis nodosum
(C) toxic epidermal necrolysis
(D) erythema multiforme major
(E) erythema nodosum

**X-8.** A homosexual male develops a violaceous nodule on his right forearm (as shown in Plate M). Biopsy reveals spindle cell infiltration in the dermis with erythrocyte-containing vascular channels. Which of the following statements about this man's condition is true?

(A) It is caused by retroviral infection of dermal mesenchymal cells.
(B) Extracutaneous involvement is uncommon.
(C) The entity is seen most frequently in association with intravenous drug abuse.
(D) Interferon-γ is a useful treatment modality.
(E) Standard cytotoxic chemotherapy is absolutely contraindicated because of the low response rate and enhancement of immunosuppression.

**X-9.** A 24-year-old man is concerned because of the appearance of several light brown spots on his trunk (Plate N). The lesions (limited to the chest, back, abdomen, and upper arms) are flat and sharply marginated and have a fine scale that is easily scraped off. The most appropriate diagnostic study is

(A) Giemsa stain of scraped material (Tzanck preparation)
(B) bacterial culture of the lesions
(C) fungal culture of the lesions
(D) microscopic examination of potassium hydroxide-treated scrapings
(E) examination of the serum for anticardiolipin antibody

**X-10.** A 39-year-old pediatrician presents with severe scaling of the hands with vesicle formation (see Plate O). She reports a long-standing history of similarly dry, somewhat painful lesions that have undergone a series of remissions and exacerbations. She denies a history of asthma, hay fever, or skin problems as a child. She also notes that the small vesicles on the sides of her fingers are quite pruritic. The most likely diagnosis is

(A) herpes zoster
(B) atopic dermatitis
(C) asteatotic eczema
(D) dyshidrotic eczema
(E) lichen planus

**X-11.** For 25 years, a 55-year-old man has had recurrent episodes of nonpruritic red patches on both elbows, typically covered with thick, white scales (see Plate P). He has one brother with a similar condition. Both siblings state that their lesions are exacerbated by stress. Physical examination reveals similar lesions on the lower legs. A biopsy of such a lesion would reveal

(A) an increased number of mitotic figures in skin cells
(B) neutrophils at the tips of follicular openings
(C) degeneration of the basal cell layer
(D) infiltration of neutrophils in small dermal vessels
(E) patchy infiltration of upper dermis with atypical lymphocytes that have convoluted nuclei

**X-12.** All of the following are associated with diffuse hyperpigmentation EXCEPT

(A) Vogt-Koyanagi-Harada syndrome
(B) hemochromatosis
(C) busulfan
(D) primary biliary cirrhosis
(E) gold

**X-13.** A 65-year-old man presents with several lesions on both thighs as well as a similar lesion in his mouth. He noted pruritus in these areas several weeks ago. The patient is generally well and on no medications. Each of the lesions (see Plate R) is approximately 1 to 4 cm in size. Thumb pressure fails to cause extension of the lesion. The most likely diagnosis is

(A) pemphigus vulgaris
(B) bullous pemphigoid
(C) herpes zoster
(D) impetigo
(E) dermatitis herpetiformis

**X-14.** A 67-year-old man presents with a history of headache for 5 days and 2 days of swelling of the right part of the forehead and right eye (see Plate S). A Tzanck preparation of the lesion reveals multinucleate giant cells on Giemsa stain. The patient was admitted to the hospital and begun on intravenous acyclovir. The most important next step would be

(A) ophthalmologic consultation
(B) administration of systemic corticosteroids to prevent postherpetic neuralgia
(C) administration of antistaphylococcal antibiotics to prevent secondary bacterial infection
(D) application of iodine-containing solution to prevent secondary bacterial infections
(E) CT scan of the brain

**X-15.** A 20-year-old woman presents with a 2-week history of facial rash, fever of 39°C (102.2°F), and progressive malaise. In addition to her dermatologic findings (Plate T), physical examination also reveals swollen and tender knees and wrists bilaterally. Additional skin lesions that may be found in patients with this disorder include

(A) silvery scales on elbows and knees
(B) ulcerative lesions of the lower extremities
(C) hemorrhagic bullae
(D) hyperkeratosis
(E) vesicles in a dermatomal distribution

**X-16.** A 25-year-old homosexual man presents with a diffuse maculopapular rash over his trunk, head, neck, palms, and soles. Generalized lymphadenopathy is also present. He has a history of 4 weeks of anal pain. Which of the following tests is likely to identify the etiologic agent?

(A) Antinuclear antibody
(B) Blood culture
(C) Serum rapid plasma reagin (RPR)
(D) Skin biopsy
(E) Serum HIV antibody

**X-17.** A 35-year-old man is noted to have multiple telangiectatic lesions on the lips, face, feet, and nail beds. When the skin is stretched over an individual lesion, an eccentrically placed central area with radiating vessels is noted. The patient states that many members of his family have similar lesions. Which of the following is likely in this patient?

(A) Consumptive coagulopathy
(B) Gastrointestinal bleeding
(C) Renal failure
(D) Joint diffusions
(E) No clinical problems

**X-18.** A 35-year-old woman visits her doctor for her yearly checkup. Physical examination is unremarkable except for white patches (as shown in Plate U) involving her face, hands, torso, anus, and genitalia. The white spots have been present for 2 years. This dermatologic condition has been associated with all of the following conditions EXCEPT

(A) folate deficiency
(B) pernicious anemia
(C) Addison's disease
(D) hyperthyroidism
(E) hypothyroidism

**X-19.** A 35-year-old man has had recurrent diarrhea for at least 5 years. About 7 years ago many reddish-brown macules appeared on his torso and extremities (see Plate V). Rubbing these lesions gently results in the formation of a wheal. He also has been bothered by severe generalized itching, which is made worse when he takes aspirin for his frequent headaches. He has lost 11.4 kg (25 lb) in the last few months. Reasonable measures in his diagnosis/management would include all of the following EXCEPT

(A) draw a line on the patient's back with the handle of your reflex hammer
(B) bone survey and liver scan for evaluation of systemic involvement
(C) prescription of oral cromolyn for diarrhea
(D) prescription of codeine for his headaches
(E) genetic counseling

**X-20.** An 18-year-old man (pictured in Plate W) presents because of unsightly facial inflammation. Which of the following statements is correct?

(A) Closed comedones (whiteheads) are less commonly associated with the inflammatory lesions than are open comedones (blackheads).

(B) Glucocorticoids, although not indicated except in the most severe cases, would likely result in improvement.

(C) Vigorous scrubbing of the face, which will eliminate surface oils, is indicated.

(D) Systemic antibiotic therapy is unlikely to be helpful.

(E) Patients on systemic retinoic acid may experience very dry skin and hypertriglyceridemia.

**X-21.** A 50-year-old female developed yellow fleshy lesions on the eyelids (Plate Q). A biopsy of one of these lesions would show

(A) immature myeloid cells
(B) birefringent crystals
(C) lipid-containing macrophages
(D) neutrophils in blood vessels
(E) a collection of epidermal neutrophils

**X-22.** A 76-year-old male has developed over the last three months a large number of occasionally pruritic lesions on his trunk (Plate X). These lesions are probably a manifestation of

(A) hypertriglyceridemia
(B) systemic vasculitis
(C) severe drug reaction
(D) disseminated candidiasis
(E) malignancy

# X. DERMATOLOGIC DISORDERS

## ANSWERS

**X-1. The answer is C.** *(Chap. 57)* Flat, brown spots, called café au lait spots, are areas of increased pigmentation produced by clones of genetically programmed melanocytes. Café au lait spots, which can vary in size from several millimeters up to 1 cm in diameter, occur in both neurofibromatosis (von Recklinghausen's disease) and Albright's disease (polyostotic fibrous dysplasia with precocious puberty in females), as well as in some normal persons. One or two spots at least 0.5 cm in diameter appear in 25 percent of normal children, but three or more spots of the same size occur in only 0.6 percent. About 9 percent of college-age persons have at least one spot 1.5 cm in size or greater. Of those persons with neurofibromatosis, 95 percent have at least one spot 1.5 cm or larger, and 78 percent have six or more spots. Because persons with Albright's disease rarely have more than four macules, the presence of six or more spots 1.5 cm or greater in size, especially in the presence of axillary freckling, is strongly suggestive of neurofibromatosis. Furthermore, the café au lait spots in Albright's disease tend to be larger and more irregular than those in neurofibromatosis.

**X-2. The answer is E.** *(Chap. 57)* Pyoderma gangrenosum is most closely associated with ulcerative colitis and regional enteritis. Its association with rheumatoid arthritis also is well recognized, and it can accompany a variety of neoplastic hematologic disorders, such as acute and chronic myelogenous leukemia, myeloma, myeloid metaplasia, and polycythemia vera. Bacterial cultures and skin biopsies should be done in an evaluation for sepsis, vasculitis, or leukemia cutis. However, diagnosis of pyoderma gangrenosum is based on the lesion's morphology, not histologic analysis.

**X-3. The answer is E.** *(Chap. 57)* Acanthosis nigricans is a skin disease associated with a number of disorders. The skin, which is thrown up into folds, appears velvety and hyperpigmented (brown to black) grossly and papillomatous microscopically. The lesions appear on the flexural areas of the neck, axillae, groin, antecubital fossae, and occasionally around the areolae, periumbilical and perianal areas, lips, buccal mucosa, and over the surfaces of the palms, elbows, knees, and interphalangeal joints. The disorder may be hereditary or appear in association with obesity or an endocrinopathy (acromegaly, polycystic ovary syndrome, diabetes mellitus, Cushing's syndrome, but not adrenal insufficiency). Drugs such as nicotinic acid also can produce the condition. When acanthosis nigricans develops in a nonobese adult, neoplasia, particularly gastric adenocarcinoma, must be suspected.

**X-4. The answer is B.** *(Chap. 55)* Predisposing factors for cutaneous candidial infection include diabetes mellitus, chronic intertrigo, oral contraceptive use, and cellular immune deficiency syndromes. Candidial infections typically occur in sites which are chronically wet and macerated such as an intertriginous areas in an individual who practices frequent washing. Particularly in those with depressed cellular immunity, the oral cavity may be involved with an infection (thrush) manifested by the appearance of white plaques. Fissured lesions appear at the corners of the mouth in patients with poorly fitting dentures also occur on the basis of candida infection. The diagnosis can be made clinically or on the basis of demonstration of yeast on KOH preparation. Treatment involves removing predisposing factors such as chronic wetness, antibiotics, or improving glucose control in diabetics and use of effective topical agents such as nystatin or azoles; occasionally, the addition of hydrocortisone cream is required to decrease the associated inflammatory response. Systemic therapy with fluconazole may be required in immunosuppressed patients or individuals whose disease fails to respond to topical therapy.

**X-5.**   **The answer is C.**  *(Chaps. 57, 150)*  The skin lesions of disseminated gonococcal infection occur on the distal extremities, usually around joints, and appear within a week of the onset of joint symptoms. The lesions, which may number as many as 20 (average: four or five), often are painful, and each crop of new lesions is associated with a temperature rise. Lesions begin as a red macule or purpuric spot and then develop into a papule, a vesicle, and, finally, a pustule. Organisms rarely are cultured from the skin lesions; they can be demonstrated occasionally on Gram stain and more regularly with immunofluorescent techniques. Herpes simplex typically occurs as grouped vesicles. Skin lesions of meningococcemia consist of red macules that quickly become petechial or purpuric; migratory polyarthralgias and tenosynovitis are atypical. Erythema multiforme requires "iris" lesions for diagnosis. Anthrax consists of a single pimple or papule on exposed parts of the body; the lesion rapidly enlarges, developing into a vesicle that is surrounded by edema and later undergoes hemorrhagic necrosis, ulceration, and eschar formation.

**X-6.**   **The answer is D.**  *(Chaps. 57, 178. Steere, N Engl J Med 321:586, 1989.)*  An expanding erythematous rash not associated with scaling is characteristic of erythema chronicum migrans. The disease first appears weeks to months after a tick bite. The lesion begins as a red macule at the site of the bite; the borders of the lesion then expand to form a red ring, with central clearing, as wide as 20 to 30 cm or more in diameter. Occasionally, secondary rings may occur within the original one. The lesion may itch or burn and may be accompanied by fever, headache, vomiting, fatigue, and regional adenopathy.

**X-7.**   **The answer is D.**  *(Chaps. 56, 57. Roujeau, N Engl J Med 331:1272, 1994.)*  Patients with erythema multiforme major have typical target lesions, usually on the extremities, which are associated with mucous membrane lesions. This syndrome usually follows mycoplasma or herpes simplex infections, has a benign course, and is not thought to be associated with drug reaction. On the other hand, the Stevens-Johnson syndrome is due to reaction to a systemically administered drug such as a sulfa, dilantan, allopurinol, penicillin, and nonsteroidal anti-inflammatory drug. Typical lesions or Stevens-Johnson's syndrome are small blisters on dusky purpuric macules. 10 to 30 percent of cases include fever, lesions of the respiratory tract, and/or gastrointestinal tract. Another related severe cutaneous reaction to drugs is toxic epidermal necrolysis; individual lesions are similar to those seen in Stevens-Johnson syndrome, but epidermal separation from the basal layer with lateral pressure (Nikolsky's sign) also occurs. These patients have systemic consequences and wide-spread injury to the skin, similar to those with extensive burns. Erythema nodosum represents painful tender lesions, usually on the legs, associated with infection or drug ingestion. Stevens-Johnson syndrome and toxic epidermal necrolysis represent two severe cutaneous reactions to drugs in which fatalities have been reported. The skin lesions usually occur 1 to 3 weeks after the initial exposure to the offending drug.

**X-8.**   **The answer is D.**  *(Chaps. 57, 308)*  AIDS-associated Kaposi's sarcoma, which is present in this man, is a much more fulminant disease than the variant of the disease seen in elderly, non-HIV-infected patients. There is no evidence to implicate direct HIV-induced transformation as the etiology. For unknown reasons, the disease is much more common in homosexuals with AIDS than in heterosexuals with AIDS. While the lesions begin as papules or plaques on the face and upper extremities, they typically evolve into nodules and may be present in any location, most commonly the lungs, lymph nodes, and gastrointestinal tract. Treatment strategies include watchful waiting in low-volume, cosmetically acceptable disease; electron-beam (superficial) radiation therapy for local disease that requires palliation; and carefully administered chemotherapy (VP-16, doxo-rubicin, vinblastine, and bleomycin have activity) for disseminated disease. A promising approach involves the use of interferon-γ, which is associated with a 30 percent rate of complete remission in those with Kaposi's sarcoma and relatively well-preserved circulating helper T cells (CD4+ cells).

**X-9.** **The answer is D.** *(Chaps. 54, 55)* A very common asymptomatic fungus infection of the skin caused by the dermatophyte *Pityrosporum orbiculare* (tinea versicolor) is often the source of a patient's concerns regarding cancer or serious infectious disease. However, this infection is easily treated by scrubbing off the scales with soap and water and with short applications of selenium sulfide (2.5%) for 12 nights. Antifungal creams, including imidazoles such as miconazole, can also be used. Lesions are sharply marginated macules with fine scaling that is easily scraped off with the edge of a microscopic glass slide. The scrapings, examined microscopically after treatment with potassium hydroxide, will reveal hyphae and spores commonly referred to as "spaghetti and meatballs." Tinea versicolor has a predilection for sites in the upper trunk and upper arms; lesions rarely appear on the face.

**X-10.** **The answer is D.** *(Chap. 55)* Hand eczema is one of the most common chronic skin disorders. This condition may or may not be associated with atopic dermatitis (based on a family history of atopy, presence of other forms of allergy such as asthma or allergic rhinitis, or a history of childhood or infantile eczema). Excessive exposure to water and detergents (such as might be experienced by pediatricians who frequently wash their hands) may initiate or aggravate this disorder. Typically, the hands are dry and cracked, but redness and swelling may also accompany the lesions. A common variant of hand dermatitis, exhibited by the patient in this question, is dyshidrotic eczema, which is characterized by multiple highly pruritic vesicles on the sides of the fingers. Lichen planus is a papulosquamous disorder in which the primary lesions are pruritic and characterized by a violaceous hue. Herpes zoster presents with grouped vesicles on an erythematous base. Asteatotic eczema develops most commonly on the lower legs of elderly persons during dry seasons and is characterized by fine cracks, with or without erythema. Therapy of hand dermatitis requires avoidance of frequent washing or harsh soaps, treatment of secondary staphylococcal and streptococcal infection if present, and application of topical steroids.

**X-11.** **The answer is A.** *(Chap. 55)* Psoriasis is a very common skin disorder that typically involves the elbows, knees, gluteal cleft, and scalp. Traumatized areas may also be involved (Kobner phenomenon). The lesions are characterized by erythematous, sharply demarcated papules and rounded plaques covered by a silvery scale. Histologically, the epidermis shows intraepidermal collections of neutrophils (microabscesses of Munro), but capillaries are usually not filled with neutrophils, a finding more characteristic of leukocytoclastic vasculitis. Infiltration of the dermis with lymphocytes that have convoluted nuclei would suggest cutaneous T-cell lymphoma (mycosis fungoides). The dermatopathology of psoriasis is characterized by inflammation and alteration of the cell cycle manifested by a marked thickening of the epidermis, increased keratinocyte mitotic figures and inflammatory cells in the dermis (usually lymphocytes and monocytes), and neutrophils in the upper dermis. Though treatment depends on the type, location, and extent of disease, localized application of glucocorticoids in conjunction with keratolytic agents such as salicylic acid may be used. If psoriasis is widespread, B spectrum ultraviolet light alone or in combination with coal tar (Goeckerman regimen) may be required.

**X-12.** **The answer is A.** *(Chap. 57)* Several systemic diseases are associated with vitiligo or localized hypopigmentation. The Vogt-Koyanagi-Harada syndrome is manifested by aseptic meningitis, uveitis, tinnitus, and hearing loss. Pigment is usually lost from areas of the face and scalp. Scleroderma and melanoma may also lead to vitiligo particularly in truncal areas. In contrast, there are many diseases that lead to hyperpigmentation, both localized and diffuse. The localized forms, due to an epidermal alteration, include seborrheic keratosis and acanthosis nigricans. Local melanocyte proliferation such as melanocytic nevus and melanoma are other examples. Patients with Peutz-Jeghers syndrome have pigmented lentingines on the hand, feet, nose, mouth, and within the oral cavity. In disorders of diffuse hyperpigmentation the skin changes may be truly diffuse or accentuated in sun-exposed areas. Endocrinopathies associated with hyperpigmentation include Addison's disease and Nelson's syndrome. In these syndromes an overproduction of any or all of the pituitary hormones alpha-MSH (melanocyte-stimulating hormone), ACTH, and ß-lipotropin can cause excess melanocytic activity. Metabolic causes of hyperpigmentation include porphyria cutaneous tardia, hemachromatosis, vitamin $B_{12}$ deficiency, folic acid deficiency, pelagra, malabsorption, and Whipple's disease. Primary biliary cirrhosis is an autoimmune disease which can lead to dark brown coloration of the skin in sun-exposed areas; the hyperpigmentation is accompanied by itching, jaundice, and xanthomas. Diffuse hyperpigmentation due to drugs or metals can result in inducation of melanin-pigment formation, complexes with melanin or deposits of the drug in the dermis. For example, busulfan induces pigment production. Gold or silver deposits directly in the skin may lead to a darkening coloration.

**X-13.** **The answer is B.** *(Chap. 57)* Bullous pemphigoid is a blistering skin disease of the elderly. Extensive blisters may appear after a prodrome of urticarial or eczematous eruption over the lower abdomen, groin, and flexor service of the extremities. Oral mucosal involvement is seen in about 10 to 40 percent of patients. Unlike pemphigus vulgaris, there is no ethnic or racial association. Nikolsky's sign (extension of the blister on pressure by the examining finger) is negative. Light microscopic examination of a lesional biopsy would reveal subepidermal bullae; immunofluorescent studies would demonstrate IgG deposits along the basement membrane zone. Bullous pemphigoid is believed to be an autoimmune disease; 70 percent of patients' serum contains circulating IgG autoantibodies capable of binding the epidermal basement membrane of normal human skin. These autoantibodies and their subsequent deposition in the skin are believed to activate complement, leading to the blister-producing inflammatory cell infiltrate. The mainstay of treatment is systemic glucocorticoids. However, minimal disease may be managed with topical steroids alone. Azathioprine is useful if alternative systemic therapy is required.

**X-14.** **The answer is A.** *(Chaps. 57, 185)* Herpes zoster, caused by the varicella zoster virus, which resides in ganglia after primary infection, usually produces a vesicular eruption limited to the dermatome innervated by the corresponding sensory ganglia. Frequently the characteristic rash, grouped vesicles on an erythematous base, is preceded by several days of pain and paresthesia in the involved area. The most common site of involvement is in thoracic dermatomes, but trigeminal, lumbar, and cervical regions may also be affected. Immunosuppressed persons may display dissemination of zoster, which certainly mandates systemic therapy. Nasociliary branch involvement is not uncommon in ophthalmic zoster and may be heralded by vesicular lesions on the side or tip of the nose. Given the possibility of associated conjunctivitis, keratitis, scleritis, or iritis, an ophthalmologist should always be consulted. Though the risk of postherpetic neuralgia is significant in patients over age 60, it is unclear if early use of steroids prevents this complication. While it is reasonable to undertake measures to contain bacterial superinfection, including the use of antibacterial compresses, administration of prophylactic systemic antibiotics is not indicated.

**X-15.** **The answer is C.** *(Chap. 57)* Systemic lupus erythematosus is a systemic multiorgan disease that involves connective tissue and blood vessels. Fever and skin lesions are the most common manifestations, while arthritis and renal pulmonary disease are also typical. The characteristic rash, as exemplified by the patient in this question, is an erythematous, confluent, macular eruption in a butterfly pattern on the face with fine scaling. Other possible skin lesions include erythematous urticarial lesions on the face and arms, hemorrhagic bullae during acute flares, and discoid plaques, which would typify chronic discoid lupus erythematosus. Lupus vasculitis may also present with palpable purpura.

Skin biopsy reveals an atrophic epidermis with liquefaction necrosis at the dermal-epidermal junction, edema of the dermis, and a lymphocytic infiltrate. Fibrinoid degeneration of the connective tissue and blood vessel walls may also be noted. Immunofluorescent studies demonstrate staining for immunoglobulins in a granular or globular pattern along the dermal-epidermal junction.

**X-16.** **The answer is C.** *(Chap. 57)* The rash of secondary syphilis is a maculopapular squamous eruption characterized by scattered reddish-brown lesions with a thin scale. The eruption often involves the palms and the soles, which is an important clue in the differential diagnosis. This rash can resemble atypical pityriasis rosea or erythema multiforme. The nontreponemal serologic tests such as the Venereal Disease Research Laboratory (VDRL) or RPR tests are positive. Patients usually give a history of a chancre at the site of the primary infection—in a heterosexual male usually the penis, but possibly the anus or pharynx. Treatment for both HIV-positive and HIV-negative adults is 2.4 million units of benzathine penicillin by intramuscular injection. If this treatment is successful, the nontreponemal serologic tests should become negative.

**X-17.** **The answer is B.** *(Chap. 57)* The shape and configuration of the dilated blood vessels are important features in distinguishing among the various types of telangiectasias. For example, linear telangiectasias are seen on the face of patients with actinically damaged skin. Broad telangiectasias are seen in scleroderma, especially that associated with the CREST variant of this disease. Periungual telangiectasias may be seen in systemic lupus, scleroderma, and dermatomyositis. Finally, spider-like telangiectasias are characteristic of hereditary hemorrhagic telangiectasia (Osler-Rendu-Weber disease). These lesions are inherited in an autosomal dominant fashion and the major symptoms are recurrent epistaxis and gastrointestinal bleeding. These mucosal abnormalities are actually arteriovenous communications and tend to bleed easily. A consumptive coagulopathy is noted in hereditary Kasabach-Merritt arteriovenous malformation but not in Osler-Rendu-Weber disease.

**X-18.** **The answer is A.** *(Chap. 57)* The photographed skin lesions are depigmented macules of vitiligo. Vitiliginous macules are completely lacking in pigment and are histologically devoid of melanocytes. This disorder is believed to be transmitted as an autosomal dominant trait with incomplete penetrance. Although the majority of cases of vitiligo are not associated with other disease processes, an association has been described between vitiligo and several disorders, including diabetes mellitus, pernicious anemia, hyperthyroidism, hypothyroidism, Addison's disease, alopecia areata, and hypoparathyroidism. The polyglandular autoimmune syndromes, which may involve several of the aforementioned endocrine abnormalities, are also associated with vitiligo.

**X-19.** **The answer is D.** *(Chap. 57)* Urticaria pigmentosa is a disorder of mast cells. The development of a wheal on gentle stroking of a pigmented macule (Darier's sign) is a useful diagnostic maneuver. Prognosis is said to worsen with age of onset: half the patients who develop multiple lesions by 4 years of age are disease-free by adolescence. Onset in adulthood is more ominous, with active lesions persisting indefinitely; systemic mastocytosis, which may have a fatal outcome, occurs frequently in affected adults. Symptomatic improvement has been reported with oral cromolyn. Affected persons should be warned to avoid substances and environmental factors known to cause mast-cell degranulation (e.g., cold, heat, trauma, or the ingestion of alcohol, aspirin, or morphine-opium alkaloid drugs). Although the disorder is usually an isolated event, familial disease occurs, indicating autosomal dominant inheritance in some cases.

**X-20.** **The answer is E.** *(Chap. 55)* Acne vulgaris is a self-limited disease mainly of young adults that causes inflamed cysts (comedones), which sometimes result in scarring. Closed comedones, or whiteheads, seen as white lesions of 1 to 2 mm, are often accompanied by inflammatory papules, pustules, or nodules as a consequence of the extrusion of oily and keratinous cyst debris. On the other hand, blackheads, or open comedones, which are filled with easily expressible dark material, do not usually cause serious problems. Vigorous facial scrubbing is contraindicated since this trauma could lead to rupture of comedones. Other predisposing factors include the use of systemic glucocorticoids, phenytoin, isoniazid, or phenobarbital. Treatment strategies include oral tetracycline or erythromycin therapy to decrease cyst colonization. Severe acne may be treated with a 20-week course of oral retinoic acid therapy, which may prevent formation of comedones by altering the pattern of epidermal desquamation. Pregnant patients should avoid retinoic acid given the teratogenic nature of this compound; this drug also causes extremely dry skin and hypertriglyceridemia.

**X-21.**  **The answer is C.**  *(Chap. 57)*  Tophaceous gout and pseudoxanthoma elasticum (PXE) are each associated with yellow lesions. Biopsies of lesions in PXE would show swollen and irregularly clumped elastic fibers and deposits of calcium. Such deposits in the coronary arteries can lead to angina; long-term administration of D-penicillamine can produce similar pathologic abnormalities. Deposits of monosodium urate cause the lesions of tophaceous gout, which are particularly firm, yellow and sometimes characterized by a discharge of a chalky material, often with telangiectasias and an irregular border. Xanthomas are yellow, which are characteristic of hypertriglyceridemia. Xanthelasmas are found on the eyelids as in this case and tendon xanthomas are frequently on the Achilles and finger tendons. Xanthomas represent collections of lipid-containing macrophages also known as foam cells.

**X-22.**  **The answer is E.**  *(Chap. 57)*  These fleshy hyperpigmented papules, seborrheic keratoses, are very common especially in older adults. They may occasionally be pruritic and tender (but only if secondarily infected). Early "flat" lesions can be confused with solar lentigo whereas larger pigmented lesions may be mistaken for pigmented basal cell carcinoma or melanoma. Either electrocautery or cryotherapy may be used to remove lesions. Usually they are quite benign and not associated with any systemic condition; however, should seborrheic keratoses appear rapidly and in large numbers, especially if associated with acrochordon (skin tags) and acanthosis nigrilons, then a suspicion for internal malignancy is raised (sign of Leser-Trelat).

# APPENDIX

# APPENDIX

**A**

## LABORATORY VALUES OF CLINICAL IMPORTANCE

### INTRODUCTORY COMMENTS

All laboratory appendices should be interpreted with caution since normal values differ widely among clinical laboratories. The values given in this Appendix are meant primarily for use with this text. In preparing the Appendix, the editors have taken into account the fact that the system of international units (SI, système international d'unités) is now used in most countries and in most medical and scientific journals.[1] However, clinical laboratories in many countries continue to report values in traditional units. Therefore, both systems are used in the Appendix. Values in SI units appear first, and traditional units appear in parentheses after the SI units. The dual system is also used in the text except for (1) those instances in which the numbers remain the same but only the terminology is changed (mmol/L for meq/L or IU/L for mIU/mL), when only the SI units are given; and (2) most pressure measurements (e.g., blood and cerebrospinal fluid pressures), when the traditional units (mmHg, mmH$_2$O) are used. In all other instances in the text the SI unit is followed by the traditional unit in parentheses. The SI base units, SI derived units, other units of measure referred to in Appendix A, and SI prefixes are listed in Tables A-1 to A-3 at the end of Appendix A. Conversions from one system to another can be made as follows:

$$mmol/L = \frac{mg/dL \times 10}{atomic\ weight}$$

$$mg/dL = \frac{mmol/L \times atomic\ weight}{10}$$

### ASCITIC FLUID

See Chapter 46

### BODY FLUIDS AND OTHER MASS DATA

Body fluid, total volume: 50 percent (in obese) to 70 percent (lean) of body weight
  Intracellular: 0.3–0.4 of body weight
  Extracellular: 0.2–0.3 of body weight
Blood
  Total volume:
    Males: 69 mL per kg body weight
    Females: 65 mL per kg body weight
  Plasma volume:
    Males: 39 mL per kg body weight
    Females: 40 mL per kg body weight
  Red blood cell volume:
    Males: 30 mL per kg body weight (1.15–1.21 L/m$^2$ of body surface area)
    Females: 25 mL per kg body weight (0.95–1.00 L/m$^2$ of body surface area)

[1] Young DS: Implementation of SI units for clinical laboratory data. Ann Intern Med 106:114, 1987

## CEREBROSPINAL FLUID[2]

| | | Conversion Factor (CF) C × CF = SI |
|---|---|---|
| Osmolarity | 292–297 mmol/kg water (292–297 mOsm/L) | — |
| Electrolytes: | | |
| Sodium | 137–145 mmol/L (137–145 meq/L) | — |
| Potassium | 2.7–3.9 mmol/L (2.7–3.9 meq/L) | — |
| Calcium | 1.0–1.5 mmol/L (2.1–3.0 meq/L) | 0.5 |
| Magnesium | 1.0–1.2 mmol/L (2.0–2.5 meq/L) | 0.5 |
| Chloride | 116–122 mmol/L (116–122 meq/L) | — |
| CO$_2$ content | 20–24 mmol/L (20–24 meq/L) | — |
| P$_{CO_2}$ | 6–7 kPa (45–49 mmHg) | 0.1333 |
| pH | 7.31–7.34 | — |
| Glucose | 2.2–3.9 mmol/L (40–70 mg/dL) | 0.05551 |
| Lactate | 1–2 mmol/L (10–20 mg/dL) | 0.1110 |
| Total protein: | 0.2–0.5 g/L (20–50 mg/dL) | 0.01 |
| Albumin | 0.066–0.442 g/L (6.6–44.2 mg/dL) | 0.01 |
| IgG | 0.009–0.057 g/L (0.9–5.7 mg/dL) | 0.01 |
| IgG index[3] | 0.29–0.59 | |
| Oligoclonal bands (OCB) | <2 bands not present in matched serum sample | |
| Ammonia | 15–47 µmol/L (25–80 µg/dL) | 0.5872 |
| Creatinine | 44–168 µmol/L (0.5–1.9 mg/dL) | 88.40 |
| Myelin basic protein | <4 µg/L | — |
| CSF pressure | 50–180 mmH$_2$O | — |
| CSF volume (adult) | ~150 mL | — |
| Leukocytes | | |
| Total | <5 per mL | — |
| Differential: | | |
| Lymphocytes | 60–70 percent | — |
| Monocytes | 30–50 percent | — |
| Neutrophils | None | — |

[2] Since cerebrospinal fluid concentrations are equilibrium values, measurements of the same parameters in blood plasma obtained at the same time are recommended. However, there is a time lag in attainment of equilibrium, and cerebrospinal levels of plasma constituents that can fluctuate rapidly (such as plasma glucose) may not achieve stable values until after a significant lag phase.

[3] $IgG\ index = \dfrac{CSF\ IgG(mg/dL) \times serum\ albumin(g/dL)}{Serum\ IgG(g/dL) \times CSF\ albumin(mg/dL)}$

## CHEMICAL CONSTITUENTS OF BLOOD

See also function tests, especially "Metabolic and Endocrine Tests."

| | Conversion Factor (CF) C × CF = SI |
|---|---|
| Acetoacetate, plasma: <100 μmol/L (<1 mg/dL) | 97.95 |
| Albumin, serum: 35–55 g/L (3.5–5.5 g/dL) | 10.00 |
| Aldolase: 0–100 nkat/L (0–6 U/L) | 16.67 |
| Alpha₁ antitrypsin, serum: 0.8–2.1 g/L (85–213 mg/dL) | 0.01 |
| Alpha fetoprotein (adult), serum: <30 μg/L (<30 ng/mL) | — |
| Aminotransferases, serum: | |
| Aspartate (AST, SGOT): 0–0.58 μkat/L (0–35 U/L) | 0.01667 |
| Alanine (ALT, SGPT): 0–0.58 μkat/L (0–35 U/L) | 0.01667 |
| Ammonia, as NH₃, plasma: 6–47 μmol/L (10–80 μg/dL) | 0.5872 |
| Amylase, serum: 0.8–3.2 μkat/L; 60–180 U/L | 0.01667 |
| Angiotensin-converting enzyme (ACE): <670 nkat/L (<40 U/L) | 16.67 |
| Anticonvulsant drug levels: see Fig. 365-8 | |
| Arterial blood gases: | |
| [HCO₃⁻]: 21–28 mmol/L (21–30 meq/L) | — |
| P_CO₂: 4.7–5.9 kPa (35–45 mmHg) | 0.1333 |
| pH: 7.38–7.44 | — |
| P_O₂: 11–13 kPa (80–100 mmHg) | 0.1333 |
| Ascorbic acid (vitamin C), serum: 23–57 μmol/L (0.4–1.0 mg/dL) | 56.78 |
| Barbiturates, serum: normal, nondetectable | |
| Phenobarbital, "potentially fatal" level: approximately 390 μmol/L (9 mg/dL) | 43.06 |
| Most short-acting barbiturates, "potentially fatal" levels: approximately 150 μmol/L (35 mg/L) | 4.419 |
| β-Hydroxybutyrate, plasma: <300 μmol/L (<3 mg/dL) | 96.05 |
| Bilirubin, total, serum (Malloy-Evelyn): 5.1–17 μmol/L (0.3–1.0 mg/dL) | 17.10 |
| Direct, serum: 1.7–5.1 μmol/L (0.1–0.3 mg/dL) | 17.10 |
| Indirect, serum: 3.4–12 μmol/L (0.2–0.7 mg/dL) | 17.10 |
| Calciferols (vitamin D), plasma: | |
| 1,25-dihydroxyvitamin D [1,25(OH)₂D]: 40–160 pmol/L (16 to 65 pg/mL) | 2.4 |
| 25-hydroxyvitamin D [25(OH)D]: 20–200 nmol/L (8–80 ng/mL) | 2.496 |
| Calcium, ionized: 1.1–1.4 mmol/L (4.5–5.6 mg/dL) | 0.2495 |
| Calcium, plasma: 2.2–2.6 mmol/L (9–10.5 mg/dL) | 0.2495 |
| Carbon dioxide content, plasma (sea level): 21–30 mmol/L (21–30 meq/L) | — |
| Carbon dioxide tension (P_CO₂), arterial blood (sea level): 4.7–5.9 kPa (35–45 mmHg) | 0.1333 |
| Carbon monoxide content, blood: symptoms with over 20 percent saturation of hemoglobin | |
| Carotenoids, serum: 0.9–5.6 μmol/L (50–300 μg/dL) | 0.01863 |
| Ceruloplasmin, serum: 270–370 mg/L (27–37 mg/dL) | 10.00 |
| Chloride, serum (as Cl⁻): 98–106 mmol/L (98–106 meq/L) | — |
| Cholesterol: see Table A-4 | |
| Complement, serum: | |
| C3: 0.55–1.20 g/L (55–120 mg/dL) | 0.01 |
| C4: 0.20–0.50 g/L (20–50 mg/dL) | 0.01 |
| Copper, serum: 11–22 μmol/L (70–140 μg/dL) | 0.1574 |

| | Conversion Factor (CF) C × CF = SI |
|---|---|
| Creatine kinase, serum (total): | |
| Females: 0.17–1.17 μkat/L (10–70 U/L) | 0.01667 |
| Males: 0.42–1.50 μkat/L (25–90 U/L) | 0.01667 |
| Creatine kinase-MB: 0–7 μg/L | — |
| Creatinine, serum: <133 μmol/L (<1.5 mg/dL) | 88.40 |
| Digoxin serum: | |
| Therapeutic level: 0.6–2.8 nmol/L (0.5–2.2 ng/mL) | 1.281 |
| Toxic level: >3.1 nmol/L (>2.4 ng/mL) | 1.281 |
| Ethanol, blood: | |
| Behavioral changes: >4.3 mmol/L (>20 mg/dL) | 0.2171 |
| Legal intoxication: >17 mmol/L (>80 mg/dL) | 0.2171 |
| Coma and death: >65 mmol/L (>300 mg/dL) | 0.2171 |
| Fatty acids, free (nonesterified), plasma: 180 mg/L (<18 mg/dL) | 10.00 |
| Ferritin, serum: | |
| Women: 10–200 μg/L (10–200 ng/ml) | — |
| Men: 15–400 μg/L (15–400 ng/ml) | |
| Fibrinogen, plasma: see "Hematologic Evaluations: Platelets and Coagulation" | — |
| Fibrinogen split products: see "Hematologic Evaluations: Platelets and Coagulation" | |
| Folic acid, red cell: 340–1020 nmol/L cells (150–450 ng/mL cells) | 2.266 |
| Folic acid, serum: 7–36 nmol/L cells (3–16 ng/mL cells) | — |
| Gastrin, serum: 40–200 ng/L (40–200 pg/mL) | — |
| Glucose (fasting), plasma: | |
| Normal: 4.2–6.4 mmol/L (75–115 mg/dL) | 0.05551 |
| Diabetes mellitus: >7.8 mmol/L [>140 mg/dL (on more than one occasion)] | 0.05551 |
| Glucose, 2 h postprandial, plasma: | |
| Normal: <7.8 mmol/L (<140 mg/dL) | 0.05551 |
| Impaired glucose tolerance: 7.8–11.1 mmol/L (140–200 mg/dL) | 0.05551 |
| Diabetes mellitus: >11.1 mmol/L on more than one occasion (>200 mg/dL) | 0.05551 |
| Hemoglobin, blood (sea level): | |
| Male: 140–180 g/L (14–18 g/dL) | 10.00 |
| Female: 120–160 g/L (12–16 g/dL) | 10.00 |
| Hemoglobin A₁c: up to 6 percent of total hemoglobin | — |
| Immunoglobulins, serum: | |
| IgA: 0.9–3.2 g/L (90–325 mg/dL) | 0.01 |
| IgD: 0–0.08 g/L (0–8 mg/dL) | 0.01 |
| IgE: <0.00025 g/L (<0.025 mg/dL) | 0.01 |
| IgG: 8.0–15.0 g/L (800–1500 mg/dL) | 0.01 |
| IgM: 0.45–1.5 g/L (45–150 mg/dL) | 0.01 |
| Iron, serum: 9–27 μmol/L (50–150 μg/dL) | 0.1791 |
| Iron-binding capacity, serum: 45–66 μmol/L (250–370 μg/dL) | 0.1791 |
| Saturation: 0.2–0.45 (20–45 percent) | |
| Lactate dehydrogenase, serum: 1.7–3.2 μkat/L (100–190 U/L) | 0.01667 |
| Lactate dehydrogenase isoenzymes, serum (agarose): | |
| Fraction 1 (of total): 0.14–0.25 (14–26 percent) | 0.01 |
| Fraction 2: 0.29–0.39 (29–39 percent) | 0.01 |
| Fraction 3: 0.20–0.25 (20–26 percent) | 0.01 |
| Fraction 4: 0.08–0.16 (8–16 percent) | 0.01 |
| Fraction 5: 0.06–0.16 (6–16 percent) | 0.01 |
| Lactate, venous plasma: 0.6–1.7 mmol/L (5–15 mg/dL) | 0.1110 |
| Lead, serum: <1.0 μmol/L (<20 μg/dL) | 0.04826 |
| Lipase, serum: 0–2.66 μkat/L (0–160 U/L) | 0.01667 |
| Lipids: see Table A-4 | — |

|  | Conversion Factor (CF) C × CF = SI |
|---|---|
| Lipids, triglyceride, serum: see "Triglycerides" | — |
| Lipoprotein: see Table A-4 | — |
| Lithium, serum: | |
| Therapeutic level: 0.6–1.2 mmol/L (0.6–1.2 meq/L) | — |
| Toxic level: >2 mmol/L (2 meq/L) | — |
| Magnesium, serum: 0.8–1.2 mmol/L (1.8–3 mg/dL) | 0.4114 |
| Osmolality, plasma: 285–295 mmol/kg serum water (285–295 mosmol/kg serum water) | — |
| Oxygen content: | |
| Arterial blood (sea level): 17–21 volume percent | — |
| Venous blood, arm (sea level): 10 to 16 volume percent | — |
| Oxygen percent saturation (sea level): | |
| Arterial blood: 0.97 mol/mol (97 percent) | 0.01 |
| Venous blood, arm: 0.60–0.85 mol/mol (60–85 percent) | 0.01 |
| Oxygen tension ($P_{O_2}$) blood: 11–13 kPa (80–100 mmHg) | 0.1333 |
| pH, blood: 7.38–7.44 | — |
| Phenytoin, plasma: See Fig. 365-8 | |
| Phosphatase, acid, serum: 0.90 nkat/L (0–5.5 U/L) | — |
| Phosphatase, alkaline, serum: 0.5–2.0 nkat/L (30–120 U/L) | — |
| Phosphorus, inorganic, serum: 1.0–1.4 mmol/L (3–4.5 mg/dL) | 0.3229 |
| Potassium, serum: 3.5–5.0 mmol/L (3.5–5.0 meq/L) | — |
| Protein, total, serum: 55–80 g/L (5.5–8.0 g/dL) | 10.00 |
| Protein fractions, serum: | |
| Albumin: 35–55 g/L [3.5–5.5 g/dL (50–60 percent)] | 10.00 |
| Globulin: 20–35 g/L [2.0–3.5 g/dL (40–50 percent)] | 10.00 |
| Alpha$_1$: 2–4 g/L [0.2–0.4 g/dL (4.2–7.2 percent)] | 10.00 |
| Alpha$_2$: 5–9 g/L [0.5–0.9 g/dL (6.8–12 percent)] | 10.00 |
| Beta: 6–11 g/L [0.6–1.1 g/dL (9.3–15 percent)] | 10.00 |
| Gamma: 7–17 g/L [0.7–1.7 g/dL (13–23 percent)] | 10.00 |
| Pyruvate, venous, plasma: 60–170 μmol/L (0.5–1.5 mg/dL) | 113.6 |
| Quinidine, serum: | |
| Therapeutic range: 4.6–9.2 μmol/L (1.5–3 mg/L) | 3.082 |
| Toxic range: 15.4–18.5 μmol/L (5–6 mg/L) | 3.082 |
| Salicylate, plasma: 0 mmol/L | — |
| Therapeutic range: 1.4–1.8 mmol/L (20–25 mg/dL) | 0.07240 |
| Toxic range: >2.2 mmol/L (>30 mg/dL) | 0.07240 |
| Sodium, serum: 136–145 mmol/L (136–145 meq/L) | — |
| Steroids: see "Metabolic and Endocrine Tests" | — |
| Transferrin, serum: 2.3–3.9 mg/L (230–390 μg/dL) | 10.00 |
| Triglycerides: <1.8 mmol/L (<160 mg/dL) | 0.01129 |
| Troponin I, serum: 0–0.4 μg/L (0–0.4 ng/mL) | — |
| Troponin T, serum: 0–0.1 μg/L (0–0.1 ng/mL) | — |
| Urea nitrogen, serum: 3.6–7.1 mmol/L (10–20 mg/dL) | 0.3570 |
| Uric acid, serum: | |
| Men: 150–480 μmol/L (2.5–8.0 mg/dL) | 59.48 |
| Women: 90–360 μmol/L (1.5–6.0 mg/dL) | 59.48 |
| Vitamin A, serum: 0.7–3.5 μmol/L (20–100 μg/dL) | 0.03491 |
| Vitamin B$_{12}$, serum: 148–443 pmol/L (200–600 pg/mL) | 0.7378 |
| Zinc, serum: 11.5–18.5 μmol/L (75–120 μg/dL) | 0.1530 |

## CIRCULATORY FUNCTION TESTS

Arteriovenous oxygen difference: 30–50 mL/L
Cardiac output (Fick): 2.5–3.6 L/m$^2$ of body surface area per minute
Contractility indexes:
  Maximum left ventricular $dp/dt$: 1650 mmHg/s (range, 1320–1880, mmHg/s)
  ($dp/dt$)/DP when DP = 40 mmHg: 37.6 ±12.2 s$^{-1}$ (DP, diastolic pressure)
  Mean normalized systolic ejection rate (angiography): 3.32 ± 0.84 end-diastolic volumes per second
  Mean velocity of circumferential fiber shortening (angiography) 1.66 ± 0.42 circumferences per second
Ejection fraction, stroke volume/end-diastolic volume (SV/EDV): normal range: 0.55–0.78; average: 0.67
End-diastolic volume: 75 mL/m$^2$ (range, 60–88 mL/m$^2$)
End-systolic volume: 25 mL/m$^2$ (range, 20–33 mL/m$^2$)
Left ventricular work:
  Stroke work index: 30–110 (g·m)/m$^2$
  Left ventricular minute work index: 1.8–6.6 [(kg·m)/m$^2$]/min
  Oxygen consumption index: 110–150 mL
Maximum oxygen uptake: normal range 20–60 mL/min; average: 35 mL/min
Pulmonary vascular resistance: 20–120 (dyn·s)/cm$^5$ (2–12 kPa·s/L)
Systemic vascular resistance: 770–1500 (dyn·s)/cm$^5$ (77–150 kPa·s/L)

## GASTROINTESTINAL TESTS

See also "Stool Analysis."

Absorption tests:
  D-Xylose absorption test: After an overnight fast, 25 g xylose is given in aqueous solution by mouth. Urine collected for the following 5 h should contain 33–53 mmol (5–8 g) (or >20 percent of ingested dose). Serum xylose should be 1.7–2.7 mmol (25–40 mg/dL) 1 h after the oral dose.
  Vitamin A absorption test: A fasting blood specimen is obtained and 200,000 units of vitamin A in oil is given by mouth. Serum vitamin A levels should rise to twice fasting level in 3–5 h.
Bentiromide test (pancreatic function): 500 mg bentiromide (chymex) orally; p-aminobenzoic acid (PABA) measured in plasma and/or urine
  Plasma: >3.6 (±1.1) μg/mL at 90 min
  Urine: >50 percent recovered as PABA in 6 h
Gastric juice:
  Volume:
    24 h: 2–3 L
    Nocturnal: 600–700 mL
    Basal, fasting: 30–70 mL/h

|  | Conversion Factor (CF) C × CF = SI |
|---|---|
| Reaction: | |
| pH: 1.6–1.8 | |
| Titratable acidity of fasting juice: 4–9 μmol/s (15–35 meq/h) | 0.261 |
| Acid output: | |
| Basal: | |
| Females (mean ± 1 SD): 0.6 ± 0.5 pmol/s (2.0 ± 1.8 meq/h) | 0.2778 |
| Males (mean ± 1 SD): 0.8 ± 0.6 μmol/s (3.0 ± 2.0 meq/h) | 0.2778 |
| Maximal (after subcutaneous histamine acid phosphate 0.004 mg/kg body weight and preceded by 50 mg promethazine or after betazole 1.7 mg/kg body wt or pentagastrin 6 μg/kg body wt): | |
| Females (mean ± 1 SD): 4.4 ± 1.4 μmol/s (16 ± 5 meq/h) | 0.2778 |
| Males (mean ± 1 SD): 6.4 ± 1.4 μmol/s (23 ± 5 meq/h) | 0.2778 |

Basal acid output/maximal acid output ratio: 0.6 or less

Gastrin, serum: 40–200 ng/L (40–200 pg/mL)   —

Secretin test (pancreatic exocrine function): 1 unit per kg body wt, intravenously

  Volume (pancreatic juice): >2.0 mL/kg in 80 min   —

  Bicarbonate concentration: >80 mmol/L (>80 meq/L)   —

  Bicarbonate output: >10 mmol in 30 min (>10 meq in 30 min)   —

# METABOLIC AND ENDOCRINE TESTS

|  | Conversion Factor (CF) $C \times CF = SI$ |
|---|---|
| Adrenocorticotropin (ACTH) plasma, 8 A.M.: 2–11 pmol/L (9–52 pg/mL) | 0.2202 |
| Adrenal cortex function tests: see Chap. 332 | — |
| Adrenal medulla function tests: see Chap. 333 | — |
| Adrenal steroids, plasma: | |
|   Aldosterone, 8 A.M.: <220 pmol/L (patient supine, 100 meq Na and 60–100 meq K intake) (<8 ng/dL) | 27.74 |
|   Cortisol: | |
|     8 A.M.: 140–690 nmol/L (5–25 μg/dL) | 27.59 |
|     4 P.M.: 80–330 nmol/L (3–12 μg/dL) | 27.59 |
|   Dehydroepiandrosterone (DHEA): 7–31 nmol/L (2–9 μg/L) | 3.467 |
|   Dehydroepiandrosterone sulfate (DHEA sulfate): 1.3–6.8 μmol/L (500–2500 μg/L) | 0.002714 |
|   11-Deoxycortisol (compound S): <30 nmol/L (<1 μg/dL) | 28.86 |
|   17-Hydroxyprogesterone: | |
|     Women: follicular phase, 0.6–3 nmol/L (0.20–1 μg/L); luteal phase 1.5–10.6 nmol/L (0.5–3.5 μg/L) | 3.026 / 3.026 |
|     Men: 0.2–9 nmol/L (0.06–3 μg/L) | 3.026 |
| Adrenal steroids, urinary excretion | |
|   Aldosterone: 14–53 nmol/d (5–19 μg/d) | 2.774 |
|   Cortisol, free: 55–275 nmol/d (20–100 μg/d) | 2.759 |
|   17-Hydroxycorticosteroids: 5.5–28 μmol/d (2–10 mg/d) | 2.759 |
|   17-Ketosteroids: | |
|     Men: 20–69 μmol/d (6–20 mg/d) | 3.467 |
|     Women: 20–59 μmol/d (6–17 mg/d) | 3.467 |
| Angiotensin II, plasma, 8 A.M.: 10–30 nmol/L (10–30 pg/mL) | — |
| Arginine vasopressin (AVP), plasma: | |
|   Random fluid intake: 1.5–5.6 pmol/L (1.5–6 ng/L) | 0.92 |
| Calcitonin, plasma: <50 ng/L (<50 pg/mL) | — |
| Catecholamines, urinary excretion: | |
|   Free catecholamines: <590 nmol/d (<100 μg/d) | 5.911 |
|   Epinephrine: <275 nmol/d (<50 μg/d) | 5.458 |
|   Metanephrines: <7 μmol/d (<1.3 mg/d) | 5.458 |
|   Norepinephrine: 89–473 nmol/d (15–80 μg/d) | 5.91 |
|   Vanillylmandelic acid (VMA): <40 μmol/d (<8 mg/d) | 5.046 |
| Glucagon, plasma: 50–100 ng/L (50–100 pg/mL) | — |
| Gonadal function tests: see Chaps. 336 and 337 | — |
| Gonadal steroids, plasma: | |
|   Androstenedione: | |
|     Women: 3.5–7.0 nmol/L (1–2 ng/mL) | 3.492 |
|     Men: 3.0–5.0 nmol/L (0.8–1.3 ng/mL) | 3.492 |

|  | Conversion Factor (CF) $C \times CF = SI$ |
|---|---|
| Estradiol: | |
|   Women: 70–220 pmol/L (20–60 pg/mL), higher at ovulation | 3.671 |
|   Men: <180 pmol/L (<50 pg/mL) | 3.671 |
| Progesterone: | |
|   Men, prepubertal girls, preovulatory women, and postmenopausal women: <6 nmol/L (<2 ng/mL) | 3.180 |
|   Women, luteal, peak: 6–60 nmol/L (2–20 ng/mL) | 3.180 |
| Testosterone: | |
|   Women: <3.5 nmol/L (<1 ng/mL) | 3.467 |
|   Men: 10–35 nmol/L (3–10 ng/mL) | 3.467 |
|   Prepubertal boys and girls: 0.17–0.7 nmol/L (0.05–0.2 ng/mL) | 3.467 |
| Gonadotropins, plasma: | |
|   Women, mature, premenopausal, except at ovulation: | |
|     FSH: 1.4–9.6 IU/L (1.4–9.6 mIU/mL) | — |
|     LH: 0.8–26 IU/L (0.8–26 mIU/mL) | — |
|   Ovulatory surge: | |
|     FSH: 2.3–21 IU/L (2.3–21 mIU/mL) | — |
|     LH: 25–57 IU/L (25–57 mIU/mL) | — |
|   Postmenopausal women: | |
|     FSH: 34–96 IU/L (34–96 mIU/mL) | — |
|     LH: 40–104 IU/L (40–104 mIU/mL) | — |
|   Men, mature: | |
|     FSH: 0.9–15 IU/L (0.9–15 mIU/mL) | — |
|     LH: 1.3–13 IU/L (1.3–13 mIU/mL) | — |
|   Children of both sexes, prepubertal: | |
|     LH: 1.0–5.9 IU/L (1.0–5.9 mIU/mL) | — |
| Growth hormone, after 100 g glucose by mouth: <2 μg/L (<2 ng/ml) | — |
| Human chorionic gonadotropin, β subunit (β-hCG), plasma: | |
|   Men and nonpregnant women: <3 IU/L (<3 mIU/mL) | — |
| Insulin, serum or plasma, fasting: 43–186 pmol/L (6–26 μU/mL) | 7.175 |
| Insulin-like growth factor I (somatomedin C, IGF-1/SM C): see Chap. 329 | — |
| Oxytocin: random 1–4 pmol/L (1.25–5 ng/L) | 0.80 |
|   Ovulatory peak in women 4–8 pmol/L (5–10 ng/L) | — |
| Pancreatic islet function tests: see Chap. 334 | — |
| Parathyroid function tests: see Chap. 354 | — |
| Pituitary function tests: see Chaps. 328 to 330 | — |
| Pregnancy tests: see Chap. 337 | — |
| Prolactin, serum: 2–15 μg/L (2–15 ng/mL) | — |
| Renin-angiotensin function tests: see Chap. 332 | — |
| Semen analysis: see Chap. 336 | — |
| Thyroid function tests: | |
|   Dynamic tests of thyroid function: see Chap. 331 | — |
|   Radioactive iodine uptake, 24 h: 5–30 percent (range varies in different areas due to variations in iodine intake) | — |
|   Resin $T_3$ uptake: 0.25–0.35 (25–35 percent) (varies among laboratories; for calculation of free T4 estimate, see Chap. 331) | 0.01 |
|   Reverse triiodothyronine ($rT_3$), plasma: 0.15–0.61 nmol/L (10–40 ng/dL) | 0.01536 |
|   Thyroid-stimulating hormone (TSH): 0.4–5 mU/L (0.4–5 μU/mL) | — |
|   Thyroxine ($T_4$), serum radioimmunoassay: 64–154 nmol/L (5–12 μg/dL) | 12.86 |
|   Triiodothyronine ($T_3$), plasma: 1.1–2.9 nmol/L (70–190 ng/dL) | 0.01536 |

## PULMONARY FUNCTION TESTS

See Table A-9

## RENAL FUNCTION TESTS

| | Conversion Factor (CF) C × CF = SI |
|---|---|
| Clearances (corrected to 1.72 m² body surface area): | |
| Measures of glomerular filtration rate: | |
| Insulin clearance (C1): | |
| Males (mean ± 1 SD): 2.1 ± 0.4 mL/s (124 ± 25.8 mL/min) | 0.01667 |
| Females (mean ± 1 SD): 2.0 ± 0.2 mL/s (119 ± 12.8 mL/min) | 0.01667 |
| Endogenous creatinine clearance: 1.5–2.2 mL/s (91–130 mL/min) | 0.01667 |
| Urea: 1.0–1.7 mL/s (60–100 mL/min) | 0.01667 |
| Measures of effective renal plasma flow and tubular function: | |
| p-Aminohippuric acid clearance (C1$_{PAH}$): | |
| Males (mean ± 1 SD): 10.9 ± 2.7 mL/s (654 ± 163 mL/min) | 0.01667 |
| Females (mean ± 1 SD): 9.9 ± 1.7 mL/s (594 ± 102 mL/min) | 0.01667 |
| Concentration and dilution test: | |
| Specific gravity of urine: | |
| After 12-h fluid restriction: 1.025 or more | — |
| After 12-h deliberate water intake: 1.003 or less | — |
| Protein excretion, urine: <0.15 g/d (<150 mg/d) | 0.01 |
| Males: 0–0.06 g/d (0–60 mg/d) | 0.01 |
| Females: 0–0.09 g/d (0–90 mg/d) | 0.01 |
| Specific gravity, maximal range: 1.002–1.028 | — |
| Tubular reabsorption, phosphorus: 79–94 percent of filtered load | — |

## HEMATOLOGIC EVALUATIONS

See also "Chemical Constituents of Blood."

| | Conversion Factor (CF) C × CF = SI |
|---|---|
| Bone marrow: see Table A-6 | — |
| Carboxyhemoglobin: | |
| Nonsmoker: 0–0.023 (0–2.3 percent) | 0.01 |
| Smoker: 0.021–0.042 (2.1–4.2 percent) | 0.01 |
| Erythrocyte: | |
| Count: 4.15–4.90 × 10¹²/L (4.15–4.90 × 10⁶/mm³) | — |
| Distribution width: 0.13–0.15 (13–15 percent) | — |
| Glucose-6-phosphate dehydrogenase: 12.1 ± 2 IU/gHb (WHO) | — |
| Life span: | |
| Normal survival: 120 days | — |
| Chromium-labeled, half-life ($t_{1/2}$): 28 days | — |
| Mean corpuscular hemoglobin (MCH): 28–33 pg/cell (28–33 pg/cell) | — |
| Mean corpuscular hemoglobin concentration (MCHC): 320–360 g/L (32–36 g/dL) | 10.00 |
| Mean corpuscular volume (MCV): 86–98 fl (86–98 μm³) | — |
| Ham's test (acid serum): negative | — |
| Haptoglobin, serum 0.5–2.2 g/L (50–220 mg/dL) | 0.01 |
| Hematocrit | |
| Males: 0.42–0.52 (42–52%) | — |
| Females: 0.37–0.48 (37–48%) | — |

| | Conversion Factor (CF) C × CF = SI |
|---|---|
| Hemoglobin: | |
| Plasma: 0.01–0.05 g/L (1–5 mg/dL) | 0.01 |
| Whole blood: | |
| Males: 8.1–11.2 mmol/L (13–18 g/dL) | — |
| Females: 7.4–9.9 mmol/L (12–16 g/dL) | — |
| Hemoglobin A₂ (HbA₂): 0.015–0.035 (1.5–3.5 percent) | 0.01 |
| Hemoglobin, fetal (HbF): <0.02 (<2 percent) | 0.01 |
| Leukocytes: | |
| Alkaline phosphatase (LAP): 0.2–1.6 μkat/L (13–100 μ/L) | — |
| Count: 4.3–10.8 × 10⁹/L (4.3–10.8 × 10³/mm³) | |
| Differential: | |
| Neutrophils: 0.45–0.74 (45–74 percent) | |
| Bands: 0–0.04 (0–4 percent) | |
| Lymphocytes: 0.16–0.45 (16–45 percent) | |
| Monocytes: 0.04–0.10 (4–10 percent) | |
| Eosinophils: 0–0.07 (0–7 percent) | |
| Basophils: 0–0.02 (0–2 percent) | |
| Methemoglobin: <2 mg/L (<2 μg/mL) | — |
| Osmotic fragility: | |
| Slight hemolysis: 0.45–0.39 percent | — |
| Complete hemolysis: 0.33–0.30 percent | — |
| Platelets and coagulation parameters: | |
| Alpha₂ antiplasmin: 70–130 percent | |
| Antithrombin III: 80–120 percent | |
| Bleeding time: | |
| Simplate: <7 min | |
| Euglobulin lysis time: >2 h | |
| Factor II: 60–100 percent | |
| Factor V: 60–100 percent | |
| Factor VII: 60–100 percent | |
| Factor IX: 60–100 percent | |
| Factor X: 60–100 percent | |
| Factor XI: 60–100 percent | |
| Factor XII: 60–100 percent | |
| Factor XIII: 60–100 percent | |
| Fibrinogen: 200–400 mg/dL | |
| Plasminogen: 2.4–4.4 CTA U/mL | |
| Protein C (antigenic assay): 58–148 percent | |
| Protein S (antigenic assay): 58–148 percent | |
| Partial thromboplastin time (activated PTT): comparable to control | |
| Prothrombin time (quick one-stage): control ± 1 s | |
| Platelets: 130–400 × 10⁹/L (130,000–400,000/mm³) | |
| Thrombin time: control ± 3 s | |
| von Willebrand's antigen: 60–150 percent | |
| Protoporphyrin, free erythrocyte (FEP): 0.28–0.64 μmol/L of red blood cells (16–36 μg/dL of red blood cells) | 0.0177 |
| Red cells: (see "Erythrocytes") | |
| Schilling test: 7–40 percent of orally administered vitamin B₁₂ excreted in urine | |
| Sedimentation rate: | |
| Westergren, <50 years of age: | |
| Males: 0–15 mm/h | |
| Females: 0–20 mm/h | |
| Westergren, >50 years of age: | |
| Males: 0–20 mm/h | |
| Females: 0–30 mm/h | |
| Sucrose hemolysis: negative | |
| Viscosity | |
| Plasma: 1.7–2.1 | |
| Serum: 1.4–1.8 | |
| White blood cells: (see "Leukocytes") | |

## STOOL ANALYSIS

Conversion
Factor (CF)
C × CF = SI

Bulk:
    Wet weight: <197.5 (115 ± 41) g/d — —
    Dry weight: <66.4 (34 ± 15) g/d — —
Alpha₁ antitrypsin: 0.98 (±0.17) mg/g dry weight stool —
Coproporphyrin: 600–1500 nmol/d (400–1000 μg/d)  1.527
Fat (on diet containing at least 50 g fat): <6.0
(4.0 ± 1.5) g/d when measured on a 3-day
(or longer) collection
    Percent of dry weight: 0.30 (<30.4 percent)  0.01
    Coefficient of fat absorption: >0.95 (>95 percent)  0.01
Fatty acid:
    Free: 0.01–0.10 (1–10 percent of dry matter)  0.01
    Combined as soap: 0.005–0.12 (0.5–12 percent of  0.01
    dry matter)
Nitrogen: <1.7 (1.4 ± 0.2) g/d —
Protein content: minimal —
Urobilinogen: 68–470 μmol/d (40–280 mg/d)  1.693
Water: 0.65 (approximately 65 percent)  0.01

## URINE ANALYSIS

See also "Metabolic and Endocrine Tests"

Conversion
Factor (CF)
C × CF = SI

Acidity, titratable: 20–40 mmol/d (20–40 meq/d) —
Ammonia: 30–50 mmol/d (30–50 meq/d) —
Amylase: 35–260 Somogyi units/h —
Amylase/creatinine clearance ratio [(Cl_am/Cl_cr) × 100]: —
  1–5
Bentiromide (pancreatic function): 50 percent excreted —
  in 6 h as *p*-amino benzoic acid (PABA) after 500 mg
  oral bentiromide
Calcium (10 meq/d or 200-mg/d calcium diet):  0.5
  <3.8 mmol/d (<7.5 meq/d)
Catecholamines: see under "Metabolic and Endocrine —
  Tests"
Copper: 0–0.4 μmol/d (0–25 μg/d)  0.01574
Coproporphyrins (types I and III): 150–460 nmol/d  1.527
  (100–300 μg/d)
Creatine, as creatinine:
    Adult males: <380 μmol/d (<50 mg/d)  7.625
    Adult females: <760 μmol/d (<100 mg/d)  7.625
Creatinine: 8.8–14 mmol/d (1.0–1.6 g/d)  8.840
Glucose, true (oxidase method): 0.3–1.7 mmol/d  0.5551
  (50–300 mg/d)
5-Hydroxyindoleacetic acid (5-HIAA): 10–47 μmol/d  5.230
  (2–9 mg/d)
Lead: <0.4 μmol/d (<80 μg/d)  0.004826
Protein: <0.15 g/d (<150 mg/d)  0.1
Porphobilinogen: none —
Potassium: 25–100 mmol/d [25–100 meq/d (varies —
  with intake)]
Sodium: 100–260 mmol/d [100–260 meq/d (varies —
  with intake)]
Urobilinogen: 1.7–5.9 μmol/d (1–3.5 mg/d)  1.693
D-Xylose excretion: 5 to 8 g within 5 h after oral dose —
  of 25 g

### Table A-1

#### SI and Other Units

| Quantity | Name of Unit | Symbol for Unit | Derivation of Units |
|---|---|---|---|
| **SI BASE UNITS** | | | |
| Length | meter | m | |
| Mass | kilogram | kg | |
| Time | second | s | |
| Thermodynamic temperature | Kelvin | K | |
| Amount of substance | mole | mol | |
| **SI DERIVED UNITS** | | | |
| Area | square meter | $m^2$ | |
| Force | newton | N | $(m \cdot kg)/s^2$ |
| Pressure | pascal | Pa | $N \cdot m^2$ |
| Work, energy | joule | J | $N \cdot m$ |
| Celsius temperature | degree Celsius | °C | K |
| **OTHER UNITS RETAINED FOR USE** | | | |
| Time | minute | min | |
| | hour | h | |
| | day | d | |
| Volume | liter | L | |

### Table A-2

#### Radiation Derived Units

| Quantity | Old Unit | SI Unit | Name for SI Unit (and Abbreviation) | Conversion |
|---|---|---|---|---|
| Activity | curie (Ci) | Disintegrations per second (dps) | becquerel (Bq) | 1 Ci = 3.7 × $10^{10}$ Bq<br>1 mCi = 37 mBq<br>1 μCi = 0.037 MBq or 37 GBq<br>1 Bq = 2.703 × $10^{-11}$ Ci |
| Absorbed dose | rad | joule per kilogram (J/kg) | gray (Gy) | 1 Gy = 100 rad<br>1 rad = 0.01 Gy<br>1 mrad = $10^{-3}$ cGy |
| Exposure | roentgen (R) | coulomb per kilogram (C/kg) | — | 1 C/kg = 3876 R<br>1 R = 2.58 × $10^{-4}$ C/kg<br>1 mR = 258 pC/kg |
| Dose equivalent | rem | joule per kilogram (J/kg) | sievert (Sv) | 1 Sv = 100 rem<br>1 rem = 0.01 Sv<br>1 mrem = 10 μSv |

### Table A-3

#### SI Prefixes and Their Symbols

| Factor | Prefix | Symbol for Prefix |
|---|---|---|
| $10^9$ | giga | G |
| $10^6$ | mega | M |
| $10^3$ | kilo | k |
| $10^2$ | hecto | h |
| $10^1$ | deka | da |
| $10^{-1}$ | deci | d |
| $10^{-2}$ | centi | c |
| $10^{-3}$ | milli | m |
| $10^{-6}$ | micro | μ |
| $10^{-9}$ | nano | n |
| $10^{-12}$ | pico | p |
| $10^{-15}$ | femto | f |
| $10^{-18}$ | alto | a |

Table A-4

## Classification of Total Cholesterol, LDL-Cholesterol, and HDL-Cholesterol Values

| | Total Plasma Cholesterol | LDL-Cholesterol | HDL-Cholesterol | Conversion Factor (C to SI) |
|---|---|---|---|---|
| Desirable | <5.20 mmol/L (<200 mg/dL) | <3.36 mmol/L (<130 mg/dL) | >1.55 mmol/L (>60 mg/dL) | 0.02586 |
| Borderline | 5.20–6.18 mmol/L (200–239 mg/dL) | 3.36–4.11 mmol/L (130–159 mg/dL) | 0.9–1.55 mmol/L (35–60 mg/dL) | 0.02586 |
| Undesirable | ≥6.21 mmol/L (≥240 mg/dL) | ≥4.14 mmol/L (≥ 160 mg/dL) | <0.9 mmol/L (<35 mg/dL) | 0.02586 |

SOURCE: Modified from the report of the Expert Panel on Detection, Evaluation, and Treatment of High Blood Cholesterol in Adults: Second Report of the National Cholesterol Education Program (NCEP) expert panel on detection, evaluation, and treatment of high blood cholesterol (Adult Treatment Panel II). Circulation 89:1329, 1994.

Table A-5

### Normal Values of Doppler Echocardiographic Measurements in Adults

| | Range | Mean |
|---|---|---|
| RVD (cm) | 0.9 to 2.6 | 1.7 |
| LVID (cm) | 3.5 to 5.7 | 4.7 |
| Posterior LV wall thickness (cm) | 0.6 to 1.1 | 0.9 |
| IVS wall thickness (cm) | 0.6 to 1.1 | 0.9 |
| Left atrial dimension (cm) | 1.9 to 4.0 | 2.9 |
| Aortic root dimension (cm) | 2.0 to 3.7 | 2.7 |
| Aortic cusps separation (cm) | 1.5 to 2.6 | 1.9 |
| Percentage of fractional shortening | 34 to 44% | 36% |
| Mitral flow (m/sec) | 0.6 to 1.3 | 0.9 |
| Tricuspid flow (m/sec) | 0.3 to 0.7 | 0.5 |
| Pulmonary artery (m/sec) | 0.6 to 0.9 | 0.75 |
| Aorta (m/sec) | 1.0 to 1.7 | 1.35 |

NOTE: RVD, right ventricular dimension; LVID, left ventricular internal dimension; LV, left ventricle; IVS, interventricular septum.
SOURCE: From H Feigenbaum, *Echocardiography*, 5th ed, Philadelphia. Lea & Febiger, 1994

Table A-6

## Differential Nucleated Cell Counts of Bone Marrow

| | Normal, Mean%* | Range, %† | | Normal, Mean%* | Range, %† |
|---|---|---|---|---|---|
| Myeloid | 56.7 | | Erythroid | 25.6 | |
| Neutrophilic series | 53.6 | | Pronormoblasts | 0.6 | 0.2–1.3 |
| Myeloblast | 0.9 | 0.2–1.5 | Basophilic normoblasts | 1.4 | 0.5–2.4 |
| Promyelocyte | 3.3 | 2.1–4.1 | Polychromatophilic normoblasts | 21.6 | 17.9–29.2 |
| Myelocyte | 12.7 | 8.2–15.7 | | | |
| Metamyelocyte | 15.9 | 9.6–24.6 | Orthochromatic normoblasts | 2.0 | 0.4–4.6 |
| Band | 12.4 | 9.5–15.3 | Megakaryocytes | <0.1 | |
| Segmented | | | Lymphoreticular | 17.8 | |
| Eosinophilic series | 3.1 | 1.2–5.3 | Lymphocytes | 16.2 | 11.1–23.2 |
| Basophilic series | <0.1 | 0–0.2 | Plasma cells | 2.3 | 0.4–3.9 |
| | | | Reticulum cells | 0.3 | 0–0.9 |

* From MM Wintrobe et al, *Clinical Hematology*, 8th ed. Philadelphia, Lea & Febiger, 1981.
† Range observed in 12 healthy men.

Table A-7

## Erythrocytes and Hemoglobin: Normal Values at Various Ages

| Age | Red Blood Cell Count,* 10¹²/L | Hemoglobin,* g/L (g/dL) | Vol. Packed RBCs,* mL/dL | MCV, fL | MCH, pg | MCHC, g/L (g/dL) | MCD, µm |
|---|---|---|---|---|---|---|---|
| Days 1–13 | 5.1 ± 1.0 | 195 ± 50 (19.5 ± 5) | 54.0 ± 10.0 | 106–98 | 38–33 | 340–360 (36–34) | 8.6 |
| Days 14–60 | 4.7 ± 0.9 | 140 ± 33 (14 ± 3.3) | 42.0 ± 7.0 | 90 | 30 | 330 (33) | 8.1 |
| 3 months to 10 years | 4.5 ± 0.7 | 122 ± 23 (12.2 ± 2.3) | 36.0 ± 5.0 | 80 | 27 | 340 (34) | 7.7 |
| 11–15 years | 4.8 | 131 (13.14) | 39.0 | 82 | 28 | 340 (34) | |
| Adults: | | | | | | | |
| Females | 4.8 ± 0.6 | 140 ± 20 (14 ± 2) | 42.0 ± 5.0 | 90 ± 7 | 29 ± 2 | 340 ± 20 (34 ± 2) | 7.5 ± 0.3 |
| Males | 5.4 ± 0.9 | 160 ± 20 (16 ± 2) | 47.0 ± 5.0 | 90 ± 7 | 29 ± 2 | 340 ± 20 (34 ± 2) | 7.5 ± 0.3 |

* The range of values represents almost the extremes of observed variations (93 percent or more) at sea level. The blood values of healthy persons should fall well within these mean ± SD figures.
NOTE: MCV, mean corpuscular volume; MCH, mean corpuscular hemoglobin; MCHC, mean corpuscular hemoglobin concentration; MCD, mean corpuscular diameter.
SOURCE: MM Wintrobe et al, *Clinical Hematology*, 8th ed, Philadelphia, Lea & Febiger, 1981.

Table A-8

Normal Leukocyte Count, Differential Count, and Hemoglobin Concentration at Various Ages

| Age | Leukocytes, Total | Neutrophils | | | Eosinophils | Basophils | Lymphocytes | Monocytes |
| | | Total | Band | Segmented | | | | |
|---|---|---|---|---|---|---|---|---|
| 12 mo | 11.4(6.0–17.5) | 3.5(1.5–8.5) *31* | 0.35 *3.1* | 3.2 *28* | 0.3(0.05–0.7) *0.4* | 0.05(0–0.20) *0.4* | 7.0(4.0–10.5) *61* | 0.55(0.05–1.1) *4.8* |
| 4 yr | 9.1(5.5–15.5) | 3.8(1.5–8.5) *42* | 0.27(0–1.0) *3.0* | 3.5(1.5–7.5) *39* | 0.25(0.02–0.65) *2.8* | 0.05(0–0.20) *0.6* | 4.5(2.0–8.0) *50* | 0.45(0–0.8) *5.0* |
| 6 yr | 4.3(1.5–8.0) | 0.25(0–1.0) *51* | 4.0(1.5–7.0) *3.0* | 4.0(1.5–7.0) *48* | 0.23(0–0.65) *2.7* | 0.05(0–0.20) *0.6* | 3.5(1.5–7.0) *42* | 0.40(0–0.8) *4.7* |
| 10 yr | 8.1(4.5–13.5) | 4.4(1.8–8.0) *54* | 0.24(0–1.0) *3.0* | 4.2(1.8–7.0) *51* | 0.20(0–0.60) *2.4* | 0.04(0–0.20) *0.5* | 3.1(1.5–6.5) *38* | 0.35(0–0.8) *4.3* |
| 21 yr | 7.4(4.5–11.0) | 4.4(1.8–7.7) *59* | 0.22(0–0.7) *3.0* | 4.2(1.8–7.0) *56* | 0.20(0–0.45) *2.7* | 0.04(0–0.20) *0.5* | 2.5(1.0–4.8) *34* | 0.30(0–0.8) *4.0* |

NOTE: Values are expressed as "cells $\times 10^9$/L." The numbers in italic are percentages.

SOURCE: E Beutler et al (eds), *Williams Hematology*, 5th ed, New York, McGraw-Hill, 1995. By permission.

Table A-9

Summary of Values Useful in Pulmonary Physiology

| | Symbol | Typical Values | |
| | | Man Aged 40, 75 kg, 175 cm Tall | Woman Aged 40, 60 kg, 160 cm Tall |
|---|---|---|---|
| **PULMONARY MECHANICS** | | | |
| Spirometry—volume-time curves: | | | |
| Forced vital capacity | FVC | 4.8 L | 3.3 L |
| Forced expiratory volume in 1 s | $FEV_1$ | 3.8 L | 2.8 L |
| $FEV_1/FVC$ | $FEV_1$% | 76% | 77% |
| Maximal midexpiratory flow | MMF (FEF 25–27) | 4.8 L/s | 3.6 L/s |
| Maximal expiratory flow rate | MEFR (FEF 200–1200) | 9.4 L/s | 6.1 L/s |
| Spirometry—flow-volume curves: | | | |
| Maximal expiratory flow at 50% of expired vital capacity | $V_{max}$ 50 (FEF 50%) | 6.1 L/s | 4.6 L/s |
| Maximal expiratory flow at 75% of expired vital capacity | $V_{max}$ 75 (FEF 75%) | 3.1 L/s | 2.5 L/s |
| Resistance to airflow: | | | |
| Pulmonary resistance | RL ($R_L$) | <3.0 (cmH$_2$O/s)/L | |
| Airway resistance | Raw | <2.5 (cmH$_2$O/s)/L | |
| Specific conductance | SGaw | >0.13 cmH$_2$O/s | |
| Pulmonary compliance: | | | |
| Static recoil pressure at total lung capacity | Pst TLC | 25 ± 5 cmH$_2$O | |
| Compliance of lungs (static) | CL | 0.2 L cmH$_2$O | |
| Compliance of lungs and thorax | C(L + T) | 0.1 L cmH$_2$O | |
| Dynamic compliance of 20 breaths per minute | C dyn 20 | 0.25 ± 0.05 L/cmH$_2$O | |
| Maximal static respiratory pressures: | | | |
| Maximal inspiratory pressure | MIP | >90 cmH$_2$O | >50 cmH$_2$O |
| Maximal expiratory pressure | MEP | >150 cmH$_2$O | >120 cmH$_2$O |
| **LUNG VOLUMES** | | | |
| Total lung capacity | TLC | 6.4 L | 4.9 L |
| Functional residual capacity | FRC | 2.2 L | 2.6 L |
| Residual volume | RV | 1.5 L | 1.2 L |
| Inspiratory capacity | IC | 4.8 L | 3.7 L |
| Expiratory reserve volume | ERV | 3.2 L | 2.3 L |
| Vital capacity | VC | 1.7 L | 1.4 L |
| **GAS EXCHANGE (SEA LEVEL)** | | | |
| Arterial O$_2$ tension | Pa$_{O_2}$ | 12.7 ± 0.7 kPa (95 ± 5 mmHg) | |
| Arterial CO$_2$ tension | Pa$_{CO_2}$ | 5.3 ± 0.3 kPa (40 ± 2 mmHg) | |
| Arterial O$_2$ saturation | Sa$_{O_2}$ | 0.97 ± 0.02 (97 ± 2%) | |
| Arterial blood pH | pH | 7.40 ± 0.02 | |
| Arterial bicarbonate | HCO$_3^-$ | 24 + 2 meq/L | |
| Base excess | BE | 0 ± 2 meq/L | |
| Diffusing capacity for carbon monoxide (single breath) | DL$_{CO}$ | 0.42 mLCO/s/mmHg (25 mL CO/min/mmHg) | |
| Dead space volume | V$_D$ | 2 ml/kg body wt | |
| Physiologic dead space; dead space-tidal volume ratio | V$_D$/V$_T$ | | |
| Rest | | ≤35% V$_T$ | |
| Exercise | | ≤20% V$_T$ | |
| Alveolar-arterial difference for O$_2$ | P(A – a)$_{O_2}$ | ≤2.7 kPa ≤20 kPa (≤20 mmHg) | |

# BIBLIOGRAPHY

# BIBLIOGRAPHY

Aaltonen LA, Peltomaki P, Leach FS, et al: Clues to the pathogenesis of familial colorectal cancer. *Science* 260:812–816, 1993.

Adelman RR, Warachs S: Magnetic resonance imaging. *N Engl J Med* 328:708–716, 1993.

Agarwal N, Pitchumoni CS: Assessment of severity in acute pancreatitis. *Am J Gastroenterol* 86:1385–1391, 1991.

Allen JN, Pacht ER, Gadek JE, et al: Acute eosinophilic pneumonia as a reversible cause of non-infectious respiratory failure. *N Engl J Med* 321:569–574, 1989.

American Society of Clinical Oncology recommendations for the use of hematopoietic colony-stimulating factors: Evidence-based, clinical practice guidelines. *J Clin Oncol* 12:2471–2508, 1994.

American Thoracic Society and Centers for Disease Control: Treatment of tuberculosis and tuberculosis infection in adults and children. *Am J Respir Crit Care Med* 149:1359, 1994.

Anderson HV, Willerson JT: Thrombolysis in acute myocardial infarction. *N Engl J Med* 329:703–709, 1993.

Andriole GL: Serum prostate-specific antigen: The most useful tumor marker. *J Clin Oncol* 10:1205–1207, 1992.

Antonucci G, Girardi E, Raviglione MC, et al: Risk factors for tuberculosis in HIV-infected persons. A prospective cohort study. The Gruppo Italiano di Studio Tuburcolosi e AIDS (GISTA). *JAMA* 274:143–148, 1995.

Armitage JO: Drug therapy. Treatment of non-Hodgkin's lymphoma. *N Engl J Med* 328:1023–1030, 1993.

Attal M, Harousseau J-L, Stoppa A-M, et al: A prospective, randomized trial of autologous bone marrow transplantation and chemotherapy in multiple myeloma. *N Engl J Med* 335:91, 1996.

Baer GM, Fishbein DB: Rabies post–exposure prophylaxis: *N Engl J Med* 316:1270–1271, 1987.

Baim DS, Grossman W (eds) *Cardiac Catheterization, Angiography and Intervention*, 5th ed Williams and Wilkins, 1996.

Baker DG, Schumacher HR: Acute monoarthritis. *N Engl J Med* 329:1013–1020, 1993.

Balow JE, Austin HA, Tsokos GC, et al: Lupus nephritis. *Ann Intern Med* 106:79–94, 1987.

Barlogie B, Epstein J, Selvanayagam P, et al: Plasma cell myeloma: New biological insights and advances in therapy. *Blood* 73:865–879, 1989.

Barnes PF, Bloch AB, Davidson PT, et al: Tuberculosis in patients with human immunodeficiency virus infection. *N Engl J Med* 324:1644–1650, 1991.

Barnes PF, DeCock KM, Reynolds TN, et al: A comparison of amoebic and pyogenic abscess of the liver. *Medicine* 66:472–483, 1987.

Benedetti J, Corey L, Ashley R: Recurrance rates in genital herpes after symptomatic first-episode infections. *Ann Intern Med* 121:847–854, 1994.

Bennet WM, Debroe ME: Analgesic nephropathy. A preventable renal disease. *N Engl J Med* 320:1269–1271, 1989.

Berkmann N, Kramer MR: Diagnostic tests in pleural effusion: An update. *Postgrad Med J* 69:12–18, 1993.

Beutler E: Gaucher's disease. *N Engl J Med* 325:1354–1360, 1991.

Beutler E: Glucose 6-phosphate dehydrogenase deficiency. *N Engl J Med* 324:169–174, 1991.

Bick RL, Strauss JF, Frankel EP: Thrombosis and hemorrage in oncology patients. *Hematol Oncol Clin North Am* 10:875–907, 1996.

Bishop JM: The molecular genetics of cancer. *Science* 235:305–311, 1987.

Black P McL: Brain tumors. *N Engl J Med* 324:1555–1564, 1991.

Black RE: Epidemiology of traveler's diarrhea and relative importance of various pathogens. *Rev Infect Dis* 12(suppl 1):S73–S79, 1990.

Bochner BS, Lichtenstein LM: Anaphylaxis. *N Engl J Med* 324:1785–1790, 1991.

Bone RC, Balk R, Slotman G, et al: Adult respiratory distress syndrome: Stage and importance of development in multiple organ failure. *Chest* 101:320–326, 1992.

Bothwell TH, Charlton RW: A general approach to the problems of iron deficiency and iron overload in the population at large. *Semin Hematol* 19:54–69, 1982.

Bravo EL, Gifford RW: Pheochromocytoma: Diagnosis, localization and management. *N Engl J Med* 311:1298–1303, 1984.

Brooks PM, Day RO: Non-steroidal anti-inflammatory drugs: Differences and similarities. *N Engl J Med* 324:1716–1725, 1991.

Brown MS, Goldstein JL: A receptor-mediated pathway for cholesterol homeostasis. *Science* 232:34–47, 1986.

Buckley RH, Schiff RI: The use of intravenous immune globulin in immunodeficiency diseases. *N Engl J Med* 325:110–117, 1991.

Burtis WJ, Brady TG, Orloff JJ, et al: Immunochemical characterization of circulating parathyroid hormone-related protein in patients with humoral hypercalcemia of cancer. *N Engl J Med* 322:1106–1112, 1990.

Calhoun DA, Oparil S: Treatment of hypertensive crisis. *N Engl J Med* 323:1177–1183, 1991.

Callahan N, Garrett A, Goggin T: Withdrawal of anticonvulsant drugs in patients free of seizures for two years: A prospective study. *N Engl J Med* 318:942–946, 1988.

Carlos TM, Harlan JM: Leukocyte-endothelial adhesion molecules. *Blood* 84:2068–2101, 1994.

Caroff SN, Mann SC: Neuroleptic malignant syndrome. *Med Clin North Am* 77:185–202, 1993.

Carpenter CC, Fischl MA, Hammer SM. Antiretroviral therapy for HIV infection in 1996 recommendations of an international panel. *JAMA* 276:146–154, 1996.

Centers for Disease Control: Policy guidelines in the prevention and management of pelvic inflammatory disease. *MMWR* 4022–4025, 1992.

Centers for Disease Control: Prevention and control of influenza. *MMWR* 40:1–2, 1991.

Chandrasekharappa SC, Guru SC, Manicham P, et al: Positional cloning of the gene for multiple endocrine neoplasia type 1. *Science* 276:404–406, 1997.

Charness ME, Simon RP, Greenberg DA, et al: Ethanol and the nervous system. *N Engl J Med* 321:442–454, 1989.

Cherubin CE, Eng RH: Quinolones for the treatment of infections due to Salmonella. *Rev Infect Dis* 13:343–344, 1991.

Chu KC, Smart CR, Tarone RE: Analysis of breast cancer mortality and stage distribution by age for the Health Insurance Plan clinical trial. *J Natl Cancer Inst* 80:1125–1132, 1988.

Coe FL, Parks JH, Asplin JR: The pathogenesis and treatment of kidney stones. *N Engl J Med* 327:1141–1152, 1992.

Cohn JN, Levine TB, Olvari MT, et al: Plasma norepinephrine as a guide to prognosis in patients with chronic congestive heart failure. *N Engl J Med* 311:819–823, 1984.

Collins FS: BRCA1—lots of mutations, lots of dilemmas. *N Engl J Med* 334:186–188, 1996

Collins FS: Cystic fibrosis: Molecular biology and therapeutic implications. *Science* 256:774–779, 1992.

Consensus Development Conference Panel: Diagnosis and management of asymptomatic primary hyperparathyroidism: Consensus Development Conference Statement. *Ann Intern Med* 114:593–597, 1991.

Coustan DR: Pregnancy in diabetic women. *N Engl J Med* 319:1663–1665, 1988.

Craven DE, Steger KA: Epidemiology of nosocomial pneumonia. New perspectives of an old disease. *Chest* 108:1s–16s, 1995.

Crawford ED, Eisenberger MA, McLeod DG, et al: A controlled trial of leuprolide with and without flutamide in prostatic carcinoma. *N Engl J Med* 321:419–424, 1989.

Crook JE, Moertel CG, Gunderson LL, et al: Effective surgical adjuvant therapy for high-risk rectal carcinoma. *N Engl J Med* 324:709–715, 1991.

Crossley IR, Williams R: Spontaneous bacterial peritonitis. *Gut* 26:325–331, 1985.

Dalakas MC: Polymyositis dermatomyositis and inclusion body myositis. *N Engl J Med* 325:1487–1498, 1991.

Daniels GH et al: Thyroid disease and pregancy: a clinical overview. *Endocrine Pract* 1:287, 1995.

DeFronzo RA, Goodman AM, and the multicenter Metformin Study Group: Efficacy of melformin in patients with Non-insulin-dependent diabetes mellitus. *N Engl J Med* 333:541–549, 1995.

Degos L, Dombret H, Chomienne C, et al: All-*trans* retinoic acid as a differentiating agent in the treatment of acute promyelocytic leukemia. *Blood* 85:2643–2653, 1995.

Department of Veterans' Affairs Laryngeal Cancer Study: Induction chemotherapy plus radiation compared with surgery plus radiation in patients with advanced laryngeal cancer. *N Engl J Med* 324:1685, 1991.

The Diabetes Control and Complications Trial Research Group: The effect of intensive treatment of diabetes on the development and progression of long-term complications in insulin-dependent diabetes mellitus. *N Engl J Med* 329:977–986, 1993.

Dinarello CA, Cannon JG, Wolff SM: New concepts on the pathogenesis of fever. *Rev Infect Dis* 10:168–189, 1988.

Domasio AR: Aphasia. *N Engl J Med* 326:531–539, 1992.

Donowitz M, Koffe FT, Saidi R: Evaluation of patients with chronic diarrhea. *N Engl J Med* 322:725–729, 1995.

Drew WL: Diagnosis of cytomegalovirus infection. *Rev Infect Dis* 10:S468–S476, 1988.

Dufont HL, Chappell CL, Sterling CR, et al: The infectivity of *Cryptosporidium parvum* in healthy volunteers. *N Engl J Med* 332:855–859, 1995.

Dupont HL, Ericsson CD: Prevention and treatment of traveler's diarrhea. *N Engl J Med* 328:1821–1827, 1993.

Early Breast Cancer Trialists' Collaborative Group: Systemic treatment of early breast cancer by hormonal, cytotoxic, or immune therapy: 133 randomized trials involving 31,000 recurrences and 24,000 deaths among 75,000 women. *Lancet* 339:71–85, 1992.

Ellerbroek N, Holmes F, Singletary E, et al: Treatment of patients with isolated axillary nodal metastases from an occult primary carconoma consistent with breast origin. *Cancer* 66:1461–1467, 1990.

Emmanuel D, Cunningham I, Jules-Elysee K, et al: Cytomegalovirus pneumonia after bone marrow transplantation successfully treated with the combination of ganciclovir and high-dose intravenous immune globulin. *Ann Intern Med* 109: 777–782, 1988.

Ernst CB: Abdominal aortic aneurysm. *N Engl J Med* 328:1167–1172, 1993.

Eschbach JW, Abdulhadi MH, Browne JK, et al: Recombinant erythropoietin in anemic patients with endstage renal disease. *Ann Intern Med* 111: 992–1000, 1989.

Estey EH, Kurzrock R, Kantarjian HM, et al: Treatment of hairy cell leukemia with 2-chlorodeoxyadenosine (2-CdA). *Blood* 79:882–887, 1992.

Fang G-D, Fine M, Orloff J, et al: New and emerging etiologies for community acquired pneumonia with implications for therapy. *Medicine* 69:307–316, 1992.

Farley MM, Stephens DS, Brachman PS Jr, et al: Invasive *Haemophilus influenzae* disease in adults. *Ann Intern Med* 116:806–812, 1992.

Feinstein DI: Lupus anticoagulant, anticardiolipin, antibodies, fetal loss, and systemic lupus erythematosus. *Blood* 80:859–862, 1992.

Fendrick AM, Chernew ME, Hirth RA, et al: Alternative management strategies for patients with suspected peptic ulcer disease. *Ann Intern Med* 123:260–269, 1995.

Field M, Rao MC, Chang EB: Intestinal electrolyte transport and diarrheal disease. *N Engl J Med* 321:879–883, 1989.

Fine H, Mayer RJ: Primary central nervous system lymphoma. *Ann Intern Med* 119:1093–1104, 1993.

Fishbein DB, Robinson LE: Rabies. *N Engl J Med* 329:1632–1638, 1993.

Fisher B, Redmond C, Poisson R, et al: Eight-year results of a randomized clinical trial comparing total mastectomy and lumpectomy with or without irradiation in the treatment of breast cancer. *N Engl J Med* 320:822–828, 1989.

Fisher CM: Lacunar strokes and infarcts: A review. *Neurology* 32:871–876, 1982.

Fitzpatrick TB, Johnson RA, Wolff K, et al: *Color Atlas and Synopsis of Clinical Dermatology*, 3d ed. New York, McGraw-Hill, 1997.

Flier JS: Syndromes of insulin resistance: From patient to gene and back again. *Diabetes* 41:1207–1219, 1992.

Fowler NO: Tuberculous pericarditis. *JAMA* 266:99–103, 1991.

Frank BB: Clinical evaluation of jaundice: A guideline of the patient care committee of the American Gastroenterological Association. *JAMA* 262: 3031–3034, 1989.

Frank MM: Complement in the pathophysiology of human disease. *N Engl J Med* 316:1525–1530, 1987.

Friedland IR, McGracken GH Jr: Management of infections caused by antibiotic-resistant Streptococcus pneuomia. *N Engl J Med* 331:377–382, 1994.

Froehling DA, Silverstein MD, Mohr DN, et al: Does this dizzy patient have a serious form of vertigo? *JAMA* 271:385–388, 1994.

Fujita S: Obstructive sleep apnea syndrome: Pathophysiology, upper-airway evaluation, and surgical treatment. *Ear Nose Throat J* 72:67–72, 75–76, 1993.

Fuster V, Badimon L, Badimon JJ, Chesebro JH: Mechanisms of disease: Pathophysiology of coronary artery disease and the acute coronary syndromes. *N Engl J Med* 326:242–250, 310–318, 1992.

Gil-Grande LA, Rodriguez-Caabeiro F, et al. Randomized controlled trial of efficacy of albendazole in intra-abdominal hydatid disease. *Lancet* 324:1269–1272, 1993.

Gilman S: Advances in neurology, part II. *N Engl J Med* 326:1671–1676, 1992.

Goodgame RW: Gastrointestinal cytomegalovirus disease. *Ann Intern Med* 119:924–935, 1993.

Graham DY, Lew GM, Klein PD, et al: Effect of treatment of *Helicobacter pylori* infection on the long-term recurrence of gastric or duodenal ulcers. *Ann Intern Med* 116:705–708, 1992.

Greenberger PA, Patterson R: Allergic bronchopulmonary aspergillosis. Model of bronchopulmonary disease with defined serologic, radiologic, pathologic and clinical findings from asthma to fatal destructive lung diseases. *Chest* 91:165S–171S, 1987.

Groop L. Sulfonyureas in NIDDM. *Diabetes Care* 15:737–747, 1992.

Grossman W: Diastolic dysfunction in congestive heart failure. *N Engl J Med* 325:1557–1564, 1991.

Grunberg SM, Hesketh PJ: Control of chemotherapy-induced emesis. *N Engl J Med* 329:1790–1796, 1993.

Grunberger G, Weiner JL, Silverman R, et al: Factitious hypoglycemia due to surreptitious administration of insulin: Diagnosis, treatment, and long-term follow-up. *Ann Intern Med* 108:252–257, 1988.

Haber DA, Mayer RJ: Primary gastrointestinal lymphoma. *Semin Oncol* 15:154–169, 1988.

Hainsworth JD, Greco FA: Treatment of patients with cancer of an unknown primary site. *N Engl J Med* 329:257–263, 1993.

Harris JR, Lippman ME, Veronesi U, et al: Breast cancer. *N Engl J Med* 327:319–328, 390–398, 473–480, 1992.

Harris NL, Jaffe ES, Stein H, et al: A revised European-American classification of lymphoid neoplasms: a proposal from the International Lymphoma Study Group. *Blood* 84:1361–1392, 1995.

Harrison LC, Campbell IL, Allison J, et al: MHC molecules and beta-cell destruction. Immune and non-immune disorders. *Diabetes* 38:815–818, 1989.

Havel RJ: Lowering cholesterol, 1988. Rationale, mechanism, and means. *J Clin Invest* 81:1653–1660, 1988.

Hayakawa H, Sato A, Toyoshima M, et al: A clincal study of idiopathic eosinophilic pneumonia. *Chest* 105:1462–1466, 1992.

Heyman MR, Schiffer CA: Platelet transfusion therapy for the cancer patient. *Semin Oncol* 17:198–209, 1990.

Hinson JR, Marini JF: Principles of mechanical ventilation in respiratory failure. *Annu Rev Med* 43: 341–361, 1992.

Hollsberg P, Hafler DA: Seminars in medicine of the Beth Israel Hospital, Boston. Pathogenesis of diseases induced by human lymphotropic virus type 1 infection. *N Engl J Med* 328:1173–1182, 1993.

Hoofnagle JH: Type D (delta): hepatitis. *JAMA* 261: 1321–1325, 1989.

Hook EW, Marra CM: Acquired syphilis in adults. *N Engl J Med* 326:1060–1069, 1992.

Hooper DC, Wolfson JS: Fluoroquinolone antimicrobial agents. *N Engl J Med* 324:384–394, 1991.

Horning SJ, Carrier EK, Rouse RV, et al: Lymphomas presenting as histologically unclassified neoplasms: Characteristics and response to treatment. *J Clin Oncol* 7:1281–1287, 1989.

Hunninghake GW, Kalica AR: Approaches to the treatment of pulmonary fibrosis. *Am J Respir Crit Care Med* 151:915–918, 1995.

Isselbacher KJ, Braunwald E, Wilson JD, Martin JB, Fauci AS, Kasper DL (eds): *Harrison's Principles of Internal Medicine*, 13th ed. New York, McGraw-Hill, 1994.

Jarcho JA, McKenna W, Pare JAP, et al: Mapping a gene for familial hypertrophic cardiomyopathy to chromosome 14q1. *N Engl J Med* 321:1372–1378, 1989.

Jensen RT, Fraken DL: Zollinger-Ellison syndrome. Advances in treatment of gastric hypersecretion and the gastrinoma. *JAMA* 271:1429–1435, 1994.

Johnston GD, Kaplan MM: Pathogenesis and treatment of gallstones. *N Engl J Med* 328:412–421, 1993.

Kaye BR: Rheumatologic manifestations of infection with human immunodeficiency virus (HIV). *Ann Intern Med* 11:158–167, 1989.

Kaye D, Abrutyn E: Prevention of bacterial endocarditis 1991. *Ann Intern Med* 114:803–804, 1991.

Kazazian HH Jr: The thalassemia syndromes: Molecular basis and prenatal diagnosis in 1990. *Semin Hematol* 27:209–228, 1990.

King DJ et al, Heparin Induced Thrombocytopenia *Ann Intern Med* 8:325–332, 1980.

Kinzler KW, Nilbert MC, Vogelstein B, et al: Identification of a gene located at chromosome 5q21 that is mutated in colorectal cancers. *Science* 251:1366–1370, 1991.

Kirchoff LV: American trypanosomiasis (Chagas' disease): A tropical disease now in the United States. *N Engl J Med* 329:639–644, 1993.

Kirkwood JM, Strawderman MH, Ernstoff MS, et al: Interferon-alpha-2b adjuvant therapy of high risk resected cutaneous melanoma: the Eastern Cooperative Oncology Group Trial Est 1684. *J Clin Oncol* 14:7–17, 1996.

Klingenberg-Knoll EC, Festen HP, Jansen JB, et al: Long-term treatment with omeprazole for refractory reflux esophagitis: efficacy and safety. *Ann Intern Med* 121:161–167, 1994.

Koenig M, Hoffman EP, Bertelson CJ, et al: Complete cloning of the Duchenne muscular dystrophy (DMD) cDNA and preliminary genomic organization of the DMD gene in normal and affected individuals. *Cell* 50:509–517, 1987.

Koh HK: Cutaneous melanoma. *N Engl J Med* 325: 171–182, 1991.

Kollef MH, Schuster DP: The acute respiratory distress syndrome. *N Engl J Med* 332:27–31, 1995.

Krawitt EL: Autoimmune hepatitis. *N Engl J Med* 334:897–903, 1996.

Kuntz RE, Tosteson AN, Berman AD, et al: Predictors of event-free survival after balloon aortic valvuloplasty. *N Engl J Med* 325:17–23, 1991.

Kupin WL, Narins RG: The hyperkalemia of renal failure: Pathophysiology, diagnosis, and therapy. *Contrib Nephrol* 102:1–22, 1993.

Laderson PW, Levin AA, Ridgway EC, et al: Complication of surgery in hyperthyroid patients. *Am J Med* 77:261–266, 1984.

Lawly TJ, Bielory L, Gascon P, et al: A prospective clinical and immunologic analysis of patients with serum sickness. *N Engl J Med* 311:1407–1413, 1984.

Lee WM: Drug-induced hepatotoxicity. *N Engl J Med* 333:1118–1127, 1995.

Lengerich EJ, Addiss DG, Juranek DD: Severe giardiasis in the United States. *Clin Infect Dis* 18:760, 1993.

Levy MH: Pharmacologic treatment of cancer pain. *N Engl J Med* 335:1124–1132, 1996.

Liberman UA, Weiss SR, Minne HW, et al. Effect of oral alendronate on bone mineral density and the incidence of fractures in postmenopausal osteoporosis. *N Engl J Med* 333:1437–1443, 1995.

Luzzatto G, Schafer AI: The prethrombotic state in cancer. *Semin Oncol* 17:147–159, 1990.

Lynn RB, Friedman LS: Irritable bowel syndrome. *N Engl J Med* 329:1940–1945, 1993.

Lynn RB, Friedman LS: Irritable bowel syndrome. Managing the patient with abdominal pain and altered bowel habits. *Med Clin North Am* 79:373–390, 1995.

Lynn WA, Cohen J: Adjunctive therapy for septic shock: a review of experimental approaches. *Clin Infect Dis* 20:143–158, 1995.

Mandel JS, Bond JH, Church TR, et al: Minnesota Colon Cancer Control Study: Reducing mortality from colorectal cancer by screening for fecal occult blood. *N Engl J Med* 328:1365–1371, 1993.

Mannheimer SB, Soave R: Protozoal infections in patients with AIDS. Cryptosporidiosis, isosporiasis, cyclosporiasis, and microsporidiosis. *Infect Dis Clin North Am* 8:483–498, 1994.

Marks AR, Choong CY, Sanfilippo AJ, et al: Identification of high-risk and low-risk subgroups of patients with a mitral valve prolapse. *N Engl J Med* 320:1031–1036, 1989.

Martin JB, Gusella JF: Huntington's disease: Pathogenesis and management. *N Engl J Med* 315: 1267–1276, 1986.

McAlister HF, Klementowicz PT, Andrews C, et al: Lyme carditis: an important cause of reversible heart block. *Ann Intern Med* 110:339–345, 1989.

McCarthy DM: Sucralfate. *N Engl J Med* 325:1017–1025, 1991.

McFadden ER Jr, Gilbert IA: Asthma. *N Engl J Med* 327:1928–1937, 1993.

McFadden ER Jr, Elsanadi N, Dixon L, et al: Protocol therapy for acute asthma: therapeutic benefits and cost savings. *Am J Med* 99:651–661, 1995.

Michels R, Marzuk PM: Progress in psychiatry. *N Engl J Med* 329:552–560, 628–638, 1993.

Mitchelson F: Pharmacologic agents affecting emesis: A review (part 1). *Drugs* 43:443–463, 1992.

Modell JH: Drowning. *N Engl J Med* 328:253–256, 1993.

Moreno S, Baraia-Etxabura J, Bouza E, et al: Risk for developing tuberculosis among anergic patients infected with HIV. *Ann Intern Med* 119:194–198, 1993.

Naclerio RM: Allergic rhinitis. *N Engl J Med* 325:860–869, 1991.

Narins RG, Jones ER, Stom MC, et al: Diagnostic strategies in disorders of fluid, electrolyte, and acid-base homeostasis. *Am J Med* 72:496–520, 1982.

Nathan DM: Long-term complications of diabetes mellitus. *N Engl J Med* 328:1676–1685, 1993.

National Institutes of Health–University of California Expert Panel for Corticosteroids as Adjunctive Therapy for Pneumocystis Pneumonia: Consensus statement on the use of corticosteroids as adjunctive therapy for Pneumocystis pneumonia in AIDS. *N Engl J Med* 323:1500–1504, 1990.

Neu HC: Ciprofloxacin: A major advance in quinolone chemotherapy. *Am J Med* 82(4A):1–2, 1987.

Niederau C, Heintges T, Lange S, et al: Long-term follow-up of HBeAg-positive patients treated with interferon alfa for chronic hepatitis B. *N Engl J Med* 334:1422, 1996.

Nienaber CA, von Kodolitsch Y, Nicolas V, et al: The prognosis of thoracic aortic dissection by noninvasive imaging procedures. *N Engl J Med* 328:1–9, 1993.

Oates JA, Wood AJJ: Adenosine and superventricular tachycardia. *N Engl J Med* 325:1621–1629, 1991.

Ochs A, Rössle M, Haag K, et al: The transjugular intrahepatic portosystemic stent-shunt procedure for refractory ascites. *N Engl J Med* 332:1192, 1995.

Okuda H: Hepatocellular carcinoma: Recent progress. *Hepatology* 15:948–963, 1992.

Oldfield EH, et al: Petronal sinus sampling with and without corticotropin-releasing hormone for the differential diagnosis of Cushings syndrome. *N Engl J Med* 325:897, 1991.

Oswald-Mammosser M, Weitzenblum E, Quoix E, et al: Prognostic factors in COPD patients receiving long-term oxygen therapy. Importance of pulmonary artery pressure. *Chest* 107:1193–1198, 1995.

Pape, JW, Jean SS, Ho JL, et al: Effect of isoniazid prophylaxis on incidence of active tuberculosis and progression of HIV infection. *Lancet* 342:268, 1993.

Peppercorn MA: Advances in drug therapy for inflammatory bowel disease. *Ann Intern Med* 112:50–60, 1990.

Perrillo RP, Schiff ER, Davis GL, et al: A randomized controlled trial of interferon, alpha-2b alone and after steroid withdrawal for treatment of chronic hepatitis B. *N Engl J Med* 323:295–301, 1990.

Pizzo PA: Management of fever in patients with cancer and treatment-induced neutropenia. *N Engl J Med* 328:1323–1332, 1993.

Podolsky DL: Inflammatory bowel disease. *N Engl J Med* 325:928–937, 1008–1016, 1991.

Popp RL: Medical progress: Echocardiography (two parts). *N Engl J Med* 323:101–108, 165–172, 1990.

Posner JB: Paraneoplastic syndromes. *Neurol Clin* 9:919–936, 1991.

Poupon RE, Poupon R, Balkau B: Ursodiol for the long-term treatment of primary biliary cirrhosis. The UDCA-PBC Study Group. *N Engl J Med* 330:1342, 1994.

Prados J, Finison L, Andres PL, et al: The natural history of amyotrophic lateral sclerosis and the use of natural history controls in therapeutic trials. *Neurology* 43:751–755, 1993.

Preston DS, Stern RS: Nonmelanoma cancers of the skin. *N Engl J Med* 327:1649–1662, 1992.

Ransohoff DF, Gracie W: Assessment of prophylactic cholecystectomy and medical therapy for diabetics with silent gallstones. *Gastroenterology* 92:1588, 1987.

Ransohoff DF, Miller GL, Forsythe SB, et al: Outcome of acute cholecystitis in patients with diabetes mellitus. *Ann Intern Med* 106:829–832, 1987.

Reed SL, Wessel DW, Davis CE: *Entamoeba histolytica* infection and AIDS. *Am J Med* 90:269–271, 1991.

Reeders S: Multilocus polycystic disease. *Nat Genetics* 1:235–237, 1992.

Relman DA, Schmidt TM, MacDermott RP, Falkow S: Identification of the uncultured bacillus of Whipple's disease. *N Engl J Med* 327:293–301, 1992.

Resnick NM, Valla SV, Laurine E: The pathophysiology of urinary incontinence among institutionalized elderly persons. *N Engl J Med* 320:1–7, 1989.

Revler JB, Broudy VC, Cooney TG: Adult scurvy. *JAMA* 253:805–807, 1985.

Rich S: Primary pulmonary hypertension. *Prog Cardiovasc Dis* 31:205–238, 1988.

Ridker PM, Hennekens CH, Lindpaintner K, et al: Mutation in the gene coding for coagulation factor V and the risk of myocardial infarction, stroke, and venous thrombosis in apparently healthy men. *N Engl J Med* 332:912–917, 1995.

Rigel DS, Rivers JK, Koff AW, et al: Dysplastic nevi: Markers for increased risk from melanoma. *Cancer* 63:386–389, 1989.

Robertson MJ, Ritz J: Biology and clinical relevance of natural killer cells. *Blood* 76:2421–2438, 1990.

Rolachon A, Cordier L, Bacq Y, et al: Ciprofloxin and long-term prevention of spontaneous bacterial peritonitis: results of a prospective controlled trial. *Hepatology* 22:1171–1174, 1995.

Rosen FS, Cooper MD, Wedgewood RJP: The primary immunodeficiencies. *N Engl J Med* 311: 235–242, 300–310, 1984.

Roth BJ, Nichols CR: Testicular cancer. *Semin Oncol* 19:117–118, 1992.

Roujeau JC, Stern RS: Severe adverse cutaneous reactions to drugs. *N Engl J Med* 331:1272, 1994.

Samuel D, Muller R, Alexander G, et al: Liver transplantation in European patients with hepatic B surface antigens. *N Engl J Med* 329:1842–1847, 1993.

Saven A, Piro LD: 2-Chlorodeoxyadenosine: a newer purine analog active in the treatment of indolent lymphoid malignancies. *Ann Intern Med* 120:784–791, 1994.

Sears DA: Anemia of chronic disease. *Med Clin North Am* 76:567–579, 1992.

Shader RI, Greenblatt DJ: Use of benzodiazepines in anxiety disorders. *N Engl J Med* 328:1398–1405, 1993.

Shapiro ED, Berg AT, Austrian R, et al: The protective efficacy of polyvalent pneumococcal vaccine. *N Engl J Med* 325:1453–1460, 1991.

Shipp MA: Prognostic factors in aggressive non-Hodgkin's lymphoma: who has "high-risk" disease? *Blood* 83:1165–1173, 1994.

Silverstien FE, Graham DY, Seniors JR, et al: Misoprostol reduces serious gastrointestinal complications in patients with rheumatoid arthritis receiving non-steroidal anti-inflammatory drugs. A randomized, double-blind, placebo-controlled trial. *Ann Intern Med* 123:241–249, 1995.

Simon HB: Hyperthermia. *N Engl J Med* 329:483–487, 1993.

Slamon DJ, Godolphin W, Jones CA, et al: Studies of the HER-2/neu proto-oncogene in human breast and ovarian cancer. *Science* 244:707–712, 1989.

Sneller MC, Strober W, Isenstein E, et al: New insights into common variable immunodeficiency. *Ann Intern Med* 118:720–730, 1993.

Snilkstein MJ, Knapp GL, Kulig KW, Rumack BH: Efficacy of oral *N*-acetylcysteine in the treatment of acetaminophen overdose: Analysis of the national multi-center study. *N Engl J Med* 319:1557–1562, 1988.

SOLVD Investigators: Effect on survival in patients with induced left ventricular ejection fractions and congestive heart failure. *N Engl J Med* 325:293–302, 1991.

Spach DH, Liles WC, Campbell GL, et al: Tick-borne diseases in the United States. *N Engl J Med* 329:936–947, 1993.

Stabler SP, Allen RH, Savage DG, et al: Clinical spectrum and diagnosis of cobalamin deficiency. *Blood* 76:871–881, 1990.

Stamm WE: Catheter-associated urinary tract infections: epidemiology, pathogenesis, and prevention. *Ann Intern Med* (Suppl)3B:65s–71s, 1991.

Standaert DG, Stern MB: Update on the management of Parkinson's disease. *Med Clin North Am* 77:169–183, 1993.

Standards and guidelines for cardiopulmonary resuscitation (CPR) in emergency cardiac care (ECC). *JAMA* 255:2905–2989, 1986.

Steer ML, Waxman I, Freedman S: Chronic pancreatitis. *N Engl J Med* 332:1482–1490, 1995.

Steinberg W, Tenner S: Acute pancreatitis. *N Engl J Med* 330:1198–1210, 1994.

Stevens DA: Coccidioidomycosis. *N Engl J Med* 332:1077–1082, 1995.

Stockley RA: Alpha-1 antitrypsin and the pathogenesis of emphysema. *Lung* 165:61–77, 1987.

Stutts, Canessa CM, Olsen JC, et al: CFTR as a cAMP-dependent regulator of sodium channels. *Science* 269:847–850, 1995.

Swenerton K, Jeffrey J, Stuart G, et al: Cisplatin-cyclophosphamide versus carboplatin-cyclophosphamide in advanced ovarian cancer: A randomized phase III study of the National Cancer Institute of Canada clinical trials group. *J Clin Oncol* 10:718–726, 1992.

Talpaz M, Kantarjian H, Kurzrock R, et al: Interferon-alpha produces sustained cytogenetic response in chronic myelogenous leukemia. *Ann Intern Med* 114:532–538, 1991.

Terblanche J, Burroughs AK, Hobbs KE: Controversies in the management of bleeding esophageal varices. *N Engl J Med* 320:1469–1475, 1989.

Thaler M, Pastakia B, Shawker TH, et al: Hepatic candidiasis in cancer patients: The evolving picture of the syndrome. *Ann Intern Med* 108:88–100, 1988.

Third International Study of Infarct Survival Collaborative Group: 1515-3: A randomized comparison of streptokinase 'vs' tissue plasminogen activator 'vs' antistreplase and of aspirin plus heparin 'vs' aspirin alone among 41,299 cases of suspected myocardial infarction. *Lancet* 339:753–770, 1992.

Thompson CE, Damon LE, Ries CA, et al: Thrombotic microorganiopathies in the 1980s. Clinical Features. *Blood* 80:1890–1895, 1992.

Tompkins LS: Use of molecular methods in infectious diseases. *N Engl J Med* 327:1290–1297, 1992.

Tong MJ, el-Farra NS, Reikes AR, et al: Clinical outcomes after infusion-associated hepatitis C. *N Engl J Med* 332:1463–1466, 1995.

Trier JS: Celiac sprue. *N Engl J Med* 325:1709–1719, 1991.

Urba WJ, Longo DL: Hodgkin's disease. *N Engl J Med* 326:678–687, 1992.

Vogelstein B, Fearon ER, Hamilton SR, et al: Genetic alterations during colorectal-tumor development. *N Engl J Med* 319:525–532, 1988.

Vokes EE, Weichselbaum RR, Lippman SM, et al: Head and neck cancer. *N Engl J Med* 328:184–194, 1993.

Walker CK, Kahn JG, Washington AE, et al: Pelvic inflammatory disease: Metaanalysis of antimicrobial regimen efficacy. *J Infect Dis* 168:969–978, 1993.

Walsh JH, Peterson WL: The treatment of *Helicobacter pylori* infection in the management of peptic ulcer disease. *N Engl J Med* 338:984–991, 1995.

Walt RP: Drug-therapy: Misoprostol for the treatment of peptic ulcer and anti-inflammatory-drug-induced gastroduodenal ulceration. *N Engl J Med* 327:1575–1580, 1992.

Warrell RP Jr, DeThe H, Wang Z-Y, et al: Acute promyelocytic leukemia. *N Engl J Med* 329:177–189, 1993.

Warshaw AL, Fernandez-del Castillo C: Pancreatic carcinoma. *N Engl J Med* 326:455–465, 1992.

Wayne AS, Kevy SV, Nathan DG: Transfusion management of sickle cell disease. *Blood* 81:1109–1123, 1993.

Weinberg RA: The retinoblastoma protein and cell cycle control. *Cell* 81:323–330, 1995.

Weinberg RA: Tumor suppressor genes. *Science* 254:1138–1146, 1991.

Weinberger SE: Recent advances in pulmonary medicine. *N Engl J Med* 328:1389–1397, 1993.

Welch KMA: Drug therapy of migraine. *N Engl J Med* 329:1476–1483, 1993.

Wetzler M, Kantarjian H, Kurzrock R, et al: Interferon alpha therapy for chronic myelogenous leukemia. *Am J Med* 99:402–411, 1995.

Wheat LJ, Connolly-Stringfield PA, Baker RL, et al: Disseminated histoplasmosis in AIDS: Clinical findings, diagnosis, treatment, and review of the literature. *Medicine* 69:361–374, 1990.

Wheats J, Hafner R, Korzun AH, et al: Itraconazole treatment of disseminated histoplasmosis in patients with the acquired immunodeficiency syndrome. AIDS Clinic Trial Group. *Am J Med* 98:336–342, 1995.

White RJ, Likavech MJ: The diagnosis in initial management of head injury. *N Engl J Med* 327:1507–1511, 1992.

Whitley RJ, Gnann JW Jr: Acyclovir: A decade later. *N Engl J Med* 327:782–789, 1992.

Willard JE, Lange RA, Hillis LD: The use of aspirin in ischemic heart disease. *N Engl J Med* 327: 175–181, 1992.

Williams GH: Converting enzyme inhibitors in the treatment of hypotension. *N Engl J Med* 319: 1517–1525, 1989.

Woolf SH: Screening for prostate cancer with prostate-specific antigen: An examination of the evidence. *N Engl J Med* 333:1401, 1995.

Wolff SM: Monoclonal antibodies and the treatment of gram-negative bacteremia and shock. *N Engl J Med* 324:486–488, 1991.

Wrenn KD, Solvis SM, Minion GE, et al: The syndrome of alcoholic ketoacidosis. *Am J Med* 91: 119–128, 1991.

Yankner BA, Mesulam M-M: Beta-amyloid and the pathogenesis of Alzheimer's disease. *N Engl J Med* 325:1849–1857, 1991.

Zangwill KM, Hamilton DH, Perkins BA, et al: Cat scratch disease in Connecticut: Epidemiology, risk factors, and evaluation of a new diagnostic test. *N Engl J Med* 329:8, 1993.

# NOTES

# NOTES

# COLOR PLATES

# Color Plates

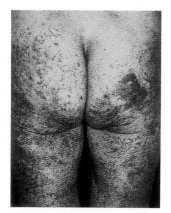

A (QUESTION VIII-44)

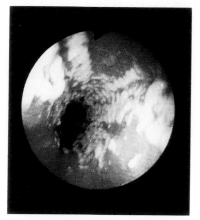

B (QUESTION VIII-45)

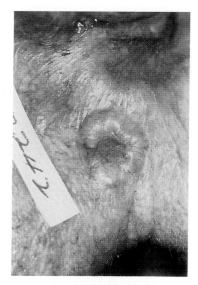

C (QUESTION IX-2)

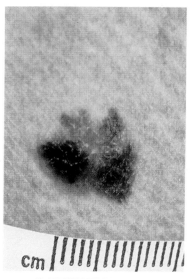

D (QUESTION IX-3)

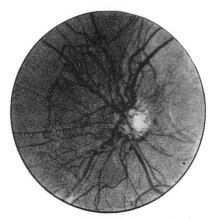

E (QUESTION V-45)

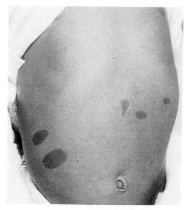

F (QUESTION X-1)

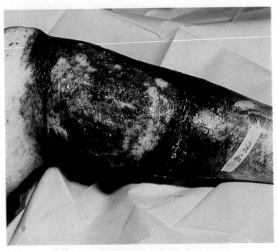

G (QUESTION X-2)

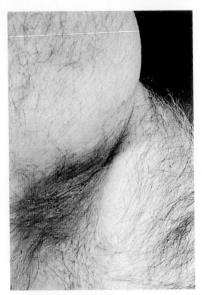

H (QUESTION X-3)

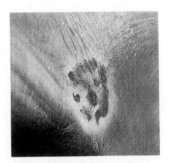

I (QUESTION X-4)

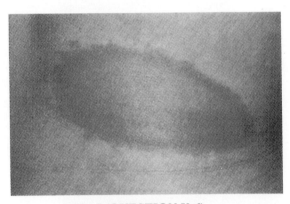

J (QUESTION X-6)

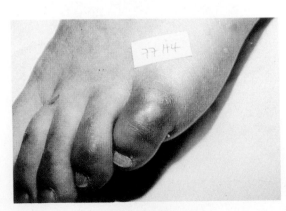

K (QUESTION X-5)

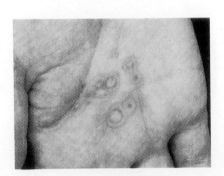

L (QUESTION X-7)

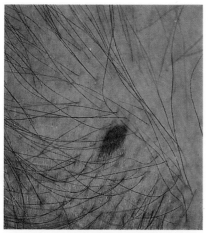

**M (QUESTION X-8)**

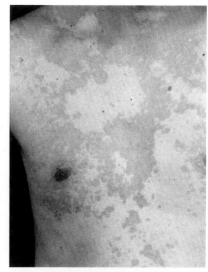

**N (QUESTION X-9)**

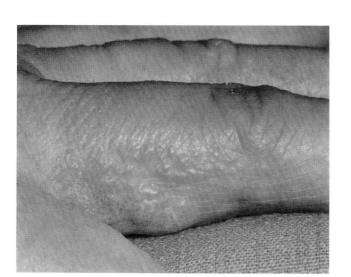

**O (QUESTION X-10)**

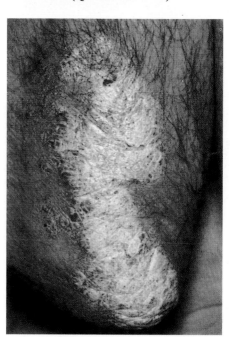

**P (QUESTION X-11)**

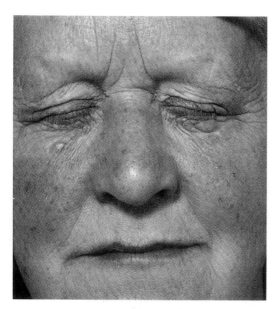

**Q (QUESTION X-21)**

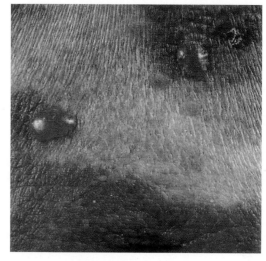

**R (QUESTION X-13)**

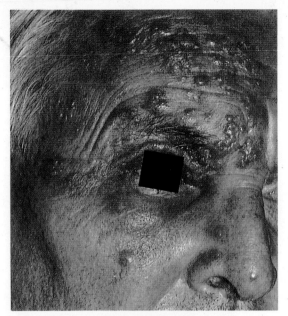

S (QUESTION X-14)

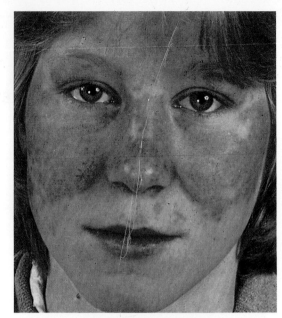

T (QUESTION X-15)

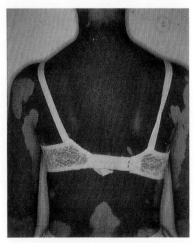

U (QUESTION X-18)

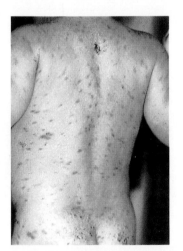

V (QUESTION X-19)

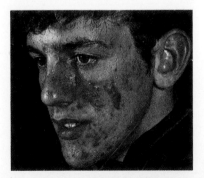

W (QUESTION X-20)

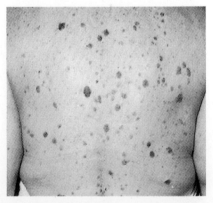

X (QUESTION X-22)